D1599924

Stress Echocardiography

Eugenio Picano

Stress Echocardiography

Fifth, Completely Revised and Updated Edition

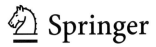 Springer

Eugenio Picano MD, PhD
Director General
Institute of Clinical Physiology of Pisa
National Research Council
1st Fisiologia Clinica
Via G. Moruzzi, 1
56124 Pisa
Italy

ISBN: 978-3-540-76465-6   e-ISBN: 978-3-540-76466-3

DOI: 10.1007/978-3-540-76466-3

Library of Congress Control Number: 2008940140

Cover design: Frido Steinen-Broo, eStudio Calamar, Spain

Printed on acid-free paper

9 8 7 6 5 4 3 2 1

springer.com

Preface

This book has a past. Its various editions parallel the growth of stress echocardiography within the scientific community and the clinical arena. The first edition in 1991 consisted of 100 pages, which increased to 200 in the second (1994), 300 in the third (1997), nearly 500 pages in the fourth, and finally more than 600 in the current fifth edition. The general perception of stress echocardiography has changed in the cardiology community. No longer a promising innovation viewed with a mixture of suspicion and attraction, it is now an established technique with the huge potential to resolve the present paradox of saving health care money while at the same time improving diagnostic standards. In a cardiological climate where inappropriate, redundant, and often risky imaging examinations proliferate, stress echocardiography offers the great advantage of being relatively low cost, free of biohazards for the patient, and causing no ecological stress on the planet. By choice and by necessity, modern, responsible diagnosis with cardiac imaging must be economical, ecological, and therefore usually echocardiographic. Another major change has taken place in stress echocardiography laboratories during the last 5 years, making a new edition of the book mandatory. For a long time, the scope and application of stress echocardiography remained focused on coronary artery disease. In the last few years, it has exploded in its breadth and variety of applications, enjoying the tremendous technological and conceptual versatility that this technique offers. Nowadays, in the stress echocardiography laboratory we assess not only left ventricular function, but also coronary artery flow, valve gradients, intraventricular pressures, and pulmonary hemodynamics. We stress not only coronary arteries, but also the valves, myocardium, vessels, alveolar–capillary barrier in the lung, and peripheral and pulmonary circulation. Ten years ago, only patients with known or suspected coronary artery disease entered the stress echocardiography laboratory, and only regional wall motion was assessed. Now, we evaluate coronary artery disease as well as cardiomyopathy, valvular heart disease, children with congenital heart disease, and patients with incipient or advanced vascular disease. For each patient, we can tailor a dedicated stress with a specific method to address a particular diagnostic question. Thirty years ago, Harvey Feigenbaum – one of the founding fathers of modern echocardiography – stated that it is not possible to understand the cardiac patient without the help of resting transthoracic echocardiography. After 30 years, we can safely state that it is not possible to understand the cardiac patient without the help of stress echocardiography. The book was single authored in the first edition, and then enjoyed many distinguished contributors in its subsequent editions, up to the record number of 29 contributors in the present edition. They come from 15 countries spanning four continents and represent, in my opinion, some of the best available knowledge and expertise in their respective fields. I am proud and honored that they accepted the invitation to be a part of this project. At the same time, I aimed to avoid the fragmentation, gaps, and inconsistencies of a multiauthor text; therefore, I painfully decided to draft the first version of each chapter – then asked for corrections, revisions, cuts, additions, and integrations from more knowledgeable contributors. To all of them and to the junior and senior colleagues who have worked with me over the last 30 years – far too many to be mentioned here – *grazie*.

Pisa, February 2009   **Eugenio Picano**

Contents

List of Contributors

Giorgio Arpesella
Dipartimento Cardiovascolare
Universitá di Bologna
Via Massarenti 9
40138 Bologna, Italy

Gigliola Bedetti
Cardiology Division
Imola Hospital
Via Montericco 4
40026 Imola, Italy

Tonino Bombardini
Associate Researcher
Istituto di Fisiologia Clinica
CNR, Via Moruzzi 1
56124 Pisa, Italy

Robert Bonow
Goldberg Professor of Medicine
Division of Cardiology
Northwestern University's Feinberg
School of Medicine
676 St., Claire St., Suite 600
Chicago, IL 60611, USA

Adrian C. Borges
Medizinische Klinik für Kardiologie
und Angiologie, Campus Mitte
Charité – Universitätsmedizin
Schumannstr 20/21
10117 Berlin, Germany

Paolo G. Camici
Division of Clinical Sciences
Hammersmith Hospital
MRC Clinical Sciences Centre
London SW7 2AZ, UK

Rodolfo Citro
Cardiology Imaging Unit
San Luca Hospital
Via F Cammarota
Vallo della Lucania
Salerno 84048, Italy

Lauro Cortigiani
Cardiac Imaging Lab, Lucca Hospital
"Campo di Marte"
Via dell'Ospedale 238
55100 Lucca, Italy

Kwan Damon
Division of Cardiology,
Department of Medicine
San Francisco Veterans Affairs Hospital
University of California San Francisco
San Francisco, CA 94143-0214, USA

Maurizio Galderisi
Department of Clinical
and Experimental Medicine
Federico II University Hospital
Cardiology Unit
Via Sergio Pansini, 5
80131 Naples Italy

Ekkehard Grünig
Pulmonary Hypertension Unit
Department of Cardiology and
Pneumology
University Hospital Heidelberg
INF 410
69120 Heidelberg, Germany

Michael Henein
Cardiology Department
Heart Centre University Hospital
90185 Umea, Sweden

Patrizio Lancellotti
Department of Cardiology
University Hospital Sart Tilman
CHU Sart Tilman B35
4000 Liège, Belgium

Jorge Lowenstein
Cardiodiagnostic Department
Investigaciones Médicas
Viamonte 1871, CP 1056
Buenos Aires, Argentina

Thomas H. Marwick
University of Queensland
Princess Alexandra Hospital
Brisbane
Queensland 4000, Australia

Mark J. Monaghan
Department of Cardiology,
King's College Hospital
Denmark Hill
London SE5 9RS, UK

Jean-Luc Monin
Department of Cardiology
Assistance Publique-Hôpitaux de Paris
Henri Mondor Hospital
51 avenue De Lattre de Tassigny
94010 Créteil, France

Miodrag Ostojic
Cardiology Department
University of Belgrade
Belgrade Medical School
Koste Todorovica 8
11000 Belgrade, Serbia

Philippe Pibarot
Laval Hospital Research Center
Québec Heart Institute
Laval University
2725, Chemin Sainte-Foy
Québec, G1V-4G5, Canada

Luc A. Piérard
Department of Cardiology
University Hospital Sart Tilman B-35
4000 Liège, Belgium

Fabio Recchia
Scuola Superiore Sant'Anna
Piazza Martiri della Libertà 33
56127 Pisa, Italy

Fausto Rigo
Dipartimento Cardiovascolare
Ospedale Civile di Mestre
Via Ospedale
30170 Venezia (VE), Italy

Alberto San Román
Department of Cardiology
Instituto de Ciencias del
Corazón (ICOCOR),
Hospital Clnico
Ramón y Cajal, 3
47005 Valladolid, Spain

Nelson B. Schiller
Division of Cardiology
Department of Medicine, Box 0214
San Francisco Veterans Affairs Hospital
University of California San Francisco
San Francisco, CA 94143-0214, USA

Juerg Schwitter
University Hospital Zurich
Clinic of Cardiology and
Cardiac MR Center
Raemistrasse 100
CH-8091 Zurich, Switzerland

Rosa Sicari
Institute of Clinical Physiology
CNR
Via Moruzzi, 1
56124 Pisa, Italy

Jae-Kwan Song
Echo Laboratory, Asan Medical Center
Department of Pulmonary and
Critical Care Medicine,
Asan Medical Center, University of Ulsan
College of Medicine, 388-1,
Pungnap-2dong, Songpa-gu
Seoul, Republic of Korea

William Wijns
Cardiovascular Center
OLV Hospital, Moorselbaan 164
9300 Aalst, Belgium

Section 1

Basic Principles, Methodology and Pathophysiology

Stress Echocardiography: A Historical and Societal Perspective

1

Eugenio Picano

Like many scientific innovations, in the last 30 years stress echocardiography has evolved from the status of "promising technique," embraced by a few enthusiastic supporters [1, 2] amid general skepticism [3], to "established technology" [4] accepted by the overwhelming majority of cardiologists [5], to finally play a pivotal role in general cardiology [6, 7] with specialty echocardiography guidelines [8, 9] (Fig. 1.1). An astounding increase in the amount of editorial space devoted to stress echocardiography in major journals and meetings testifies to its greater acceptance by cardiologists (Fig. 1.1) and to the progressive expansion of the diagnostic domain, from coronary artery disease to its currently increasing role in the characterization of cardiomyopathy and valvular heart disease patients [10] (Fig. 1.2). The growth of this technique can be schematically staged by decade, grossly corresponding to three major technological step-ups: its infancy, as a monodimensional approach only applied with exercise during the 1970s; adolescence, characterized by two-dimensional echocardiography technology also applied with pharmacological stresses in the 1980s; young adulthood, when the methodology was reshaped with the addition of coronary flow reserve to standard wall motion analysis; and full maturity today, with deployment of the technique in the clinical arena to minimize the iatrogenic, legal, and social burdens that accompany the use of complementary and competing ionizing techniques such as scintigraphy and multislice computed tomography (MSCT) (Fig. 1.3).

1.1
Dawn of the Stress Echocardiography Era: From Experimental Studies to the Monodimensional Approach

In 1935, Tennant and Wiggers showed that coronary occlusion resulted in almost instantaneous abnormality of wall motion [11]. Experimental studies performed some 40 years later with ultrasonic crystals [12] and two-dimensional echocardiography [13] on a canine model proved that during acute ischemia [12] and infarction [13] reductions in regional flow are closely mirrored by reductions in contractile function, setting the stage for the clinical use of ultrasonic methods in ischemic heart disease. The monodimensional (*M*-mode) technique

E. Picano, *Stress Echocardiography*,
© Springer-Verlag Berlin Heidelberg 2009

1

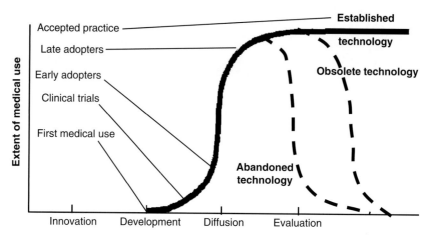

Fig. 1.1 The life cycle of a medical innovation, from promising technique (stress echocardiography in the 1980s) to established technology (stress echocardiography in the last 10 years). Various applications of stress echocardiography are all simultaneously present in today's stress echocardiography laboratory, but at different stages of maturity. The qualitative assessment of regional wall motion abnormalities for detection of coronary artery disease is clearly "established", but coronary flow reserve is still in the "early adopter" phase, while other applications (such as tissue characterization or myocardial velocity imaging with tissue Doppler or strain rate) have been discarded after the validation process and are now obsolete or have been abandoned for current clinical applications of stress echocardiography

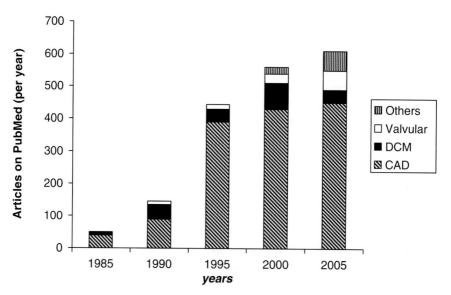

Fig. 1.2 Stress echocardiography vital signs: the editorial golden age. *y-axis* indicates the number of published articles on stress echo; the *x-axis* indicates the year. DCM=dilated cardiomyopathy; CAD=coronary artery disease (From Medline Healthgate)

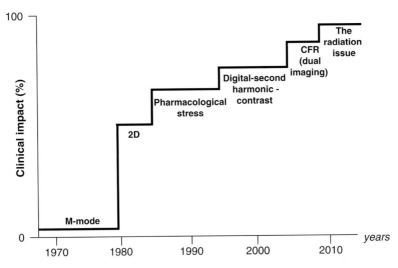

Fig. 1.3 The timeline of innovation in stress echocardiography. Quantum leaps in clinical impact are linked to technological improvements and cultural advancement. CFR=coronary flow reserve

was the only one available to cardiologists in the 1970s and nowadays appears largely inadequate for providing quality information when diagnosing myocardial ischemia. The time-motion technique sampling, according to an "ice-pick" view, greatly limited exploration to a small region on the left ventricle. Although this feature could hardly be reconciled with the strict regional nature of acute and chronic manifestations of ischemic heart disease, for the first time the monodimensional technique outlined echocardiography's potential in diagnosing transient ischemia. The very first reports describing echocardiographic changes during ischemia dealt with the use of *M*-mode in two different models of exercise-induced ischemia [14] and spontaneous vasospastic angina [15]. Landmark studies by Alessandro Distante of the Pisa echo laboratory recognized transient dyssynergy to be an early, sensitive, specific marker of transient ischemia, clearly more accurate than electrocardiogram (ECG) changes and pain (Fig. 1.4). The potential clinical impact of these observations became more obvious with the advent of the two-dimensional technique, which allowed exploration of all segments of the left ventricle with excellent spatial and temporal resolution, and was, therefore, ideally suited for searching for the regional and transient manifestations of myocardial ischemia. If the monodimensional technique was a bludgeon, then the two-dimensional technique was a bow – a more potent weapon, and much easier to use.

1.2
Second-Generation Stress Echocardiography: Pharmacological Stresses in the 2D Era

Once armed with the bow – the 2D technique – stress echocardiographers now had to find the arrows – the proper stresses. Exercise, although already on hand, was soon revealed to be a blunt arrow: what was the "mother of all tests" for the cardiologist was

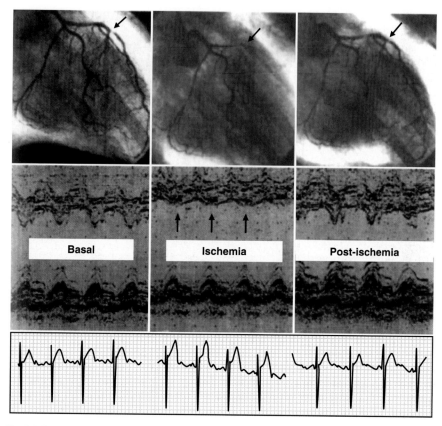

Fig. 1.4 Coronary angiographic (*upper panels*) and echocardiographic monodimensional tracings (*lower panels*) during attacks of variant angina induced by ergonovine maleate. At baseline, left anterior descending coronary artery shows a tight stenosis (*left panel*); the artery is totally occluded by a complete vasospasm during ischemia (*middle panel*); and it is again open in the recovery phase (*right panel*). The corresponding three frames of an original *M*-mode recording document a fully reversible sequence of myocardial ischemia. The septum moves normally at rest (*left panel*) and is obviously akinetic during ischemia (*middle panel*). During the recovery phase (*right panel*), the previously ischemic wall exhibits a significant overshoot in motion and systolic thickening. (From [15])

at that time a disagreeable "stepmother" for the echocardiographer due to the technical difficulties and degraded quality of echocardiographic imaging during exercise. The problem was minimized with posttreadmill imaging, still the standard in the USA today [16]. An alternative approach, more popular in Europe, was the introduction of pharmacological stress echocardiography detecting myocardial ischemia [17] and viability [18].

In the late 1980s, multiple generations of ultrasound equipment evolved very rapidly, boosting image quality and offering the ability to image almost any patient. In two-dimensional exercise echocardiography, stress echocardiography sometimes was a "guess gram" (Fig. 1.5) and torture for the eyes. It was often repeated by eminent opinion leaders that you needed "magic eyes" and "magic machines" to obtain good results. The technique divided the echocardiographic community into two camps, "believers" and "skeptics"

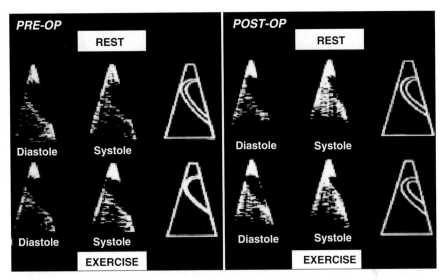

Fig. 1.5 Stress echocardiography in its infancy: not easy on the eyes. Exercise echocardiograms are shown before (*left panel*) and after (*right panel*) coronary artery bypass surgery. At that time (1979), image quality was so poor that even obtaining a single "typical example" for publication purposes was a challenge. (From [16])

[3, 4], and never attained extensive clinical application. Things changed rapidly in the mid-1980s, with the evolution of imaging technology and the advent of pharmacological stresses, which were less technically challenging than exercise. In the 1990s, thanks to this methodological evolution, the technique was upgraded from research toy to clinical tool. The widespread use of this technique received wide-scale support and credibility; prospective multicenter studies provided effectiveness [19] and safety [20] data with pharmacological stress echocardiography. The same groups that proposed stress echocardiography in journals and meetings now introduced the technique into their clinical practice. Rather than the number of published articles, it was this compelling argument that convinced most laboratories to implement stress echocardiography in their own practice as well; the world described in journals eventually came to resemble real-life cardiology (Fig. 1.6).

1.3
Third-Generation Stress Echocardiography Today: Coronary Flow Reserve and Dual Imaging

For 20 years, throughout the 1980s and the 1990s, stress echocardiography remained virtually unchanged [1, 4, 5]. Certainly, there were obvious, continuous, subtle improvements in imaging technology. Digital echocardiographic techniques permitted the capture and synchronized display of the same view at different stages. The introduction of native tissue harmonic imaging, which increases lateral resolution and signal-to-noise ratio, clearly improved endocardial border detection. Intravenous contrast echocardiography with second-generation lung-crossing agents for endocardial border recognition allowed

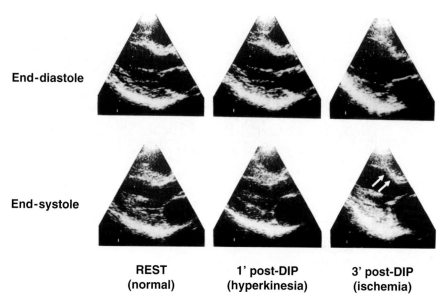

End-diastole

End-systole

REST	**1' post-DIP**	**3' post-DIP**
(normal)	**(hyperkinesia)**	**(ischemia)**

Fig. 1.6 The birth of pharmacological stress echo. End-diastolic (*upper panels*) and end-systolic (*lower panels*) frames at baseline (*left panel*), during early hyperkinetic phase (*middle panel*, 1 min postdipyridamole infusion), and 3 min postdipyridamole infusion at peak ischemic effect (*right panel*) showing septal akinesia. The quality of the image (compared to Fig. 1.5) is dramatically improved thanks to the evolution of technology and the use of pharmacological instead of posttreadmill exercise echo. (Original images from [17])

cardiologists to study otherwise "acoustically hostile" patients and segments [8, 9]. To be honest, however, the last 20 years were also disappointing with regard to the three great unfulfilled promises of stress echocardiography: tissue characterization of the myocardial structure (scar vs. normal tissue); myocardial perfusion with myocardial contrast echocardiography (allowing perfusion to be coupled with function in the same stress); regional wall motion quantification with myocardial velocity imaging methods (turning the diagnosis of regional wall motion from an opinion into a quantifiable unit). At first, each of these targets appeared to be within reach, based on strong experimental data and encouraging clinical experiences, but they did not pass the test of multicenter studies and to date have not revealed any valuable clinic impact [8, 9]. Each of these objectives – tissue structure, myocardial perfusion, and regional function quantification – can be realized in a more effective and reproducible way with cardiovascular magnetic resonance (CMR) – with delayed contrast enhancement for scar detection, contrast imaging for myocardial perfusion, and tagging for wall motion objective quantification [5]. However, in the last 5 years, a major innovation changed the face and the diagnostic content of stress echocardiography: dual imaging of wall motion and coronary flow reserve with pulsed-Doppler imaging of the middistal left anterior descending coronary artery [21–23]. Imaging coronary flow reserve dramatically expands the prognostic potential of stress echocardiography, since in the absence of wall motion negativity, the patient subset with reduced coronary flow reserve has a less benign outcome and in patients with wall motion abnormality, those with reduced coronary flow reserve also have a more malignant prognosis (Fig. 1.7) [22, 23]. In the same

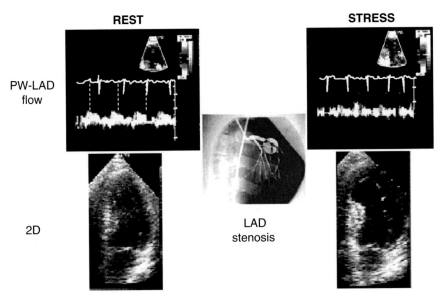

Fig. 1.7 The magical world of coronary flow reserve enters the stress echocardiography laboratory with pulsed Doppler, which allows assessment of coronary flow reserve on the middistal left anterior descending artery (visualized by color Doppler on *upper panel*). In this case, there is a normal coronary flow reserve, with a >2.5-fold increase in coronary flow velocity during stress (*right lower panel*) compared with rest (*left lower panel*). LAD, left anterior descending; PW, Pulsed Wave Doppler. (By courtesy of Fausto Rigo, Venice-Mestre [21])

setting, with the same stress, it is now possible to image function and flow simultaneously, and therefore catch two "birds" (flow and function) with one "stone" (vasodilator stress). Although coronary flow reserve is a technology-in-progress and has yet to reach its full maturity, it is now considered a new standard in the clinical application of stress echocardiography [24]. However, once again this quantum leap in the impact of stress echocardiography was the result of a conceptual rather than a technological step-up during the last 5 years: that is, the need to incorporate long-term radiation risk in the risk–benefit assessment of competing imaging techniques [5]. Medical, legal, and social arguments have boosted the use of stress echocardiography as the best way to optimize the risk–benefit ratio for the individual patient, minimize the risk of litigation due to unjustified long-term cancer risk, and nullify the oncological population burden of cardiac stress testing [5].

1.4
Cardiac Imaging and Its Guidelines

After 30 years of evolution, in the last 10 years stress echocardiography has reached its established rank in the diagnosis and prognosis of coronary artery disease, as officially certified by general cardiology [6, 7] and specialist guidelines [8, 9]. These guidelines unanimously conclude that nuclear cardiology and stress echocardiography provide comparable information on key issues such as diagnostic accuracy for noninvasive detection of coronary artery disease, identification of myocardial viability, and prognostic stratification. In the recent American College of Cardiology (ACC)/American Heart Association (AHA) guidelines, the advantages listed for stress echocardiography include higher specificity, versatility, greater convenience, and lower cost. The advantages of stress perfusion imaging include higher technical success rate, higher sensitivity (especially for single-vessel disease involving the left circumflex artery), better accuracy when multiple resting left ventricular wall motion abnormalities are present, and a more extensive database in evaluation of the prognosis [6]. The European Society of Cardiology guidelines (2006) on stable angina conclude that "on the whole, stress echocardiography and stress perfusion scintigraphy, whether using exercise or pharmacological stress (inotropic or vasodilation), have very similar applications" [7]. However, the certified, comparable clinical performance cannot be construed as an argument for an opinion-driven choice of one technique over the other. The ACC/AHA Task Force (Committee on Management of Patients with Chronic Stable Angina) concluded that "the choice of which test to perform depends on issues of local expertise, available facilities and considerations of cost-effectiveness" [6]. The European Society of Cardiology concluded that "the choice as to which test is employed depends largely on local facilities and expertise." In the present era characterized by a quest for sustainability, the issues of relative cost (Fig. 1.8) [25], biological risk, and

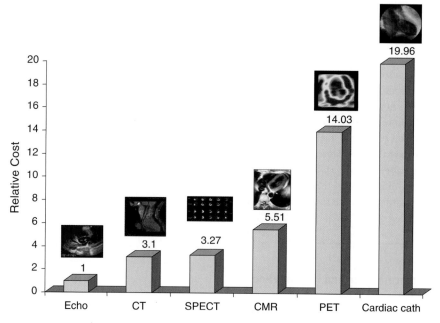

Fig. 1.8 Relative costs of cardiac imaging. CT = cardiac tomography; SPECT = single photon emission computed tomography; CMR = cardiac magnetic resonance; PET = positron emission tomography (Adapted and modified from [25])

environmental impact of stress-testing procedures – not even mentioned in the guidelines – should be included in the decision-making process, not only for cardiac stress testing, but for every imaging test in all branches of medicine, as clearly recommended by the European Commission Medical Imaging guidelines [26].

1.5
Cardiac Imaging and the Radiation-Induced Biorisks

Small individual risks multiplied by billions of examinations become significant population risks [27–31]. At least 10% of all cancers are due to diagnostic imaging, and at least half of them come from cardiac examinations (Fig. 1.9). Cardiac stress imaging contributes to these individual and population biorisks. On the individual level, the effective dose is expressed in millisievert (mSv). It provides an estimate of the whole-body dose and a measure of the biological effects. The dose of a single nuclear cardiology procedure ranges from 27 mSv (>1,500 chest X-rays) from a thallium scan to 10 mSv (500 chest X-rays) from a technetium-MIBI scan [32–34]. One millisievert corresponds to the dose equivalent of 50 chest X-rays (single postero–anterior projection = 0.02 mSv). According to the latest estimation of BEIR VII (2006), this exposure dose corresponds to an extra-lifetime risk of cancer per examination ranging from 1 in 500 (thallium) to 1 in 1,000 (sestamibi) [35, 36]. The typical effective dose of several common diagnostic procedures is reported in Table 1.1

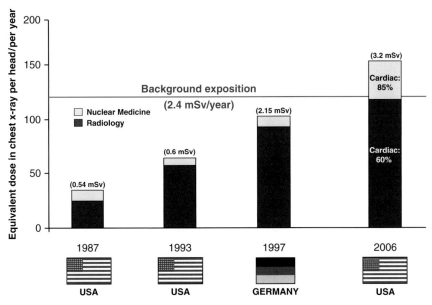

Fig. 1.9 Annual effective dose received by an average US inhabitant (from [23], National Council on Radiation Protection and Measurements). The total dose is of 3.2 mSv per year: 2.4 mSv from natural and 0.4 mSv from man-made sources. (Updated from [27])

Table 1.1 Doses in cardiology

Examination	Effective dose (mSv)	Equivalent no. of chest X-rays
Conventional radiology		
■ Chest X-ray (single postero–anterior)	0.02	1
Nuclear medicine		
■ Tc-99 m tetrafosmin cardiac rest–stress (10 mCi + 30 mCi)[a]	10.6	530
■ Tc-99 m sestamibi cardiac 1-day rest–stress (10 mCi + 30 mCi)[a]	12	600
■ Tc-99 m sestamibi cardiac 2-day stress–rest (30 mCi + 30 mCi)[a]	17.5	775
■ Tl-201 cardiac stress and reinjection (3.0 mCi + 1.0 mCi)[a]	25	1,250
■ Dual isotope cardiac (3.0 mCi Tl201 + 30 mCi Tc-99 m)[a]	27	1,350
64-Slice *Cardiac computed tomography*		
■ ECG pulsing, no aorta[b]	9	450
■ No ECG pulsing, yes aorta[b]	29	1,450
Interventional radiology		
■ Conventional rhythm device[c]	1.4	70
■ Cardiac resynchronization device[c]	5.5	275
■ Cerebral angiography[c]	1.6–10.6	80–530
■ Coronary angiography[c]	3.1–10.6	155–555
■ Abdominal angiography[c]	6–23	300–1,150
■ Peripheral angiography[c]	2.7–14	135–700
■ Coronary angioplasty[c]	6.8–28.9	340–1,445
■ Peripheral angioplasty[c]	10–12	500–600
■ Radiofrequency ablation[c]	17–25	850–1,250
■ Valvuloplasty[c]	29	1,450

[a]From [26], [33]
[b]From [34]
[c]From [35]
CT protocols that rescan the same region of interest (e.g., noncontrast and contrast-enhanced scans) impart two to three times the radiation dose

and translated into the corresponding additional lifetime risk of cancer per examination in Fig. 1.10 [35, 36]. The risk is cumulative, and the dose exposure of an average adult cardiology patient easily reaches 100 mSv, corresponding to 5,000 chest X-rays and an additional risk of 1 cancer in 100 [37]. This threshold can be reached, for instance, by summing up dose exposures of four thallium or dual isotope stress perfusion scintigraphy studies – still the preferred protocol for radionuclide stress imaging in the USA in spite of the unfavorable dosimetry [33, 35]. With the current best (BEIR VII) risk estimates, the 10 million stress perfusion studies per year lead to an estimated 20,000 new cancers each year in the USA alone (Table 1.2). The estimated 10 million cardiac CT studies per year yield an

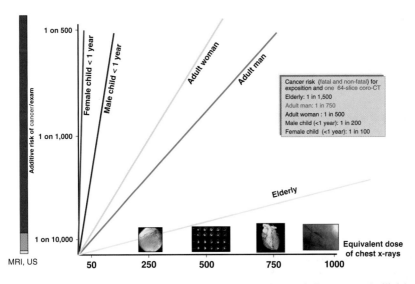

Fig. 1.10 Population risk of radiation-induced cancer, today around 10% of all cancers and still rising. (From [29])

Table 1.2 Cardiac imaging for detection of coronary artery disease: population impact

	Dose per examination (CXRs)	Risk per examination	Examinations per year	New cancers per year
MPI	1,000 (500–1,500)	1 in 500	10 million	20,000
MSCT	750 (500–1,500)	1 in 750	10 million	15,000
CMR	0	0	10 million	0
Stress echocardiography	0	0	10 million	0

CXR, chest X-ray; *MPI*, myocardial perfusion imaging; *MSCT*, multislice computed tomography; *CMR*, cardiovascular magnetic resonance

additional 15,000 new cancers per year in the USA alone (Fig. 1.11) [30]. Obviously this has raised public health concerns in regulating bodies and scientific societies. As stated in the recent White Paper of the ACR (American College of Radiology), "the expanding use of imaging modalities using ionizing radiation may eventually result in an increased incidence of cancer in the exposed population" [31]. If stress echocardiography and CMR are employed instead of perfusion imaging and MSCT, no known individual or population oncological burden is observed (Table 1.2).

1

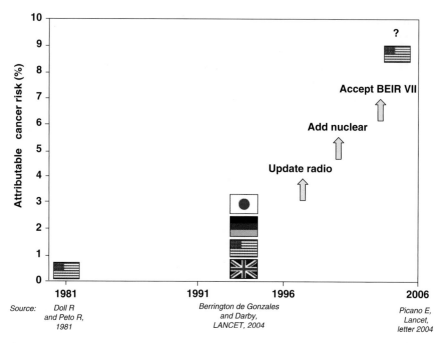

Fig. 1.11 Simplified effective dose ranges of some common medical procedures involving exposure to ionizing radiations in diagnostic nuclear medicine and radiological procedures. The reference unit is one chest X-ray (postero–anterior projection), equal to an effective dose of 0.02 mSv. There is a linear relationship between dose (*x*-axis) and risk (*y*-axis), with no safe dose (the risk line starts from zero). Ultrasound and MRI have zero dose and zero risk. (Adapted from [32])

1.6
Cardiac Imaging and the Regulatory Framework

The abovementioned environmental, population, and biological burdens are fully acceptable when there is no substitute or alternative for information provided by the imaging technique, in a proper risk–benefit assessment that includes long-term risks in the balance. The same burden may become too heavy, and the risks offset the benefits, when comparable diagnostic information can be obtained using widely available alternative techniques, with no known biohazards and no environmental impact. In cardiology, the frequent need for serial repeated stress imaging testing in the same patient amplifies the biohazard, since radiological risk is cumulative [38]. These obvious considerations have left a mark on the regulatory framework governing the use of cardiac imaging in medical guidelines, and – at least in Europe – in federal, national, and regional laws regulating cardiac imaging prescriptions. In the European Union [39], a 97/43 EURATOM directive establishes that indication and execution of diagnostic procedures should follow three basic principles: the justification principle (article 3: "if an exposure cannot be justified, it should be prohibited"), the optimization principle (article 4: "according to the ALARA principle, all doses due to medical exposures must be kept As Low As Reasonably Achievable"), and the responsibility principle (article 5: "both the referring physician ordering the test – the prescriber – and the physician – the practitioner – are responsible for the justification of the test exposing the patient to ionizing radiations"). These principles have been reinforced on the national level. In Italy [40], a recent law (DL 187, 26 May 2000) states that an ionizing examination can only be performed when "it cannot be replaced by other techniques which do not employ ionizing radiation." In the same law, article 14 sanctions the inappropriate use of ionizing tests with fines up to €5,000 and jail for a period up to 3 months. These laws are not so strictly implemented in clinical practice, where at least 1 out of 3 imaging tests is inappropriate [41, 42] and both doctors [43–46] and patients [46] are largely unaware of doses and risks, setting the stage for a perfect medicolegal storm [38].

1.7
Cardiac Imaging in the Age of Sustainability: The "Eco-Eco-Echo" Diagnosis

In today's cost-environment – and risk-conscious climate, the prescribing physician must be aware that his/her choice places economic and biohazard burdens upon the planet, society, and the individual. Ours was the last generation of prescribers and practitioners that could afford to neglect costs and environmental impact, ignore radiological doses, and deny the risks of our often inappropriate imaging testing. Society, the government, patients, and the law will rightfully demand accountability for our acts. It is entirely likely that our increased awareness of the doses, risks, and environmental impact of imaging methods will profoundly reshape the way cardiology (and medicine in general) is taught, learned, and practiced. A cost-environment – and risk-conscious algorithm should follow simple rules. Faced with comparable or largely similar information, non-ionizing testing should be chosen: echo instead of nuclear, and MRI instead of CT. For any given ionizing test, the one with a lower dose should be chosen. For similar doses and accuracy, the test with less environmental impact should be chosen [for instance, CT rather than positron emission tomography (PET)]. This simple, common sense-driven algorithm could revolutionize the current practice of medicine. Today, the cardiac imaging community is gratified by the huge rise of imaging numbers, on the order of magnitude of +4,800% for CT, +2,800% for stress echocardiography, +100% for CMR, and +300% for stress perfusion imaging projected from 2006 to 2020 [47]. It does not matter that nearly half of these examinations [41, 42] are inappropriate – even when long-term risks are not considered [48].

In this societal perspective, sensitive to the environmental, economic, and societal milieu, a virtuous attempt to keep to the highest diagnostic standards while minimizing the economic and biological footprint of our medical acts will inevitably lead to a growing role for stress echocardiography in cardiac imaging practice.

References

1. Picano E (1989) Dipyridamole-echocardiography test: historical background and physiologic basis. Eur Heart J 10:365–76
2. Armstrong WF (1991) Stress echocardiography for detection of coronary artery disease. Circulation 84:I43–9
3. Bairey CN, Rozanski A, Berman DS (1988) Exercise echocardiography: ready or not? J Am Coll Cardiol 11:1355–8
4. Picano E (1992) Stress echocardiography. From pathophysiological toy to diagnostic tool. Point of view. Circulation 85:1604–12
5. Picano E (2003) Stress echocardiography: the historical background. (Special article). Am J Med 114:1–6
6. Gibbons RJ, Chatterjee K, Daley J, et al (1999) ACC/AHA/ACP-ASIM guidelines for the management of patients with chronic stable angina: a report of the American College of Cardiology/American Heart Association Task Force on Practice Guidelines (Committee on Management of Patients With Chronic Stable Angina). J Am Coll Cardiol 33:2092–197
7. Fox K, Garcia MA, Ardissino D, Task force on the management of stable angina pectoris of the european society of cardiology; ESC Committee for Practice Guidelines (CPG), et al (2006) Guidelines on the management of stable angina pectoris: executive summary: the task force on the management of stable angina pectoris of the european society of cardiology. Eur Heart J 27:1341–81
8. Pellikka PA, Nagueh SF, Elhendy AA, American Society of Echocardiography, et al (2007) American Society of Echocardiography recommendations for performance, interpretation, and application of stress echocardiography. J Am Soc Echocardiogr 20:1021–41
9. Sicari R, Nihoyannopoulos P, Evangelista A, European Association of Echocardiography et al (2008) Stress echocardiography expert consensus statement: European Association of Echocardiography (EAE) (a registered branch of the ESC). Eur J Echocardiogr 9:415–37
10. Picano E (2009) Stress echocardiography in valvular heart disease. In: Henein M (ed): Valvular Heart Disease in Clinical Practice. Springer Verlag, Berlin
11. Tennant R, Wiggers CJ (1935) The effects of coronary occlusion on myocardial contraction. Am J Physiol 112:351–61
12. Theroux P, Franklin D, Ross J jr, et al (1974) Regional myocardial function during acute coronary artery occlusion and its modification by pharmacologic agents in the dog. Circ Res 34:896–908
13. Kerber RE, Abboud FM (1973) Echocardiographic detection of regional myocardial infarction. An experimental study. Circulation 47:997–1005
14. Sugishita Y, Koseki S, Matsuda M, et al (1983) Dissociation between regional myocardial dysfunction and ECG changes during myocardial ischemia induced by exercise in patients with angina pectoris. Am Heart J 106:1–8
15. Distante A, Rovai D, Picano E, et al (1984) Transient changes in left ventricular mechanics during attacks of Prinzmetal's angina: an M-mode echocardiographic study. Am Heart J 107:465–70
16. Wann LS, Faris JV, Childress RH, et al (1979) Exercise cross-sectional echocardiography in ischemic heart disease. Circulation 60:1300–8
17. Picano E, Distante A, Masini M, et al (1985) Dipyridamole-echocardiography test in effort angina pectoris. Am J Cardiol 56:452–56
18. Pierard LA, De Landsheere CM, Berthe C, et al (1990) Identification of viable myocardium by echocardiography during dobutamine infusion in patients with myocardial infarction

after thrombolytic therapy: comparison with positron emission tomography. J Am Coll Cardiol 15:1021–31

19. Picano E, Landi P, Bolognese L, et al (1993) Prognostic value of dipyridamole echocardiography early after uncomplicated myocardial infarction: a large-scale, multicenter trial. The EPIC Study Group. Am J Med 95:608–18

20. Picano E, Mathias W Jr, Pingitore A, et al (1994) Safety and tolerability of dobutamine-atropine stress echocardiography: a prospective, multicentre study. Echo Dobutamine International Cooperative Study Group. Lancet 344:1190–2

21. Rigo F, Richieri M, Pasanisi E, et al (2003) Usefulness of coronary flow reserve over regional wall motion when added to dual-imaging dipyridamole echocardiography. Am J Cardiol 91:269–73

22. Cortigiani L, Rigo F, Gherardi S, et al (2007) Additional prognostic value of coronary flow reserve in diabetic and nondiabetic patients with negative dipyridamole stress echocardiography by wall motion criteria. J Am Coll Cardiol 50:1354–61

23. Rigo F, Sicari R, Gherardi S, et al (2008) The additive prognostic value of wall motion abnormalities and coronary flow reserve during dipyridamole stress echo. Eur Heart J. 29:79–88

24. Rigo F, Murer B, Ossena G, et al (2008) Transthoracic echocardiographic imaging of coronary arteries: tips, traps, and pitfalls. Cardiovasc Ultrasound 6:7

25. Pennell DJ, Sechtem UP, Higgins CB, Society for Cardiovascular Magnetic Resonance; Working Group on Cardiovascular Magnetic Resonance of the European Society of Cardiology et al (2004) Clinical indications for cardiovascular magnetic resonance (CMR): Consensus Panel report. Eur Heart J 25:1940–65

26. European Commission. Radiation protection 118: referral guidelines for imaging. http://europa.eu.int/comm/environment/radprot/118/rp-118-en.pdf (accessed 10 January 2006)

27. Picano E (2004) Sustainability of medical imaging. Educational and Debate. BMJ. 328: 578–80

28. Berrington de Gonzales A, Darby S (2004) Risk of cancer from diagnostic X-rays: estimates for the UK and 14 other countries. Lancet 363:345–51

29. Picano E (2004) Risk of cancer from diagnostic X-rays. Letter. Lancet 363:1909–10

30. Brenner DJ, Hall EJ (2007) Computed tomography–an increasing source of radiation exposure. N Engl J Med 357:2277–84

31. Amis ES Jr, Butler PF, Applegate KE, et al; American College of Radiology (2007) American College of Radiology white paper on radiation dose in medicine. J Am Coll Radiol 4:272–84

32. Picano E (2004) Informed consent and communication of risk from radiological and nuclear medicine examinations: how to escape from a communication inferno. BMJ 329:849–851

33. Einstein AJ, Henzlova MJ, Rajagopalan S. (2007) Estimating risk of cancer associated with radiation exposure from 64-slice computed tomography coronary angiography. JAMA 298:317–23

34. Einstein AJ, Moser KW, Thompson RC, et al (2007) Radiation dose to patients from cardiac diagnostic imaging. Circulation 116:1290–305

35. Italian Health Ministry Medical Imaging Guidelines. Linea guida Agenzia Servizi Sanitari Regionali e Istituto Superiore Sanità sulla diagnostica per immagini. 2004 http://www.sirm.org/professione/pdf_lineeguida/linee_diag_x_img.pdf

36. Picano E, Vano E, Semelka R, et al (2007) The American College of Radiology white paper on radiation dose in medicine: deep impact on the practice of cardiovascular imaging. Cardiovasc Ultrasound 5:37

37. Bedetti G, Pizzi C, Gavaruzzi G, et al (2008) Suboptimal awareness of radiologic dose among patients undergoing cardiac stress scintigraphy. J Am Coll Radiol 5:126–31

38. Bedetti G, Loré C (2007) Radiological informed consent in cardiovascular imaging: towards the medico-legal perfect storm? Cardiovasc Ultrasound 5:35

39. Council Directive 97/43/EURATOM of 30 June 1997 on health protection of individuals against the dangers of ionizing radiation in relation to medical exposure and repealing Directive84/466/Euratomhttp://ec.europa.eu/energy/nuclear/radioprotection/doc/legislation/9743_en.pdf

40. Decreto Legislativo 26 maggio 2000, n. 187, Attuazione della direttiva 97/43/Euratom in materia di protezione sanitaria delle persone contro i pericoli delle radiazioni ionizzanti connesse a esposizioni mediche

41. Picano E, Pasanisi E, Brown J et al (2007) A gatekeeper for the gatekeeper: inappropriate referrals to stress echocardiography. Am Heart J 154:285–90

42. Gibbons RJ, Miller TD, Hodge D, et al (2008) Application of appropriateness criteria to stress single-photon emission computed tomography sestamibi studies and stress echocardiograms in an academic medical center. J Am Coll Cardiol 51:1283–9

43. Shiralkar S, Rennie A, Snow M, et al (2003) Doctors' knowledge of radiation exposure: questionnaire study. BMJ 327:371–2

44. Correia MJ, Hellies A, Andreassi MG, et al (2005) Lack of radiological awareness among physicians working in a tertiary-care cardiological centre. Int J Cardiol 105:307–11

45. Lee CI, Haims AH, Monico EP et al (2004) Diagnostic CT scans: assessment of patient, physician, and radiologist awareness of radiation dose and possible risks. Radiology 231:393–8

46. Thomas KE, Parnell-Parmely JE, Haidar S, et al (2006) Assessment of radiation dose awareness among pediatricians. Pediatric Radiol 36:823–32

47. Gershlick AH, de Belder M, Chambers J, et al (2007) Role of non-invasive imaging in the management of coronary artery disease: an assessment of likely change over the next 10 years. A report from the British Cardiovascular Society Working Group. Heart 93:423–31

48. Redberg RF (2007) The appropriateness imperative. Am Heart J 154:201–2

Anatomical and Functional Targets of Stress Testing

2

Eugenio Picano

The principle of stress under controlled conditions derives from the Industrial Revolution: metallic materials undergo endurance tests to identify the breaking load. This approach identifies structural defects, which – although occult in the resting or static state – might show up under real-life loading conditions, leading to a dysfunction of the industrial product. In the same way, a patient with normal findings at rest undergoes a stress test to identify any potential vulnerability of the myocardium to ischemia, if there is clinical suspicion of ischemic heart disease.

2.1
Pathways of Ischemia

Myocardial ischemia is the final common pathway of various morphological and functional substrates. In order to describe the pathways of ischemia, the normal heart can be conveniently schematized into its three fundamental anatomical components, each a potential target of pathological conditions leading to ischemia: epicardial coronary arteries, myocardium, and small coronary vessels (Fig. 2.1).

2.2
Epicardial Coronary Arteries

The alterations of epicardial coronary arteries can be either fixed or dynamic. Fixed epicardial artery stenosis is the target of functional stress testing, but we also know from pathology studies that the degree and number of coronary artery stenoses do not predict onset, course, complications, infarct size, and death in ischemic heart disease [1].

E. Picano, *Stress Echocardiography*,
© Springer-Verlag Berlin Heidelberg 2009

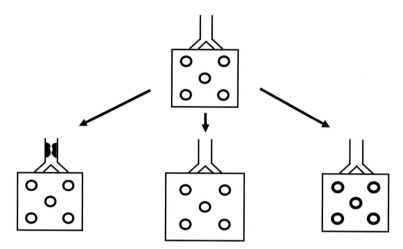

Fig. 2.1 The pathways of ischemia. *Upper panel*: The fundamental anatomical components of the normal heart are shown: epicardial coronary arteries (*parallel lines*), myocardium (*square box*), small vessels (*circles*). *Lower panel*: The three main pathophysiological conditions that may provoke myocardial ischemia. *Left to right*: coronary stenosis (either fixed or dynamic); myocardial hypertrophy; small vessel disease. (Redrawn and modified from [2])

2.3
Fixed Stenosis

The human body incorporates a functional reserve, which allows it to cope with the physiological emergencies and dangers of pathological states. By exploiting its functional reserve, each organ can – for a certain amount of time – play a role that is much more demanding than the usual one or, when a pathological process develops, it can maintain normal function in resting conditions. Coronary circulation is no exception to this rule. Coronary reserve is the ability of the coronary arteriolar bed to dilate in response to increased cardiac metabolic demands [2]. It is fully exhausted when maximal vasodilation is reached, corresponding to about four times the resting coronary blood flow in the normal subject (Fig. 2.2). A fixed atherosclerotic stenosis reduces the coronary reserve in a predictable way according to the curve described in Fig. 2.2 [3]. In this curve four separate segments can be identified: (a) the hemodynamically silent zone, where stenoses ranging from 0 to 40% do not affect the coronary flow reserve to any detectable extent; (b) the clinically silent zone, where stenoses ranging from 40 to 70% reduce the flow reserve without reaching the critical threshold required to provoke ischemia with the usual stresses; (c) the zone potentially capable of inducing ischemia, where stenoses exceeding the critical level of 70% elicit myocardial ischemia when stress is applied, but not in resting conditions; and (d) the zone provoking ischemia at rest, where tight stenoses (>90%) completely abolish the flow reserve and may critically reduce coronary blood flow even in resting conditions.

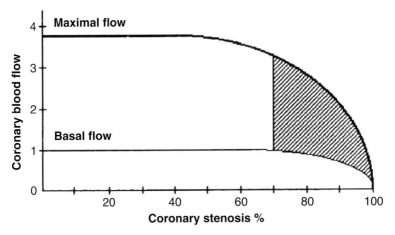

Fig. 2.2 Coronary blood flow curve (*on the ordinate*) for increasing levels of coronary stenosis (*on the abscissa*) experimentally obtained in resting conditions (*lower curve*) and at maximal postischemic vasodilation (*upper curve*). Coronary reserve – i.e., the capacity of the coronary circulation to dilate following increased myocardial metabolic demands – is expressed as the difference between hyperemic flow and the resting flow curve. The *dashed area* between the two curves identifies a critical value of coronary stenosis (70%) beyond which the flow reduction is so severe as to make the myocardium vulnerable to ischemia in the presence of increased oxygen consumption. (Modified from [3])

2.4
Dynamic Stenosis

From a theoretical point of view, dynamic stenoses may be the consequence of three different conditions: increased tone at the level of an eccentric coronary plaque, complete vasospasm caused by local hyperreactivity of the coronary smooth muscle cells, or intravascular thrombosis. The first mechanism can significantly modulate the anginal threshold in patients with chronic stable angina [4], while vasospasm is responsible for variant angina. All three mechanisms coexist in unstable angina [5]. The biochemical mechanisms of coronary vasoconstriction remain somewhat elusive; however, we know that coronary vasoconstriction can be superimposed on any degree of anatomical stenosis and that functional and organic (fixed and dynamic) stenoses can be associated to a variable extent over time, transiently lowering exercise tolerance in the individual patient (Fig. 2.3). Organic stenosis determines the fixed ceiling of flow reserve which cannot be exceeded without eliciting ischemia, whereas dynamic stenosis can modulate exercise capacity in a given patient in a transient, reversible, and unpredictable way [4].

2.5
Myocardium and Small Coronary Vessels

Even in the presence of normal epicardial arteries, myocardial hypertrophy can lower coronary reserve through several mechanisms: vascular growth that is inadequate with

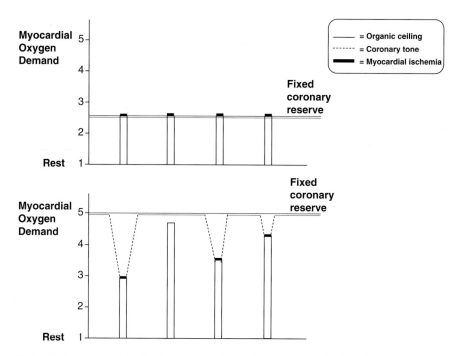

Fig. 2.3 In the presence of a fixed hemodynamically significant stenosis, there is a pathologically reduced "ceiling" of flow reserve (*continuous transverse line*) which induces ischemia when myocardial oxygen demand exceeds a definite threshold (*upper panel*). In the presence of a dynamic stenosis (*lower panel*) the effort tolerance is modulated – in an intermittent, unpredictable way – by fluctuations of coronary tone (*dashed line*), which may reduce the oxygen supply even in the presence of a normal organic ceiling of flow reserve. (Modified from [4])

respect to myocardial growth; a reduction of the cross-sectional area of resistance of a vessel caused by vascular hypertrophy; and compression of intramural coronary vessels by increased extravascular resistance [2]. Furthermore, hypertrophy determines increased oxygen consumption in resting conditions: the resting flow curve shifts upward with a consequent reduction in coronary reserve (Fig. 2.2). Due to myocardial hypertrophy, as well as accompanying small vessel disease, coronary reserve may also be reduced in both dilated and hypertrophic cardiomyopathy. With normal epicardial coronary arteries and myocardial mass, coronary reserve can still be reduced following increased resistance at the level of the small prearteriolar vessels, which are too small to be imaged by coronary angiography [6].

Small vessel disease can be either primary (as in syndrome X) or secondary (as in arterial hypertension [2]). The decreased flow reserve may be related to a functional and/ or an organic factor of the coronary microcirculation. In the former situation, one must assume the inability of the microcirculation to vasodilate appropriately, due to errors in the decoding or transmission of the myocardial metabolic message. In the latter case, anatomical reduction of the microvascular cross-sectional area is likely to occur for medial hyperplasia, which determines an increased wall-to-lumen ratio (Fig. 2.1). This anatomical phenomenon may also determine hyperreactivity to functional stimuli for purely geometric reasons, since minimal caliber reductions cause a marked increase in resistances, with a consequently exaggerated response to normal vasoconstrictive stimuli.

2.6
The Target of Ischemia: The Subendocardial Layer

The many functional and anatomical pathways of ischemia share a common pathophysiological mechanism: the reduction of coronary reserve. This makes the myocardium vulnerable to ischemia during stress. Regardless of the stress employed and the morphological substrate, ischemia tends to propagate centrifugally with respect to the ventricular cavity [7, 8]: it involves the subendocardial layer, whereas the subepicardial layer is affected only at a later stage if the ischemia persists (Fig. 2.4). In fact, extravascular pressure is higher in the subendocardial than in the subepicardial layer; this provokes a higher metabolic demand (wall tension being among the main determinants of myocardial oxygen consumption) and an increased resistance to flow. Selective stress-induced hypoperfusion is especially important for stress echocardiography applications, since regional systolic thickening is linearly and closely related to subendocardial perfusion and only loosely related to subepicardial perfusion [8, 9] (Fig. 2.5).

2.7
The Diagnostic "Gold Standard": Pure Gold?

The results of noninvasive diagnostic tests (Table 2.1) are usually compared with a "gold standard," that is, angiographically assessed coronary artery disease. Although generally accepted, the gold standard has some limitations of both a theoretical and a practical nature [10] (Table 2.2).

First, coronary stenosis is assessed by angiography through the visually assessed percentage reduction of the vessel lumen. The percent of stenosis is a reliable index of severity only if the vascular segment immediately proximal and distal to the stenotic segment is normal and the lesion concentric and symmetrical. Both assumptions are valid in only a very limited number of cases: atherosclerotic involvement usually extends beyond the point of maximum lumen reduction, and the most frequent type of lesion is eccentric. Second, coronary angiography represents only the vessel lumen, an innocent bystander of atherosclerotic disease, rather than the vessel wall, which is the real victim. Minimal, "nonsignificant" lesions at angiography can harbor a diffuse severe atherosclerotic process [2]. The close correlation between coronary stenosis and coronary flow reserve found in the experimental animal [3] is replaced in the clinical setting by an impressive scatter of data [11]. It is impossible to predict the physiological meaning of a stenosis solely on the basis of its angiographic appearance – unless selected patients with single vessel disease, no previous myocardial infarction, no collateral circulation, and no left ventricular hypertrophy are enrolled [12]. Coronary stenosis provokes ischemia as a result of

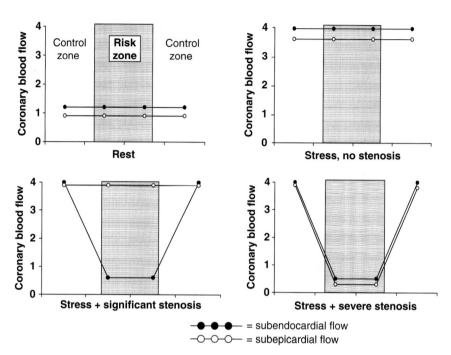

Fig. 2.4 Distribution of flow in the subendocardial and subepicardial layers under different hemodynamic conditions. *Upper left panel*: In resting conditions the subendocardial and subepicardial flows overlap. *Upper right panel*: During stress, the flow increases homogeneously in both layers without affecting the transmural distribution. In the presence of a coronary stenosis, the resting flow is similar to that under normal conditions (*upper left panel*); however, during stress (*lower left panel*) flow remains elevated in the subepicardial layer but falls precipitously in the subendocardium, within the region supplied by the stenotic artery. In the presence of a severe stenosis (*lower right panel*), stress provokes a fall in the subendocardial as well as the subepicardial layer, therefore determining a transmural ischemia. (Redrawn and modified from [7])

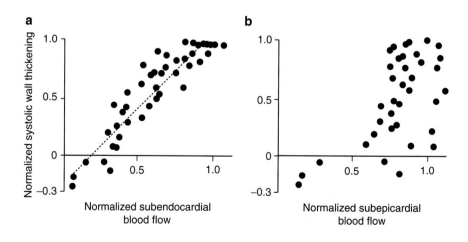

Table 2.1 Standard terminology in diagnostic testing

True positive = Abnormal test result in individual with disease

False positive = Abnormal test result in individual without disease

True negative = Normal test result in individual without disease

False negative = Normal test result in individual with disease

Sensitivity = True positives/True positives + False negatives

Specificity = True negatives/True negatives + False positives

Accuracy = True positives + True negatives/Total number of tests performed

Positive predictive value = True positives/True positives + False positives

Negative predictive value = True negatives/True negatives + False negatives

Table 2.2 Limitations of the coronary angiographic gold standard

	Practical	Theoretical
Limited reproducibility % stenosis	++	
% stenosis unrelated to CFR		+++
Underestimation of diffuse disease	++	
Infarct-producing plaques often noncritical		++
Static luminogram	++	
Thrombus, spasm, inflammation, rupture, and embolization unrelated to plaque size		+++

CFR coronary flow reserve

hemodynamic consequences on the coronary reserve; however, the two parameters (anatomical and pathophysiological) can diverge, and the individual values of coronary flow reserve vary substantially for stenoses of intermediate (40–80%) angiographic severity. In these patients, positive stress test results are more frequently found in patients with depressed coronary flow reserve (<2.0) than in patients with preserved flow reserve (>2.0). This is true for all forms of stress testing, including exercise electrocardiography [13–17] and, to a greater extent, stress perfusion scintigraphy [18–21] and stress echocardiography [22–24]. Third, coronary angiography evaluates the anatomical component of myocardial ischemia, while stress tests can induce ischemia through mechanisms that are totally

Fig. 2.5 The relationship between regional blood flow and systolic wall thickening in resting conscious dogs subjected to various degrees of circumflex coronary artery stenosis. Flow is expressed as a decimal fraction of that in a normal region of the ventricle, and percentage wall thickening (*%WTh*) is expressed as a fraction of the resting value prior to coronary stenosis. **a** Subendocardial blood flow vs. wall thickening, showing a nearly linear relationship (*solid line*). **b** Subepicardial blood flow vs. wall thickening, showing considerable scatter and no change in subepicardial flow until function is reduced by more than 50%. (Modified from [9])

2

different from the organic stenosis (such as dynamic vasoconstriction) and cannot be assessed by means of a purely morphological, static evaluation of the coronary tree [25]. Extra-coronary factors such as myocardial hypertrophy can also reduce coronary flow reserve and therefore make the myocardium potentially vulnerable to ischemia during stress tests [26, 27]. Finally, the commonly employed visual and subjective assessment of stenosis is burdened by a marked intra- and interobserver variability, and arbitrary threshold criteria (such as the presence of a 50% diameter stenosis in at least one major coronary vessel) are introduced to distinguish between "normal" and "sick" patients, when in fact the severity of the atherosclerotic disease ranges over a continuous spectrum. Anatomical coronary artery disease can be assessed much more accurately by intracoronary ultrasound (Fig. 2.6), which substantially improves the representation of atherosclerosis compared with coronary angiography [28]. This improvement is comparable to that achieved in left ventricular imaging when moving from chest X-ray to transthoracic echocardiography. Chest X-ray outlines external profiles and provides a rough index of cardiac volumes, whereas transthoracic echocardiography describes tomographically the various heart chambers and

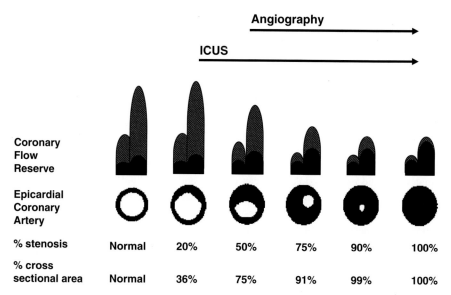

Fig. 2.6 Invasive diagnostic tests for the detection of coronary artery disease. Invasive tests include the luminogram of coronary angiography and the direct visualization of the coronary arterial wall by intracoronary ultrasound (*ICUS*). The percentage of a stenosis can be expressed in angiographic studies as a percentage reduction in diameter and as a percentage reduction in cross-sectional area. The percentage reduction is greater for area than for diameter because of the quadratic relationship between the diameter ($2r$) and area (πr^2) of a circle. The two estimates of stenosis correspond perfectly only for zero stenosis and for 100% stenosis. For each level of stenosis severity, the coronary flow reserve is expressed with a Doppler tracing before and after a coronary vasodilator (adenosine or dipyridamole). Stenoses of less than 50% diameter reduction are not hyperemic flow limiting. (Redrawn and modified from [29])

the thickness of the walls, and identifies within each segment the different layers (endo-cardium, myocardium, and pericardium). In a similar fashion, coronary angiography offers only a luminogram of the vessel, whereas intracoronary ultrasound imaging provides an assessment of the lumen and of the vessel wall thickness [29]. In addition, at each site, the different layers (intima, media, and adventitia) can also be evaluated. Angiography and intracoronary ultrasound correlate closely in healthy vessels with a nearly circular lumen shape. However, as the lumen becomes progressively more irregular, the correlation between a silhouette imaging method (angiography) and a tomographic modality (ultra-sound) diverges significantly. The most substantial disagreement is found in status after angioplasty in which angiography cannot accurately depict the true size of the complex and distorted luminal shape commonly encountered after interventions. Abnormal stress test results can be found in patients with nonsignificant coronary angiographic findings in whom intracoronary sonography may show angiographically unrecognized atheroscle-rotic changes [30], as typically happens in cardiac allograft vasculopathy [31]. Invasive angiographic gold standards are the obligatory reference for noninvasive stress testing procedures, but not all that glitters is gold [32]. In several conditions, coronary arteries are perfectly smooth, even with intracoronary ultrasound, and the coronary flow reserve is impaired by transthoracic stress echocardiography, for instance, in aortic stenosis, syndrome X, or dilated cardiomyopathy [33] (Fig. 2.7). A "false-positive" result by ana-tomic criteria (i.e., a reduced coronary flow reserve with angiographically normal coronary arteries) can became a "true-positive" prognostic response in the long run, and patients with reduced coronary flow reserve – assessed by complex techniques such as positron emission tomography or simple methods such as transthoracic vasodilatory stress echocar-diography – are more likely to experience adverse events in a variety of clinical conditions such as chest pain with normal coronary arteries [34], dilated cardiomyopathy [35, 36], and hypertrophic cardiomyopathy [37, 38].

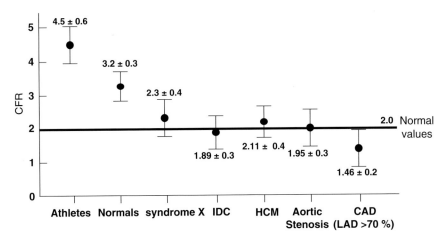

Fig. 2.7 The spectrum of clinical conditions with normal coronary arteries and reduced coronary flow reserve on the left anterior descending artery by transthoracic vasodilatory stress echocardiography. (Redrawn and modified from [33])

References

1. Baroldi G, Bigi R, Cortigiani L (2004) Ultrasound imaging versus morphopathology in cardio-vascular diseases. Coronary atherosclerotic plaque. Cardiovasc Ultrasound 2:29
2. Marcus ML (1983) The coronary circulation in health and disease. McGraw Hill, New York, pp 65–92
3. Gould KL, Lipscomb K (1974) Effects of coronary stenoses on coronary flow reserve and resistance. Am J Cardiol 34:48–55
4. Maseri A (1987) Role of coronary artery spasm in symptomatic and silent myocardial ischemia. J Am Coll Cardiol 9:249–262
5. Gorlin R, Fuster V, Ambrose JA (1986) Anatomic-physiologic links between acute coronary syndromes. Circulation 74:6–9
6. Epstein SE, Cannon RO 3rd (1986) Site of increased resistance to coronary flow in patients with angina pectoris and normal epicardial coronary arteries. J Am Coll Cardiol 8:459–461
7. L'Abbate A, Marzilli M, Ballestra AM, et al (1980) Opposite transmural gradients of coronary resistance and extravascular pressure in the working dog's heart. Cardiovasc Res 14:21–29
8. Ross J Jr (1989) Mechanisms of regional ischemia and antianginal drug action durin exercise. Prog Cardiovasc Dis 31:455–466
9. Gallagher KP, Matsuzaki M, Koziol JA, et al (1984) Regional myocardial perfusion and wall thickening during ischemia in conscious dogs. Am J Physiol 247:H727–H738
10. Marcus ML, White CW, Kirchner PT (1986) Isn't it time to reevaluate the sensitivity of noninva-sive approaches for the diagnosis of coronary artery disease? J Am Coll Cardiol 8:1033–1034
11. White CW, Wright CB, Doty DB, et al (1984) Does visual interpretation of the coronary arteriogram predict the physiologic importance of a coronary stenosis? N Engl J Med 310:819–824
12. Uren NG, Melin JA, De Bruyne B, et al (1994) Relation between myocardial blood flow and the severity of coronary-artery stenosis. N Engl J Med 330:1782–1788
13. Legrand V, Mancini GB, Bates ER, et al (1986) Comparative study of coronary flow reserve, coronary anatomy and results of radionuclide exercise tests in patients with coronary artery disease. J Am Coll Cardiol 8:1022–1032
14. Wilson RF, Marcus ML, Christensen BV, et al (1991) Accuracy of exercise electrocardiography in detecting physiologically significant coronary arterial lesions. Circulation 83:412–421
15. De Bruyne B, Bartunek J, Sys SU, et al (1995) Relation between myocardial fractional flow reserve calculated from coronary pressure measurements and exercise-induced myocardial ischemia. Circulation 92:39–46
16. Schulman DS, Lasorda D, Farah T, et al (1997) Correlations between coronary flow reserve measured with a Doppler guide wire and treadmill exercise testing. Am Heart J 134:99–104
17. Piek JJ, Boersma E, Di Mario C, et al (2000) Angiographical and Doppler flow-derived parameters for assessment of coronary lesion severity and its relation to the result of exercise electrocardiography. DEBATE study group. Doppler Endpoints Balloon Angioplasty Trial Europe. Eur Heart J 21:466–474
18. Joye JD, Schulman DS, Lasorda D, et al (1994) Intracoronary Doppler guide wire versus stress single-photon emission computed tomographic thallium-201 imaging in assessment of intermediate coronary stenoses. J Am Coll Cardiol 24:940–947
19. Daimon M, Watanabe H, Yamagishi H, et al (2001) Physiologic assessment of coronary artery stenosis by coronary flow reserve measurements with transthoracic Doppler echocardiogra-phy: comparison with exercise thallium-201 single photon emission computed tomography. J Am Coll Cardiol 37:1310–1315

20. Heller LI, Cates C, Popma J, et al (1997) Intracoronary Doppler assessment of moderate coronary artery disease: comparison with 201Tl imaging and coronary angiography. FACTS Study Group. Circulation 96:484–490

21. El-Shafei A, Chiravuri R, Stikovac MM, et al (2001) Comparison of relative coronary Doppler flow velocity reserve to stress myocardial perfusion imaging in patients with coronary artery disease. Catheter Cardiovasc Interv 53:193–201

22. Picano E, Parodi O, Lattanzi F, et al (1994) Assessment of anatomic and physiological severity of single-vessel coronary artery lesions by dipyridamole echocardiography. Comparison with positron emission tomography and quantitative arteriography. Circulation 89:753–761

23. Pijls NH, De Bruyne B, Peels K, et al (1996) Measurement of fractional flow reserve to assess the functional severity of coronary-artery stenoses. N Engl J Med 334:1703–1708

24. Bartunek J, Marwick TH, Rodrigues AC, et al (1996) Dobutamine-induced wall motion abnormalities: correlations with myocardial fractional flow reserve and quantitative coronary angiography. J Am Coll Cardiol 27:1429–1436

25. Bortone AS, Hess OM, Eberli FR, et al (1989) Abnormal coronary vasomotion during exercise in patients with normal coronary arteries and reduced coronary flow reserve. Circulation 79:516–527

26. Scheler S, Motz W, Strauer BE (1992) Transient myocardial ischemia in hypertensives: missing link with left ventricular hypertrophy. Eur Heart J 13(Suppl D):62–65

27. Motz W, Strauer BE (1996) Improvement of coronary flow reserve after long-term therapy with enalapril. Hypertension 27:1031–1038

28. Di Mario C, Gorge G, Peters R, et al (1998) Clinical application and image interpretation in intracoronary ultrasound. Study Group on Intracoronary Imaging of the Working Group of Coronary Circulation and of the Subgroup on Intravascular Ultrasound of the Working Group of Echocardiography of the European Society of Cardiology. Eur Heart J 19:207–229

29. Erbel R (1996) The dawn of a new era – non-invasive coronary imaging. Herz 21:75–77

30. Verna E, Ceriani L, Giovanella L, et al (2000) "False-positive" myocardial perfusion scintigraphy findings in patients with angiographically normal coronary arteries: insights from intravascular sonography studies. J Nucl Med 41:1935–1940

31. Spes CH, Klauss V, Rieber J, et al (1999) Functional and morphological findings in heart transplant recipients with a normal coronary angiogram: an analysis by dobutamine stress echocardiography, intracoronary Doppler and intravascular ultrasound. J Heart Lung Transplant 18:391–398

32. Topol EJ, Nissen SE (1992) Our preoccupation with coronary luminology. The dissociation between clinical and angiographic findings in ischemic heart disease. Circulation 92:2333–2342

33. Rigo F (2005) Coronary flow reserve in stress-echo lab. From pathophysiologic toy to diagnostic tool. Cardiovasc Ultrasound 3:8

34. Rigo F, Cortigiani L, Pasanisi E, et al (2006) The additional prognostic value of coronary flow reserve on left anterior descending artery in patients with negative stress echo by wall motion criteria. A transthoracic vasodilator stress echocardiography study. Am Heart J 151:124–30

35. Neglia D, Michelassi C, Trivieri MG, et al (2002) Prognostic role of myocardial blood flow impairment in idiopathic left ventricular dysfunction. Circulation 105:186–93

36. Rigo F, Gherardi S, Galderisi M, et al (2006) The prognostic impact of coronary flow-reserve assessed by Doppler echocardiography in non-ischaemic dilated cardiomyopathy. Eur Heart J 27:1319–23

37. Cecchi F, Olivotto I, Gistri R, et al (2003) Coronary microvascular dysfunction and prognosis in hypertrophic cardiomyopathy. N Engl J Med 349:1027–35

38. Cortigiani L, Rigo F, Gherardi S et al (2009) Prognostic implications of coronary flow reserve in hypertrophic cardiomyopathy. A Doppler echocardiographyc study. Am J Cardiol 1:36–41

Symptoms and Signs of Myocardial Ischemia

3

Eugenio Picano

A transient regional imbalance between oxygen supply and demand usually results in myocardial ischemia, the signs and symptoms of which can be used as a diagnostic tool [1]. Myocardial ischemia results in a typical "cascade" of events in which the various markers are hierarchically ranked in a well-defined time sequence [2]. Flow heterogeneity, especially between the subendocardial and subepicardial perfusion, is the forerunner of ischemia, followed by regional dyssynergy, and only at a later stage by electrocardiographic changes, global left ventricular dysfunction, and pain (Fig. 3.1). The ideal marker of ischemia should provide absolute values of sensitivity and specificity, as well as a diagnosis of the site and severity of ischemia. Unfortunately, such a marker does not exist; in contrast, we have a number if imperfect markers that it associated can provide a reasonably good noninvasive estimation of the presence, extent, and severity of myocardial ischemia. The pathophysiological concept of the ischemic cascade is translated into a gradient of sensitivity of different available clinical markers of ischemia, with chest pain being the least sensitive and regional malperfusion the most sensitive (Fig. 3.2).

3.1
Chest Pain

Chest pain is, in general, the reason the patient seeks medical care. However, many chest pain syndromes are not ischemic in origin and are due to extracardiac causes (such as anxiety or reflux esophagitis), and about 25% of deaths due to coronary artery disease are observed to occur in patients who had never complained of chest pain. Ischemia is "silent" when diagnostic electrocardiographic changes are not associated with symptoms; it is "supersilent" when mechanic and/or metabolic alterations are not associated with either chest pain or electrocardiographic signs (Fig. 3.3). More than 60% of ischemic episodes observed on Holter monitoring are silent, and about 20% of transient dyssynergies detected by echocardiography are supersilent. Thus, chest pain is an important clinical symptom, but it is also a simple diagnostic optional feature [3].

E. Picano, *Stress Echocardiography*,
© Springer-Verlag Berlin Heidelberg 2009

3

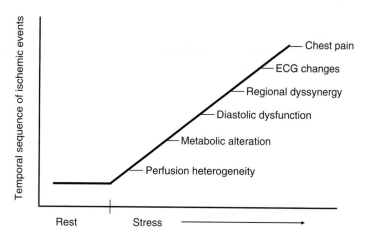

Fig. 3.1 The classical ischemic cascade, triggered by coronary vasospasm and/or epicardial stenosis. The various markers are usually ranked according to a well-defined time sequence

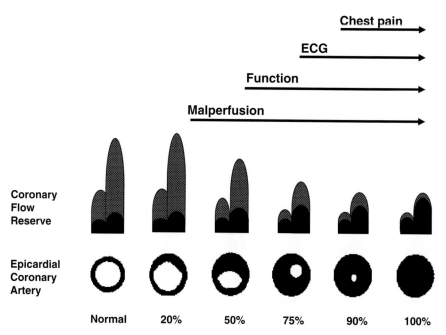

Fig. 3.2 The sensitivity of different diagnostic markers of ischemia ranked according to the underlying coronary anatomy and physiological impairment in coronary flow reserve. Electrocardiographic changes appear late during stress testing and provide only a modest sensitivity, barely superior to that of chest pain. The sensitivity of wall motion abnormalities is markedly superior to that of ECG changes. Malperfusion is more sensitive than wall motion abnormalities in detecting minor, but flow-limiting, levels of coronary artery stenosis

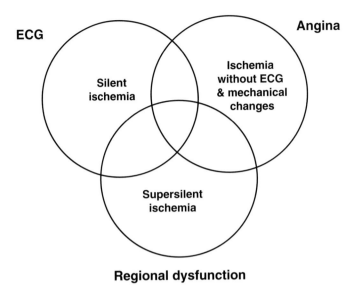

Fig. 3.3 Relative sensitivity of electrocardiography, pain, and echocardiography in diagnosing myocardial ischemia. In the domain of electrocardiography there is the entity of silent ischemia; in the domain of echocardiography there is the entity of so-called supersilent ischemia

3.2
Electrocardiographic Changes

Electrical alterations provoked by ischemia can easily be detected by the 12-lead electrocardiogram (ECG). The electrocardiographic signs of subendocardial ischemia are represented by ST-segment shift or T-wave changes; by contrast, transmural ischemia is generally associated with transient ST-segment elevation. The site of ST-segment elevation is correlated with the site of ischemia, while this agreement does not hold in the more frequently found ST-segment depression. However, ST-segment shifts and T-wave changes are often an equivocal marker of ischemia because the line dividing normal from abnormal is not sharp, and a series of factors (electrical, metabolic, pharmacological, neurohumoral, hemodynamic) can induce ischemia-like ST–T changes [4]. Therefore, the electrocardiographic marker – alone or associated with chest pain – is not always capable of detecting the presence of myocardial ischemia and usually cannot predict its site and extent. The ECG is no longer the definitive proof in the diagnostic process of myocardial ischemia, but only one of the clues.

3.3
Alterations in Left Ventricular Function

Myocardial ischemia causes left ventricular regional dyssynergy (an early, sensitive, and specific marker of ischemia) and global dysfunction (a late and nonsensitive sign). Various techniques have been proposed for the imaging of left ventricular function: echocardiography, radioisotopic ventriculography (at first pass or equilibrium), fast computed tomography, and magnetic resonance imaging [5]. To date, echocardiography has been the technique of choice for the assessment of ventricular function, both in resting conditions and even more so during stress, in spite of the dependence of echocardiographic imaging on the patient's acoustic window and on the experience of the cardiologist interpreting the study. The advantages of feasibility, safety, reliability, and unsurpassed temporal and spatial resolution allow the documentation under optimal conditions of a regional dysfunction which can be extremely localized in space and transient in time.

3.4
Perfusion Abnormalities

An epicardial coronary artery stenosis reduces the maximal flow achievable in the related territory, although the blood flow in resting condition can be equal to that observed in regions supplied by normal coronary arteries. During hyperemia (either during exercise or after dipyridamole or adenosine) a perfusion heterogeneity will occur with lower blood flow increase in the regions supplied by the stenotic artery, even in the absence of regional ischemia [6]. The criterion of positivity is the presence of a regional flow heterogeneity or malperfusion between different zones of the left ventricle (Fig. 3.4). Perfusion imaging is routinely performed with gamma-camera scintigraphy, but it can be also obtained – with

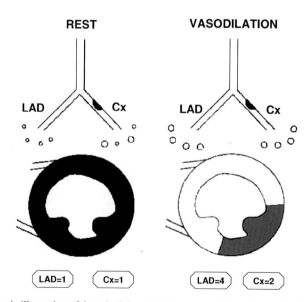

Fig. 3.4 Schematic illustration of the principle underlying myocardial perfusion imaging for the diagnosis of coronary artery disease. At rest, myocardial perfusion is homogeneous, with no differences between the territory of the normal coronary artery (*LAD*, left anterior descending artery) and that of the diseased coronary artery (*Cx*, left circumflex, with 80% stenosis). The resting flow image (obtained, for instance, with thallium-201 scintigraphy or with contrast echocardiography) does not

higher accuracy and at substantially greater cost – by means of positron emission tomography. Other techniques with potential for perfusion imaging are contrast echocardiography and magnetic resonance imaging with injection of specific contrast agents.

3.5
The Paradigm Challenged: The Alternative Ischemic Cascade

In diagnostic practice with stress imaging, not all patients follow the reassuring paradigm proposed by the "ischemic cascade." ECG changes may often occur with typical chest pain, in the absence of echocardiographic changes, and are often accompanied by real, not artifactual [6], reversible perfusion defects. In fact, the typical behavior of microvascular disease during stress testing is the frequent induction of chest pain, ST-segment depression, and also perfusion abnormalities without regional or global wall motion changes [7]. The sequence of events is therefore strikingly different from the classical ischemic cascade described in Fig. 3.1 and in the right panels of Fig. 3.5 as well as from that found during stress testing in the presence of a coronary stenosis. This alternative ischemic cascade is illustrated in the left panel of Fig. 3.5 and derives from real clinical experience [8]. The classical ischemic cascade was a clear laboratory phenomenon described as early as 1935 by Tennant and Wiggers [9], who demonstrated that the immediate result of a coronary occlusion was an instantaneous abnormality of wall motion. The alternative ischemic cascade was a clear clinical finding disclosed by cardiac imaging techniques and it still requires a good laboratory model. It was initially described in cardiac syndrome X by Kemp et al. in 1973 with pacing left ventriculography [10], and later observed with stress echocardiography [11–13]. The left ventricle is hyperdynamic during stress, in spite of the frequent occurrence of chest pain and ST-segment depression: it is "too good to be ischemic," [14] at least when the usual pattern of classic ischemia due to coronary artery stenosis is considered. The alternative cascade refers to a sequence of clinical events, during which the occurrence of ischemia usually cannot be proven [15], although in a subset of patients a reduction in coronary flow reserve [16, 17], and/or a metabolic evidence of inducible ischemia [18, 19], and/or a strictly subendocardial stress-induced hypoperfusion [20] have

---

Fig. 3.4 (continued) show any interregion variation. However, perfusion in the territory of the stenotic coronary artery is maintained at the price of a partial exhaustion of coronary reserve, with partial dilatation of the arteriolar bed – represented by *larger circles* located downstream from the epicardial coronary arteries. The normal arteriolar tone is represented by *smaller circles* (normally vasoconstricted arterioles). During vasodilation obtained with a metabolic stimulus, such as exercise, or with a pharmacological stimulus, such as dipyridamole, the arteriolar tone is lost determining an increase in flow that will be greater in the normal coronary artery (which, at rest, has a preserved tone in the entire arteriolar district) than in the stenotic coronary artery (with lower coronary reserve). Perfusion imaging will show the stenosis "mirrored" in the myocardium as a region with relative underconcentration of flow tracer when compared with the normal contralateral region. The septal and anterior wall appear "*brighter*" (due to greater echocontrast concentration) when compared with the "*darker*" inferoposterior wall (lower echocontrast concentration)

3

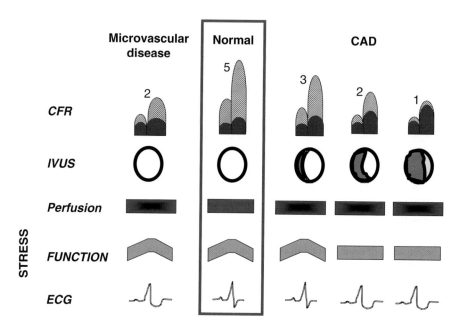

Fig. 3.5 A concise view of the different pathophysiological situations of the classic (*CAD*) and alternative (microvascular) ischemic cascade. In normal conditions (*framed, second column from left*) there is a normal coronary flow reserve (*CFR, first row, with intracoronary Doppler ultrasound*), normal coronary anatomy (*IVUS, second row, with intravascular ultrasound*), normal perfusion pattern with scintigraphy (*Perfusion, third row*), and normal contraction during stress (*Function, fourth row*). ECG is shown in the *last row*. Coronary flow reserve is pictorially expressed with a Doppler tracing before, during, and after a coronary occlusion. With the classic ischemic cascade, perfusion defects are present with mild (*third column from the right*), moderate (*second column from the right*), and severe (*first column from the right*) coronary stenosis, mirroring reductions in coronary flow reserve and accompanied (for moderate-to-severe stenoses) by regional wall motion abnormalities, which are usually absent for mild degrees of stenosis, capable of limiting coronary flow reserve without inducing ischemia. In microvascular disease (*first column from the left*) the depressed coronary flow reserve is associated with a normal coronary anatomy, the frequent occurrence of stress-induced perfusion defects (often with ST-segment depression), and normal left ventricular function. (Modified from [8])

been described. Thus, while few would argue that induced myocardial dysfunction is an accurate marker of regional ischemia, the occurrence of ECG changes and demonstration of regional abnormal vasodilator reserve may or may not be associated with ischemia [8]. In this debate, one should consider that the absence of stress-induced dysfunction does not rule out the ischemic nature of the electrocardiographic abnormalities. It is well known that under ideal imaging conditions even a subendocardial infarction characterized by prolonged chest pain, a rise in serum enzymes, and ST-segment and T-wave changes can be accompanied in 20% of cases by a perfectly normal echocardiogram [21]. Several conditions can be clustered together with cardiac syndrome X in coronary microvascular disease, characterized by normal coronary arteries and reduced coronary flow reserve, without epicardial coronary artery vasospasm [14]. In each of them, an echocardiographically silent ST-segment depression has been described as the typical pattern during stress testing. Among others, they include arterial hypertension (with normal coronary arteries, with or without left ventricular hypertrophy), hypertrophic cardiomyopathy [22], and diabetes [23]. It is entirely likely that our monolithic view of ischemia mirrored in the classical ischemic cascade should integrate awareness of the reverse or alternative ischemic cascade best describing microvascular disease, with ECG changes coming first, perfusion abnormalities second, and with echocardiographic changes usually absent during physical or pharmacological stress. Not all forms of myocardial ischemia are the same, and milder, patchy degrees of myocardial ischemia – like those possibly induced in microvascular angina – remain silent in its mechanical functional manifestations and may represent a physiological scotoma of stress echocardiography (Fig. 3.5). The typical stress imaging pattern of a hypertensive patient with epicardial coronary artery stenosis is displayed in Fig. 3.6: perfusion defect with wall motion abnormality. The typical stress imaging pattern of a patient with normal coronary arteries is displayed in Fig. 3.7: perfusion defect without wall motion abnormality. "Anatomic lies" on the ECG may well be turned into "physiologic truths," when coronary flow reserve or systemic endothelial function are considered, or even into correct prognostic predictions – possibly identifying troublemakers in the long run [22].

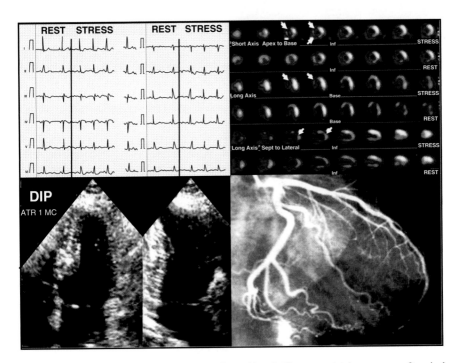

Fig. 3.6 Positive ECG response (*left upper panel*), positive thallium scan (*right upper panel*), apical 4- and 2-chamber view of end-systolic frames at peak stress with apical akinesis (*indicated by arrows, left lower panel*) of a patient with significant left anterior descending coronary artery stenosis (*right lower panel*). (From [13])

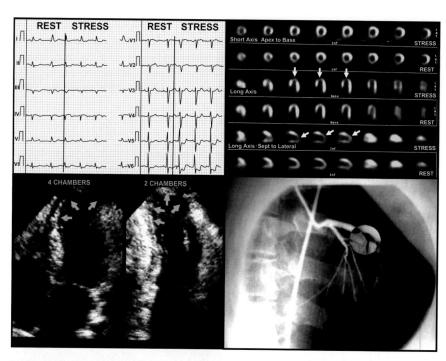

Fig. 3.7 Positive ECG response (*left upper panel*), positive thallium scan (*right upper panel*), apical 4- and 2-chamber view of end-systolic frames at peak stress with normal left ventricular motion of a patient without significant coronary artery disease (*right lower panel*). (From [13])

3.6
Equations in the Diagnosis of Ischemia

On the basis of the classical markers of ischemia, i.e., chest pain and ECG changes, diagnostic equations have been proposed, and are reported in Table 3.1. In view of the limitations of these traditional hallmarks of acute transient myocardial ischemia, "new practical objective criteria (other than ECG changes and pain) for the diagnosis of transient myocardial ischemia are needed" as pointed out by Maseri in 1980 [24]. The classic equations ignore the variable of mechanical changes. However, it is known that the three most commonly used markers of ischemia (chest pain, electrocardiographic changes, mechanical abnormalities) identify at least partially superimposed diagnostic fields (Fig. 3.3). In the absence of concomitant electrocardiographic changes, one is reluctant to affirm the ischemic nature of chest pain; however, ischemic processes resulting in angina pectoris may occur without significant alteration of the ECG [25], as shown by angiographic [26], hemodynamic [27], scintigraphic [28], and echocardiographic [29] studies. It is also well known that asymptomatic myocardial ischemia, as detected by ECG changes and wall motion abnormalities, is a frequent finding during daily activity and during stress testing [30]. The diagnostic accuracy of chest pain and ECG changes is markedly lower than that of echocardiographic changes during all forms of stress [31]. In terms of prognostic impact, the stress-induced echocardiographically recognized dysfunction matters independently of the associated induced chest pain [32, 33]. Considering the low diagnostic and prognostic accuracy of the traditional hallmarks of acute transient ischemia, namely, pain and ST-segment depression, the standard diagnostic equations can be profoundly remodeled by introducing a new variable, such as transient mechanical changes detected by two-dimensional (2D) echocardiography, during spontaneously occurring chest pain or during stress (Table 3.2). Being highly specific for an ischemic event, the mechanical marker is the only "stand-alone" criterion (justifying even the equation "asynergy – ST change–pain = supersilent ischemia"). However, such a statement, although sound from the conceptual point of view, should be applied with caution to daily clinical practice when hypokinesis is involved, since at present we lack reliable quantitative criteria for the detection of hypokinesis with echocardiographic techniques. In clinical practice things are more complicated and the good old ECG can offer surprisingly important information in the imaging era. During stress testing, ECG changes can occur without scintigraphic abnormalities (which are more sensitive than echocardiographic changes) and are associated with poor long-term prognosis [34]. In patients with positive stress echocardiography results and underlying coronary artery disease, a concomitant ST-segment depression identifies a group at higher prognostic risk [35]. In patients with negative stress echocardiography results and normal coronary arteries, stress-induced ST-segment depression identifies patients with endothelial dysfunction [36]. Patients with positive stress echocardiography results may have no ST-segment changes, but have an increase in QT dispersion, which may be a marker of electrical instability and represents an electrocardiographic sign of ischemia different from the ST-segment shift [37, 38]. In conclusion, no diagnostic marker is perfect, but some are more imperfect than others.

3.7
A New Diagnostic Variable: Coronary Flow Reserve

The diagnostic equations based on ECG and wall motion abnormalities have been further remodeled in the last 5 years with the advent of coronary flow reserve evaluated by pulsed Doppler transthoracic echocardiography in the stress echocardiography laboratory [39]. It represents an ideal complement of regional wall motion in the stress echocardiography diagnostic one-stop shop [40]. The equations of ischemia become more robust with the integration of the two markers, one (regional wall motion) assessing mainly anatomic epicardial coronary artery disease, the other (reduced coronary flow reserve) also mirroring the functional condition of coronary microcirculation. The spectrum of responses will range anywhere from very abnormal (induced wall motion abnormalities and reduced coronary flow reserve, indicating epicardial stenosis and abnormal microcirculatory response) to completely normal (no inducible wall motion abnormalities and normal coronary flow reserve), indicating absence of hemodynamically significant macroepicardial upstream, and micro, distal, downstream arteriolar coronary alterations. The stress response can be stratified into a severity code, mirroring the experimental ischemic cascade: no evidence of abnormality (normal wall motion and normal coronary flow reserve) associated with very low risk; isolated perfusion or coronary flow reserve abnormality (without inducible wall motion) associated with intermediate risk; and inducible wall motion abnormalities (usually with a perfusion or coronary flow reserve reduction) associated with the highest risk, in patients who will benefit most from ischemia-driven revascularization. When handling in clinical terms this exciting additional information, rich in novel diagnostic [41] and prognostic [42–44] dividends, we should be always aware that – as smart clinicians said already 25 years ago, at the very beginning of the cardiac imaging explosion – *"our surprise in finding out that a new approach gives information that the old methods do not give, in detecting myocardial ischemia, does not differ from the surprise that an intelligent primitive human would experience if he were suddenly confronted with the problem of understanding what makes a car run. After a short observation he would probably first conclude that if you smash your car probably it will not run any more. Then he will discover that even an intact car will not run if its engine is broken. With time he will come to the astonishing discovery that even intact cars with intact engines may not run if they run out of gasoline and, furthermore, that some will not run even when full of gasoline. This, they would probably classify as super-silent trouble."* [45].

References

1. Ross J Jr (1991) Myocardial perfusion-contraction matching. Implications for coronary heart disease and hibernation. Circulation 83:1076–1083
2. Nesto RW, Kowalchuk GJ (1987) The ischemic cascade: temporal sequence of hemodynamic, electrocardiographic and symptomatic expressions of ischemia. Am J Cardiol 59:23C–30C
3. Malliani A (1986) The elusive link between transient myocardial ischemia and pain. Circulation 73:201–204
4. Surawicz B (1986) ST-segment, T-wave, and U-wave changes during myocardial ischemia and after myocardial infarction. Can J Cardiol(Suppl A):71A–84A
5. Keenan NG, Pennell DJ (2007) CMR of ventricular function. Echocardiography. 24:185–193
6. Gould KL (2006) Physiological severity of coronary artery stenosis. Am J Physiol Heart Circ Physiol 291:H2583–H2585
7. Picano E (1992) Stress echocardiography: from pathophysiological toy to diagnostic tool. Point of view. Circulation 85:1604–1612
8. Picano E, Palinkas A, Amyot R (2001) Diagnosis of myocardial ischemia in hypertensive patients. J Hypertension 19:1177–1183
9. Tennant R, Wiggers CJ (1935) The effects of coronary occlusion on myocardial contraction. Am J Physiol 112:351–361
10. Kemp HG (1973) Left ventricular function in patients with the anginal syndrome and normal coronary angiograms. Am J Cardiol 32:375–380
11. Picano E, Lattanzi F, Masini M, et al (1987) Usefulness of dipyridamole-echocardiography test for the diagnosis of syndrome X. Am J Cardiol 60:508–512
12. Panza JA, Laurienzo JM, Curiel RV, et al (1997) Investigation of the mechanism of chest pain in patients with angiographically normal coronary arteries using transesophageal dobutamine stress echocardiography. J Am Coll Cardiol 29:293–301
13. Astarita C, Palinkas A, Nicolai E, et al (2001) Dipyridamole-atropine stress echocardiography versus exercise SPECT scintigraphy for detection of coronary artery disease in hypertensives with positive exercise test. J Hypertens 19:495–502

14. Lucarini AR, Picano E, Lattanzi F, et al (1991) Dipyridamole echocardiography testing in essential hypertensive patients. Targets and tools. Circulation 83(Suppl III):III68–III72
15. Maseri A, Crea F, Kaski JC, et al (1991) Mechanisms of angina pectoris in syndrome X. J Am Coll Cardiol 17:499–506
16. Chauhan A, Mullins PA, Petch MC, et al (1994) Is coronary flow reserve in response to papaverine really normal in syndrome X? Circulation 89:1998–2004
17. Legrand V, Hodgson JM, Bates ER, et al (1985) Abnormal coronary flow reserve and abnormal radionuclide exercise test results in patients with normal coronary angiograms. J Am Coll Cardiol 6:1245–1253
18. Buchthal SD, Den Hollander JA, Merz NB, et al (2000) Abnormal myocardial phosphorus-31 nuclear magnetic resonance spectroscopy in women with chest pain but normal coronary angiograms. N Engl J Med 324:829–835
19. Crake T, Canepa-Anson R, Shapiro LM, et al (1987) Continuous recording of coronary sinus saturation during atrial pacing in patients with and without coronary artery disease or with syndrome X. Br Heart J 57:67–72
20. Panting JR, Gatehouse PD, Yang GZ, et al (2002) Abnormal subendocardial perfusion in cardiac syndrome X detected by cardiovascular magnetic resonance imaging. N Engl J Med 346:1948–1953
21. Carpeggiani C, L'Abbate A, Marzullo P, et al (1998) Multiparametric approach to diagnosis of non-Q wave acute myocardial infarction. Am J Cardiol 63:404–408
22. Lazzeroni E, Picano E, Morozzi L, et al (1997) Dipyridamole-induced ischemia as a prognostic marker of future adverse cardiac events in adult patients with hypertrophic cardiomyopathy. Echo Persantine Italian Cooperative (EPIC) Study Group, subproject hypertrophic cardiomyopathy. Circulation 96:4268–4272
23. Gaddi O, Tortorella G, Picano E, et al (1999) Diagnostic and prognostic value of vasodilator stress echocardiography in asymptomatic type-2 diabetic patients with positive exercise Thallium scintigraphy: a pilot study. Diabet Med 16:762–766
24. Maseri A (1980) Pathogenetic mechanisms of angina pectoris: expanding views. Br Heart J 43:648–660
25. Haiat R, Desoutter P, Stoltz JP (1983) Angina pectoris without ST-T changes in patients with documented coronary heart disease. Am Heart J 105:883–884
26. Maseri A, Mimmo R, Chierchia S, et al (1975) Coronary spasm as a cause of acute myocardial ischemia in man. Chest 68:625–633
27. Distante A, Picano E, Moscarelli E, et al (1985) Echocardiographic versus hemodynamic monitorino during attacks of variant angina pectoris. Am J Cardiol 55:1319–1322
28. Parodi O, Uthurralt N, Severi S, et al (1981) Transient reduction of regional myocardial perfusion during angina at rest with ST-segment depression or normalization of negative T waves. Circulation 63:1238–1347
29. Rovai D, Distante A, Moscarelli E, et al (1985) Transient myocardial ischemia with minimal electrocardiographic changes: an echocardiographic study in patients with Prinzmetal's angina. Am Heart J 109:78–83
30. Picano E, Distante A, Masini M, et al (1986) Echocardiographic documentation of myocardial ischemia in presence of angina pectoris without ST-T changes. Can J Cardiol 1(Suppl A):67A–70A
31. Picano E, Masini M, Lattanzi F, et al (1986) Role of dipyridamole-echocardiography test in electrocardiographically silent effort myocardial ischemia. Am J Cardiol 58:235–237
32. Bolognese L, Rossi L, Sarasso G, et al (1992) Silent versus symptomatic dipyridamole induced ischemia after myocardial infarction: clinical and prognostic significance. J Am Coll Cardiol 19:953–959

33. Cohn PF (1992) Silent left ventricular dysfunction during dipyridamole echocardiography: a new prognostic marker. J Am Coll Cardiol 19:960–961
34. Klodas E, Miller TD, Christian TF, et al (2003) Prognostic significance of ischemic electrocardiographic changes during vasodilator stress testing in patients with normal spect images J Nuclear Cardiol 10:4–8
35. Cortigiani L, Lombardi M, Michelassi C, et al (1998) Significance of myocardial ischemic electrocardiographic changes during dipyridamole stress echocardiography. Am J Cardiol 82:1008–1012
36. Palinkas A, Toth E, Amyot R et al (2002) The value of ECG and echocardiography during stress testing for identifying systemic endothelial dysfunction and epicardial artery stenosis. Eur Heart J 23:1587–1595
37. Carluccio E, Biagioli P, Bentivoglio M et al (2003) Effects of acute myocardial ischemia on QT dispersion by dipyridamole stress echocardiography. Am J Cardiol 91:385–390
38. Preda I (2002) Differentiation between endothelial dysfunction and epicardial coronary artery stenosis with the aid of stress ECG and echocardiography. A novel return of the old ECG! Eur Heart J 23:1561–1562
39. Rigo F (2005). Coronary flow reserve in stress-echo lab. From pathophysiologic toy to diagnostic tool. Cardiovasc Ultrasound 3:8
40. Rigo F, Murer B, Ossena G, et al (2008). Transthoracic echocardiographic imaging of coronary arteries: tips, traps, and pitfalls. Cardiovasc Ultrasound 6:7
41. Rigo F, Richieri M, Pasanisi E, et al (2003). Usefulness of coronary flow reserve over regional wall motion when added to dual-imaging dipyridamole echocardiography. Am J Cardiol 91:269–273
42. Rigo F, Gherardi S, Galderisi M, et al (2006). The prognostic impact of coronary flow-reserve assessed by Doppler echocardiography in non-ischaemic dilated cardiomyopathy. Eur Heart J. 27:1319–1323
43. Rigo F, Sicari R, Gherardi S, et al (2008). The additive prognostic value of wall motion abnormalities and coronary flow reserve during dipyridamole stress echo. Eur Heart J. 29:79–88
44. Bodi V, Sanchis J, Lopez-Lereu MP, et al (2009) Prognostic and therapeutic implications of dipyridamole stress cardiovascular magnetic resonance on the basis of the ischemic cascade. Heart 95:49–55
45. Donato L (1986) Concluding remarks: the "stunned" cardiologist. Can J Cardiol(Suppl A): 260A–262A

Rational Basis of Stress Echocardiography

4

Fabio Recchia and Eugenio Picano

Stress echocardiography stems from three lines of evidence placed at three different levels: biochemical, pathophysiological, and clinical. The pathophysiological hallmark of stress echocardiography positivity is myocardial ischemia: when the stress echocardiography study shows abnormalities, myocardial ischemia is present. The presence of regional dysfunction requires ischemia, and – in the words of John Ross Jr. – the very definition of ischemia requires an alteration of myocardial function: *"Ischemia is a reduction in myocardial blood flow sufficient to cause a decrease in myocardial contraction"* [1]. In considering this definition, however, one must consider that "decrease in myocardial contraction" is not synonymous with "reduction in visually assessed regional systolic thickening," which expresses only one dimension (radial strain) of the complex three-dimensional event of myocardial contraction. This latter also includes circumferential and longitudinal strain, all contributing to changes in ejection fraction and to the pump function. In addition, systolic thickening is evaluated in a subjective and qualitative, not objective and quantitative, way and reflects the average transmural function, without discriminating between the subendocardium (highly vulnerable to ischemia) and subepicardium (more resistant to ischemia) [2]. The clinical world is not the experimental laboratory, stress echocardiography is not equivalent to implanted sonomicrometry, and therefore the fundamental parameter of regional systolic thickening by two-dimensional (2D) echocardiography should be integrated with information derived from clinical presentation, patient specificity, and information provided by other markers of ischemia.

4.1
Biochemical Basis

At rest, about 60% of the high-energy phosphates produced by cell metabolism is used for development of contractile force, about 15% for relaxation, 3–5% for maintenance of electrical activity, and the remaining 20% for "wear and repair" [3]. The cell's top priority

4

is to repair itself. During ischemia, therefore, the cell minimizes its expenditure of energy on cardiac work and utilizes whatever is left for maintenance of cell integrity. In the normal heart at rest intracellular calcium is sequestered mostly in the sarcoplasmic reticulum, where it cannot be used for myocardial contraction (mediated by the actin–myosin system). Cell membrane excitation and depolarization are followed by a rapid "downhill" (i.e., along the concentration gradient) influx of extracellular calcium, triggering the release of intracellular calcium from sarcoplasmic reticulum; this activates the contraction following the calcium–troponin interaction, which exposes myosin to the binding site of actin. For relaxation to occur, intracellular calcium must be sequestered back "uphill" (i.e., with energy expenditure against a concentration gradient) to the sarcoplasmic reticulum; in this phase, a calcium efflux through the plasma membrane also takes place. When ischemia occurs, the process of contraction and relaxation is slowed by two main intracellular biochemical events: the reduction of high-energy phosphates, due to the blockade of mitochondrial aerobic metabolism, which requires oxygen, and the increased concentration of hydrogen ions, due to the activation of anaerobic glycolysis. Hydrogen ions compete with calcium ions for the troponin activation sites – thereby slowing the actin–myosin interaction. The reduction of intracellular high-energy phosphates in turn reduces the rate of the energy-dependent active reuptake of calcium into the sarcoplasmic reticulum, thus determining an impairment of relaxation [3].

4.2
Physiological Heterogeneity of Myocardial Function

The contraction of the heart is a complex phenomenon involving a deformation (strain) along three coordinates: radial thickening; longitudinal contraction; and circumferential contraction (torsional twist): Fig. 4.1. In addition, the normal adult left ventricle is characterized both morphologically and functionally by a high degree of regional nonuniformity [4]. Myocardial strain is defined as the difference between any end-systolic and end-diastolic dimension divided by the reference end-diastolic dimension and is, as such, dimensionless and presented as percent values. Positive radial strains represent wall thickening, whereas negative strains represent segment shortening (e.g., circumferential shortening). In the clinical assessment of myocardial function, all three types of strain can be measured – at least in principle: systolic thickening with M-mode and 2D echocardiography (by far the most used and the only one adequately validated for clinical applications); longitudinal contraction with myocardial velocity imaging; and circumferential shortening with 2D speckle tracking (Table 4.1). In addition, regional ejection fraction can now also be measured with real-time 3D echocardiography. The inward motion and deformation (circumferentially and longitudinally) of the endocardium determine the changes in intracavitary volume, and endocardial regional ejection fraction can thus be viewed as a composite measure of the local contribution to ejection. The regional ejection fraction increases significantly from base to apex, and remarkably the regions with the highest ejection fraction show the least wall thickening (Fig. 4.2). There is some degree of horizontal (intersegment) variation of myocardial function, but it is less marked than in the vertical (base-to-apex) and transmural (subendocardium-to-subepicardium) direction (Fig. 4.3).

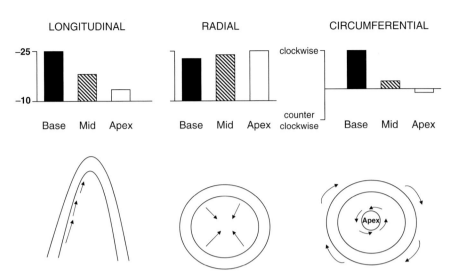

Fig. 4.1 Base-to-apex heterogeneity in radial (*left panel*), longitudinal (*middle panel*), and circumferential (*right panel*) function

Table 4.1 Physiological heterogeneity of myocardial functions

	Transmural gradient	Base-to-apex	Horizontal gradient	Echocardio-graphy method	Alternative method
% Systolic thickening (radial strain)	+++	++	±	*M*-mode 2D	MRI
Longitudinal strain	++	+++	±	Myocardial velocity imaging	MRI tagging
Circumferential strain	+	+++	±	Speckle tracking	MRI tagging
Regional ejection fraction	+	++	±	Real time (RT3D)	MRI tagging

RT real time

This gradient is magnified by stress also in healthy normal subjects, suggesting that a "relative" hyperkinesia during stress is a normal warrant which should imply a conservative reading of stress echocardiograms, to avoid an exorbitant number of false-positive responses [5] (Fig. 4.4). The normal myocardial function is rather heterogeneous at different levels (base to apex) since the relative contribution to ejection increases towards the apex and, within the same segment, at different layers (subendocardium–subepicardium) of the left ventricular walls (Fig. 4.5). Measurements of intramyocardial thickening demonstrate that normally 67% of thickening occurs in the inner half of the wall [7]. Thus, normally there is only a small contribution of the subepicardium to the overall thickening (Fig. 4.6). A "functional" gradient, although less significant, also exists at the various levels of the left ventricle, with greater systolic thickening in the apical than in the basal segments (6–9).

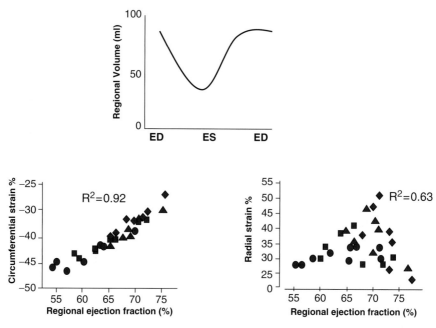

Fig. 4.2 Regional ejection fraction can be obtained with real-time 3D imaging in the echocardiography laboratory (*upper panel*). It is correlated only weakly with % systolic thickening (*lower right panel*) and tightly with circumferential strain (*lower left panel*). (Redrawn and adapted from original MRI tagging data from [3])

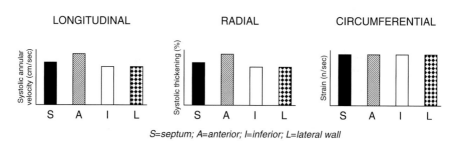

Fig. 4.3 Heterogeneity of radial, longitudinal and strain in septal (*S*), anterior (*A*), inferior (*I*), and lateral (*L*) walls. (Adapted from [10])

This heterogeneity of function is mirrored by perfusion, since contractility is a major determinant of myocardial oxygen consumption and there is a tight beat-by-beat coupling between myocardial oxygen consumption and coronary blood flow [8]. Thus, coronary flow is greater in the subendocardium than in the subepicardium, and greater at the apex than at the base, whereas no significant interregional variations can be observed. Flow and

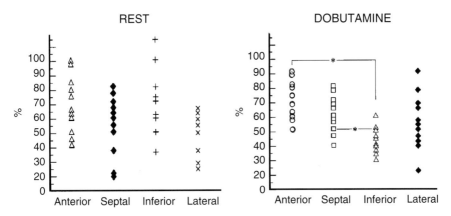

Fig. 4.4 Circumferential heterogeneity in radial strain (% systolic thickening) magnified during stress (*right panel*). (From [6])

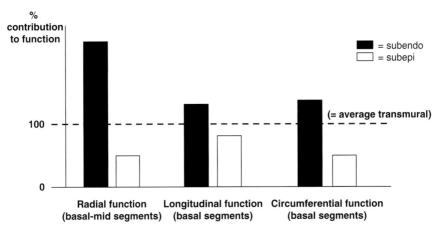

Fig. 4.5 Physiologic, transmural heterogeneity determined as % systolic thickening (radial strain, *left panel*), longitudinal strain (*middle panel*), and circumferential strain (*right panel*). (Adapted from [7, 11])

function tend to show a physiological variability not only in space but also over time with minimal, continuous variations in contractility and perfusion. The relationship between regional flow and function holds true not only in physiological states, when by definition there is a perfect coupling between oxygen supply and demand, but also in pathological conditions determining a mismatch between these two parameters.

4

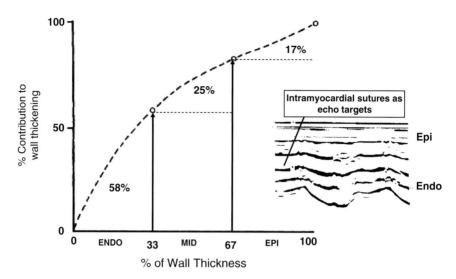

Fig. 4.6 A gradient of thickening (radial function) exists across the myocardial wall, with the inner, middle, and outer thirds of the myocardial wall contributing to 50, 25, and 17% of total wall thickening, respectively. In the *right part* of the graph, the echocardiographic tracing obtained with an epicardial *M*-mode echocardiographic transducer and a suture inserted in the wall of an open-chest dog and used as an intramural echocardiography target. (Adapted from original data from [7])

4.3
Regional Flow–Function Relationship in Myocardial Ischemia

Ischemia may occur either at rest for a progressive coronary stenosis or during stress in the presence of a critical obstruction. A close association between mean transmural blood flow and regional wall thickening can be observed (Fig. 4.7). Above normal perfusion levels, the functional response to a two- to four-fold increase in flow is flat [8]. Conversely, when perfusion is below normal values, regional thickening appears to be almost linearly related to flow: in particular, the subendocardial flow determines regional thickening, which is mainly due to the subendocardial layer. On average, a reduction in subendocardial blood flow of about 20% produces a 15–20% decrease in left ventricular wall thickening; a 50% reduction in subendocardial blood flow decreases regional wall thickening by about 40%, and when subendocardial blood flow is reduced by 80%, akinesia occurs. When the flow deficit is extended to the subepicardial layer, dyskinesia occurs [8]. For minimal flow reductions, abnormalities of regional systolic function are subtle and certainly below the threshold of detection by echocardiography. The detection of a regional dysfunction by 2D echocardiography requires a "critical ischemic mass" of at least 20% of transmural wall thickness and about 5% of the total myocardial mass [9]. Thus, relatively milder and more localized forms of myocardial ischemia do not leave echocardiographic fingerprints and represent the physiological scotoma of the echocardiographic eye when compared with

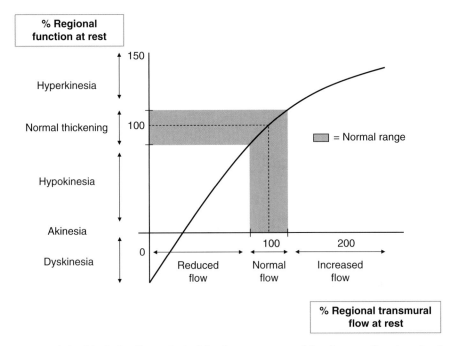

Fig. 4.7 Relationship obtained in anesthetized dogs between transmural flow (measured by microsphere) and regional function (assessed with 2D echocardiography). (Redrawn and modified from [7])

ischemia – at least when radial strain and regional systolic thickening or (regional or global) ejection fraction are considered. Initial forms of contractile dysfunction can, however, more selectively affect longitudinal and circumferential strain, both at baseline [10] and during stress-induced ischemia of mild degree [11].

4.4
Postischemic Recovery of Contractile Function

The postischemic recovery of myocardial function is related to two main variables: the duration of the ischemic attack and the efficacy of postischemic reperfusion. In animals, doubling ischemia time quadruplicates recovery time. For a given duration and severity of ischemia, the recovery of contractile function will be faster with a more complete coronary reflow. In the experimental model, the reopening of a coronary artery previously occluded for a few seconds or minutes is followed by a complete reactive hyperemia and a prompt recovery of contractile function, transiently even above baseline levels. In man, the resolution of transient transmural ischemia is also accompanied by a short postischemic rebound in the previously ischemic areas [12]. In contrast, a severe coronary stenosis will significantly slow reperfusion and, therefore, the recovery of contractile function (Fig. 4.8). Thus, the experimental evidence confirms that a slower, at times partial, recovery of

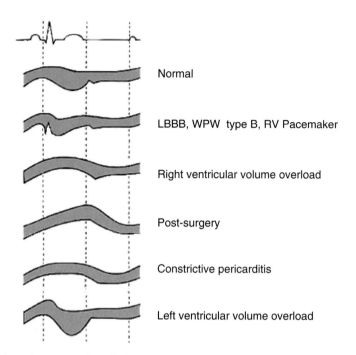

Normal

LBBB, WPW type B, RV Pacemaker

Right ventricular volume overload

Post-surgery

Constrictive pericarditis

Left ventricular volume overload

Fig. 4.8 Schematic representation of ischemia, repetitive stunning, hibernation, and scar as points of a spectrum of myocardial dysfunction. In the *upper panel*, myocardial blood flow (*MBF*). In the *lower panel*, the corresponding regional contractile function at baseline (rest) and during stress. (Adapted and modified from [20])

regional function may be associated with a longer period of ischemia and/or with markedly diseased coronary vessels. In all these conditions, flow and function vary symmetrically in rest, ischemia, and recovery states. There is, however, a "point of no return," beyond which the restoration of flow is unable to restore regional function due to irreversible myocardial cell damage. There is a blurred transition zone between fully reversible ischemia and ischemia lasting more than 20 min and invariably associated with necrotic phenomena. In this border zone, ischemia is too short to cause myocardial necrosis, but long enough to induce a persistent contractile dysfunction (lasting for hours, days, and even weeks) after flow restoration – the so-called myocardial stunning [13]. The stunned myocardium is different from "hibernated" myocardium, where the myocardial perfusion is chronically reduced (for months or years), but remains above the critical threshold indispensable to keep the tissue viable (although with depressed performance) [14]. While in the stunned myocardium a metabolic alteration causes an imbalance between energy supply and the work produced, the hibernating myocardial cell adapts itself to a chronically reduced energy supply and its survival is guaranteed by a reduced or abolished contractile function. This adaptation is incomplete, and degeneration of terminally differentiated myocytes occurs, with loss of contractile proteins and deposition of glycogen granules. Over time, apoptotic cell death eventually occurs with replacement fibrosis and, therefore, progressive loss of potential for contractile function recovery. The ventricular dysfunction persists until the flow is restored but, if revascularization is delayed by several months, left ventricular function no longer improves [14]. Unlike the infarcted myocardium, the postischemic viable tissue retains a contractile reserve. The necrotic myocardium is unresponsive to any inotropic stimulus, whereas the viable myocardium typically responds with a transient increase in regional function which predicts the functional recovery [15].

4.5
Determinants of Regional Dysfunction

In chronic infarction the transmural extent of myocardial damage is correlated to the severity of the regional dyssynergy. A necrosis confined to less than 20% of myocardial thickness is associated with only mild hypokinesia [16]. Dyskinesia is associated with a more transmural extent of necrosis, involving at least 30–40% of myocardial thickness in the vertical (endocardium–epicardium) direction. These experimental data have a clinical correlate: in non-Q myocardial infarction, stable changes of the ST–T segment, with prolonged chest pain and an increase of necrosis enzymes, can be accompanied in 20% of cases by a perfectly normal echocardiogram [17].

Ischemia, infarction, stunning, and hibernation are not the only possible causes of regional asynergy [18]. A series of other factors, both intrinsic and extrinsic to the ischemic region (Table 4.1), can mimic or mask the signs of ischemia on the myocardial wall or disrupt the linearity of the regional flow–function relationship. Fibrosis of nonischemic origin obviously induces a stable regional dysfunction, for instance, in dilated cardiomyopathy. Septal wall motion abnormalities – usually with normal systolic thickening – can be observed in conditions associated with abnormal ventricular depolarization, such as left bundle branch block, Wolff–Parkinson–White type B syndrome, and right ventricular paced rhythm [19] (Fig. 4.9). Following onset of electrical depolarization, there is a downward motion of the interventricular septum or early systolic downward dip or beaking. The abnormal early systolic septal motion with left bundle branch block [6] and with ventricular pacing [21] is secondary to an early rise in pressure in the right ventricle. The abnormal depolarization produces contraction of the right ventricular chamber prior to the left ventricular chamber, thus producing an earlier rise in right ventricular pressure. This differential in pressure then produces the abnormal septal motion. The download displacement is reversed as soon as the left ventricle begins to contract and raises the left ventricular pressure. Almost all patients with left bundle branch block and right ventricular paced rhythm have the early beaking of interventricular septum, but septal motion is paradoxic only in some of them. In left bundle branch block, the paradoxical wall motion is more frequent with markedly abnormal activation sequence (QRS>150 ms) and/or septal fibrosis (see also Chap. 29) [22]. In right ventricular pacing, a paradoxical septal motion is more frequent with pacing from right ventricular outflow or right ventricular inflow [22, 23] (see also Chap. 14). Other nonischemic causes of altered septal motion include right ventricular volume overload and/or elevated right ventricular end-diastolic pressure and postoperative status [16]. A septal "bounce" is consistent with constriction [19].

4

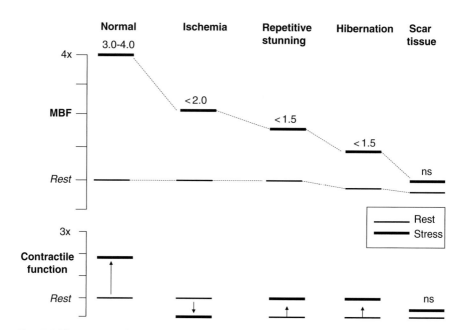

Fig. 4.9 Different types of nonischemic septal wall motion changes. Abnormal (paradoxical) septal motion can be found in a variety of conditions, including (*from top to bottom*) abnormal electrical activation (left bundle branch block, Wolff–Parkinson–White type B, paced right ventricular rhythm), right ventricular volume overload, and/or elevated right ventricular end-diastolic pressure, postoperative status. A septal "bounce" is consistent with constriction. On the other hand, left ventricular volume overload may cause vigorous, supernormal septal motion. (Adapted and modified from [20])

The regional function can be modulated by factors extrinsic to the wall. In left ventricular volume overload, septal motion is exaggerated (Fig. 4.9) and might mask signs of ischemic dysfunction. Two potentially important causes of "normal" wall motion following acute myocardial infarction are the ventricular septal rupture and acute mitral insufficiency: the hemodynamic unloading of the left ventricle tends to lessen the regional abnormality induced by ischemia or infarction. The increase in heart rate and systolic blood pressure can reduce regional systolic thickening independently of ischemia [24, 25]. At high heart rate and high blood pressure values, regional function may also decrease in normal healthy subjects [20]. Finally, during acute ischemia, the extent of mechanical alterations exceeds that of metabolic or flow abnormalities. In fact, there is a border zone where the muscle is normally perfused but shows reduced thickening, representing the continuity between ischemic and hypercontractile myocardium. The phenomenon of adjacent dysfunction is spatially limited to the regions immediately close to the ischemic area and seems to be due to a purely passive mechanism (tethering) by which the ischemic region acts as a parallel resistance, limiting the function of the contiguous myocardium (Table 4.2).

Table 4.2 Coronary and noncoronary causes of regional dysfunction

Coronary	Noncoronary
Ischemia	Myocardial fibrosis
Infarction	Systolic blood pressure and heart rate increase
Stunning	Electrical activation (LBBB, WPW, RV pacing)
Hibernation	Right ventricular overload, cardiac surgery

LBBB left bundle branch block, *RV* Right ventricular, *WPW* Wolff–Parkinson–White

4.6
Clinical Basis

Regional or global mechanical dysfunction as markers of ischemia gained clinical recognition in the preechocardiographic era through exercise radionuclide ventriculography. Although this technique was based on a less than perfect detector of mechanical dysfunction, with limited spatial and temporal resolution, it clearly showed the advantages of the new, mechanical marker over the old electrocardiographic one. With the development of ultrasound imaging it was natural to exploit the mechanical marker of ischemia through the echocardiographic probe. A series of studies established a conceptual framework for the future and extensive applications of stress echocardiography. During ischemia, the regional echocardiographic changes usually occur earlier than the electrocardiographic ones, which can even be totally absent in the presence of obvious regional dyssynergy [14, 20]. Wall motion changes are as reliable as the most sensitive invasive indexes of left ventricular performance, such as left ventricular dP/dt of contraction [26]. The capability of regional systolic dysfunction to detect the presence, site, and extent of ischemia obviously cleared the way to extensive clinical applications of stress echocardiography for the diagnosis and risk stratification of coronary artery disease [27, 28]. In the future, the challenge ahead will be to implement – with the help of new technologies – a more comprehensive assessment of cardiac function during stress, incorporating a more quantitative assessment of not only radial, but also circumferential and longitudinal function at baseline and during stress, possibly not only in a regional transmural but also strictly subendocardial function.

References

1. Hearse DJ (1994) Myocardial ischemia: can we agree on a definition for the 21st century? Cardiovasc Res 28:1737–1744
2. Ross J Jr (1986) Assessment of ischemic regional myocardial dysfunction and its reversibility. Circulation 74:1186–1190
3. Bogaert J, Rademakers FE (2001) Regional nonuniformity of normal adult human left ventricle. Am J Physiol Heart Circ Physiol 280:H610–H620
4. Stein PD, Marzilli M, Sabbah HN, et al (1980) Systolic and diastolic pressure gradients within the left ventricular wall. Am J Physiol 238:H625–H630

4

5. Borges AC, Pingitore A, Cordovil A, et al (1995). Heterogeneity of left ventricular regional wall thickening following dobutamine infusion in normal human subjects. Eur Heart J 16: 1726–1730
6. Gomes JA, Damato AN, Akhtar M, et al (1977) Ventricular septal motion and left ventricular dimensions during abnormal ventricular activation. Am J Cardiol 39:641–650
7. Myers JH, Stirling MC, Choy M, et al (1986). Direct measurement of inner and outer wall thickening dynamics with epicardial echocardiography. Circulation 74:164–172
8. Kaul S (1990) Echocardiography in coronary artery disease. Curr Probl Cardiol 15:233–298
9. Armstrong WF (1988) Echocardiography in coronary artery disease. Prog Cardiovasc Dis 30:267–288
10. Mondillo S, Galderisi M, Ballo P, Study Group of Echocardiography of the Italian Society of Cardiology, et al (2006) Left ventricular systolic longitudinal function: comparison among simple M-mode, pulsed, and M-mode color tissue Doppler of mitral annulus in healthy individuals. J Am Soc Echocardiogr 19:1085–1091
11. Reant P, Labrousse L, Lafitte S, et al (2008) Experimental validation of circumferential, longitudinal, and radial 2-dimensional strain during dobutamine stress echocardiography in ischemic conditions. J Am Coll Cardiol. 51:149–157
12. Braunwald E, Kloner RA (1982) The stunned myocardium: prolonged, postischemic ventricular dysfunction. Circulation 66:1146–1149
13. Braunwald E, Rutherford JD (1986) Reversible ischemic left ventricular dysfunction: evidence for the "hibernating myocardium". J Am Coll Cardiol 8:1467–1470
14. Vanoverschelde JL, Melin JA (2001) The pathophysiology of myocardial hibernation: current controversies and future directions. Prog Cardiovasc Dis 43:387–398
15. Pierard LA, De Landsheere CM, Berthe C, et al (1990) Identification of viable myocardium by echocardiography during dobutamine infusion in patients with myocardial infarction after thrombolytic therapy: comparison with positron emission tomography. J Am Coll Cardiol 15: 1021–1031
16. Lieberman AN, Weiss JL, Jugdutt BI, et al (1981) Two-dimensional echocardiography and infarct size: relationship of regional wall motion and thickening to the extent of myocardial infarction in the dog. Circulation 63:739–746
17. Carpeggiani C, L'Abbate A, Marzullo P, et al (1989) Multiparametric approach to diagnosis of non-Q-wave acute myocardial infarction. Am J Cardiol 63:404–408
18. Gardin JM, Adams DB, Douglas PS et al, on behalf of American Society of Echocardiography (2002) Recommendations for a standardized report for adult transthoracic echocardiography: a report from the American Society of Echocardiography's Nomenclature and Standards Committee and Task Force for a Standardized Echocardiography Report. J Am Soc Echocardiogr 15:275–290
19. Little WC, Reeves RC, Arciniegas J, et al (1982) Mechanism of abnormal interventricular septal motion during delayed left ventricular activation. Circulation 65:1486–1491
20. De Castro S, Pandian NG (eds) (2000) Manual of clinical echocardiography. Time-Science
21. Geleijnse ML, Vigna C, Kasprzak JD, et al (2000) Usefulness and limitations of dobutamine atropine stress echocardiography for the diagnosis of coronary artery disease in patients with left bundle branch block. A multicentre study. Eur Heart J 21:1666–1673
22. Stojnic BB, Stojanov PL, Angelkov L, et al (1996) Evaluation of asynchronous left ventricular relaxation by Doppler echocardiography during ventricular pacing with AV synchrony (VDD): comparison with atrial pacing (AAI). Pacing Clin Electrophysiol 19:940–944
23. Beker B, Vered Z, Bloom NV, et al (1994) Decreased thickening of normal myocardium with transient increased wall thickness during stress echocardiography with atrial pacing. J Am Soc Echocardiogr 7:381–387

24. Hirshleifer J, Crawford M, O'Rourke RA, et al (1975) Influence of acute alterations in heart rate and systemic arterial pressure on echocardiographic measures of left ventricular performance in normal human subjects. Circulation 52:835–841

25. Carstensen S, Ali SM, Stensgaard-Hansen FV, et al (1995) Dobutamine-atropine stress echocardiography in asymptomatic healthy individuals. The relativity of stress-induced hyperkinesia. Circulation 92:3453–3463

26. Distante A, Picano E, Moscarelli E, et al (1985) Echocardiographic versus hemodynamic monitorino during attacks of variant angina pectoris. Am J Cardiol 55:1319–1322

27. Pellikka PA, Nagueh SF, Elhendy AA, et al; American Society of Echocardiography (2007). American Society of Echocardiography recommendations for performance, interpretation, and application of stress echocardiography. J Am Soc Echocardiogr. 20:1021–1041

28. Sicari R, Nihoyannopoulos P, Evangelista A, et al (2008). Stress echocardiography consensus statement of the European Association of Echocardiography. Eur J Echocardiogr 9:415–437

Pathogenetic Mechanisms of Stress

5

Eugenio Picano

For a rational use of stress tests and an appropriate interpretation of their results, it may be useful to adopt a pathogenetic classification, taking into account the diagnostic end point of the test. Tests inducing vasospasm (ergonovine infusion and hyperventilation) explore the functional component. Tests trying to unmask coronary stenosis (exercise, dipyridamole, adenosine, dobutamine, pacing) mostly explore the ceiling of coronary reserve as defined by organic factors (Fig. 5.1). Some of these stressors (such as exercise) may also induce variations in coronary tone which can be superimposed on the organic factors, thus blurring the correlation between coronary anatomy and test positivity.

5.1
Ischemia and Vasospasm

Since coronary vasospasm can coexist with any degree of coronary stenosis, the presence of angiographically normal coronary arteries does not rule out the possibility of vasospastic myocardial ischemia; on the other hand, a "significant" coronary stenosis at angiography does not automatically establish a cause–effect relationship between organic disease and myocardial ischemia. In the past 20 years, we have come to appreciate the fact that the endothelium serves not only as a nonthrombogenic diffusion barrier to the migration of substances into and out of the blood stream, but also as the largest and most active paracrine organ in the body, producing potent vasoactive, anticoagulant, procoagulant, and fibrinolytic substances. Normal endothelium produces two vasoactive and platelet-active products, prostacyclin and EDRF, which act in concert to inhibit platelet adhesion and aggregation and relax vascular smooth muscle [1]. Normal endothelium also opposes a variety of vasoconstrictive stimuli, including catecholamines, acetylcholine, and serotonin, and it enhances the vasorelaxant effects of dilators, such as adenosine nucleotides. In the presence of a dysfunctional endothelium, vasodilatory stimuli – such as adenosine or dipyridamole – may become less potent, and vasoconstrictive stimuli much more effective [1] (Fig. 5.2). The mechanisms of coronary spasm are still unclear. No specific receptor subtypes appear to be involved, since a variety of physical and pharmacological stimuli

E. Picano, *Stress Echocardiography*,
© Springer-Verlag Berlin Heidelberg 2009

5

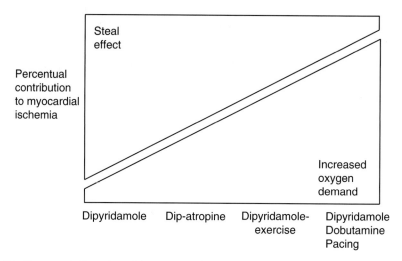

Fig. 5.1 Conceptual allocation of the tests employed in combination with echocardiography to induce ischemia via coronary vasospasm (*left*), coronary stenosis (*right*), or both mechanisms

can provoke spasm and no specific antagonist has proved capable of preventing it. The smooth muscle cell in the medial layer of coronary epicardial arteries reacts to several vasoconstrictive stimuli, coming centripetally from the adventitial layer (such as α-mediated vasoconstriction), or centrifugally from the intima–blood interface (such as endothelin and serotonin). In fact, serotonin has a vasodilatory effect on normal human myocardial arteries, which is mediated by endothelium-derived relaxing factors; when the endothelium is damaged, as in coronary artery disease, serotonin has a direct, unopposed vasoconstrictive effect [1]. Clinically, coronary vasospasm can be elicited by ergonovine maleate, an ergot alkaloid which stimulates both β-adrenergic and serotonergic receptors, and therefore exerts a direct constrictive effect on vascular smooth muscle. Hyperventilation induces spasm through systemic alkalosis. Physiologically, a powerful calcium-antagonistic action is exerted by hydrogen ions, which appear to compete with calcium ions for the same active sites both in the transmembrane calcium transport system and in the myofibrillar ATPase. Thus, vasoconstriction occurs if either calcium ion concentration increases or hydrogen ion concentration decreases. Exercise can also induce an increase in coronary tone, up to complete vasospasm, through α-sympathetic stimulation [2]. Dobutamine has a vasospastic and coronary vasoconstrictive effect mediated by α-adrenergic stimulation [3, 4]. Dipyridamole has no coronary constrictive effects per se; however, interruption of the test by aminophylline (which blocks adenosine receptors but also stimulates α-adrenoreceptors) can evoke coronary vasospasm in one-third of patients with variant angina [5]. Tests exploring organic coronary stenosis can induce ischemia by means of two basic mechanisms: (a) an increase in oxygen demand, exceeding the fixed supply and (b) flow maldistribution due to inappropriate coronary arteriolar vasodilation triggered by a metabolic/pharmacological stimulus. The main pharmacodynamic actions of dobutamine and dipyridamole stresses are summarized in Tables 5.1 and 5.2, respectively. Dobutamine

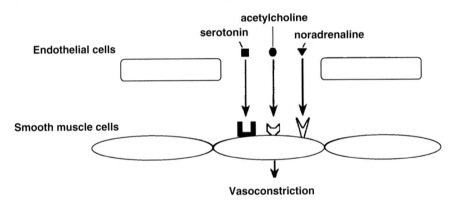

Fig. 5.2 *Top*: endothelial and smooth muscle cells in coronary vessels in the presence of intact endothelium. Mediators such as serotonin, acetylcholine, and noradrenaline stimulate the corresponding receptors present on the endothelial surface, which induce smooth muscle cell relaxation and vasodilation via EDRF release. *Bottom*: when endothelium is damaged, the same mediators act directly on the corresponding receptors present on the smooth muscle membrane, causing vasoconstriction

has complex dose-dependent effects on β_1-, β_2-, and α_1-adrenoreceptors [6], whereas the principal target of adenosine and dipyridamole are adenosine receptors, both A_1 and A_2, present both in myocardium and in coronary vessels [7]. In particular, stimulation of A_2a receptors produces marked dilation of coronary resistance vessels, determining arteriolar vasodilation, whereas A_2b receptors mediate vasodilation in conductance vessels. Myocardial A1 adenosine receptors mediate the negative chronotropic and dromotropic effects of

Table 5.1 Pharmacodynamics of dobutamine

	Receptor populations		
	α_1	β_1	β_1
Myocardium	Increased inotropy	Increased chronotropy, Increased inotropy	–
Vasculature	Vasoconstriction	–	Vasodilation

Table 5.2 Pharmacodynamics of adenosine and dipyridamole

	Receptor populations			
	A_1	A_2a	A_2b	A_3
Myocardium	Decreased chronotropy Decreased dromotropy Chest pain ? Preconditioning			
Vasculature		Coronary arteriolar vasodilation	Conductance vessel vasodilation	
Mast cells				? Bronchospasm ? Hypotension ? Preconditioning

adenosine and the direct algogenic effect. A_3 receptors are found on the surface of mast cells and may play a role in mediating bronchospasm and hypotension. Exogenous and endogenous adenosine may profoundly dilate coronary arterioles with minimal effect, if any, on systemic circulation, probably because A_2a receptors are more abundant in coronary arterioles than in any other vascular area [7]. A_1 and A_3 receptors also have a potential role in mediating preconditioning [7].

Adenosine is produced intracellularly via two pathways (Fig. 5.3), but it does not exert its effects until it leaves the intracellular environment and interacts with A_1 and A_2 adenosine receptors on the cell membrane [8]. As illustrated by the scheme in Fig. 5.3, dipyridamole acts by blocking the uptake and transport of adenosine into the cells, thereby resulting in a greater availability of adenosine at the receptor site. Both these mechanisms can provoke myocardial ischemia in the presence of a fixed reduction in coronary flow reserve due to organic factors (involving the epicardial coronary arteries and/or myocardium and/or microvasculature).

5.2
Increased Demand

This mechanism can be easily fitted into the familiar concept framework of ischemia as a supply–demand mismatch, deriving from an increase in oxygen requirements in the presence of a fixed reduction in coronary flow reserve. The different stresses can determine increases in demand through different mechanisms (Fig. 5.4).

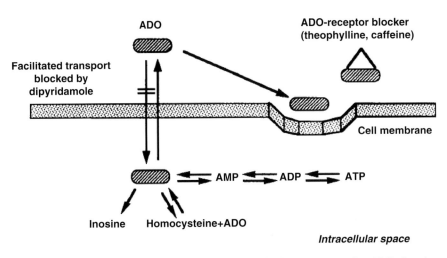

Fig. 5.3 Metabolism and mechanisms of action of adenosine in the coronary arteries. *ADO* adenosine, *AMP* adenosine monophosphate, *ADP* adenosine diphosphate, *ATP* adenosine triphosphate. (Modified from [8])

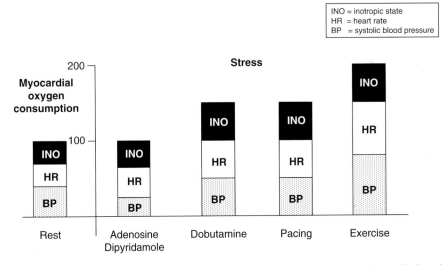

Fig. 5.4 Major determinants of myocardial oxygen consumption in resting conditions (*left*) and during some stresses (*right*) commonly employed with echocardiography. The relative contributions of systolic blood pressure, heart rate, and inotropic state to myocardial oxygen demand are represented. During dipyridamole or adenosine stress there is a mild increase in oxygen consumption, due to the increase in the inotropic state or heart rate, respectively. The rise in oxygen demand is even more marked during exercise, which causes an increased heart rate as well as increased inotropic state and systolic pressure. (Redrawn and modified from [9])

5

In resting conditions, myocardial oxygen consumption is dependent mainly on heart rate, inotropic state, and the left ventricular wall stress (which is proportional to the systolic blood pressure) [9]. Following dipyridamole or adenosine administration, a slight increase in myocardial function, a modest decrease in blood pressure, and mild tachycardia can be observed, overall determining only a trivial increase in myocardial oxygen demand [10].

During exercise, the increase in heart rate, blood pressure, and inotropic state accounts for the overall increase in myocardial oxygen consumption (Fig. 5.2) [11]. To a lesser degree, pacing and dobutamine also increase myocardial oxygen demand [12]. During pacing, the increase is mainly due to the increased heart rate. Dobutamine markedly increases contractility and heart rate (Fig. 5.2). Greater myocardial oxygen consumption due to heart rate increase occurs with the coadministration of atropine with dobutamine [13] and dipyridamole [14].

5.3
Flow Maldistribution

In the presence of coronary atherosclerosis, appropriate arteriolar dilation can paradoxically exert detrimental effects on regional myocardial perfusion, causing overperfusion of myocardial layers or regions already well perfused in resting conditions at the expense of regions or layers with a precarious flow balance in resting conditions [15].

In "vertical steal," the anatomical requisite is the presence of an epicardial coronary artery stenosis, and the subepicardium "steals" blood from the subendocardial layers. The mechanism underlying vertical steal is a fall in poststenotic pressure secondary to the increase in flow across the stenosis [16]. From the hydraulic viewpoint, it is well known that even in the presence of a fixed anatomical stenosis, resistance is not fixed. After administration of dipyridamole the arterioles dilate, thereby increasing flow across the stenotic lesion. This increased flow may lead to a greater drop in pressure, the magnitude of which is related to the severity of the stenosis and to the increase in flow. In the presence of a coronary stenosis, the administration of a coronary vasodilator causes a fall in poststenotic pressure, and therefore a critical fall in subendocardial perfusion pressure (Fig. 5.5), which in turn provokes a fall in absolute subendocardial flow, even with subepicardial overperfusion. In fact, the coronary autoregulation curve can be broken into two different curves (Fig. 5.5), with the subendocardium more vulnerable than the subepicardium to lowering of coronary perfusion pressure. Regional thickening is closely related to subendocardial rather than transmural flow, and this explains the "paradox" of a regional asynergy, with ischemia in spite of regionally increased transmural flow. Because endocardial oxygen demands are greater than epicardial ones, the resistance vessels of the endocardium are more dilated than those of the subepicardium, ultimately resulting in selective subendocardial hypoperfusion (Fig. 5.5).

"Horizontal steal" requires the presence of collateral circulation between two vascular beds (Fig. 5.6); the victim of the steal is the myocardium fed by the more stenotic vessel. The arteriolar vasodilatory reserve must be at least partially preserved in the

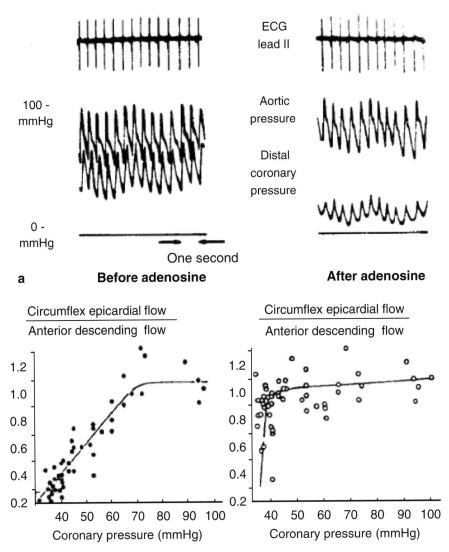

Fig. 5.5 *Upper panel*: The mechanisms of vertical steal, effect of adenosine infusion in an experimental model of severe coronary stenosis. (From [16]). *Lower panel*: Coronary autoregulation curve in the subendocardial and subepicardial layers. (From [17])

donor vessel and abolished in the vessel receiving collateral flow [17, 18]. After vasodilation, the flow in the collateral circulation is reduced relative to resting conditions, since the arteriolar bed of the donor vessel "competes" with the arteriolar bed of the receiving vessel, whose vasodilatory reserve was already exhausted in resting conditions (Figs. 5.6, 5.7).

5

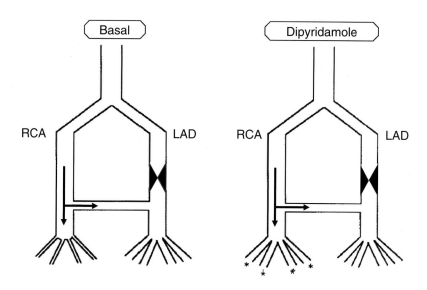

Fig. 5.6 Hydraulic model illustrating coronary horizontal steal. For this example, the right coronary artery (*RCA*) is the supply artery, with the vascular distribution of the severely stenotic left anterior descending (*LAD*) artery supplied by collaterals from the right coronary artery. Coronary steal following coronary arteriolar vasodilation refers to a decrease in absolute forward flow through collateral channels to the collateral-dependent vascular bed. With vasodilation of distal coronary arteriolar beds there is a flow-related drop in pressure along the supply artery. Therefore, distal perfusion pressure to the collateral vessels falls since collateral flow depends primarily on the driving pressure gradient (between distal perfusion pressure of the supply and collateralized vascular bed). (Redrawn and modified from [17])

The stresses provoking this flow maldistribution act through a "reverse Robin Hood effect" [19]; unlike the hero who stole from the rich to give to the poor [20, 21], they steal from the poor (myocardial regions or layers dependent on a critically stenosed coronary artery) and give to the rich (regions or layers already well nourished in resting conditions). The biochemical effector of this hemodynamic mechanism is the inappropriate accumulation of adenosine, which is the main physiological modulator of coronary arteriolar vasodilation. Inappropriate adenosine accumulation can be triggered either by a metabolic stimulus (such as exercise or pacing) or by a pharmacological one (such as exogenous adenosine or dipyridamole, which inhibits the cellular reuptake of endogenously produced adenosine) [22]. It is certainly difficult to quantify the relevance of flow maldistribution in inducing ischemia, but this mechanism is likely to play a key role in adenosine- or dipyridamole-induced ischemia and a relatively minor, although significant, role in exercise- or pacing-induced ischemia [20–23]. Theoretically, dobutamine might also induce a moderate degree of flow maldistribution by stimulating β-adrenergic receptors, which mediate coronary arteriolar vasodilation [24] (Fig. 5.8).

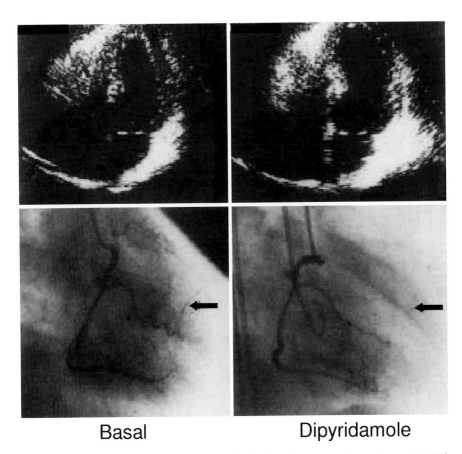

Basal   Dipyridamole

Fig. 5.7 An example in which collaterals were supplied by the right coronary artery to the occluded left anterior descending artery. Two-dimensional echocardiographic frames, taken at end-systole (*top*); and coronary angiographic images (*bottom*), obtained in basal conditions and after dipyridamole administration. After dipyridamole, the apex is dyskinetic; the coronary angiography shows almost total disappearance of the collateral vessels (*arrows*). (Modified from [15])

5.4
Exercise-Simulating Agents: Scientific Fact or Fancy Definition?

Among stresses, a currently used differentiation is between "exercise-simulating agents," such as dobutamine or arbutamine, and vasodilator stressors, such as dipyridamole or adenosine. It is important to emphasize that none of the pharmacological stresses are "exercise simulating" in a strict sense. Only exercise offers complex information not only on coronary flow reserve, but also on cardiac reserve and cardiovascular efficiency (i.e., how the coronary reserve is translated into external work). Coronary reserve and cardiovascular efficiency are codeterminants of exercise tolerance and therefore of

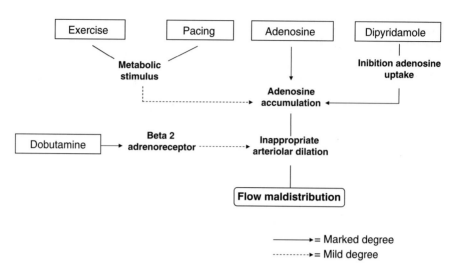

Fig. 5.8 The biochemical pathways leading to inappropriate arteriolar vasodilation under different stresses

the quality of life for the individual patient. No pharmacological stress can mimic the complex hemodynamic, neural, and hormonal adaptations triggered by exercise, nor can they offer information on cardiovascular efficiency. Exercise explores the entire physiological chain supporting external work: psychological motivation, central and peripheral nervous system, lungs, myocardium, coronary circulation, peripheral blood circulation and skeletal muscle, down to cell respiration and mitochondrial oxygen utilization [25]. Of this chain, pharmacological stresses only test the "coronary" ring. From the echocardiographic viewpoint, the mechanical pattern of stress-induced function increase differs between exercise and pharmacological stresses – including dobutamine, which affects regional wall function in a manner similar to atrial pacing rather than dynamic exercise [26]. From the clinical viewpoint, changes in rate–pressure product can stratify disease severity with exercise, not with pharmacological stresses. Antianginal therapy affects pharmacological stress results – and especially dobutamine results (as discussed in more detail in Chap. 18) in a manner largely unrelated to the effects of the same therapy on exercise. Finally, arrhythmias, heart rate, and blood pressure response enrich the diagnostic information obtainable with exercise stress testing, not with pharmacological testing. On the other hand, all stresses can be considered "exercise simulating" for the purpose of diagnosing coronary artery disease. Their mechanism of action is the extreme exaggeration of a biochemical and hemodynamic mechanism actually operating during exercise, such as adrenergic stimulation with dobutamine or adenosinergic stimulation with dipyridamole [20–22].

Last but not least, from a less physiological but more pragmatic point of view, all stresses should be considered exercise simulating since they induce ischemia with similar frequency, in the same region, and to a comparable degree as exercise. They also titrate the positive response, but the equivalent of the ischemic workload is the drug dose (the "pharmacological dose load") sufficient to elicit ischemia.

5.5
New Pharmacological Stresses

The family of pharmacological stresses is rapidly expanding, due to the combined pressure of scientific and economic motivations. In the family of catecholaminic stresses, arbutamine is characterized by a potent β-agonist effect, with a stronger chronotropic and a milder inotropic action than dobutamine. It might be considered conceptually similar to a pacing test, since it stresses the myocardium mainly through an increase in heart rate [27]. However, differently from pacing, arbutamine stress is noninvasive rather than semiinvasive; it is pharmacological rather than electrical; it is a flexible stress, tailored to the patient's response, rather than fixed and standard like electrical pacing. It is also highly expensive and no longer commercially available in most countries. For vasodilator stresses as well, new drugs are on the horizon, such as new selective adenosine A_2 receptor agonists with short half-lives [28].

5.6
The Atropine Factor in Pharmacological Stress Echocardiography

Atropine is a naturally occurring antimuscarinic drug consisting of an alkaloid of the belladonna plants. During the time of the Roman Empire the plant was frequently used to produce poison. This prompted Linnaeus to name the shrub *Atropa belladonna*, after Atrops, the eldest of the Three Fates, who cuts the thread of life. The name belladonna (i.e., "beautiful woman") derives from the alleged use of this preparation by Italian women to dilate their pupils [29]. Atropine is the prototype of antimuscarinic drugs, which inhibit the actions of acetylcholine on anatomical effectors innervated by postganglionic cholinergic nerves. The main effect of atropine on the heart is to induce tachycardia by blocking vagal effects on the M2 receptors on the seno-atrial nodal pacemaker. Atropine also enhances atrioventricular conduction, and for this reason it is usually given before pacing stress (see Chap. 14). Atropine-induced mydriasis may occasionally raise the intraocular pressure in patients with glaucoma, which is therefore a contraindication to atropine administration. Atropine also decreases the normal amplitude of bladder contraction, and severe prostatic disease is thus another contraindication to atropine administration. Finally, atropine reduces gastrointestinal tract motility and secretion and for this reason can be given before transesophageal stress. Administration of atropine on top of dobutamine [13] vasodilators [14–30], or exercise [31, 32] improves diagnostic sensitivity. Not surprisingly, however, the risk of resistant ischemia increases with atropine [33, 34], along with nonischemic side effects, including (as described in dobutamine plus atropine) atropine intoxication [35], consisting of restlessness, irritability, disorientation, hallucinations, or delirium, usually disappearing spontaneously over a few hours [2].

5.7
The Combined Stress Approach

The combined stress can be either dipyridamole–exercise or dipyridamole–dobutamine. Dipyridamole causes only a trivial increase in myocardial oxygen demand, provoking ischemia mainly through flow maldistribution phenomena triggered by endogenous adenosine accumulation. The flow increase achieved by a high dipyridamole dose lasts for a relatively long time, remaining at plateau for about 30 min and, therefore, representing an ideal "flow maldistribution" background over which another stress can be superimposed. It has previously been shown that dipyridamole does not block the hemodynamic response of exercise [36] or dobutamine [37], and that it potentiates the ischemic potential of both exercise and dobutamine. The underlying hypothesis is that a stepwise increment of myocardial oxygen consumption – unable per se to elicit ischemia in the presence of mild coronary artery disease – might reach the critical threshold when the ischemic ceiling is lowered by concomitant flow maldistribution triggered by dipyridamole infusion [36] (Fig. 5.9). The clinical fact is that the combined stress test can detect anatomically milder forms of coronary disease missed by either test used separately [36–38].

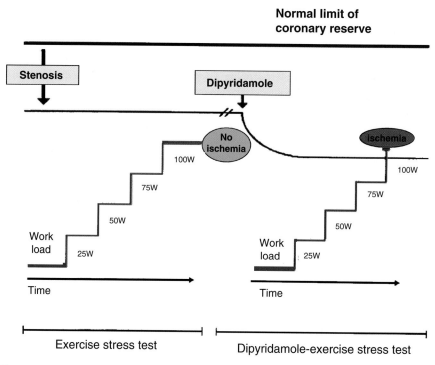

Fig. 5.9 Dipyridamole sensitization of the ischemic potential of exercise. Coronary stenosis (*thick arrow*) may permanently although not severely lower the maximal flow availability (coronary reserve), so that the myocardial ischemic threshold is not reached with an "ordinary" exercise stress test. With dipyridamole premedication (*thin arrow*), the hemodynamic response to exercise is not prevented (normal stepwise increase in workload), but the maximal flow availability is significantly lowered for the occurrence of flow maldistribution phenomena. (From [36] with permission)

5.8
Vasodilatory Power and the Hierarchy of Testing

Each of the prototype stresses for the detection of coronary artery disease can induce ischemia through either one of the two main pathophysiological pathways: "steal effect" (also named flow maldistribution) and increased oxygen demand (Fig. 5.10).

No stress is 100% "pure," since adenosine and dipyridamole also slightly increase heart rate, and exercise and dobutamine also induce a certain (mild) degree of flow maldistribution. Both families of stresses are more or less equally effective as ischemic stressors in the presence of significant coronary artery disease (Fig. 5.11). For a given ischemic diagnostic marker (for instance, regional wall motion abnormalities with stress echocardiography), sensitivity is higher for tests combining the two pathways (such as dipyridamole–exercise, dipyridamole–dobutamine, or dipyridamole atropine) when compared with tests based on one pathway (dipyridamole or dobutamine or exercise) alone. The relevance of the steal effect is also directly mirrored by the stress capacity to recruit coronary flow reserve. Adenosinergic stresses are ideally suited for this, since – unlike dobutamine or exercise associated with a threefold flow increase – they determine a fivefold increase in coronary blood flow with a full recruitment of pharmacological flow reserve [39]. The greater the vasodilation, the higher the potential for inappropriate steal phenomena in the presence of coronary artery disease. In recent years, the two different sides of the coin of the stress test, vasodilatory and ischemic stress, merged in the dual imaging of coronary flow reserve and wall motion during vasodilatory stress echocardiography [40–42].

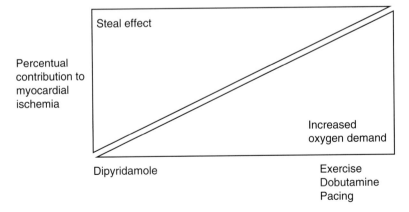

Fig. 5.10 Conceptual allocation of tests employed in combination with echocardiography to detect coronary artery stenosis inducing ischemia via steal effect (*left*) or increased myocardial oxygen demand (*right*), or both mechanisms

5

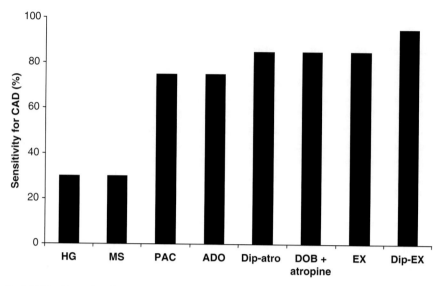

Fig. 5.11 The hierarchy of test sensitivity for the diagnosis of coronary artery disease. The sensitivity is highest for tests combining the two main mechanisms of increased oxygen consumption and steal phenomena. On the *far left* of the *x-axis*, tests that are below the threshold of clinical value, such as handgrip and mental stress. *Dip-Ex* dipyridamole exercise, *Dip* dipyridamole, *Ado* adenosine, *HG* handgrip, *MS* mental stress, *PAC* pacing

5.9
The Fosbury Flop and the Classic Straddle in the Stress Echocardiography Laboratory

The use of stress to increase myocardial oxygen demand in order to provoke ischemia is like the classic straddle method in the high jump: it is conceptually familiar to everybody (everyone has tried it at least once) and it is pushed forward by the force of tradition. The steal effect is like the "Fosbury flop": it is more recent, may appear counterintuitive, but works at least as well as the straddle method. As a young high jumper in the early 1960s, Dick Fosbury had trouble mastering the standard technique, called the straddle, so he began doing the high jump by approaching the bar with his back to it instead, doing a modified scissor kick and going over the bar backwards and horizontal to the ground. As goofy as it looked, it worked. Similarly, as strange as it may look within the supply–demand mismatch framework, the concept of inducing ischemia through a vasodilator instead of by increasing myocardial oxygen demand has worked. Fosbury caused a sensation when he won the gold medal in the 1968 Olympics. The Fosbury flop has since become a standard technique for high jumpers – whether Olympic champions pushing forward the limits of the specialty, or lazy, fat, chubby kids trying to satisfy the coach in gym class at elementary school. Twenty years after the initial proposal in 1985, vasodilatory stress echocardiography is the convenient option for primary care stress echocardiographers, who will benefit from a stress that pollutes the image quality very little, reducing the problems of interpretation. It is also a good option for stress echocardiographers with top level expertise and technology, since it allows one to combine wall motion and coronary flow imaging in the same stress [40, 41]. Dual imaging is currently recommended by European guidelines as the state-of-the-art approach along with pharmacological stress echocardiography [42]. The force of innovation sets new standards – impossible to accept if one ignores the pathophysiological basis of the technique.

References

1. Bonetti PO, Lerman LO, Lerman A (2003) Endothelial dysfunction: a marker of atherosclerotic risk. Arterioscler Thromb Vasc Biol 23:168–175
2. Feigl EO (1987) The paradox of adrenergic coronary vasoconstriction. Circulation 76:737–745
3. Kawano H, Fujii H, Motoyama T, et al (2000) Myocardial ischemia due to coronary artery spasm during dobutamine stress echocardiography. Am J Cardiol 85:26–30
4. Roffi M, Meier B, Allemann Y (2000) Angiographic documented coronary arterial spasm in absence of critical coronary artery stenoses in a patient with variant angina episodes during exercise and dobutamine stress echocardiography. Heart 83:E4
5. Picano E, Lattanzi F, Masini M, et al (1988) Aminophylline termination of dipyridamole stress as a trigger of coronary vasospasm in variant angina. Am J Cardiol 62:694–697
6. Ruffolo RR Jr, Spradlin TA, Pollock GD, et al (1981) Alpha- and -adrenergic effects of the stereoisomers of dobutamine. J Pharmacol Exp Ther 219:447–452
7. Fredholm BB, Abbracchio MP, Burnstock G, et al (1994) Nomenclature and classification of purinoceptors. Pharmacol Rev 46:143–156
8. Verani MS (1991) Adenosine thallium 201 myocardial perfusion scintigraphy. Am Heart J 122:269–278
9. Ross J Jr (1972) Factors regulating the oxygen consumption of the heart. In: Russek HI, Zoham BL (eds) Changing concepts in cardiovascular disease. Williams and Wilkins, Baltimore, pp 20–31
10. Picano E, Simonetti I, Carpeggiani C, et al (1989) Regional and global biventricular function during dipyridamole stress testing. Am J Cardiol 63:429–432
11. Beleslin BD, Ostojic M, Stepanovic J, et al (1994) Stress echocardiography in the detection of myocardial ischemia.Head-to-head comparison of exercise, dobutamine, and dipyridamole tests. Circulation 90:1168–1176
12. Picano E (2002) Dipyridamole in myocardial ischemia: Good Samaritan or Terminator? Int J Cardiol 83:215–216
13. McNeill AJ, Fioretti PM, el-Said SM, et al (1992) Enhanced sensitivity for detection of coronary artery disease by addition of atropine to dobutamine stress echocardiography. Am J Cardiol 70:41–46
14. Picano E, Pingitore A, Conti U, et al (1993) Enhanced sensitivity for detection of coronary artery disease by addition of atropine to dipyridamole echocardiography. Eur Heart J 14:1216–1222
15. Picano E (1989) Dipyridamole-echocardiography test: historical background and physiologic basis. Eur Heart J 10:365–376
16. Bove AA, Santamore WP, Carey RA (1983) Reduced myocardial blood flow resulting from dynamic changes in coronary artery stenosis. Int J Cardiol 4:301–317

17. Guyton RA, McClenathan JH, Newman GE, et al (1977) Significance of subendocardial S-T segment elevation caused by coronary stenosis in the dog. Epicardial S-T segment depression, local ischemia and subsequent necrosis. Am J Cardiol 40:373–380
18. Demer L, Gould KL, Kirkeeide R (1988) Assessing stenosis severity: coronary flow reserve, collateral function, quantitative coronary arteriography, positron imaging, and digital subtraction angiography. A review and analysis. Prog Cardiovasc Dis 30:307–322
19. Picano E, Lattanzi F (1991) Dipyridamole echocardiography. A new diagnostic window on coronary artery disease. Circulation 83:III19–III26
20. Crea F, Pupita G, Galassi AR, et al (1989) Effect of theophylline on exercise-induced myocardial ischaemia. Lancet 1:683–686
21. Emdin M, Picano E, Lattanzi F, et al (1989) Improved exercise capacity with acute aminophylline administration in patients with syndrome X. J Am Coll Cardiol 14:1450–1453
22. Cannon RO 3rd (1989) Aminophylline for angina: the "Robin Hood" effect? J Am Coll Cardiol 14:1454–1455
23. Picano E, Pogliani M, Lattanzi F, et al (1989) Exercise capacity after acute aminophylline administration in angina pectoris. Am J Cardiol 63:14–16
24. Waltier DC, Ziwoloski M, Gross FJ, et al (1981) Redistribution of myocardial blood flow distal to a dynamic coronary artery stenosis by sympathomimetic amines. Am J Cardiol 48:269–279
25. Varga A, Preda I (1997) Pharmacological stress echocardiography for exercise independent assessment of anti-ischaemic therapy. Eur Heart J 18:180–181
26. Carstensen S, Ali SM, Stensgaard-Hansen FV, et al (1995) Dobutamine-atropine stress echocardiography in asymptomatic healthy individuals. The relativity of stress-induced hyperkinesia. Circulation 92:3453–3463
27. Hammond HK, McKirnan D (1994) Effects of dobutamine and arbutamine on regional myocardial function in a porcine model of myocardial ischemia. J Am Coll Cardiol 23:475–482
28. Glover DK, Ruiz M, Yang JY, et al (1996) Pharmacological stress thallium scintigraphy with 2- cyclohexylmethylidenehydrazino adenosine (WRC-0470). A novel, short-acting adenosine A2A receptor agonist. Circulation 94:1726–1732
29. Brown JH (1992) Atropine, scopolamine and related antimuscarinic drugs. In: Goodman A, Gilman G (eds) The pharmacologic basis of therapeutics, 8th edn, vol 1. McGraw Hill, New York, pp 150–165
30. Miyazono Y, Kisanuki A, Toyonaga K, et al (1998) Usefulness of adenosine triphosphate atropine stress echocardiography for detecting coronary artery stenosis. Am J Cardiol 82:290–294
31. Attenhofer CH, Pellikka PA,Roger VL, et al (2000) Impact of atropine injection on heart rate response during treadmill exercise echocardiography: a double-blind randomized pilot study. Echocardiography 17:221–227
32. Banerjee S, Yalamanchili VS, Abdul-Baki T, et al (2002) Use of atropine to maintain higher heart rate after exercise during treadmill stress echocardiography. J Am Soc Echocardiogr 15:43–45
33. Nedeljkovic MA, Ostojic M, Beleslin B, et al (2001) Dipyridamole-atropine-induced myocardial infarction in a patient with patent epicardial coronary arteries. Herz 26:485–488
34. Erdogan O, Altun A, Akdemir O, et al (2001) Unexpected occurrence of ST segment elevation during administration of intravenous atropine. Cardiovasc Drugs Ther 15:367–368
35. Mathias W Jr, Arruda A, Santos FC, et al (1999) Safety of dobutamine-atropine stress echocardiography: a prospective experience of 4,033 consecutive studies. J Am Soc Echocardiogr 12:785–791
36. Picano E, Lattanzi F, Masini M, et al (1988) Usefulness of the dipyridamole-exercise echocardiography test for diagnosis of coronary artery disease. Am J Cardiol 62:67–70

37. Ostojic M, Picano E, Beleslin B, et al (1994) Dipyridamole-dobutamine echocardiography: a novel test for the detection of milder forms of coronary artery disease. J Am Coll Cardiol 23:1115–1122

38. Marwick TH (1997) Use of stress echocardiography for the prognostic assessment of patients with stable chronic coronary artery disease. Eur Heart J 18(Suppl D):D97–D101

39. Iskandrian AS, Verani MS, Heo J (1994) Pharmacologic stress testing: mechanism of action, hemodynamic responses, and results in detection of coronary artery disease. J Nucl Cardiol 1:94–111

40. Rigo F, Richieri M, Pasanisi E et al (2003) Usefulness of coronary flow reserve over regional wall motion when added to dual-imaging dipyridamole echocardiography. Am J Cardiol 91:269–273

41. Rigo F, Sicari R, Gherardi S, et al (2008) The additive prognostic value of wall motion abnormalities and coronary flow reserve during dipyridamole stress echo. Eur Heart J 29:79–88

42. Sicari R, Nihoyannopoulos P, Evangelista A, on behalf of the European Association of Echocardiography, et al (2008) Stress echocardiography expert consensus statement: European Association of Echocardiography (EAE) (a registered branch of the ESC). Eur J Echocardiogr 9:415–437

Echocardiographic Signs of Ischemia

6

Eugenio Picano

The response of left ventricular function to ischemia is monotonous and independent of the employed stress [1]. The same echocardiographic signs can be found in transient ischemia and acute infarction. The difference is in the time sequence, and from an echocardiographic viewpoint myocardial ischemia is a "reversible" myocardial infarction. The cardinal sign of ischemia is the transient, regional wall motion abnormality – the cornerstone of diagnosis. There are other ancillary signs of severity which may occasionally help in disease severity stratification, such as left ventricular cavity dilation, acute severe mitral insufficiency, fall of stroke volume, or appearance of ultrasound lung comets on the chest (Table 6.1). In leading-edge stress echocardiography environments, wall motion analysis can be coupled today during vasodilator stress with assessment of coronary flow reserve– which further expands the diagnostic and prognostic information during stress echocardiography.

6.1
The Main Sign of Ischemia with 2D Echocardiography:

6.1.1
Regional Asynergy

The normal myocardium shows systolic thickening and endocardial movement toward the center of the cavity. The hyperkinesia indicates an increase of normal movement and thickening (Table 6.2).

The hallmark of transient myocardial ischemia is regional asynergy (or dyssynergy) in its three degrees: hypokinesia (decrease of movement and systolic thickening); akinesia (absence of movement and systolic thickening); dyskinesia (paradoxical outward movement and possible systolic thinning). Obviously, this description is arbitrarily focused on three points of a continuous spectrum of mechanical modifications induced by ischemia. From a clinical point of view, the reliability of hypokinesia is reduced because of a greater intra- and interobserver variability. In contrast, akinesia and dyskinesia reflect more marked modifications of regional mechanics with smaller interobserver discordance. From

E. Picano, *Stress Echocardiography*,
© Springer-Verlag Berlin Heidelberg 2009

6

Table 6.1 Signs of ischemia

	Simplicity	Usefulness	Meaning
Regional wall motion	++	+++	Diagnosis/Prognosis
Ancillary signs:			
LV cavity dilation	+++	±	Prognosis
• *Severe MI*			
• *ULC*			
• *Stroke volume fall*			
CFR	+	++	Prognosis/Diagnosis

LV left ventricular; *MI* mitral insufficiency; *ULC* ultrasound lung comets

Table 6.2 Regional wall function

	Systolic thickening	Endocardial motion
Hyperkinesis	Increased	Increased
Normokinesis	10–80 (%)	4–10 mm
Hypokinesis	Reduced	Reduced
Akinesis	Abolished	Abolished
Dyskinesis	Systolic thinning	Outward systolic movement

a pathophysiological viewpoint, the severity of dyssynergy is correlated to the severity and transmural extension of the flow deficit [2]. Virtually all approaches and all projections can be utilized to document regional dyssynergy. From each projection, an *M*-mode line of view can help document the asynergy, thanks to the better axial resolution and the easier quantification of the time–motion tracings when compared with the bidimensional images. The *M*-mode tracing must be perpendicular to the ischemic region and geometrically controlled from the bidimensional image. The evaluation of a segmentary dyssynergy is easier in a ventricle with normal baseline function than in a ventricle with a resting asynergy. In the latter case, the stress can induce a homozonal ischemia in the infarcted area: for instance, a hypokinetic zone becomes akinetic. The stress-induced worsening of a baseline dysfunction (so-called homozonal ischemia) indicates a residual critical stenosis in the infarct-related coronary artery and the presence of jeopardized myocardium in the infarcted area. Homozonal residual ischemia may also involve a segment adjacent to the necrotic area but belonging to the distribution territory of the same coronary artery. In contrast, heterozonal ischemia develops in an area remote from the necrotic segment and supplied by a different coronary artery. Heterozonal ischemia is very specific for multivessel coronary disease. The reduced regional systolic thickening is theoretically more sensitive and specific than wall motion [2]. In fact, the latter – unlike the thickening – can remain unmodified during ischemia because of a passive movement transmitted by neighboring regions where perfusion and contraction are normal. In practice, regional movement and

systolic thickening tend to be symmetrically affected with the exception of a few pathological situations (i.e., postsurgical septum after bypass intervention, left bundle branch
block, or right ventricular pacing) in which the two parameters may dissociate, with alterations of movement and normal thickening. In these cases it is essential to evaluate only the
systolic thickening both in resting conditions and during stress.

6.2
Stress Echocardiography in Four Equations

All stress echocardiographic diagnoses can be easily summarized into four equations centered on regional wall function and describing the fundamental response patterns: normal;
ischemic; viable; necrotic (Table 6.3). The possible mechanical patterns are schematically
shown in Fig. 6.1 together with their myocardial and coronary correlates. The corresponding stress echocardiography patterns are displayed in Fig. 6.2.

In the normal response, a segment is normokinetic at rest and normal–hyperkinetic
during stress. In the ischemic response, the function of a segment worsens during stress
from normokinesis to dyssynergy. In the viable response, a segment with resting dysfunction improves during stress. In the necrotic response, a segment with resting dysfunction
remains fixed during stress. A resting akinesia which becomes dyskinesia during stress
reflects a purely passive, mechanical phenomenon of increased intraventricular pressure developed by normally contracting walls and should not be considered a true active
ischemia [3]. It is conceptually similar to the increase of ST-segment elevation during
exercise in patients with resting Q waves.

In the jeopardized pattern, a segment with resting hypokinesis becomes akinetic or
dyskinetic during stress (Chap. 1, Fig. 6.3). A viable response at low dose can be followed
by an ischemic response at high dose; the "biphasic" response is suggestive of viability and
ischemia, with jeopardized myocardium fed by a critically stenosed coronary artery [4].

Table 6.3 Stress echocardiography in four equations

Rest	+	Stress	=	Diagnosis
Normokinesis	+	Normo–hyperkinesis	=	Normal
Normokinesis	+	Hypo-, a-, dyskinesia	=	Ischemia
Akinesis	+	Hypo-, normokinesis	=	Viable
A-, dyskinesis	+	A-, dyskinesis	=	Necrosis

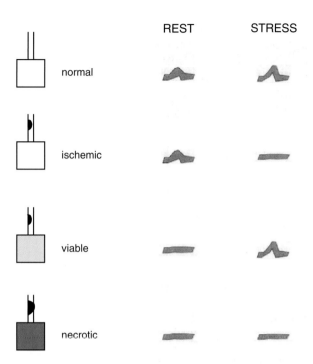

Fig. 6.1 Stress echographic pattern of normal (*upper row*), ischemic (*second row*), viable (*third row*), and necrotic (*fourth row*) responses are schematically represented. On the *left side*, the corresponding schemes of the coronary artery (*parallel lines*) and the myocardium (*box*) are shown. A normal myocardium is represented as a *white box*; a necrotic myocardium as a *black box*; a viable myocardium as a *gray box*. In a normal segment fed by a normal coronary artery, the segment is normokinetic at rest and normal–hyperkinetic during stress (*upper row*). In a normal myocardium fed by a critically stenosed coronary artery, the segment is normokinetic at rest and hypo, a-, or dyskinetic during stress (*second row*). A viable segment (*third row*) is akinetic at rest and normal during stress. A necrotic segment shows a fixed wall motion abnormality at rest and during stress (*lower row*)

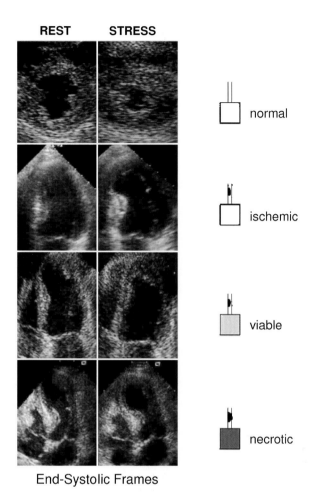

Fig. 6.2 Echocardiographic examples of normal (*upper row*), ischemic (*second row*), viable (*third row*), and necrotic (*fourth row*) responses. On the *left side*, the end-systolic frames of a rest (*left part*) and stress (*right part*) study are shown. In a viable myocardium with resting dysfunction and fed by a coronary artery with noncritical coronary stenosis, the segment is hypo-, akinetic at rest and normokinetic during stress (*third row*). Necrotic tissue shows unchanged function throughout the test, regardless of the underlying anatomical condition of the infarct-related vessel (*fourth row*)

6.2.1
False-Negative Results

A stress echocardiography examination can be normal in the presence of angiographically assessed coronary artery disease (Table 6.4). This more frequently happens with submaximal stresses which do not test efficiently the coronary circulation. With maximal stress,

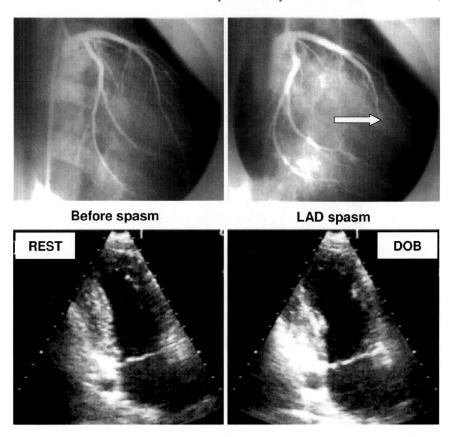

Before spasm   **LAD spasm**

Fig. 6.3 Normal coronary angiogram (*left upper panel*), spontaneous spasm of the left anterior descending coronary artery of the same patient (*right upper panel, indicated by arrow*), end-systolic frames of the patient in 2-chamber view at rest (*left lower panel*), and at peak stress (*right lower panel*) with clear akinesia of the apex. (Modified from [16])

Table 6.4 Sources of false-negative results

1. Submaximal stress
2. Limited (single vessel) coronary artery disease
3. Mild (50–75%) coronary artery disease
4. Left circumflex coronary artery disease
5. Patients studied under antiischemic therapy
6. Inadequate imaging/inadequate reading

a false-negative response is found more frequently in the presence of less extensive (single-vessel disease) or less severe (50–75% stenosis) coronary disease, and especially on the left circumflex coronary artery [5]. Not all coronary stenoses were created equal and – when a maximal stress is administered – those with negative stress echocardiography response are less severe from the anatomic [6], functional [7], and prognostic [8] viewpoint. Antianginal therapy lowers the sensitivity of exercise echocardiography as it does with vasodilator stresses [9, 10]. Dobutamine stress results are much less affected by calcium-channel blockers and nitrate therapy [11, 12]. In some cases, true ischemia occurs but may go undetected by stress echocardiography, especially in less well-imaged segments, such as the inferior wall, because of the inherent limitations of subjective analysis and lack of quantitative criteria. In these cases, cine-magnetic resonance imaging (MRI) documents a true impairment in regional systolic thickening [13].

6.3
False-Positive Responses

A transient alteration of regional function represents a very specific sign of myocardial ischemia. Nevertheless, false-positive results in stress echocardiography do exist and occur with (Table 6.5) or without (Table 6.6) true induced ischemia. Even with a nonsignificant stenosis at coronary angiography, a stress test for coronary artery disease can induce true ischemia and asynergy by triggering a coronary vasospasm in susceptible patients. Stress-induced coronary vasospasm has been described with exercise [14], dobutamine [15–16] (Fig. 6.3), or dipyridamole (more frequently following aminophylline) [17]. Coronary spasm is easily recognized when it is associated with transient ST-segment elevation during

Table 6.5 Sources of false-positive results (with true ischemia)

1. Spasm on a nonsignificant fixed stenosis
2. Inadequate angiographic imaging of a fixed, significant stenosis
3. Severe reduction in flow reserve with mild, nonsignificant stenosis
4. Occult, or unrecognized, cardiomyopathy
5. Hemodynamic changes (excessive increase in systolic blood pressure and/or heart rate)

Table 6.6 Sources of false-positive results (without true ischemia)

1. Human error
2. Heterogeneity of contraction
3. Artifactual asynergies
4. Occult, or unrecognized, cardiomyopathy
5. Hemodynamic changes (excessive increase in systolic blood pressure and/or heart rate)

6

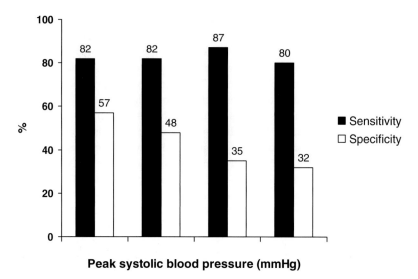

Fig. 6.4 Sensitivity (*empty bars*) and specificity (*full bars*) of exercise echocardiography according to peak systolic blood pressure response during exercise. (Modified from [24])

stress, but frequently it also occurs with ST-segment depression or even with no obvious changes on the ECG. True ischemia can also be found in patients with an angiographic stenosis below the "magic" 50%, but with a physiologically important reduction in flow reserve. In this case, the regional dysfunction during stress echocardiography is a "false negative" versus the angiographic standard, but a "true positive" versus a more accurate descriptor of anatomy such as intracoronary ultrasound [18]. True stress-induced ischemia may occur in the presence of occult cardiomyopathy [19]. The incipient muscle disease cannot be overt at rest, but a chronotropic and afterload challenge associated with stress can unmask a true regional dysfunction – destined to progress over time to frank cardiomyopathy. An extreme reduction in coronary flow reserve usually associated with left ventricular hypertrophy [20, 21] may also provoke stress-induced ischemia. As described pathophysi-ologically in Chap. 2, and clinically in Chap. 31, microvascular angina typically occurs with chest pain, ST-segment depression, and perfusion abnormalities without wall motion change [22]. However, in extreme left ventricular hypertrophy and especially in aortic stenosis, in which there is a critical contribution of increased end-systolic wall stress of the left ventricle, true extensive subendocardial hypoperfusion can develop [23] with real wall motion abnormalities [21]. Finally, an excessive systolic blood pressure rise during exercise may increase disproportionately the afterload determining a wall motion abnormality [24] – often severe and in multiple regions – in the left ventricle (Fig. 6.4). Stress-induced high heart rate [25] and high blood pressure [26] may reduce regional systolic thickening also in normal subjects. False-positive results may occur in the absence of a true ischemic asynergy, because of a mistake in the acquisition and/or interpretation and/or analysis. The human error determining a false-positive result is more frequent with aggressive reading

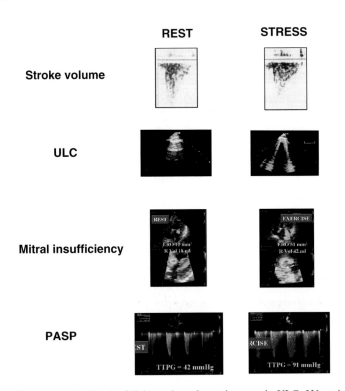

Fig. 6.5 Ancillary signs of ischemia: fall in stroke volume; increase in ULC; LV cavity dilation; decrease in S wave at tissue Doppler imaging; rise in pulmonary artery systolic pressure; acute severe mitral insufficiency. Each of these signs has an ominous prognostic meaning

criteria (for instance, lack of hyperkinesia) and with stressors polluting image quality and determining marked increase in heart rate and contractility, which inflate the number of indeterminate or ambiguous results. In fact, a relative lack of hyperkinesis, or even a true hypokinesia, can be a part of the physiological response by a completely normal ventricle to an inotropic stress [27, 28].

Last but not least, no left ventricle can be called free of artifactual asynergies. Spurious off-axis projections can create artifactual asynergies – more frequent in basal and infero-posterior regions.

6.3.1
"False" Stress Echocardiography Results: Anatomic Lies and Prognostic Truths?

Even the best laboratory will have a "physiological" percentage of false-positive and false-negative results. Obviously, this percentage of stress echocardiography "lies" will be higher with inexperienced readers and with stresses polluting image quality (exercise and dobutamine more than dipyridamole). Patients with variant angina, severe left ventricular hypertrophy, and uncontrolled hypertension have a higher chance of false-positive responses; patients studied under full antiischemic therapy will have a higher chance of false-negative responses. If the rate of false responses exceeds the expected average of 20%, the method should be reassessed. The "angiographic lies" of stress echocardiography can turn out to be striking "prognostic truths" in the long-run, over-ruling the prognostic stratification provided by the anatomic gold standard of coronary angiography. Thereby, in the anatomically defined subset of patients with single-vessel disease, patients with negative stress echocardiography findings ("false negative") have an excellent prognosis, better with medical therapy rather than with anatomy-guided revascularization [8]. In patients with angiographically normal coronary arteries, patients with stress echocardiography positivity (false-positive result) have higher chances of adverse events in the long run [29].

6.3.1.1
Ancillary Signs of Ischemia

With stress scintigraphy, left ventricular cavity dilation and lung tracer uptake reflect late signs of global pump dysfunction and increase in pulmonary wedge pressure with interstitial lung edema. Also during stress echocardiography, we can sometimes observe poorly sensitive but highly specific signs of extensive ischemia, severe underlying coronary artery disease, and ominous prognostic outcome (Fig. 6.6): a stroke volume fall [30, 31]; a transient dilation of the left ventricular cavity (>20% from baseline of end-systolic diameter) [32]; the development of acute mitral insufficiency [33, 34]; an increase in ultrasound lung comets, a sign of extravascular lung water accumulation (detectable by chest sonography by placing the cardiac echocardiography probe on the third right intercostal space) [35, 36]; the reduction in amplitude of the S wave by strain rate Doppler imaging [37].

6.3.1.2
Beyond Regional Wall Motion: Coronary Flow Reserve

In the last decade, the old dream to combine wall motion with a simultaneous assessment of coronary flow reserve became a reality in the echocardiography laboratory. There are conceptual and methodological differences between myocardial perfusion and coronary flow reserve, since perfusion requires contrast opacification of the myocardium and coronary flow reserve assesses the vasodilating capacity of the coronary artery (Table 6.7). However, both mirror information on coronary vasodilating capability, which requires full integrity of the epicardial (proximal, upstream) and microcirculatory (distal, downstream) component of the coronary circulation. In the nuclear medicine and cardiovascular magnetic resonance stress laboratory, perfusion is usually evaluated. In the stress echocardiography laboratory, decades of attempts with myocardial contrast echocardiography led to disappointing and inconclusive results [38]. On the contrary, the diffusion of assessment of coronary flow reserve in the left anterior descending coronary artery was rapidly accepted

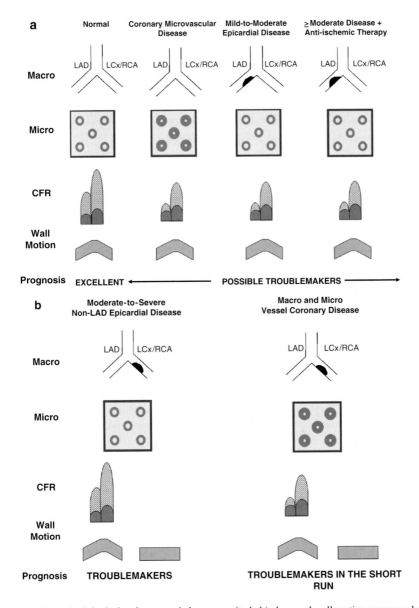

Fig. 6.6 a Pathophysiological and prognostic heterogeneity behind normal wall motion response during stress. In the *upper panel*, we show epicardial coronary arteries: normal in the *first two columns*, with moderate disease in the *third column*, and moderate-to-severe disease but concomitant, effective antiischemic therapy in the *last column*. The myocardium is shown as a *square box,* with small vessels as *circles.* Coronary small vessel disease is shown (*second column*) as *bold circles* (structural or functional impairment). All four very different pathophysiological conditions show the negativity of wall motion response. The abnormal coronary flow reserve (*CFR*) response is present in the *last three columns*, with abnormality of micro- or macrocirculation. **b** Pathophysiological and prognostic heterogeneity behind abnormal wall motion response during stress. Symbols as in **a**. The CFR can be normal in spite of wall motion abnormality when the LAD is not significantly involved and the microcirculatory level is not impaired (*left panel*). (Modified from [38])

6

Table 6.7 Myocardial perfusion of coronary flow reserve in the stress echocardiography laboratory

	Perfusion	Coronary flow reserve
Target	Myocardium	Coronary arteries
Contrast	Mandatory	Not needed
Coronary artery territories	All three	LAD (and RCA)

LAD left anterior descending, *RCA* right coronary artery

Table 6.8 Two birds with one stone: wall motion and coronary flow reserve

	Wall motion	Coronary flow reserve
Technique	2D	Color pulsed-wave Doppler
Ischemia required	Yes	No
Antianginal therapy reduces sensitivity	Yes	No
Sensitivity	++	+++
Specificity	+++	++
Prognostic value	+++	++
Troublemakers	Short run	Long run

in the clinical arena and led to a remodeling of our diagnostic equations. There are differences between wall motion and reduction of coronary flow reserve as diagnostic markers, since only the former requires true ischemia, is affected by antianginal therapy, and is sensitive to epicardial stenosis and much less sensitive to purely microvascular coronary impairment (Table 6.8). As a consequence, the diagnostic semiotics shown in Fig. 6.1 can be remodeled as shown in Fig. 6.6. Normal function with normal coronary flow reserve (in the left anterior descending and right coronary artery) express absence of anatomic and functionally significant stenosis of the epicardial artery and microcirculatory integrity. On the contrary, a normal wall motion with abnormal coronary flow reserve is associated with either a mild-to-moderate hemodynamically significant epicardial stenosis or significant microcirculatory disease [39]. The two markers are also prognostically complementary, since wall motion abnormalities identify troublemakers in the short run (months); and coronary flow reserve reduction – in the absence of wall motion disturbances – identifies troublemakers in the long run (years).

References

1. Picano E (1992) Stress echocardiography. From pathophysiological toy to diagnostic tool. Circulation 85:1604–12
2. Ross J Jr (1991) Myocardial perfusion-contraction matching. Implications for coronary heart disease and hibernation. Circulation 83:1076–83

3. Arnese M, Fioretti PM, Cornel JH, et al (1994) Akinesis becoming dyskinesis during high-dose dobutamine stress echocardiography: a marker of myocardial ischemia or a mechanical phenomenon? Am J Cardiol 73:896–9

4. Chen C, Li L, Chen LL, et al (1995) Incremental doses of dobutamine induce a biphasic response in dysfunctional left ventricular regions subtending coronary stenoses. Circulation 92:756–66

5. Gibbons RJ, Chatterjee K, Daley J, et al (1999) ACC/AHA/ACP-ASIM guidelines for the management of patients with chronic stable angina: a report of the American College of Cardiology/American Heart Association Task Force on Practice Guidelines (Committee on Management of Patients With Chronic Stable Angina). J Am Coll Cardiol 33:2092–197

6. Sheikh KH, Bengtson JR, Helmy S, et al (1990) Relation of quantitative coronary lesion measurements to the development of exercise-induced ischemia assessed by exercise echocardiography. J Am Coll Cardiol 15:1043–51

7. Picano E, Parodi O, Lattanzi F et al (1994) Assessment of anatomic and physiological severity of single-vessel coronary artery lesions by dipyridamole echocardiography. Comparison with positron emission tomography and quantitative arteriography. Circulation 89:753–61

8. Cortigiani L, Picano E, Landi P, et al (1998) Value of pharmacologic stress echocardiography in risk stratification of patients with single-vessel disease: a report from the Echo-Persantine and Echo-Dobutamine International Cooperative Studies. J Am Coll Cardiol 32:69–74

9. Lattanzi F, Picano E, Bolognese L, et al (1991) Inhibition of dipyridamole-induced ischemia by antianginal therapy in humans. Correlation with exercise electrocardiography. Circulation 83:1256–62

10. Ferrara N, Longobardi G, Nicolino A, et al (1992) Effect of beta-adrenoceptor blockade on dipyridamole-induced myocardial asynergies in coronary artery disease. Am J Cardiol 70:724–7

11. Dodi C, Pingitore A, Sicari R, et al (1997) Effects of antianginal therapy with a calcium antagonist and nitrates on dobutamine-atropine stress echocardiography. Comparison with exercise electrocardiography. Eur Heart J 18:242–7

12. San Roman JA, Vilacosta I, Castillo JA, et al (1996) Dipyridamole and dobutamine-atropine stress echocardiography in the diagnosis of coronary artery disease. Comparison with exercise stress test, analysis of agreement, and impact of antianginal treatment. Chest 110:1248–54

13. Nagel E, Lehmkuhl HB, Bocksch W, et al (1999) Noninvasive diagnosis of ischemia-induced wall motion abnormalities with the use of high-dose dobutamine stress MRI: comparison with dobutamine stress echocardiography. Circulation 99:763–70

14. Specchia G, de Servi S, Falcone C, et al (1981) Significance of exercise-induced ST-segment elevation in patients without myocardial infarction. Circulation 63:46–53

15. Kawano H, Fuji H (1995) Induction of coronary spasm during dobutamine stress echocardiography. Circulation 92:1–89

16. Varga A, Cortigiani L, Rossi PC, et al (1999) Coronary vasospasm as a source of false positive results during dobutamine echocardiography. Cardiologia 44:907–12

17. Picano E, Lattanzi F, Masini M, et al (1988) Aminophylline termination of dipyridamole stress as a trigger of coronary vasospasm in variant angina. Am J Cardiol 62:694–7

18. Spes CH, Mudra H, Schnaack SD, et al (1996) Dobutamine stress echocardiography for noninvasive diagnosis of cardiac allograft vasculopathy: a comparison with angiography and intravascular ultrasound. Am J Cardiol 78:168–74

19. Franchini M, Traversi E, Cannizzaro G, et al (2000) Dobutamine stress echocardiography and thallium-201 SPECT for detecting ischaemic dilated cardiomyopathy in patients with heart failure. Eur J Echocardiogr 1:109–15

20. Bach DS, Muller DW, Gros BJ et al(1994) False positive dobutamine stress echocardiograms: characterization of clinical, echocardiographic and angiographic findings. J Am Coll Cardiol 24:928–33

21. Baroni M, Maffei S, Terrazzi M, et al (1996) Mechanisms of regional ischaemic changes during dipyridamole echocardiography in patients with severe aortic valve stenosis and normal coronary arteries. Heart 75:492–7

22. Picano E, Palinkas A, Amyot R (2001) Diagnosis of myocardial ischemia in hypertensive patients. J Hypertens 19:1177–83

23. Rajappan K, Rimoldi OE, Dutka DP et al (2002) Mechanisms of coronary microcirculatory dysfunction in patients with aortic stenosis and angiographically normal coronary arteries. Circulation 105:470–6

24. Ha JW, Juracan EM, Mahoney DW, et al (2002) Hypertensive response to exercise: a potential cause for new wall motion abnormality in the absence of coronary artery disease. J Am Coll Cardiol 39:323–7

25. Beker B, Vered Z, Bloom NV, et al (1994) Decreased thickening of normal myocardium with transient increased wall thickness during stress echocardiography with atrial pacing. J Am Soc Echocardiogr 7:381–7

26. Hirshleifer J, Crawford M, O'Rourke RA, et al (1975) Influence of acute alterations in heart rate and systemic arterial pressure on echocardiographic measures of left ventricular performance in normal human subjects. Circulation 52:835–41

27. Borges AC, Pingitore A, Cordovil A, et al (1995) Heterogeneity of left ventricular regional wall thickening following dobutamine infusion in normal human subjects. Eur Heart J 16:1726–30

28. Carstensen S, Ali SM, Stensgaard-Hansen FV, et al (1995) Dobutamine-atropine stress echocardiography in asymptomatic healthy individuals. The relativity of stress-induced hyperkinesia. Circulation 92:3453–63

29. Sicari R, Palinkas A, Pasanisi E et al (2005) Long-term survival of patients with chest pain syndrome and angiographically normal or near-normal coronary arteries: the additional prognostic value of dipyridamole echocardiography test (DET). Eur Heart J. 26:2136–41

30. Harrison MR, Smith MD, Friedman BJ, et al (1987) Uses and limitations of exercise Doppler echocardiography in the diagnosis of ischemic heart disease. J Am Coll Cardiol 10:809–17

31. Agati L, Arata L, Neja CP, et al (1990) Usefulness of the dipyridamole-Doppler test for diagnosis of coronary artery disease. Am J Cardiol 65:829–34

32. Olson CE, Porter TR, Deligonul U, et al (1994) Left ventricular volume changes during dobutamine stress echocardiography identify patients with more extensive coronary artery disease. J Am Coll Cardiol 24:1268–73

33. Zachariah ZP, Hsiung MC, Nanda NC, et al (1987) Color Doppler assessment of mitral regurgitation induced by supine exercise in patients with coronary artery disease. Am J Cardiol 59:1266–70

34. Pierard LA, Lancellotti P (2006) Dyspnea and stress testing. N Engl J Med. 354:871–3

35. Picano E, Frassi F, Agricola E et al (2006) Ultrasound lung comets: a clinically useful sign of extravascular lung water. J Am Soc Echocardiogr. 19:356–63

36. Agricola E, Picano E, Oppizzi M, et al (2006) Assessment of stress-induced pulmonary interstitial edema by chest ultrasound during exercise echocardiography and its correlation with left ventricular function. J Am Soc Echocardiogr. 19:457–63

37. Bjork Ingul C, Rozis E, Slordahl SA, et al (2007) Incremental value of strain rate imaging to wall motion analysis for prediction of outcome in patients undergoing dobutamine stress echocardiography. Circulation. 115:1252–9

38. Sicari R, Nihoyannopoulos P, Evangelista A, et al (2008) Stress echocardiography expert consensus statement: European Association of Echocardiography (EAE) (a registered branch of the ESC). Eur J Echocardiogr 9:415–37
39. Rigo F, Sicari R, Gherardi S, et al (2008) The additive prognostic value of wall motion abnormalities and coronary flow reserve during dipyridamole stress echo. Eur Heart J 29:79–88

Segmentation of the Left Ventricle

7

Eugenio Picano

As with all methods of cardiac imaging, from ventriculography to scintigraphy, the left ventricle can be subdivided into a series of slices or segments also for the purposes of echocardiographic examination. The resolution of the segmental approach is a function of the number of segments; thus it can range from 20% (in the 5-segment model) to 5% (in the 20-segment model). However, increasing the number of segments, and thus reducing their size, leads to an unacceptable complication in the analysis with a greater need for approximation and interpolation. A reasonable trade-off between accuracy and feasibility is represented by the 16-segment model proposed by the American Society of Echocardiography [1], recently modified to include the 17th segment, i.e., the true apex [2]. The wall segments are identified according to internal anatomical landmarks of the left ventricle, in the standard parasternal (long axis and short axis at the mitral, papillary, apical levels), apical (5-, 4-, 3-, and 2-chamber), and subcostal (long axis and short axis) views (Fig. 7.1). Each segment can usually be visualized in more than one echocardiographic section and from different approaches for a more reliable and complete evaluation of wall motion. As a rule, segmental wall motion can be safely assessed when the endocardial contour is clearly visualized for at least 50% of its length. The 17-segment model meets the basic requirements of any reasonable segmentation: it is simple enough to be employed in practice; it has an anatomical basis; segments can be easily identified on the basis of obvious echocardiographic landmarks; there is good correspondence with the distribution of coronary arteries; and the model has stood the test of multicenter studies [3].

There are at least two good reasons to accept the 17-segment system, updating the 16-segment system. First, the 16-segment system did not include a true apical myocardial segment devoid of cavity – with the development of echocardiographic contrast agents for the assessment of myocardial perfusion, the myocardial apex segment or apical cap beyond the left ventricular cavity becomes pertinent, and a 17-segment model may become more appropriate for both the assessment of wall motion and myocardial perfusion with echocardiography [2]. The 16-segment model can still be appropriate for studies assessing wall motion abnormalities, as the tip of the normal apex (segment 17) does not move [3].

E. Picano, *Stress Echocardiography*,
© Springer-Verlag Berlin Heidelberg 2009

7

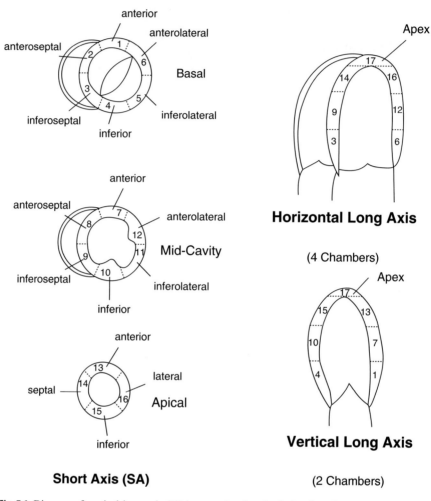

Fig. 7.1 Diagram of vertical long-axis (*VLA*, approximating the 2-chamber view), horizontal long-axis (*HLA*, approximating the 4-chamber view), and short-axis (*SA*) planes. The name, location, and anatomic landmarks for selection of the basal (tips of the mitral valve leaflets), midcavity (papillary muscles), and apical (beyond papillary muscles but before cavity ends) short-axis slices for the recommended 17-segment system are shown. All imaging modalities should use these same landmarks, when available, for slice selection

The second – and more important – reason to adopt the 17-segment model is that it proposes a standardized myocardial segmentation and nomenclature for tomographic imaging of the heart that is shared by all imaging modalities: nuclear cardiology, cardiovascular magnetic resonance, cardiac computed tomography, positron emission tomography, and coronary angiography. This consensus effort will lead to improved standardization and will make accurate intra- and cross-modality comparisons for clinical patient management and research possible, at last [2].

7.1
The 17-Segment Model

Autopsy studies provide precise data on the mass and size of the myocardium, which sets the basis for division of the heart. In adults without cardiac disease, the heart was sectioned into apical, midcavity, and basal thirds perpendicular to the left ventricular long axis, and the measured myocardial mass for each of these ventricular thirds was 42% from the base, 36% for the midcavity, and 21% for the apex [4]. The 17-segment model, shown in Fig. 7.1, creates a distribution of 35, 35, and 30% for the basal, midcavity, and apical thirds of the heart, which is close to the observed autopsy data [2].

Myocardial segments are named and localized with reference to both the long axes of the ventricle and the 360° circumferential locations on the short-axis views. Using basal, midcavity, and apical as part of the name defines the location along the long axis of the ventricle from the apex to the base. With regard to the circumferential location, the basal and midcavity slices should be divided into six segments of 60° each, as shown in Fig. 7.1. The attachment of the right ventricular wall to the left ventricle should be used to identify and separate the septum from the left ventricular anterior and inferior free walls. Figure 7.2 shows the location and the recommended names for the 17 myocardial segments on

Left Ventricular Segmentation

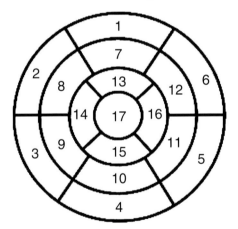

1. basal anterior	7. mid anterior	13. apical anterior
2. basal anteroseptal	8. mid anteroseptal	14. apical septal
3. basal inferoseptal	9. mid inferoseptal	15. apical inferior
4. basal inferior	10. mid inferior	16. apical lateral
5. basal inferolateral	11. mid inferolateral	17. apex
6. basal anterolateral	12. mid anterolateral	

Fig. 7.2 A circumferential polar plot display of the 17 myocardial segments and the recommended nomenclature for tomographic imaging of the heart. (Modified from [5])

a bull's-eye display. The names basal, midcavity, and apical identify the location on the long axis of the left ventricle. The circumferential locations in the basal and midcavity are anterior, anteroseptal, inferoseptal, inferior, inferolateral, and anterolateral.

Using this system, segments 1 and 7 identify the locations of the anterior wall at the base and midcavity. The appropriate names are basal anterior and midanterior segments. The septum, delineated by the attachment of the right ventricle, is divided into anterior and inferior segments. Segments 2 and 3 are named basal anteroseptal and basal inferoseptal. Continuing this approach, segment 4 is the basal inferior, segment 5 is the basal inferolateral, and segment 6 is the basal anterolateral. Similar names are used for the six segments, 7–12, at the midcavity level. The left ventricle tapers as it approaches the true apex, and it was believed appropriate to use just four segments. The names for segments 13–16 are apical anterior, apical septal, apical inferior, and apical lateral, respectively. The apical cap represents the true muscle at the extreme tip of the ventricle where the cavity disappears, and this is defined as segment 17, called the apex. Although in echocardiography the term posterior is sometimes used, for consistency, the term inferior is recommended.

7.2
Assignment of Segments to Coronary Arterial Territories

There is tremendous variability in the coronary artery blood supply to myocardial segments. Nevertheless, it was agreed to assign individual segments to specific coronary artery territories. The assignment of the 17 segments to one of the three major coronary arteries is shown in Fig. 7.3. The greatest variability in myocardial blood supply occurs at the apical

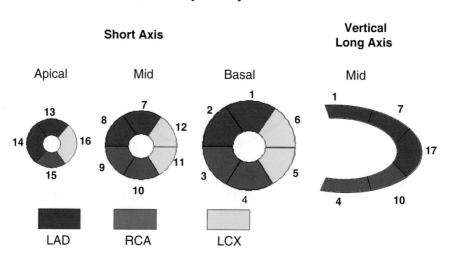

Fig. 7.3 Assignment of the 17 myocardial segments to the territories of the left anterior descending (*LAD*), right coronary artery (*RCA*), and the left circumflex coronary artery (*LCX*). (Modified from [5])

cap, segment 17, which can be supplied by any of the three arteries. Segments 1, 2, 7, 8, 13, 14, and 17 are assigned to the left anterior descending coronary artery distribution. Segments 3, 4, 9, 10, and 15 are assigned to the right coronary artery when it is dominant. Segments 5, 6, 11, 12, and 16 are generally assigned to the left circumflex artery. Individual myocardial segments can be assigned to the three major coronary arteries with the recognition that there is anatomic variability (Fig. 7.4). In the parasternal long-axis view, the inferior wall is supplied by either the left circumflex or right coronary artery, depending on dominance of the system. The most proximal portion of the interventricular septum (segment number 2) is perfused by the first septal perforator, and with a high-grade left anterior descending obstruction the proximal portion of the interventricular septum may be involved. The parasternal short-axis view of the myocardium is the most suitable for assessing the distribution of the three main arteries. The posterior descending coronary artery supplies the posterior portion of the interventricular septum as well as the inferior wall. If the proximal portion of the anterior wall (segment number 1) is affected, a high-grade proximal stenosis of the left anterior descending artery before the origin of the first septal perforator can be suspected. The anatomical relationship described above, although frequent, is by no means uniform: different anatomical patterns may be found in different patients [5]. In particular, the assignment of myocardial regions to coronary artery territories may change substantially with a dominant right coronary artery (Fig. 7.4) or with a less frequent dominant left circumflex artery (Fig. 7.4). The apex is a heterogeneous

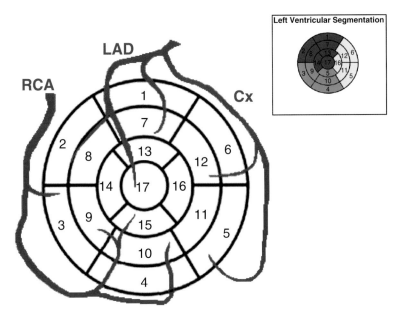

Fig. 7.4 Assignment of myocardial segments to coronary artery territories in the presence of a dominant right coronary artery (*upper panel*). The *lower panel* shows the borders of the coronary artery perfusion fields. (Adapted and modified from [6])

territory for coronary perfusion, and its infero–apical segment quite often pertains to the right coronary artery. However, as a rule, the presence of a clearly visualized stress-induced dyssynergy reliably predicts the presence and location of a coronary stenosis, especially when the left anterior descending artery is affected.

The 4-chamber subxiphoidal view closely parallels the image obtained with the apical 4-chamber view; short-axis views are similar to the short-axis parasternal ones. The main advantage is that this acoustic window remains "open" in patients in whom the ultrasonic study would otherwise be difficult, such as those who are obese or bronchopneumopathic. This projection is certainly useful for assessing a right ventricular dyssynergy, which is usually accompanied by acute dilation of the right ventricle.

Multiple projections can, and should, be employed in stress echocardiography: they guarantee a very high feasibility of the procedure with interpretable images in over 95% of patients studied and a complete, integrated assessment of all left ventricular segments.

7.3
Left Ventricular Function in a Number

The segmentation of the left ventricle also represents the anatomical background for rapid (real-time) semiquantitative assessment of wall motion. Numerical values can be given to any segment corresponding to the degree of wall motion abnormality: for instance, according to the recommendations of the American Society of Echocardiography [7], 1 is given for normokinesis or hyperkinesis, 2 for hypokinesis, 3 for akinesis, and 4 for dyskinesis (Table 7.1). The values for all segments are summed to yield the left ventricular wall motion score, and the total is divided by the number of segments studied to obtain a wall motion score index. For instance, in the 17-segment model, a normal left ventricle has an index of 1 (17 points/17 segments); hypokinesia of two segments will give an index of 1.12 (19 points/17 segments); dyskinesia of three segments will correspond to an index of 1.53 (26 points/17 segments). The wall motion score index can be calculated both in resting conditions and during stress and represents an integrated – although simple and easy to obtain – measurement of the extent and severity of ischemia; it is computer independent and obtainable within a few seconds. An example of a stress echocardiography report from our laboratory is shown in Fig. 7.5.

The assessment of ejection fraction – different from wall motion score index – requires a computer, geometric assumptions about left ventricular shape, and stop-frames to trace

Table 7.1 The segmental scoring system

Score:
1 = Normal/hyperkinetic: normal/increased systolic wall motion and thickening
2 = Hypokinetic: decreased systolic wall motion and thickening
3 = Akinetic: absent systolic wall motion and thickening
4 = Dyskinetic: outward systolic wall motion and thickening

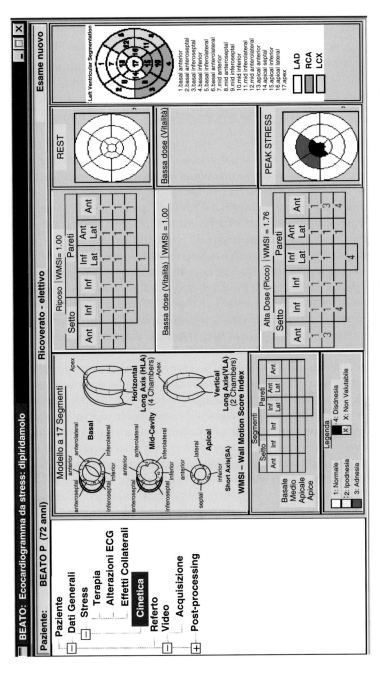

Fig. 7.5 Report from a positive stress echocardiography response from our laboratory. The bull's eye representation of the left ventricle at baseline and during stress allows one to transfer the integrated view of baseline (*upper panel*, normal function, resting wall motion score index = 1) and stress function (*lower panel*, extensive ischemia, peak wall motion score index = 1.56)

7

Table 7.2 Indices of global left ventricular function

	Wall motion score index	Ejection fraction
Nature of parameter	Semiquantitative	Quantitative
Time required	Seconds	Minutes
Geometric assumptions	No	Yes
Analysis	Real time	Still frames
Computer facilities required	No	Yes
Audience	Echocardiographers	Cardiologists

endocardial borders (Table 7.2). However, the ejection fraction has unquestionable advantages over other left ventricular global function indices used in echocardiography, such as the mean velocity of circumferential shortening, fractional shortening, or the wall motion score index. The ejection fraction – as an index of global function – is a term unrelated to the jargon (known by echocardiographers only); rather, it belongs to the Esperanto of the cardiological community at large, being a parameter common to all imaging methods and one that is used in angiographic, nuclear, and echocardiographic techniques. It has a very wide range of values, from below 10% to above 80%, and it has been extensively validated in its prognostic value.

The use of ejection fraction entails limitations, too: it is a global index which does not provide information on the segmental or diffuse nature of the myocardial abnormality; it is affected by a number of parameters besides ventricular function (preload, afterload, heart rate), and it remains insensitive to mild or limited regional abnormalities. Being a ratio, it offers no information on left ventricular volumes. Echocardiographic ejection fraction may be calculated during the study of regional wall motion, by integrating the information on regional function, with no need for dedicated imaging during the acquisition, as in the case with Doppler ultrasound. The same advantages are shared by wall motion score index, which is, however, sensitive to even the slightest abnormalities in regional function. For instance, the hypokinesia of one segment does not significantly affect the ejection fraction, but it does generate an abnormal wall motion score index. Furthermore, the wall motion score index does not require the recordings of all possible section planes but only that each segment be visualized in at least one projection. This is a great advantage for clinical studies, when the full visualization of the entire ventricular silhouette in a given plane can be problematic in resting conditions and even more so during stress. The major limitations to the widespread use of the wall motion score index are the lack of standardization and its unfamiliarity to many cardiologists. The wall motion score index stands for global left ventricular function exclusively in the slang of echocardiographers. Furthermore, even with the echocardiographic community there is no consensus as to the number of segments and the scoring criteria that should be used. Some authors use values that are more positive with increasing severity of wall motion abnormality, whereas others apply the reverse criterion. Some distinguish different degrees of hypokinesia (mild = 1.5; severe = 2), while others extend the range by taking hyperkinesia (=0) and aneurysmal dilation (=5) into account. Once necessary standardization (projections, segments, score) was accomplished [6], the wall motion score index gained increasing acceptance in stress echocardiography for both clinical and research purposes.

7.4
Artifactual Pseudoasynergies

Each of the projections employed has its own merits and limitations for the assessment of regional wall motion. The resolution of bidimensional echocardiography is optimal in the axial direction of the ultrasonic beam. A regional dyssynergy can be artifactually "created" by incorrect positioning of the transducer; thus the presence of a transient asynergy should be assessed in several projections, the same region being imaged from different angles of incidence. The long-axis parasternal view allows optimal visualization of the anterior septum and of the inferior wall, since endocardium is perpendicular to the ultrasonic beam. This projection, however, can be limited by the susceptibility to respiratory interference induced by the hyperventilation associated with some stresses. A foreshortened long axis creates a false hyperkinesis (and can mask a true hypokinesia) of apical segments and creates a false hypokinesis of the proximal septal and inferior segments.

The short-axis view at the papillary level allows a simultaneous assessment of the walls belonging to the distribution territories of all three coronary arteries; it is particularly suited for quantitative wall motion analysis, although difficult to obtain in patients with relatively advanced age, such as those with coronary artery disease. Even less frequently utilized is the short-axis view at the mitral level, where a spurious transient dyssynergy of the inferobasal segment is common. The cause of this pseudoasynergy is the physiological systolic shortening of the left ventricle in a base-to-apex direction, so that in diastole the left ventricular wall is imaged while in systole the left atrium enters the image plane. A further drawback is that during many stresses the base-to-apex shortening is more marked than at rest. Thus if only the short-axis projection at the mitral level is employed the finding of posterobasal asynergy should be judged with caution unless the inferobasal segment can be shown to be asynergic in another projection. The perfect short axis must be round. An elliptic shape can mask an anterior asynergy and mimic an inferolateral hypokinesis (Fig. 7.6). The apical (4- and 2-chamber) view is the most used and most useful projection in stress echocardiography. The apical 2-chamber view, if properly applied, should not visualize the aortic root [6]; it is analogous to the right anterior oblique projection employed in ventriculography and clearly shows the inferior and anterior walls. A foreshortened 2-chamber can mask a hypokinesia of the apex and mimic a hypokinesia of the basal inferior wall. A foreshortened 4-chamber view can mask a hypokinesia of the apex (which is created falsely hyperkinetic) and can mimic a hypokinesia of the laterobasal and septobasal wall.

7.5
Matching Between TTE and TEE Segments

Transesophageal stress echocardiography can be performed in patients with limited transthoracic echocardiography image quality. The semiinvasive nature of the technique makes it more unpleasant for the patient [8], as stated by conventional wisdom that "transesophageal echocardiography can be considered a noninvasive examination if you do it,

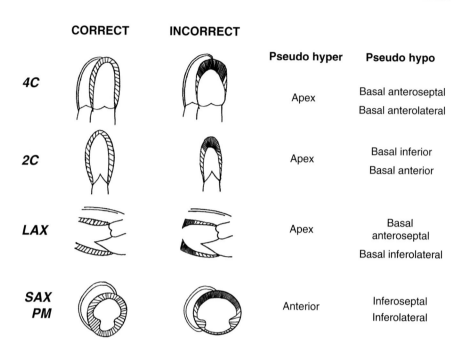

Fig. 7.6 Stress echocardiographic iatrogenesis. The *left panel* shows the correct imaging for each of the main projections; the *right panel* shows the incorrect imaging which may mask or mimic regional dysfunction during stress

and an invasive examination if others do it on you." Excellent results have been obtained with pharmacological transesophageal stress echocardiography for the assessment of myocardial ischemia (with dobutamine or dipyridamole) [9–11], myocardial viability (with dobutamine) [12], coronary flow reserve (with dipyridamole or adenosine) [13–17], and prognostic stratification on the basis of inducible wall motion abnormalities [18, 19]. Segmental analysis is generally performed using the 17-segment model modified for transesophageal echocardiography (Fig. 7.7) – although the last official recommendations of the American Society of Echocardiography date back to 1999 and therefore refer to 16 segments [8]. Intraoperatively, however, monitoring of regional function is generally restricted to the six segments of the transgastric papillary view; in this view, areas of myocardium subtended by the three major coronary arteries are present [20]. In spite of its undisputed accuracy, the clinical role of transesophageal stress echocardiography is decreasing because of the emerging use of cardiac stress magnetic resonance imaging for nonionizing stress testing in patients with difficult acoustic windows who do not improve after native second harmonic imaging and contrast-enhanced echocardiography. It remains the first choice stress test in patients in the operating room (for early assessment of functional results of revascularization) or in the intensive care unit (for instance, for recruitment of heart donors).

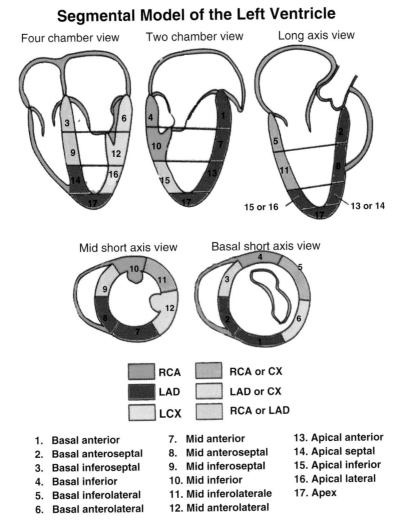

Segmental Model of the Left Ventricle

RCA
RCA or CX
LAD
LAD or CX
LCX
RCA or LAD

1. Basal anterior
2. Basal anteroseptal
3. Basal inferoseptal
4. Basal inferior
5. Basal inferolateral
6. Basal anterolateral
7. Mid anterior
8. Mid anteroseptal
9. Mid inferoseptal
10. Mid inferior
11. Mid inferolaterale
12. Mid anterolateral
13. Apical anterior
14. Apical septal
15. Apical inferior
16. Apical lateral
17. Apex

Fig. 7.7 Model of left ventricular segmentation using transesophageal echocardiographic images. The short-axis view (**a**) is obtained from the stomach, and 4-chamber (**b**) and 2-chamber (**c**) views are recorded from the esophagus. *Ant* anterior, *ao* aortic root, *inf* inferior, *LA* left atrium, *lat* lateral, *inf-lat* inferior–lateral, *RV* right ventricle, *sept* septum. (Modified from [20], with permission)

7.6
Left Ventricular Segments: Matching Between 2D and 3D Imaging

Real-time three-dimensional echocardiography (RT3DE) is an attractive clinical tool for improving the technical difficulty and the diagnostic accuracy of the 2D technique, given the theoretical opportunity of overcoming most of the shortcomings of

Table 7.3 Ejection fraction: from 2D to 3D in the echocardiography laboratory

	2D	3D
Foreshortening artifacts	Yes	No
Geometric assumption	Yes	No
Accuracy	Good	Excellent
Reproducibility	Good	Excellent
Imaging time	Minutes	Seconds
Analysis time	Minutes	Minutes

2D stress echocardiography. In fact, the fast and almost instantaneous imaging of the entire heart from a single acoustic window, avoiding foreshortening and geometric assumptions inherent to the 2D approach, makes stress echocardiography less problematic and provides true volumetric data that allow any cardiac plane to be visualized off-line/postacquisition [21]. At present, there is no evidence of a clear advantage of 3D or 2D beyond the considerably shorter acquisition time – mostly due to the limited endocardial resolution and limited frame rate of the 3D image. However, there is little doubt that RT3D has great potential to make stress echocardiography more quantitative and less technically demanding, and is now already the gold standard for assessment of cardiac volumes, left ventricular mass, and ejection fraction at baseline and during stress (3), with accuracy and reproducibility comparable to cardiovascular magnetic resonance (Table 7.3). From RT3D, much ancillary information can be derived during stress that may be important: the stroke volume (relevant, for instance, during dobutamine stress echocardiography in low flow, low gradient aortic stenosis); the end-systolic volume (relevant, for instance, to measure the pressure–volume relationship during stress as an index of contractile reserve in heart failure); the mean diastolic filling rate (potentially important for the characterization of the diastolic function, and which can be derived from stroke volume and duration of cardiological diastole); vascular impedance (expressed as the ratio of stroke volume/arterial systolic pressure).

References

1. Schiller NB, Shah PM, Crawford M, et al (1989) Recommendations for quantitation of the left ventricle by two-dimensional echocardiography. American Society of Echocardiography Committee on Standards, Subcommittee on Quantitation of Two-Dimensional Echocardiograms. J Am Soc Echocardiogr 2:358–67
2. Cerqueira MD, Weissman NJ, Dilsizian V, et al (2002) Standardized myocardial segmentation and nomenclature for tomographic imaging of the heart: a statement for healthcare professionals from the Cardiac Imaging Committee of the Council on Clinical Cardiology of the American Heart Association. Circulation 105:539–42
3. Lang RM, Bierig M, Devereux RB, et al; Chamber Quantification Writing Group; American Society of Echocardiography's Guidelines and Standards Committee; European Association of Echocardiography (2005) Recommendations for chamber quantification: a report from the

American Society of Echocardiography's Guidelines and Standards Committee and the Chamber Quantification Writing Group, developed in conjunction with the European Association of Echocardiography, a branch of the European Society of Cardiology. J Am Soc Echocardiogr 18:1440–63

4. Edwards WD, Tajik AJ, Seward JB (1981) Standardized nomenclature and anatomic basis for regional tomographic analysis of the heart. Mayo Clin Proc 56:479–97

5. Feigenbaum H (1994) Echocardiography. 5th edn. Lea and Febiger, Philadelphia

6. Sensky PR, Samani NJ, Reek C, et al (2002) Magnetic resonance perfusion imaging in patients with coronary artery disease: a qualitative approach. Int J Cardiac Imag 18:373–83

7. Armstrong WF, Pellikka PA, Ryan T, et al (1998) Stress echocardiography: recommendations for performance and interpretation of stress echocardiography. Stress Echocardiography Task Force of the Nomenclature and Standards Committee of the American Society of Echocardiography. J Am Soc Echocardiogr 11:97–104

8. Shanewise JS, Cheung AT, Aronson S, et al (1999) ASE/SCA guidelines for performing a comprehensive intraoperative multiplane transesophageal echocardiography examination: recommendations of the American Society of Echocardiography Council for Intraoperative Echocardiography and the Society of Cardiovascular Anesthesiologists Task Force for Certification in Perioperative Transesophageal Echocardiography. Anesth Analg 89:870–84

9. Panza JA, Laurienzo JM, Curiel RV, et al (1994) Transesophageal dobutamine stress echocardiography for evaluation of patients with coronary artery disease. J Am Coll Cardiol 24:1260–7

10. Chaudhry FA, Tauke JT, Alessandrini RS, et al (2000) Enhanced detection of ischemia myocardium by transesophageal dobutamine stress echocardiography: comparison with simultaneous transthoracic echocardiography. Echocardiography 17:241–53

11. Agati L, Renzi M, Sciomer S, et al (1992) Transesophageal dipyridamole echocardiography for diagnosis of coronary artery disease. J Am Coll Cardiol 19:765–70

12. Baer FM, Voth E, Deutsch HJ, et al (1994) Assessment of viable myocardium by dobutamine transesophageal echocardiography and comparison with fluorine-18 fluorodeoxyglucose positron emission tomography. J Am Coll Cardiol 24:343–53

13. Iliceto S, Marangelli V, Memmola C, et al (1991) Transesophageal Doppler echocardiography evaluation of coronary blood flow velocity in baseline conditions and during dipyridamole-induced coronary vasodilation. Circulation 83:61–9

14. Redberg RF, Sobol Y, Chou TM, et al (1995) Adenosine-induced coronary vasodilation during transesophageal Doppler echocardiography. Rapid and safe measurement of coronary flow reserve ratio can predict significant left anterior descending coronary stenosis. Circulation 92:190–6

15. Radvan J, Marwick TH, Williams MJ, et al (1995) Evaluation of the extent and timing of the coronary hyperemic response to dipyridamole: a study with transesophageal echocardiography and positron emission tomography with oxygen 15 water. J Am Soc Echocardiogr 8:864–73

16. Hutchinson SJ, Shen A, Soldo S, et al (1996) Transesophageal assessment of coronary flow velocity reserve during "regular" and "high"-dose dipyridamole stress testing. Am J Cardiol 77:1164–8

17. Coletta C, Galati A, Ricci R, et al (1999) Coronary flow reserve of normal left anterior descending artery in patients with ischemic heart disease: a transesophageal Doppler study. J Am Soc Echocardiogr 12:720–8

18. Panza JA, Curiel RV, Laurienzo JM, et al (1995) Relation between ischemic threshold measured during dobutamine stress echocardiography and known indices of poor prognosis in patients with coronary artery disease. Circulation 92:2095–101

19. Biagini A, Maffei S, Baroni M, et al (1990) Early assessment of coronary reserve after bypass surgery by dipyridamole transesophageal echocardiographic stress test. Am Heart J 120:1097–101

20. American Society of Echocardiography (2008) Guidelines for performing multiplane transesophageal echocardiography. New guidelines Poster. J Am Soc Echocardiogr 21 (poster Suppl)

21. Takeuchi M, Lang RM (2007) Three-dimensional stress testing: volumetric acquisitions. Cardiol Clin. 25:267–72

Dynamic and Pharmacologic Right Heart Stress Echocardiography: Right Ventricular Function, Right Coronary Artery Flow, Pulmonary Pressure, and Alveolar–Capillary Membrane Testing in the Echocardiography Laboratory

8

Eugenio Picano, Ekkehard Grünig, Alberto San Román, Kwan Damon, and Nelson B. Schiller

The behavior of the right side of the heart during stress has been underemphasized and sparsely investigated by cardiologists and pneumologists. Reasons vary, but the right ventricle has traditionally been considered a passive conduit between the venous system and the lungs largely because of early animal experiments showing no increase of central venous pressure after the free wall of the right ventricle had been destroyed [1–3]. In addition, ultrasound systems are generally optimized for imaging of the left ventricle. Recent pathophysiological, clinical, and prognostic data have defined an important role for the right ventricle in many conditions, including ischemic heart disease and heart failure. Given that the right ventricle and the left ventricle share a common septum, have an overlapping blood supply, and are bound together by the pericardium, changes induced by myocardial ischemia and/or heart failure are reflected in pulmonary hemodynamics and right ventricular function [4]. Modern Doppler echocardiography allows a systematic evaluation of five key aspects of cardiopulmonary pathophysiology during stress: segmental right ventricular function; global right ventricular longitudinal function; coronary flow reserve in the posterior descending of the right coronary artery; indices of pulmonary hemodynamics, namely, pulmonary artery systolic pressure, pulmonary velocity time integrals, and pulmonary vascular resistances; and extravascular lung water in the lung, mirroring the distress of the alveolar–capillary membrane. Technical improvements were also matched by a greater understanding of the complexity and the clinical relevance of the adaptation of the right heart (functionally including pulmonary circulation and lung alveolar–capillary membrane) in several pathological conditions, from coronary artery disease to heart failure [4]. In many situations, it is not possible to fully understand heart disease if we do not look at the right heart and pulmonary stress hemodynamics.

E. Picano, *Stress Echocardiography*,
© Springer-Verlag Berlin Heidelberg 2009

8

8.1
Regional Right Ventricular Function in Coronary Artery Disease

The right ventricle is less vulnerable to ischemia than the left ventricle for several anatomic and functional factors, including the rich system of thebesian veins in the right ventricle (allowing perfusion of the papillary muscles of the right ventricle), the dual anatomic supply system (in which the left coronary branches perfuse almost one-third of the right ventricle), the rapid development of collateral vessels to the right ventricle given the lower resistance that favors a left-to-right transcoronary pressure gradient, and the relatively thin walls and lower stroke work and wall tension (with lower oxygen demand and less vulnerability to transmural perfusion heterogeneity during stress) [4]. Blood supply of the right ventricle is characterized by a rich collateral system and a perfusion during diastole and systole. The perfusion rate of the right ventricle at rest is $50\,ml\,min^{-1}\,100\,g^{-1}$, much lower than that of the left ventricle ($120\,ml\,min^{-1}\,100\,g^{-1}$). However, right ventricular ischemia occurs during stress and occasionally as an isolated finding, without concomitant left ventricular ischemia, and must be recognized. The contractile reserve of the right ventricle is low. Small changes of afterload and/or reduction in contractility are followed by a dilatation of the right ventricle. Elevation of the preload activates the Frank–Starling mechanism that can increase contractility and stroke volume of the right ventricle. Beside the Frank–Starling mechanism, the active contraction of the interventricular septum increases the right ventricular pump function especially during exercise and is one of the main mechanisms of compensation. Right ventricular infarction is followed by right heart failure only when the contractility of the septum has been reduced [5–8]. Thus, septal motion should be closely assessed during stress.

The evaluation of right ventricular size and function is made difficult by the retrosternal position, complex geometry, and heavy trabeculation of the right ventricle, which also partially overlaps with the silhouettes of the left ventricle. There is not one single echocardiographic view in which the complete right ventricle can be seen. For purposes of echocardiographic analysis, the right ventricle can be divided into four segments [9]: anterior wall, lateral wall, inferior wall, and wall of the outflow tract (Fig. 8.1). Schematically, the right ventricle is composed of an inflow and an outflow tract. The former has an anterior and an inferior (also named diaphragmatic) wall. The inferior wall lies over the diaphragm. The acute margin of the heart is formed by the external edge of the right ventricle. From an echocardiographic perspective it is called the lateral wall and it borders anteriorly with the anterior wall and posteriorly with the inferior wall. The outflow portion of the right ventricle is limited upward by the pulmonary valve and downward by the crista supraventricularis, the septal papillary muscle (Luschka's muscle), the anterior leaflet of the tricuspid valve, and the septal band. The outflow tract has an anterior wall (echocardiographically named wall of the outflow tract) and a posterior wall that is part of the interventricular septum. The inferior wall is irrigated by the marginal branches and the posterior descending artery, the lateral wall by the marginal branches, and the outflow tract and the anterior wall by the posterior and anterior descending artery. Although the interventricular septum is part of the right ventricle, the evaluation of its function is usually included in the analysis of the left ventricle. In right dominant hearts (85% of cases), the

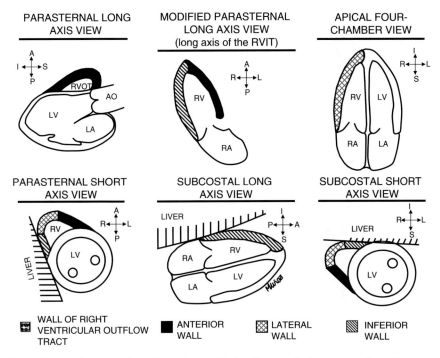

Fig. 8.1 Systematic approach to the right ventricular function during stress echocardiography. *A* anterior, *AO* aorta, *I* inferior, *L* left, *LA* left atrium, *LV* left ventricle, *P* posterior, *R* right, *RA* right atrium, *RV* right ventricle, *RVOT* right ventricular outflow tract, *S* superior

Table 8.1 Differences between right and left ventricular ischemia during stress echocardiography

	Right	Left
Prevalence in RCA disease	40–60%	70–90%
Prevalence in LCA disease	0–20%	70–90%
ECG abnormalities	Right precordial leads	Standard leads
Isolated presentation	Rare	Frequent
Feasibility to be detected	60–80%	90–98%
Prognostic value	Additive to left	Established

right ventricle is nourished by the right coronary artery. The development of contraction abnormalities of the right ventricle (more often lateral and inferior segments) is a hallmark of coronary artery involvement by coronary vasospasm in ergonovine-induced [10] or tight stenosis in dobutamine-induced ischemia [11] (Table 8.1). These alterations appear later than in the left ventricle [9], are best recognized from a modified parasternal and subcostal long-axis view (Fig. 8.2), and can be accompanied by severe right ventricular and right atrial enlargement [12, 13], sometimes with reduction of the right atrioventricular

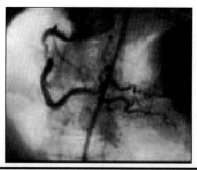

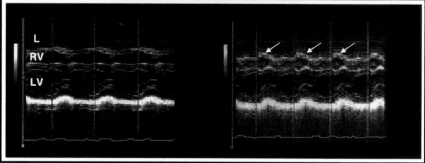

Fig. 8.2 *M*-mode study from the subcostal window. Resting exam (*left*) shows normal right ventricular wall motion. During dobutamine infusion (*right*) dyskinesis of the inferior wall of the right ventricle is clearly seen (*arrows*). *Vertical lines* correspond to ventricular systole. *L* liver, *LV* left ventricle, *RV* right ventricle

plane displacement with *M*-mode, which is an index of global longitudinal right ventricular function. Rest or stress-induced right ventricular enlargement is not necessarily due to coronary artery disease but can be due to other conditions such as stress-induced pulmonary hypertension which may nevertheless be of prognostic significance. Isolated right ventricular ischemia occurs in 2% of patients with right coronary artery stenosis when assessed by wall motion abnormalities [13], but increases to 5–10% if assessed by tricuspid plane displacement [14], and in 20% of patients with concomitant inferior wall ischemia, in whom it contributes to a negative prognostic outlook [13].

8.2
Measurement of Global Right Ventricular Function by Planimetry and Descent of the Right Ventricular Base

The global inotropic reserve of the right ventricle can be measured as the increase in ejection fraction, or in fractional area change, or in a simpler and at least equally accurate way as augmented descent of the right ventricular base or tricuspid annular plane systolic

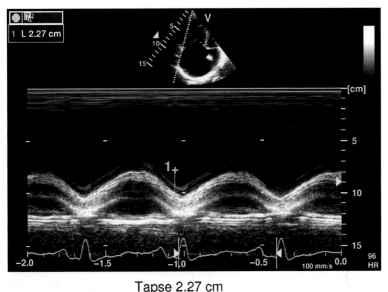

Tapse 2.27 cm

Fig. 8.3 The evaluation of TAPSE (tricuspid annulus plane systolic excursion) as a quantitative index of global longitudinal right ventricular function

excursion (TAPSE). The latter index of global right ventricular function can be calculated from the apical 4-chamber view, and 2D-targeted M-mode tracings (Fig. 8.3) by recording the free wall long-axis amplitude of movement (normally 15–20 mm). A good relationship has been reported between TAPSE and the right ventricular ejection function measured by radionuclide ventriculography in a manner independent of geometric assumptions [15]. Conceptually, TAPSE (or, if available, peak systolic velocity of Doppler tissue imaging of the lateral tricuspid annular motion) assesses longitudinal function of the right ventricle in the same way as MAPSE (mitral annular plane systolic excursion) by simple M-mode or myocardial velocity imaging does of the left ventricle [16]. The assessment of TAPSE avoids the approximation, mistakes, and computational burden inherent to the calculation of ejection fraction in the right ventricle, whose crescentic and irregular shape eludes any geometric modeling [17], although real-time 3D echocardiography has potential to solve or at least limit this problem. Moreover, its simplicity makes it easy to calculate, and translates into a very low-intra- and interobserver variability [18], an important issue when searching for end points in clinical trials. A reduced TAPSE (<1.5 cm) has a strong predictive value for exercise tolerance and clinical outcome in different cardiac conditions, including ischemic and nonischemic dilated cardiomyopathy [19], independent and additive over left ventricular systolic function. In patients with dilated cardiomyopathy, three basic responses can be identified by dobutamine stress: a low risk pattern, with preserved left and right ventricular contractile reserve; an intermediate risk pattern, with no left ventricular and preserved right ventricular contractile reserve; and a high risk pattern with abolished left and right ventricular contractility reserve (Fig. 8.4) [20]. To date, there

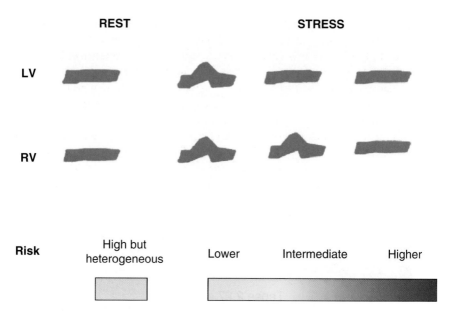

Fig. 8.4 The three patterns of response to dobutamine stress. The same resting pattern of depressed left (*upper row*) and right (*lower row*) ventricular function (*left panel*) may correspond to a profoundly heterogeneous prognostic spectrum: low risk (*second column*), with preserved biventricular contractile reserve; intermediate (*third column*) with only right ventricular reserve (*fourth column*); and high risk (*fourth column*) with lack of biventricular contractile reserve

have been no echocardiographic studies of the dynamic effect of exercise on these parameters. However, from nuclear studies, we can expect that a preserved right ventricular function at rest and during exercise is a potent predictor of exercise capacity and survival in advanced heart failure [21], as well as in patients evaluated after an acute myocardial infarction [22].

8.3
Coronary Flow Reserve of the Right Coronary Artery

Stress testing of coronary flow reserve has now become a clinical reality with last-generation, fast, high-dose vasodilatory stress echocardiography coupled with second harmonic imaging technology and pulsed Doppler of the middistal left anterior descending coronary artery [23, 24]. Under normal conditions, in the absence of stenosis, coronary blood flow can increase at least threefold over resting values when hyperemia is induced pharmacologically, for instance, with administration of exogenous adenosine or dipyridamole, which accumulates endogenous adenosine. Coronary flow reserve is the capacity of the coronary circulation to dilate and can be expressed by the difference between the hyperemic flow and the resting flow curve. This pathophysiological concept recently entered the stress echocardiography laboratory, and the combined assessment of regional wall motion by 2D echocardiography and pulsed Doppler imaging of the left anterior descending coronary artery is the recommended state-of-the-art stress echocardiography protocol in the latest recommendations (2008) of the European Association of Echocardiography [25]. More recently, the posterior descending artery of the right coronary artery has been consistently imaged, with a success rate around 75% [26, 27], usually from a modified apical 2-chamber view with counter-clockwise rotation and anterior angulations of the probe [28] (Fig. 8.5). The information of right coronary artery flow reserve is derived as the ratio of peak diastolic flow velocity during stress over rest. A concordant reduction in both left anterior descending and posterior descending arteries is associated with a worse prognosis than a reduction in either one coronary artery – both in coronary artery disease [29] and in dilated cardiomyopathy patients [30]. In addition, a reduction in right coronary artery reserve is associated with conditions of right ventricular pressure overload, and may help in the functional characterization, for instance, of congenital heart disease patients [31].

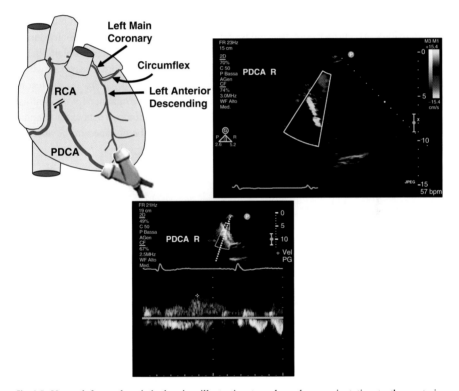

Fig. 8.5 *Upper left panel*: artist's drawing illustrating transducer beam orientation to the posterior descending coronary artery. The middistal tract is imaged from a modified apical 2-chamber view with counterclockwise rotation and anterior angulations of the probe. *Upper right panel*: The corresponding echocardiographic image of posterior descending color flow. *Lower panel*: the corresponding pulsed Doppler flow signal at rest, on which the peak diastolic flow velocity is measured. The variation in diastolic flow velocity between rest and peak vasodilation (following adenosine or dipyridamole infusion) gives an index of coronary flow reserve

8

8.4
Pulmonary Hemodynamics

Pulmonary artery systolic pressure can be estimated from peak tricuspid regurgitation (TR) jet velocities according to the well-validated modified Bernoulli's equation [32]: pulmonary artery systolic pressure = $4(V)^2$ + right atrial pressure, where V is the peak velocity (in m/s) of the tricuspid valve regurgitant jet (Table 8.2), and right atrial pressure is estimated from inferior vena cava diameter and respiratory changes, yielding a value from 5 (inferior vena cava diameter <17 mm, >50% reduction with inspiration) to 20 mmHg (inferior vena cava diameter >17 mm, no reduction with inspiration) [17] (Table 8.3). Technically adequate signals have complete envelopes with well-defined borders, a sweep velocity of at least 100–200 mm s^{-1}, and can be obtained (often without need of contrast) at baseline and at peak exercise stress in the majority of patients (Fig. 8.6). The assessment of pulmonary artery systolic pressure (PASP) depends on the presence of an at least trivial TR, which is found in about 40–85% of normal subjects [33] and 80–90% of patients with pulmonary hypertension [34]. Furthermore, training is required to be able to assess TR velocity during exercise correctly. Over- and underestimation of TR velocity is a frequent problem. In the case of missing TR, subjects can be asked to drink 500–1,000 ml before assessment which increases the preload and the size of the right atrial area and usually helps for the test to be successful. The quality of the TR velocity recording may be enhanced with contrast echocardiography by injecting agitated saline solution or other contrast echocardiographic agents intravenously [35]. However, an estimate of PASP can be obtained in the absence

Table 8.2 Noninvasive assessment of pulmonary pressure by Doppler echocardiography

		Normal values (rest)
PASP	4 × TR peak velocity^2 + RAP	<35
PAP m	79–0.45 (RVOT AT) 4 × peak pulmonary regurgitation velocity	<25
PEDP	4 × (pulmonary regurgitation end-diastolic velocity) + RAP	<15
PVR	10 × TR velocity/RVOT$_{TVI}$	<2.0

PASP pulmonary artery systolic pressures, *PVR* pulmonary vascular resistances, *PEDP* pulmonary end-diastolic pressure, *PAP* pulmonary artery pressure, *TR* tricuspid regurgitation

Table 8.3 Echocardiographic estimation of the right atrial pressure (*RAP*) by measuring the diameter of the inferior vena cava and the respiratory motion of the inferior vena cava (from [17])

Inferior vena cava diameter (cm)	Respiratory collapse (%)	RAP (mmHg)
<1.7	≥50%	5
>1.7	≥50%	10
>1.7	≤50%	15
>1.7	0	20

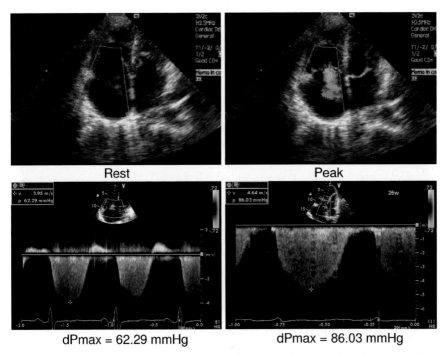

Rest   Peak

dPmax = 62.29 mmHg   dPmax = 86.03 mmHg

Fig. 8.6 Patients with resting pulmonary artery systolic pressure (estimated from jet velocity of tricuspid regurgitation) of 64 mmHg. During mild exercise, the patient experiences severe dyspnea and dramatic rise in pulmonary artery systolic pressure

of TR from the blood-pool and – more simply – with pulsed-wave Doppler tissue imaging, the isovolumic relaxation time of the tricuspid annulus of the right ventricle can be derived [36, 37]. Pulmonary hypertension causes a significant delay in the onset of right ventricular filling. A third approach is based on the assessment of pulmonary forward flow [38]. Generally, the shorter the acceleration time (measured from the onset of Q wave on ECG to the onset of pulmonary flow velocity) the higher the pulmonary vascular resistance and hence the pulmonary arterial pressure. However, assessment of acceleration time especially during exercise has a high inter- and intraobserver variability.

Notably, the pulmonary artery diastolic pressure (PADP) can be estimated at rest from the velocity of the end-diastolic pulmonary regurgitant jet (Vedpr) (Fig. 8.7), using the modified Bernoulli's equation [PADP = 4 * (Vedpr)^2 + right atrial pressure [39] (Table 8.2). When used with the tricuspid regurgitant jet to estimate pulmonary artery systolic pressure, the yield for direct information on pulmonary artery pressures increases to 90% [40].

The simple ratio of peak TR velocity (in m/s) to RVOT VTI (in cm) multiplied by 10 allows for the evaluation of pulmonary artery pressures in hemodynamic terms, namely, the basic relationship of Δpressure = flow * resistance [41] (Table 8.2). A ratio greater than 1.8 resistance units is predictive of an abnormal pulmonary vascular resistance by cardiac catheterization and may predict which pre-liver transplant patients, who often have elevated pulmonary artery pressures due to increased cardiac output with or without

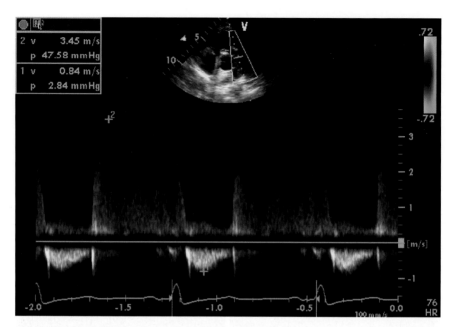

Fig. 8.7 From the peak velocity of regurgitant pulmonary flow jet of 3.45 m s⁻¹, a mean pulmonary pressure of 47.58 mmHg can be derived. The end-diastolic jet velocity plus the estimated right atrial pressure corresponds to the end-diastolic pulmonary pressure

pulmonary vascular changes that results in portopulmonary hypertension, need catheter-based evaluation [42]. The method is easy to incorporate into a standard echocardiography exam, and helps to identify a group of patients with apparently increased PASP (which may be influenced by right ventricular stroke volume) as normal [43]. This method does have an inability to replicate higher values of Wood's units, and may be further limited in patients with very dilated pulmonary arteries or RVOTs and with severe pulmonic regurgitation. Overall, the most reliable method to measure PASP or mean pulmonary artery pressure during exercise is to use continuous-wave Doppler echocardiography.

Pulmonary arterial hypertension is defined as a group of diseases characterized by a progressive increase of pulmonary vascular resistances leading to right ventricular failure and death [44]. Pulmonary hypertension is defined by a mean pulmonary arterial pressure over 25 mmHg at rest and over 30 mmHg during activity with accompanying increase of pulmonary vascular resistances over 3 Wood's units [45]. Transthoracic echocardiography is a key screening tool in the diagnostic algorithm [46]. It not only provides an estimate of pulmonary artery pressure at rest and during exercise, but it may also help to exclude any secondary causes of pulmonary hypertension, predict the prognosis, monitor the efficacy of specific therapeutic interventions, and detect the preclinical stage of disease [46]. By transthoracic echocardiography, normal values are defined by pulmonary artery systolic pressure of less than 35 mmHg at rest and less than 40 mmHg during exercise [47, 48]. However, there is no firm consensus on which PASP threshold is diagnostic for exercise-induced pulmonary hypertension, particularly if stress echocardiography is applied. There are only few invasive and noninvasive studies analyzing the normal values for pulmonary artery pressures during exercise [47–49]. Usually, in healthy subjects the systolic pressures do not exceed 40 mmHg even during heavy exercise [50, 51]. However, in well-trained athletes [48, 49] and those older than 55 years, systolic pressures as high as 55–60 mmHg are encountered [34]. Pulmonary hypertensive response during exercise (as shown in Fig. 8.6) can be clinically important in several conditions, including pulmonary hypertension due to mitral valve disease (regurgitation or stenosis) [52], heart failure [53, 54], congenital heart disease, connective tissue diseases, autoimmune diseases (e.g., lupus or systemic sclerosis) [49, 55, 56], after lung transplantation [57] and, possibly, in healthy subjects with susceptibility to high altitude pulmonary edema [58]. The assessment of PASP or mean pulmonary artery pressure during exercise by exercise Doppler echocardiography may help to identify asymptomatic gene carriers in families with pulmonary arterial hypertension who may be at risk of developing clinically overt disease over the years [59]. Also in patients with systemic sclerosis, the abnormal pulmonary pressure response to exercise has been identified as a risk factor for the development of a manifest pulmonary hypertension [56]. Only out of the group of systemic sclerosis patients with elevated pressures during exercise, did some (10%) develop manifest pulmonary hypertension within a 3-year period. Unfortunately, at present using echocardiography and right heart catheterization at rest, more than 80% of patients with pulmonary hypertension will not be diagnosed until right heart failure has occurred with the consequence of a markedly impaired life span. Thus, the assessment of PASP during stress echocardiography may be a promising method for detecting pulmonary hypertension at an early stage. Furthermore, stress echocardiography may also be useful in detecting subjects susceptible to pulmonary hypertension in special environmental and physical conditions [60]. Subjects susceptible to high-altitude pulmonary edema showed similar abnormal PASP response to exercise in normoxia and during prolonged hypoxia (12% volumes of oxygen corresponding to a 4,500-m altitude) [60]. Although echocardiography during exercise may be a promising approach for detecting early stages of pulmonary hypertension, most guidelines recommend echocardiography at rest only [61]. The accuracy of stress Doppler echocardiography for this indication has not been assessed in a larger group of patients and/or susceptible subjects.

From the pathophysiological viewpoint, on the basis of the fundamental equation of flow ($F = \Delta/R$), the abnormal exercise-induced increase in pressure can be linked to a supernormal increase in flow (e.g., in athletes), or to a normal increase in flow but with a subnormal fall in resistances due to a limited capability of pulmonary vessel recruitment and vasodilation (e.g., in chronic obstruction pulmonary disease with parenchymal pulmonary hypertension or congenital heart disease). In normal subjects, pulmonary vascular resistance falls with exercise [62–65], possibly due to pulmonary vessel recruitment, as a physiologic response that allows the thin-walled right ventricle to increase pulmonary blood flow [34]. In a clinical setting, given the absence of any specific symptoms or signs, exercise pulmonary hypertension is rarely considered, and a high degree of clinical suspicion is necessary in certain subsets of patients, such as those with a history of pulmonary thromboemboli, mitral valve disease, the sclerodermia spectrum of disorders, and familial pulmonary arterial hypertension. The potential applications of the PASP test are summarized in Table 8.4.

Table 8.4 The clinical applications of PASP stress test

Disease	Level of evidence		
	Appropriate	Uncertain	Investigational
Symptomatic, mild mitral stenosis	√		
Asymptomatic, severe mitral insufficiency	√		
Heart failure		√	
PAH		√	
SSc-PAH		√	
HAPE			√

PASP pulmonary artery systolic pressure, *HAPE* high-altitude pulmonary edema, *PAH* pulmonary arterial hypertension, *SSc-PAH* systemic sclerosis–pulmonary arterial hypertension

At present, the only application officially endorsed by general cardiology guidelines [52] is the exercise Doppler study in symptomatic individuals with mild mitral stenosis, and asymptomatic severe aortic insufficiency and mitral regurgitation [52]. In these patients, valve surgery is considered reasonable (class IIa, level of evidence C) for asymptomatic patients with preserved left ventricular function and pulmonary artery systolic pressure greater than 60 mmHg during exercise [52]. The indication to perform the study on patients with suspected pulmonary hypertension and normal or indeterminate findings after resting echocardiography study [66] remains uncertain. Other promising indications remain investigational at present.

8.5
Ultrasound Lung Comets

Ultrasound lung comets (ULCs) represent a useful, practical, appealingly simple way to image directly the extravascular lung water [67]. Because the current technology for measuring pulmonary edema can be inaccurate (chest X-rays), cumbersome (nuclear medicine or radiology techniques), or invasive (indicator dilution), there is a great potential for technology that could quantify lung edema noninvasively in real time [68, 69] with a simple, semi-quantitative, user-friendly, radiation-free direct imaging of extravascular lung water (Fig. 8.8). The cardiac transducer is employed to scan the anterior chest and the number of ULCs in each intercostal space is summed up to generate a simple score. This can be extremely important in intensive care, for instance, in detecting acute respiratory distress syndrome [70], or in cardiology departments for identifying a cardiogenic cause of dyspnea, but also in the stress testing laboratory. In fact, membrane alveolar–capillary distress is a recognized adverse prognostic determinant in patients with heart failure. Indeed, a nonphysiologic abrupt increase in pulmonary capillary wedge pressure can cause ultrastructural changes in the wall of pulmonary capillaries resulting in interstitial and alveolar edema. Particularly in patients with heart failure, a marked increase in pulmonary artery pressure and pulmonary capillary wedge pressure is observed during exercise even at very low levels creating an alveolar–capillary membrane dysfunction that contributes to symptom exacerbations and exercise intolerance (Fig. 8.9). Exercise may in fact determine the sudden appearance of

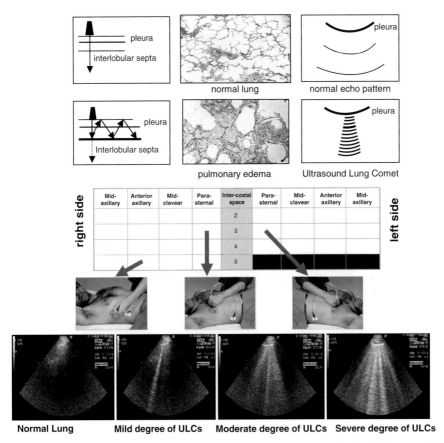

Fig. 8.8 How ULCs are generated (*upper panel*), counted (*middle panel*), and displayed (*lower panel*). The normal lung is "black" (no signal); the abnormal wet lung is "*black and white*" (with *white rockets* departing from the pleural line); and the lung with overt pulmonary edema is "*white*" (increase of coalescing comets on chest sonography)

ULC on the chest – usually on the right lung and more frequently on the midaxillary third intercostal space, which is therefore the "hot spot" for imaging in the poststress phase, when an extensive scan of the anterior chest is not always possible [67]. ULCs can be observed in heart failure patients, in whom an increase in capillary wedge pressure may occur with absence of inducible ischemia, or in patients with extensive induced ischemia, in whom ULC increase has the same conceptual meaning of the increased lung-to-heart ratio observed during sestamibi or thallium stress scan [70]. ULCs are usually accompanied by a marked stress-induced rise in E/e', which is a marker of raised left ventricular filling pressures, and/or of PASP [71]. Another interesting model is an environmental stress-induced pulmonary edema. Both in recreational climbers and in healthy elite apnea divers [72], ULCs can be detected in the presence of and, more often, in the absence of symptoms of pulmonary edema. ULCs may arise not only from water-thickened but also from fibrous-thickened subpleural septa, which are an important sign of alveolar–interstitial syndrome, for instance, in interstitial lung disease of systemic sclerosis [73]. Fibrotic ULCs are diuretic-resistant, whereas watery ULCs of pulmonary edema are reduced by diuretics [67].

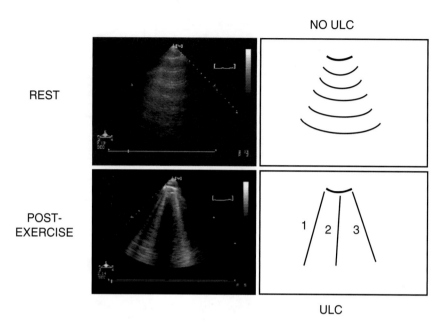

Fig. 8.9 Chest sonography (third right intercostal space) at rest (*left panel*), immediately after exercise (*middle panel*), and 15 min after the end of exercise (*right panel*). The exercise-induced appearance of ultrasound lung comets reflects the increase of extravascular lung water due to distress of the alveolar–capillary membrane

8.6
Conclusion

It is now time to remember, also in the stress echocardiography laboratory, the "forgotten" right heart, which can be extensively studied in its regional and global, segmental and longitudinal function, as well as in the novel dimension of coronary flow reserve of the right coronary artery, and pulmonary hemodynamic and alveolar–capillary membrane response. The versatility of this information can help to better characterize a variety of patients, from coronary artery disease to dilated cardiomyopathy, from valvular heart disease to pulmonary hypertension, from systemic sclerosis to healthy subjects suscep- tible to high-altitude pulmonary edema [74]. From a practical viewpoint, it is certainly not feasible to do everything to all patients, since there is so little time during stress and so many things to see. Therefore, the variable of potential diagnostic interest should be strategically tailored to the individual patient (Table 8.5). The integration of right heart evaluation (including right ventricle, right coronary artery, pulmonary hemodynamics, and alveolar–capillary membrane) will allow the characterization of an exciting new target to be included in stress echocardiography [75]. It was said 15 years ago that "*the pulmonary circulation in patients with chronic pulmonary disease is often considered a no-man's*

Table 8.5 Right heart stress echocardiography: targets and tools

	Method	Disease	Stress
Segmental function	2D	CAD	Any
Global function	*M*-mode	DCM	Dob (ex)
RCA coronary flow reserve	Color (PW) Doppler	CAD/DCM	Dip (ado)
PASP	CW Doppler (TR)	Primary or secondary pulmonary hypertension	Ex
ULC	Chest sonography	Heart failure, HAPE	Hypoxia (ex)

PASP pulmonary artery systolic pressure, *ULC* ultrasound lung comet, *CAD* coronary artery disease, *DCM* dilated cardiomyopathy, *PW* pulsed wave, *CW* continuous wave, *TR* tricuspid regurgitation, *Dob* dobutamine, *Dip* dipyridamole, *Ex* exercise

hand, falling between the domains of the respirologist and the cardiologist and understood only by the physiologist!" [76]. It can be said today that a functional dynamic evaluation of right ventricular function, right coronary artery flow reserve, pulmonary hemodynamics, and extravascular lung water can offer a unique opportunity to the cardiologist and the pneumologist to better understand the cardiovascular physiology in a variety of cardiovascular and lung diseases.

References

1. Starr I (1943) Clinical studies on incoordination of the circulation, as determined by the response of arising. J Clin Invest 22:813–26
2. Kagan A (1952) Dynamic responses of the right ventricle following extensive damage by cauterization. Circulation 5:816–23
3. Donald DE, Essex HE (1954) Massive destruction of the myocardium of the canine right ventricle; a study of the early and late effects. Am J Physiol 177:477–88
4. Rigolin VH, Robiolio PA, Wilson JS, et al (1995) The forgotten chamber: the importance of the right ventricle. Cathet Cardiovasc Diagn 35:18–28
5. MacNee W (1994) Pathophysiology of cor pulmonale in chronic obstructive pulmonary disease. Part two. Am J Respir Crit Care Med 150:1158–68
6. Armour JA, Lippincott DB, Randall WC (1973) Regional dynamic behaviour of the total right ventricle. Proc Soc Exp Biol Med 142:703–11
7. Brooks H, Holland R, Al-Sadir J (1977) Right ventricular performance during ischemia: an anatomic and hemodynamic analysis. Am J Physiol 233:H505–13
8. Zwissler B, Schosser R, Schwickert C, et al (1991) Perfusion of the interventricular septum during ventilation with positive end-expiratory pressure. Crit Care Med 19:1414–24
9. San Román JA, Vilacosta I, Rollán MJ, et al (1997) Right ventricular asynergy during dobutamine-atropine echocardiography. J Am Coll Cardiol 30:430–435
10. Parodi O, Marzullo P, Neglia D, et al (1984) Transient predominant right ventricular ischemia caused by coronary vasospasm. Circulation 70:170–7

8

11. Maurer G, Nanda NC (1981) Two dimensional echocardiographic evaluation of exercise induced left and right ventricular asynergy: correlation with thallium scanning. Am J Cardiol 48:720–727
12. Obeid AI, Battaglia J, Lozner E (1998) Right ventricular dysfunction secondary to myocardial ischemia provoked by stress testing. Echocardiography 15:451–457
13. Bangalore S, Yao SS, Chaudhry FA (2007) Role of right ventricular wall motion abnormalities in risk stratification and prognosis of patients referred for stress echocardiography. J Am Coll Cardiol 50:1981–9
14. Shah AR, Grodman R, Salazar MF, et al (2000) Assessment of acute right ventricular dysfunction induced by right coronary artery occlusion using echocardiographic atrio-ventricular plane displacement. Echocardiography 17:513–9
15. Kaul S, Tei C, Hopkins JM, Shah PM (1984) Assessment of right ventricular function using two-dimensional echocardiography. Am Heart J 107:526–31
16. Mondillo S, Galderisi M, Ballo P, et al; Study Group of Echocardiography of the Italian Society of Cardiology. (2006) Left ventricular systolic longitudinal function: comparison among simple M-mode, pulsed, and M-mode color tissue Doppler of mitral annulus in healthy individuals. J Am Soc Echocardiogr 19:1085–91
17. Lang RM, Bierig M, Devereux RB, et al; Chamber Quantification Writing Group; American Society of Echocardiography's Guidelines and Standards Committee; European Association of Echocardiography (2005) Recommendations for chamber quantification: a report from the American Society of Echocardiography's Guidelines and Standards Committee and the Chamber Quantification Writing Group, developed in conjunction with the European Association of Echocardiography, a branch of the European Society of Cardiology. J Am Soc Echocardiogr 18:1440–63
18. Pinedo M, Villacosta E, Tapia C et al (2008) Inter and intraobserver variability in echocardiographic evaluation of right ventricular function. Eur Heart J 29, Suppl 1
19. Ghio S, Recusani F, Klersy C, et al (2000) Prognostic usefulness of the tricuspid annular plane systolic excursion in patients with congestive heart failure secondary to idiopathic or ischemic dilated cardiomyopathy. Am J Cardiol 85:837–42
20. Otasević P, Popović Z, Pratali L, et al (2005) Right vs. left ventricular contractile reserve in one-year prognosis of patients with idiopathic dilated cardiomyopathy: assessment by dobutamine stress echocardiography. Eur J Echocardiogr 6:429–34
21. Di Salvo TG, Mathier M, Semigran MJ, et al (1995) Preserved right ventricular ejection fraction predicts exercise capacity and survival in advanced heart failure. J Am Coll Cardiol 25:1143–53
22. Fridrich L (1989) Prognostic significance of postinfarction arrhythmias and biventricular dysfunction under stress. Clin Cardiol 12:645–55
23. Rigo F, Richieri M, Pasanisi E, et al (2003) Usefulness of coronary flow reserve over regional wall motion when added to dual-imaging dipyridamole echocardiography. Am J Cardiol 91:269–73
24. Rigo F, Sicari R, Gherardi S, et al (2008) The additive prognostic value of wall motion abnormalities and coronary flow reserve during dipyridamole stress echo. Eur Heart J 29:79–88
25. Sicari R, Nihoyannopoulos P, Evangelista A, et al; European Association of Echocardiography (2008) Stress echocardiography expert consensus statement of European Association of Echocardiography. Eur J Echocardiogr 9:415–37
26. Ueno Y, Nakamura Y, Takashima H (2002) Noninvasive assessment of coronary flow velocity and coronary flow velocity reserve in the right coronary artery by transthoracic Doppler echocardiography: comparison with intracoronary Doppler guidewire. J Am Soc Echocardiogr 15:1074–9

27. Lethen H, P Tries H, Kersting S, Lambertz H (2003) Validation of non-invasive assessment of coronary flow velocity reserve in the right coronary artery. A comparison of transthoracic echocardiographic results with intracoronary Doppler flow wire measurements. Eur Heart J 24:1567–75

28. Rigo F, Murer B, Ossena G, et al (2008) Transthoracic echocardiographic imaging of coronary arteries: tips, traps, and pitfalls. Cardiovasc Ultrasound 6:7

29. Cortigiani L, Rigo F, Gherardi S, et al (2008) Angiographic and prognostic correlates of combined coronary flow reserve assessment in left anterior descending and right coronary artery. Eur Heart J 29, Suppl 1

30. Rigo F, Ciampi Q, Ossena G, et al (2008) Prognostic value of combined left and right coronary flow reserve assessment in non-ischemic dilated cardiomyopathy: a vasodilator stress echo study. Eur Heart J 29, Suppl 1

31. Aoki M, Harada K, Tamura M, et al (2004) Posterior descending coronary artery flow reserve assessment by Doppler echocardiography in children with and without congenital heart defect: comparison with invasive technique. Pediatr Cardiol 25:647–53

32. Yock PG, Popp RL (1984) Non-invasive estimation of right ventricular systolic pressure by Doppler ultrasound in patients with tricuspid regurgitation. Circulation 70:657–662

33. McQuillan BM, Picard MH, Leavitt M, et al (2001) Clinical correlates and reference intervals for pulmonary artery systolic pressure among echocardiographically normal subjects. Circulation 104:2797–802

34. Bossone E, Bodini BD, Mazza A, et al (2005) Pulmonary arterial hypertension: the key role of echocardiography. Chest. 127:1836–43

35. Himelman RB, Stulbarg MS, Lee E, et al (1990) Noninvasive evaluation of pulmonary artery systolic pressures during dynamic exercise by saline-enhanced Doppler echocardiography. Am Heart J 119:685–8

36. Chan KL, Currie PJ, Seward JB, et al (1987) Comparison of three Doppler ultrasound methods in the prediction of pulmonary artery pressure. J Am Coll Cardiol 9:549–54

37. Dambrauskaite V, Delcroix M, Claus P, et al (2005) The evaluation of pulmonary hypertension using right ventricular myocardial isovolumic relaxation time. J Am Soc Echocardiogr 18:1113–20

38. Tramarin R, Torbicki A, Marchandise B, et al (1991) Doppler echocardiographic evaluation of pulmonary artery pressure in chronic obstructive pulmonary disease. A European multicentre study. Working Group on Noninvasive Evaluation of Pulmonary Artery Pressure. European Office of the World Health Organization, Copenhagen. Eur Heart J 12:103–11

39. Masuyama T, Kodama K, Kitabatake A, et al (1986) Continuous-wave Doppler echocardiographic detection of pulmonary regurgitation and its application to noninvasive estimation of pulmonary artery pressure. Circulation 74:484–92

40. Ristow B, Ali S, Ren X, et al (2007) Elevated pulmonary artery pressure by Doppler echocardiography predicts hospitalization for heart failure and mortality in ambulatory stable coronary artery disease: the Heart and Soul Study. J Am Coll Cardiol 49:43–49

41. Abbas AE, Fortuin FD, Schiller NB, et al (2003) A simple method for non-invasive estimation of pulmonary vascular resistance. J Am Coll Cardiol 19:1021–1027

42. Farzaneh-Far R, McKeown BH, Dang D, et al (2008) Accuracy of Doppler-estimated pulmonary vascular resistance in patients before liver transplantation. Am J Cardiol 101:259–62

43. Ulett KB, Marwick TH (2007) Incorporation of pulmonary vascular resistance measurement into standard echocardiography: implications for assessment of pulmonary hypertension. Echocardiography 24:1020–2

44. Hatano S, Strasser T (1975) World Health organization 1975 primary pulmonary hypertension. WHO, Geneva

45. Galie N, Torbicki A, Barst R et al (2004) Guidelines on diagnosis and treatment of pulmonary arterial hypertension. The task force on diagnosis and treatment of pulmonary arterial hypertension of the European society of cardiology. Eur Heart 25:2243–2278
46. Schannwell CM, Steiner S, Strauer BE (2007) Diagnostics in pulmonary hypertension. J Physiol Pharmacol 58:591–602
47. Himelman RB, Schiller NB (1992) Exercise Doppler: functional evaluation of right heart hemodynamics. Echocardiography 9:225–33
48. Bossone E, Rubenfire M, Bach DS, et al (1999) Range of tricuspid regurgitation velocity at rest and during exercise in normal adult men: implications for the diagnosis of pulmonary hypertension. J Am Coll Cardiol 33:1662–6
49. Collins N, Bastian B, Quiqueree L, et al (2006) Abnormal pulmonary vascular responses in patients registered with a systemic autoimmunity database: pulmonary hypertension assessment and screening evaluation using stress echocardiography (PHASE-I). Eur J Echocardiogr 7:439–46
50. Bidart CM, Abbas AE, Parish JM, et al (2007) The noninvasive evaluation of exercise-induced changes in pulmonary artery pressure and pulmonary vascular resistance. J Am Soc Echocardiogr 20:270–5
51. Janosi A, Apor P, Hankoczy J, et al (1988) Pulmonary artery pressure and oxygen consumption measurement during supine bicycle exercise. Chest 93:419–21
52. American College of Cardiology/American Heart Association Task Force on Practice Guidelines; Society of Cardiovascular Anesthesiologists; Society for Cardiovascular Angiography and Interventions; Society of Thoracic Surgeons, Bonow RO, Carabello BA, Kanu C, et al (2006) ACC/AHA 2006 guidelines for the management of patients with valvular heart disease: a report of the American College of Cardiology/American Heart Association Task Force on Practice Guidelines (writing committee to revise the 1998 Guidelines for the Management of Patients With Valvular Heart Disease): developed in collaboration with the Society of Cardiovascular Anesthesiologists: endorsed by the Society for Cardiovascular Angiography and Interventions and the Society of Thoracic Surgeons. Circulation. 114:e84–231
53. Kuecherer HF, Will M, da Silva KG (1996) Contrast enhanced Doppler ultrasound for noninvasive assessment of pulmonary artery pressure during exercise in patients with chronic congestive heart failure. Am J Cardiol 78:229–32
54. Tumminello G, Lancellotti P, Lempereur M, et al (2007) Determinants of pulmonary artery hypertension at rest and during exercise in patients with heart failure. Eur Heart J. 28:569–74
55. Alkotob ML, Soltani P, Sheatt MA, et al (2006) Reduced exercise capacity and stress-induced pulmonary hypertension in patients with scleroderma. Chest 130:176–81
56. Pignone A, Mori F, Pieri F, Oddo A, et al (2007) Exercise Doppler echocardiography identifies preclinic asymptomatic pulmonary hypertension in systemic sclerosis. Ann N Y Acad Sci 1108:291–304
57. Kasimir MT, Mereles D, Aigner C, et al. (2008) Assessment of pulmonary artery systolic pressures by stress Doppler echocardiography after bilateral lung transplantation. J Heart Lung Transplant. 27:66–71
58. Grünig E, Mereles D, Hildebrandt W, et al (2000) Stress Doppler echocardiography for identification of susceptibility to high altitude pulmonary edema. J Am Coll Cardiol 35:980–7
59. Grünig E, Janssen B, Mereles D, et al (2000) Abnormal pulmonary artery pressure response in asymptomatic carriers of primary pulmonary hypertension gene. Circulation 102:1145–50
60. Grünig E, Dehnert C, Mereles D, et al (2005) Enhanced hypoxic pulmonary vasoconstriction in families of adults or children with idiopathic pulmonary arterial hypertension. Chest 128:630S–3

61. Olschewski H (2006) Current recommendations for the diagnosis and treatment of pulmonary hypertension. Dtsch Med Wochenschr 131:S334–7

62. Holmegren A, Jonsson B, Sjostarnd T (1960) Circulatory data in normal subjects at rest and during exercise in recumbent position, with special reference to the stroke volume at different work intensities. Acta Physiol Scand 49:343–346

63. Granath A, Jonsson B, Strandell T (1964) Circulation in healthy old men studied by right heart catheterization at rest and during exercise in supine and sitting position. Acta Med Scand 176:425–446

64. Ekelund LG, Holmgren A (1967) Central hemodynamics during exercise. Circ Res 30:133–143

65. Ellestad MH (1996) Cardiovascular and pulmonary responses to exercise. In: Ellestad MH (ed) Stress testing: principles and practice, 4th edn. Davis, Philadelphia, pp 11–41

66. Douglas PS, Khandheria B, Stainback RF, et al (2008) American College of Cardiology Foundation Appropriateness Criteria Task Force; American Society of Echocardiography; American College of Emergency Physicians; American Heart Association; American Society of Nuclear Cardiology; Society for Cardiovascular Angiography and Interventions; Society of Cardiovascular Computed Tomography; Society for Cardiovascular Magnetic Resonance. ACCF/ASE/ACEP/AHA/ASNC/SCAI/SCCT/SCMR 2008 appropriateness criteria for stress echocardiography: a report of the American College of Cardiology Foundation Appropriateness Criteria Task Force, American Society of Echocardiography, American College of Emergency Physicians, American Heart Association, American Society of Nuclear Cardiology, Society for Cardiovascular Angiography and Interventions, Society of Cardiovascular Computed Tomography, and Society for Cardiovascular Magnetic Resonance: endorsed by the Heart Rhythm Society and the Society of Critical Care Medicine. Circulation 117:1478–97

67. Picano E, Frassi F, Agricola E (2006) Ultrasound lung comets: a clinically useful sign of extravascular lung water. J Am Soc Echocardiogr 19:356–63

68. Jambrik Z, Monti S, Coppola V, et al (2004) Usefulness of ultrasound lung comets as a nonradiologic sign of extravascular lung water. Am J Cardiol 93:1265–70

69. Gargani L, Lionetti V, Di Cristofano C, et al (2007) Early detection of acute lung injury uncoupled to hypoxemia in pigs using ultrasound lung comets. Crit Care Med 35:2769–74

70. Agricola E, Picano E, Oppizzi M, et al (2006) Assessment of stress-induced pulmonary interstitial edema by chest ultrasound during exercise echocardiography and its correlation with left ventricular function. J Am Soc Echocardiogr19:457–63

71. Fagenholz PJ, Gutman JA, Murray AF, et al (2007) Chest ultrasonography for the diagnosis and monitoring of high-altitude pulmonary edema. Chest 131:1013–8

72. Frassi F, Pingitore A, Cialoni D, et al (2008) Chest sonography detects lung water accumulation in healthy elite apnea divers. Eur J Echocardiogr 21:1150–55

73. Gargani L, Frassi F, Doveri M, et al (2009) Ultrasound lung comets in systemic sclerosis: a chest sonography hallmark of pulmonary interstitial fibrosis. Reumatology 49:210–213

74. Picano E (2003) Stress echocardiography: a historical perspective. Special article. Am J Med 114:126–30

75. Pellikka PA, Nagueh SF, Elhendy AA, et al, American Society of Echocardiography (2007) American Society of Echocardiography recommendations for performance, interpretation, and application of stress echocardiography. J Am Soc Echocardiogr 20:1021–41

76. MacNee W (1994) Pathophysiology of cor pulmonale in chronic obstructive pulmonary disease. Part One. Am J Respir Crit Care Med 150:833–852

Fausto Rigo, Jorge Lowenstein, and Eugenio Picano

9.1
Historical Background and Physiological Basis

The seminal concept of coronary flow reserve was proposed experimentally by Lance K. Gould in 1974 [1]. Under normal conditions, in the absence of stenosis, coronary blood flow can increase approximately four- to sixfold to meet increasing myocardial oxygen demands. This effect is mediated by vasodilation at the arteriolar bed, which reduces vascular resistance, thereby augmenting flow. Coronary reserve is the capacity of the coronary circulation to dilate following an increase in myocardial metabolic demand and can be expressed by the difference between the hyperemic flow and the resting flow curve. In most clinical applications, hyperemia is induced pharmacologically, not via an increase in oxygen demand. A combined anatomical and physiological classification can ideally identify four separate segments in the hyperemic curve (Fig. 9.1): (1) The hemodynamically silent range of 0–40% stenosis, which does not affect coronary flow reserve (>2.5) to any detectable extent. (2) The clinically silent zone, where stenosis ranging from 40 to 70% may marginally reduce the coronary flow reserve without reaching the critical threshold required to provoke ischemia with the usual stresses. (3) The severe stenosis range (70–90%), where critical stenosis reduces coronary flow reserve less than 2.0, and myocardial ischemia is usually elicited when a stress is applied. (4) The very severe stenosis range (>90%), producing a marked transstenotic pressure drop at rest, with a reduction of baseline myocardial blood flow and a coronary flow reserve close to 1, or even less; in these patients, the administration of a coronary vasodilator actually decreases the poststenotic flow for steal phenomena. This experimental paradigm can be accurately reproduced clinically in highly selected series of patients with single-vessel disease, no myocardial infarction, no coronary collateral circulation, normal baseline function, no left ventricular hypertrophy, with no evidence of coronary vasospasm, and who are off therapy at the time of testing. In these patients, the more severe the stenosis, the more profound the impairment in

E. Picano, *Stress Echocardiography*,
© Springer-Verlag Berlin Heidelberg 2009

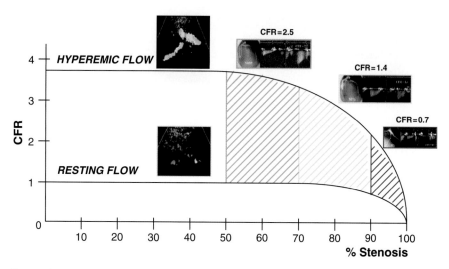

Fig. 9.1 The curve of coronary flow reserve with the four segments: hemodynamically silent (0–40% stenosis); clinically silent (40–70% stenosis); hemodynamically significant (70–90% with CFR<2.0); and very severe stenosis (>90%, with CFR<1.0). (Redrawn and adapted from [1] and [17])

coronary flow reserve. The correction of the stenosis improves coronary flow reserve, and perfect dilation normalizes the coronary flow reserve. The perfect, predictable relationship found in the experimental animal and in a very selected patient population [2] falls apart in the clinical arena [3], where many variables can modulate the imperfect match between epicardial coronary artery stenosis and coronary flow reserve. Among others, these variables include:

1. The geometric characteristics of the stenosis
2. The presence of coronary collateral circulation
3. The microvascular component of coronary resistance
4. Left ventricular hypertrophy modulating the myocardial extravascular component of coronary resistance
5. The viable or necrotic state of the myocardium distal to the stenosis
6. The presence of coronary macrovascular or microvascular spasm
7. The presence of concomitant antiischemic therapy

In fact, this impressive scatter of data leads to the need to reconsider our original stenoticocentric view of ischemic heart disease [4]. According to that view, each level of stenosis precisely predicts the level of impairment in coronary blood flow. This concept has some corollaries: stenosis is the disease and dilating the stenosis means curing the disease; the probability of subsequent occlusion depends on the severity of the stenosis; the stress test accurately maps the area at risk for subsequent infarction. Although reasonable, all these corollaries are at least partially wrong; the stenosis is only the fruit of the atherosclerotic plant, which has deep genetic, metabolic, and hemodynamic roots that must be identified and treated in order to better cure this disease. Critical stenosis may occlude, but the majority of clinically catastrophic occlusions occur in previously noncritical stenosis; the stress test accurately identifies the area at risk of subsequent infarction in only a minority (four out of ten) of patients. In two out of ten patients, the stress test is right for the wrong reason (the test results are positive and the patient develops infarction, but in an area different from the induced ischemia), and in four out of ten, the test is wrong (normal findings in a patient who subsequently develops infarction) [5]. The appeal of coronary flow reserve is to gain insight into a key physiological variable that integrates functional assessment during a stress [6]. This assessment can be obtained clinically, with six different basic approaches (Table 9.1): positron emission tomography (PET), myocardial scintigraphy, magnetic resonance perfusion imaging; intracoronary Doppler flow wire, transesophageal echocardiography, and transthoracic echocardiography. PET is highly accurate, allows a quantitative assessment of absolute myocardial blood flow, but is exorbitantly expensive, technically demanding, available in very few centers, and exposes the patient to radiation biohazards. Single-photon emission computed tomography (SPECT) is less expensive, and is also less accurate than PET, with a high radiation burden of 500–1,500 chest X-rays for a sestamibi or thallium scan, respectively). Intracoronary Doppler flow wire is invasive, risky, and expensive, requiring intracoronary catheterization; radiation exposure is required for intracoronary catheter placement, although not directly for coronary flow reserve measurement. Instead, transesophageal echocardiography has the limitation of being semiinvasive, while transthoracic echocardiography has the merit of being noninvasive, nonionizing, and compatible with other forms of functional testing for induction of wall motion abnormalities in the echocardiography laboratory. All these approaches are based on the theoretical prerequisite that the imaging technique combined with hyperemic stress will generate a signal whose intensity is correlated (possibly in a linear, direct fashion) with coronary

Table 9.1 Methods of assessing coronary flow reserve

	Measurements of flow	Radiation exposure (CXr)	Cost	Availability	Accuracy	Interest
PET	Absolute		Very high	–	+++	Research
SPECT	Relative	(500–1500)	High	++	++	Clinical cardiology
CMR	Relative	0	High	±	++	Clinical cardiology
Intracoronary Doppler	Relative	++	High	±	+++	Cath lab
Transesophageal Doppler	Relative	–	Low	+	++(+)	Echo lab
Transthoracic echocardiography	Relative	–	Very low	+++	++(+)	Clinical cardiology

CXr chest radiograph, *PET* positron emission tomography, *SPECT* single-photon emission computed tomography, *CMR* cardiovascular magnetic resonance

9

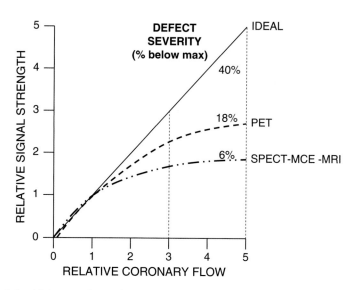

Fig. 9.2 Relationship between the true increments of coronary flow and the flow signal strength obtained with the currently available imaging techniques. All techniques, including the most sophisticated and expensive ones, are considerably far from the ideal, in which the signal increases in a linear and direct fashion with flow. In the high flow range – the most important one following a vasodilatory stimulus – the relationship between flow and signal tends toward a plateau, implying only minimal (if any) signal differences. For instance, if the flow is fivefold higher in the normal coronary vessel and only three-fold in the stenotic vessel, the recorded flow difference will be 18% by positron emission tomography (*PET*), and around 10% by SPECT, myocardial contrast echocardiography (*MCE*), transthoracic echo Doppler flowmetry, and magnetic resonance imaging (*MRI*). (Adapted and modified from [7])

flow, especially in the high-flow range that is the most important one for diagnostic purposes. Unfortunately, none of the available techniques for noninvasive assessment of
coronary flow reserve allows a truly accurate quantitative assessment of coronary flow
reserve [7] (Fig. 9.2). For instance, a 40% reduction in coronary flow reserve compared
with normal values (i.e., a flow reserve of 3 in diseased myocardium compared to a flow
reserve of 5 in the normal myocardium) will yield a difference in signal intensity of only
6% with SPECT (comparable to myocardial contrast echocardiography) and of 18% with
PET, whose results correlate well with intracoronary, transesophageal, and transthoracic
echocardiography Doppler techniques [8]. We are still far from the ideal test of coronary
flow reserve. Nevertheless, the possibility of a reasonably accurate estimation of coronary
flow reserve during a stress targeted on functional testing for wall motion analysis opens
new, exciting clinical and research opportunities.

9.2
Coronary Flow Reserve in the Echocardiography Laboratory

With either transesophageal (sampling the proximal tract) or transthoracic echocardiography (exploring the middistal tract), the left anterior descending coronary blood flow velocity profile recorded with pulsed-wave Doppler is consistent with the pathophysiological

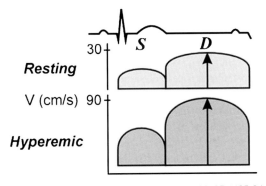

Ono S et al Circulation 19992; 85:1125-31

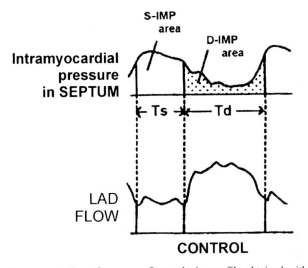

CONTROL

Fig. 9.3 Schematic representation of coronary flow velocity profile obtained with transthoracic Doppler of the middistal left anterior descending coronary artery and measurement of the coronary flow reserve through peak diastolic flow velocity. The coronary blood flow velocity is higher in diastole. The *lower panel* shows the experimental data obtained with intramyocardial pressure monitoring and left anterior descending flowmetry in the dog. (From [9], with permission)

premises. Coronary flow velocity by Doppler assessment appears to be biphasic, with a lower peak during systole and a higher peak during diastole. Myocardial extravascular resistance in fact is higher in systole and lower in diastole due to the effect of myocardial contraction (Fig. 9.3) [9]. The flow velocity variations are proportional to the total blood flow if the diameter of the vessel lumen is kept constant. In reality, the diameter of epicardial coronary arteries increases by an average of 30% in healthy subjects following adenosine infusion [10]. Therefore, failure to take into account epicardial coronary artery vasodilation during hyperemia may cause a nonsystematic underestimation of coronary flow reserve, which can be more accurately calculated as velocity time integral cross-sectional area [10]. In practice, and with an unavoidable approximation, the coronary flow

9

velocity variation between baseline and peak effect of a coronary vasodilator makes it possible to derive an index of coronary flow reserve in the left anterior descending artery territory. Several parameters might be measured from Doppler tracings of left anterior descending artery flow, including systolic flows, time–velocity integrals, and mean flows [8]. However, the best parameter is peak diastolic flow; it is not only the simplest parameter to be measured and the easiest to obtain, but also the most reproducible and the one with the closest correlation with coronary perfusion reserve measured with Doppler flow wire [11] and PET [12]. The signal of coronary flow on the left anterior descending coronary artery was first made possible by transesophageal echocardiography, with excellent diagnostic results [11, 12], but only recently has there been increased clinical interest in the development of the transthoracic method [13–17]. There were technological factors that allowed the totally noninvasive transthoracic imaging of the middistal left anterior descending coronary artery: second-harmonic imaging, which provides better definition of smaller structures such as the left anterior descending coronary artery, and high-frequency transducers (up to 8 MHz), which provide improved resolution imaging of near-field structures (Fig. 9.4). The availability of contrast agents also improved the signal-to-noise ratio, increasing the feasibility of transthoracic imaging of the left anterior descending coronary artery above the threshold of potential clinical impact.

The Doppler assessment of coronary flow reserve has some limitations. The assessment of absolute blood velocity can be limited in some patients by the large incident angle between the Doppler beam and blood flow. However, calculation of the flow reserve allows

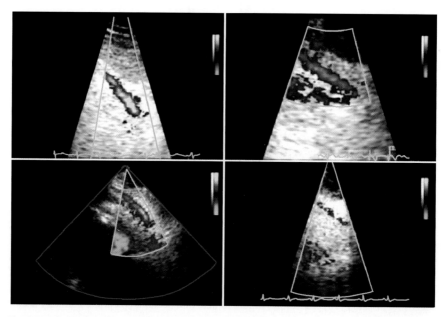

Fig. 9.4 Color Doppler flow imaging of the left anterior descending artery, visualized in its middle-to-distal portion to a variable extent in four different patients. (Courtesy of Dr. Jorge Lowenstein)

assessment of flow patterns without the need for absolute values. More importantly, the velocity ratio is used as a surrogate of flow reserve; flow within the coronary artery is not calculated because cross-sectional visualization of the vessel does not accurately measure the diameter of the vessel. The estimated flow reserve can be accurate if the coronary artery functions only as a conduit, with no change in its diameter during drug infusion. The variability and heterogeneity in coronary artery diameter response following administration of adenosine [10] or dobutamine introduce a remarkable source of error, which is amenable to correction only through direct measurement of epicardial vessel diameter changes with high-resolution imaging [10]. However, the positive correlation between true coronary flow reserve and coronary flow velocity changes, together with the lower method variability of the latter, makes it suitable for a robust assessment of coronary flow reserve in most experimental and clinical settings [19].

9.3
Methodology of Coronary Flow Reserve Testing

Stress testing of coronary flow reserve introduces a change in the choice of the stress, the use of transducers, and the methodology of testing.

After stress, the balance between exercise, dobutamine, and vasodilators clearly goes in the direction of vasodilators (Fig. 9.5), which fully recruit coronary flow reserve [20] (Fig. 9.6) and minimize the factors polluting image quality [21]. Among vasodilators, dipyridamole is better tolerated subjectively than adenosine [22], it induces less hyperventilation

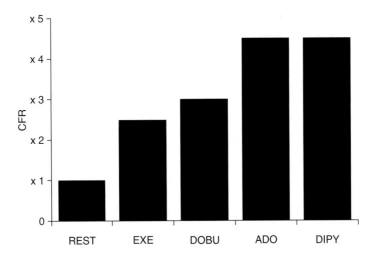

Fig. 9.5 Coronary flow reserve and stresses: vasodilators [adenosine (*ADO*) or dipyridamole (*DIPY*)] evoke a greater recruitment of coronary flow reserve, substantially higher than dobutamine (*DOB*) and exercise (*EXE*). They are more appropriate stressors for testing coronary flow reserve. (Modified from [20], with permission)

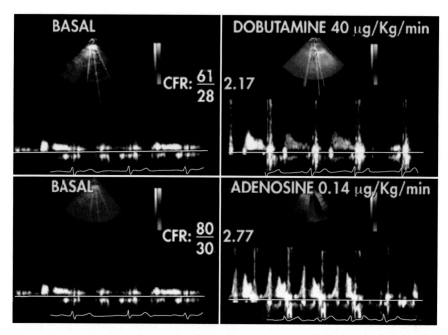

Fig. 9.6 Coronary flow reserve assessed in the same patient with transthoracic echocardiography by dobutamine (*upper panels*) and adenosine (*lower panels*). *Left panels*, baseline signal. *Right panels*, peak stress signals. The increase in coronary flow reserve is substantially higher with adenosine than with dobutamine. (Courtesy of Dr. Jorge Lowenstein)

(which may pollute the echocardiography images), costs much less in most countries, and has a longer-lasting vasodilatory effect [23] (Fig. 9.7), which is more convenient for dual flow and function imaging (Table 9.2).

A broadband transducer (2–7 MHz) or two transducers (with low-frequency imaging of wall motion and high-frequency imaging of left anterior descending coronary artery flow) must be used, allowing alternative opening of imaging windows on coronary flow and left ventricular function [24, 25]. Besides the classic projections for stress echocardiography testing, specific projection for left anterior descending coronary artery imaging should be integrated into the cardiac imaging sequence (Fig. 9.8). The posterior descending artery (Fig. 9.9) and the left circumflex artery (Fig. 9.10) can be imaged with dedicated imaging projections, but with greater difficulty and a lower success rate. The imaging protocol methodology also changes, with a shift from left anterior descending coronary artery flow to left ventricular function. This is more technically demanding, but also more thrilling for the skilled stress echocardiographer, as it combines the two different aspects of flow and functional imaging into a single test [24–26]; the split brain of imaging formally finds its conceptual corpus callosum in the echocardiography laboratory (Figs. 9.11, 9.12). The normal values are quite similar for all three coronary arteries, and are clearly normal when above 2.5, borderline between 2.0 and 2.5, and clearly abnormal below 2.0. Athletes show supernormal values (above 4.0). A reduction in coronary flow reserve can be linked to

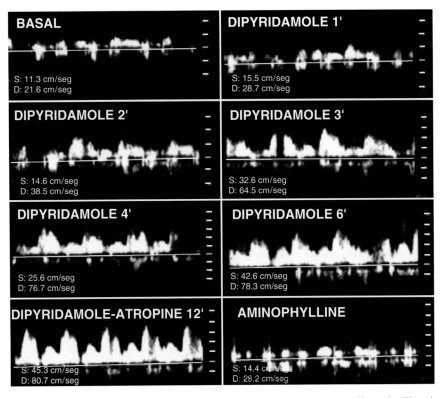

Fig. 9.7 The temporal sampling of coronary flow reserve by transthoracic echocardiography. There is a progressive, stepwise increase in coronary flow reserve peaking after the high dose and immediately reversed upon administration of aminophylline

Table 9.2 Vasodilator stress imaging

Drug	Adenosine	Dipyridamole
Patient tolerance	Lower	Higher
Vasodilator effect onset	Seconds	Minutes
Multiple coronary imaging	Difficult	Possible
Combined wall motion and CFR	Difficult	Possible

CFR coronary flow reserve

a significant epicardial coronary artery stenosis, but also to microvascular disease or to factors increasing extravascular resistance and endoluminal compressive forces with normal coronary arteries, as happens in syndrome X, dilated or hypertrophic cardiomyopathy, and aortic stenosis [27].

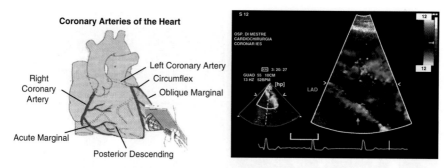

Fig. 9.8 *Left panel*: Artist's drawing illustrating transducer beam orientation to the left anterior descending coronary artery. The middistal tract is imaged from a modified apical 2-chamber view. *Right panel*: The corresponding echocardiographic image of left anterior descending color flow

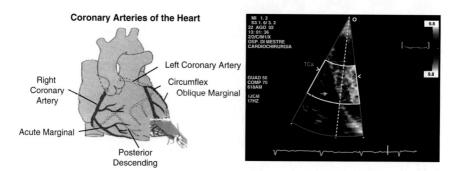

Fig. 9.9 *Left panel*: Artist's drawing illustrating transducer beam orientation to the posterior descending coronary artery. The middistal tract is imaged from a modified apical 2-chamber view with counter-clockwise rotation and anterior angulation of the probe. *Right panel*: The corresponding echocardiographic image of posterior descending color flow

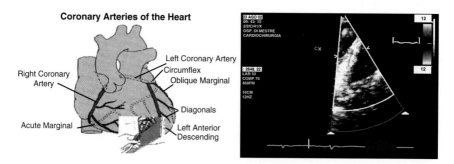

Fig. 9.10 *Left panel*: Artist's drawing illustrating transducer beam orientation to the left circumflex coronary artery. The midproximal tract of the left circumflex artery is imaged from a modified apical 4-chamber view with 50–80° clockwise rotation and posterior angulation of the probe. *Right panel*: The corresponding echocardiographic image of left circumflex color flow

REST **STRESS**

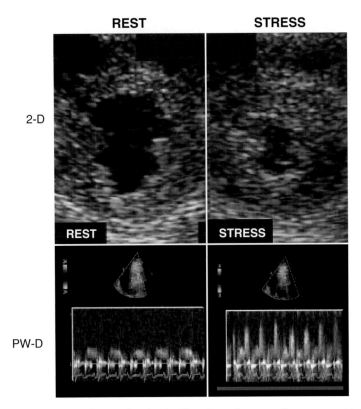

2-D

PW-D

Fig. 9.11 A typical example of a normal regional wall motion and coronary flow reserve pattern from a patient with normal coronary arteries. The end-systolic frames from parasternal short-axis view show a normal thickening at rest (*left upper panel*) and during stress (*right upper panel*). On the *left*, pulsed Doppler shows a threefold increase in Doppler peak diastolic flow velocity from baseline (*left lower panel*) to peak dipyridamole (*right lower panel*)

9.4
Coronary Flow Reserve: The Diagnostic Results

Good results have been reported with coronary flow reserve evaluation during transesophageal [11, 12] or transthoracic echocardiography [13–17] for noninvasive diagnosis of coronary artery disease (Fig. 9.13). Nevertheless, the use of coronary flow reserve as a standalone diagnostic criterion suffers from so many practical problems: first of all, only the left anterior descending coronary artery is sampled; second, coronary flow reserve cannot distinguish between microvascular and macrovascular coronary disease [27]. Therefore, it is much more interesting (and clinically realistic) to evaluate the additive value over conventional wall motion for left anterior descending coronary artery detection. The assessment of coronary flow reserve adds sensitivity for left anterior descending

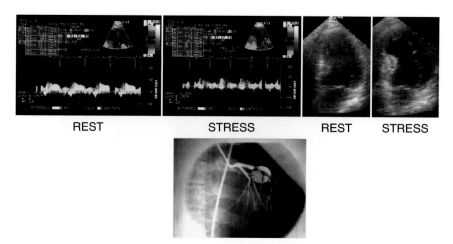

Fig. 9.12 A typical example of a regional wall motion (*right upper panel*) and coronary flow reserve (*left upper panel*) pattern from a patient with a tight proximal stenosis of the left anterior descending artery (*lower panel*). On the *right*, the end-systolic frames from the apical 4-chamber view show a normal thickening at rest and akinesia of the apex during stress. On the *left*, pulsed Doppler shows no significant increase in Doppler peak diastolic flow velocity from baseline (*left*) to peak dipyridamole (*right*)

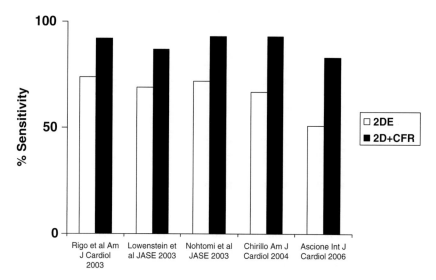

Fig. 9.13 The sensitivity for noninvasive detection of anatomic disease of the left anterior descending coronary artery on the basis of wall motion (2D echocardiography) and coronary flow reserve (CFR) criteria in five different studies, all consistently showing the higher sensitivity achieved with the contribution of 2D echocardiography and CFR criterion versus 2D echocardiography alone. (Redrawn and adapted from original data of [28–32])

Table 9.3 The two faces of stress echocardiography testing

	Wall motion	Coronary flow reserve
Specificity	Higher	Lower
Sensitivity	Lower	Higher
Technical difficulty	Lower	Higher
Interpretation	Difficult	Easier
Prognostic value	High	Unknown
Segmental positivity response	All-or-one	Continuous
Coronary arteries explored	All territories	Mostly LAD

LAD left anterior descending artery

coronary artery disease, with a modest loss of specificity [28–32]. In some ways, coronary flow reserve and wall motion analysis offer complementary information during stress echocardiography (Table 9.3). From the pathophysiological viewpoint, wall motion positivity requires ischemia as a necessary prerequisite, whereas coronary flow reserve can be impaired in the absence of induced ischemia. Wall motion is easy to acquire but can be difficult to analyze. Coronary flow reserve can be difficult to acquire, but it is usually straightforward in its quantitative interpretation of a Doppler signal. In the interpretation phase, a regional wall motion abnormality has higher positive predictive value for predicting the presence of epicardial coronary artery stenosis. A normal coronary flow reserve has a higher negative predictive value. Therefore, the two pieces of information on flow and function can complement each other since a wall motion abnormality is highly specific and a normal coronary flow reserve is highly sensitive for coronary artery disease [28–32]. In addition, the flow information is relatively unaffected by concomitant antianginal therapy, which markedly reduces sensitivity of ischemia-dependent regional wall motion abnormality [33] and does not influence coronary flow reserve except to a limited extent, if at all [34]. In this way, the coronary flow reserve can already help in the difficult task of identifying patients with coronary artery disease. Obviously, such help will be greater with the potential of imaging all three major coronary arteries, with segments of the posterior descending and left circumflex coronary artery [35, 36] being more difficult for ultrasonic imaging at present.

9.5
The Prognostic Value of Coronary Flow Reserve

In patients with idiopathic dilated cardiomyopathy [37] or hypertrophic cardiomyopathy [38] and in patients with normal to nonsignificant coronary artery disease [39, 40], a severely depressed coronary flow reserve is a predictor of poor prognosis. These studies were performed on small patient series, with a limited number of events, and employed highly academic (complex, expensive, time-consuming) techniques such as PET [37, 38] or the intracoronary Doppler flow wire technique [39, 40]. With the advent of coronary

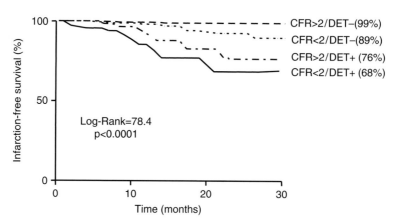

Fig. 9.14 Kaplan–Meier survival curves (considering only death and myocardial infarction as end points) in patients stratified according to normal (CFR>2.0) or abnormal (CFR<2.0) coronary flow reserve at Doppler echocardiography, and presence or absence of wall motion abnormalities by 2D echocardiography

flow reserve in the stress echocardiography laboratory, in a few years a striking amount of information became available through large-scale multicenter studies, showing the impressive prognostic value of coronary flow reserve. This value has been proven in patients with stable angina [41, 42], patients with intermediate stenosis of single-vessel disease [43, 44], and in several other challenging subsets characterized by negative wall motion response during stress echocardiography, such as patients with diabetes [45] under antianginal therapy at the time of testing [46], dilated cardiomyopathy [47], hypertrophic cardiomyopathy [48], or heart transplant [49]. The prognostic value has also been shown for hard end points only, and adds incremental information over the value of inducible wall motion abnormalities (Fig. 9.14). At this point, an evidence-based use of coronary flow reserve in clinically driven decision-making is possible and fully justified. Similar diagnostic and prognostic results can be obtained in the assessment of left ventricular wall motion and coronary flow reserve in left internal mammary artery and right internal mammary artery grafts [50–53].

9.6
Targets, Tips, and Traps in Coronary Flow Reserve

At present, different segments of native or grafted coronary arteries can be imaged transthoracically in the echocardiography laboratory. The feasibility and clinical impact are highest for the middistal native left anterior descending coronary artery and the left internal mammary artery graft, while it is lowest (albeit still feasible) for posterior descending and left circumflex arteries, and intermediate for saphenous vein grafts. Each of the segments has different transducer frequency windows, different initial velocity range, different

Table 9.4 Coronary flow reserve in the echocardiography laboratory: technicalities and targets

Vein graft	LAD	LCx	PD	LIMA	RIMA	Saphenous
Success rate	90%	50%	60%	90–100%	90–100%	80–90%
Transducer position	Modified apical	Modified apical 4-chamber	Modified apical 2-chamber	Left supra-clavicular area	Right supraclavi-cular area	Modified parasternal
Transducer frequency (MHz)	5–7	3.5	3.5	5–7	5–7	3–5
Best CFR cut-off for stenosis detection	<2.0	<2.0	<2.0	<1.9	<1.9	<1.6

CFR coronary flow reserve, *LAD* left anterior descending artery, *LCx* left circumflex artery, *PD* posterior descending artery, *LIMA* left internal mammary artery, *RIMA* right internal mammary artery

projections, and different technical difficulties (Table 9.4). There are biological and technical problems with coronary flow reserve assessment. The coronary flow reserve depends on a coronary as well as a myocardial component. Patent native arteries or graft with a low flow reserve supply myocardium that is partially scarred from previous infarction. Under these conditions, the vasodilating capacity of the recipient myocardium is probably reduced independently of any stenosis. In diagnostic terms, this may account for a reduced specificity of coronary flow reserve (abnormal with patent arteries). Poststenotic coronary flow reserve accurately reflects the residual vasodilatory capacity of that vascular bed which is specifically affected by the stenosis [24–27]. Prestenotic coronary flow reserve can be diagnostically unreliable, since the abnormal response in the poststenotic territory can be pseudonormalized by the normal vasodilatory response in the territories supplied by the branching vessels stemming off the main trunk between the sampling zone and the stenosis. Coronary flow reserve will yield the greatest information when combined with wall motion imaging. Contrast agent injection is sometimes – although not often – needed, and this will impact favorably on the cost-effectiveness profile of the method.

9.7 Coronary Flow Reserve in the Stress Echocardiography Laboratory: Here to Stay

Assessment of coronary flow reserve integrates and complements classic stress echocardiography founded on regional wall motion analysis. With the addition of coronary flow reserve to wall motion, the stress echocardiography response can be stratified into a severity code mirroring the ischemic cascade. On one end of the spectrum, there is the totally normal pattern, with hyperdynamic left ventricular function and preserved coronary flow reserve, which is highly predictive of normal coronary anatomy and normal physiological response of coronary micro- and macrocirculation. At the opposite end of the spectrum,

9

there is the totally abnormal pattern with regional wall motion abnormalities and abnormal coronary flow response, which is highly predictive of diseased epicardial coronary anatomy and impaired flow reserve. In between these extreme "black and white" responses, a gray zone can be found, more often with prognostically meaningful mild to moderate abnormal coronary flow reserve and normal function (Fig. 9.15). At present, coronary flow reserve in coronary artery disease is a feasible, useful, and prognostically validated tool to be considered with standard wall motion analysis for the "two birds with one stone" approach of dual imaging in stress echocardiography. As such, it is currently recommended as the state-of-the art method with vasodilatory stress echocardiography when adequate technology and expertise are available [54]. Its noninvasive, radiation-free nature also make it ideally suited for ethically immaculate, radiation-free research-oriented studies, especially when each subject or patient acts as his/her own control, allowing establishment of acute

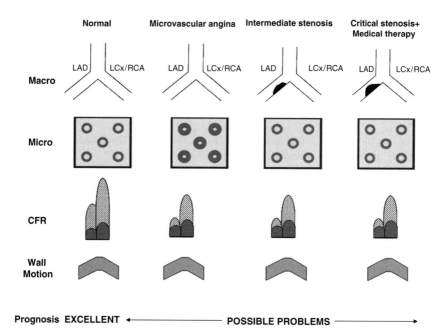

Fig. 9.15 Pathophysiological and prognostic heterogeneity behind normal wall motion response during stress. In the *upper panel*, we show epicardial coronary arteries: normal in the *first two columns*, with moderate disease in the *third column*, and moderate-to-severe disease but concomitant, effective antiischemic therapy in the *last column*. The myocardium is shown as a *square box*, with small vessels as *circles*. Coronary small vessel disease is shown (*second columns*) as bold circles (structural or functional impairment). All four very different pathophysiological conditions show the negativity of wall motion response. The abnormal CFR response is present in the *last three columns*, with abnormality of micro- or macrocirculation. *Panel B*: Pathophysiological and prognostic heterogeneity behind abnormal wall motion response during stress. Symbols as in *Panel A*. The CFR can be normal in spite of wall motion abnormality when the left anterior descending artery is not significantly involved and the microcirculatory level is not impaired (*left panel*)

or chronic changes in coronary flow reserve, induced, for instance, by acute food or beverage intake (such as alcohol or chocolate) or ingestion of medication in chronic therapeutic interventions, for instance, statins or antihypertensive drugs [55–60]. Although substantial technological and conceptual refinements are expected in the near future, for instance, with 3D imaging and the possibility of accurately assessing coronary flow reserve with simultaneous evaluation of coronary flow velocity profiles and stress-induced changes in coronary diameter, there is little doubt that the technique is here to stay.

References

1. Gould KL, Lipscomb K (1974) Effects of coronary stenosis on coronary flow reserve and resistance. Am J Cardiol 34:48–55
2. Uren NG, Melin JA, De Bruyne B, et al (1994) Relation between myocardial blood flow and the severity of coronary artery stenosis. N Engl J Med 330:1782–1788
3. White CW, Wright CB, Doty DB, et al (1984) Does visual interpretation of the coronary arteriogram predict the physiologic importance of a coronary stenosis? N Engl J Med 310:819–824
4. Topol EJ, Nissen SE (1995) Our preoccupation with coronary luminology. The dissociation between clinical and angiographic findings in ischemic heart disease. Circulation 92:2333–2342
5. Varga A, Picano E, Cortigiani L, et al (1996) Does stress echocardiography predict the site of future myocardial infarction? A large-scale multicenter study. J Am Coll Cardiol 28:45–51
6. Strauer BE (1990) The significance of coronary reserve in clinical heart disease. J Am Coll Cardiol 15:775–783
7. Gould KL (1991) Comparison of PET and other imaging techniques. In: Gould KL (ed) Coronary artery stenosis. Elsevier, Amsterdam
8. Saraste M, Koskenvuo J, Knuuti J, et al (2001) Coronary flow reserve: measurement with transthoracic Doppler echocardiography is reproducible and comparable with positron emission tomography. Clin Physiol 21:114–122
9. Ono S, Nohara R, Kambara H, Okuda K, Kawai C (1992) Regional myocardial perfusion and glucose metabolism in experimental left bundle branch block. Circulation. 85:1125–1131
10. Kiviniemi TO, Toikka JO, Koskenvuo JW, et al (2007) Vasodilation of epicardial coronary artery can be measured with transthoracic echocardiography. Ultrasound Med Biol. 33:362–370
11. Iliceto S, Marangelli V, Memmola C, et al (1991) Transesophageal Doppler echocardiography evaluation of coronary blood flow velocity in baseline conditions and during dipyridamole-induced coronary vasodilation. Circulation 83:61–69
12. Radvan J, Marwick TH, Williams MJ, et al (1995) Evaluation of the extent and timing of the coronary hyperemic response to dipyridamole: a study with transesophageal echocardiography and positron emission tomography with oxygen 15 water. J Am Soc Echocardiogr. 8:864–873
13. Hozumi T, Yoshida K, Ogata Y, et al (1998) Noninvasive assessment of significant left anterior descending coronary artery stenosis by coronary flow velocity reserve with transthoracic color Doppler echocardiography. Circulation 97:1557–1562
14. Caiati C, Montaldo C, Zedda N, et al (1999) New noninvasive method for coronary flow reserve assessment: contrast-enhanced transthoracic second harmonic echo Doppler. Circulation 99:771–778
15. Lim HE, Shim WJ, Rhee H, et al (2000) Assessment of coronary flow reserve with transthoracic Doppler echocardiography: comparison among adenosine, standard-dose dipyridamole, and high-dose dipyridamole. J Am Soc Echocardiogr 13:264–270

9

16. Daimon M, Watanabe H, Yamagishi H, et al (2001) Physiologic assessment of coronary artery stenosis by coronary flow reserve measurements with transthoracic Doppler echocardiography: comparison with exercise thallium-201 single photon emission computed tomography. J Am Coll Cardiol 37:1310–1315

17. Pizzuto F, Voci P, Mariano E, et al (2001) Assessment of flow velocity reserve by transthoracic Doppler echocardiography and venous adenosine infusion before and after left anterior descending coronary artery stenting. J Am Coll Cardiol 38:155–162

18. Barbato E, Bartunek J, Wyffels E, et al (2003) Effects of intravenous dobutamine on coronary vasomotion in humans. J Am Coll Cardiol 42:1596–1601

19. Wikström J, Grönros J, Gan LM (2008) Adenosine induces dilation of epicardial coronary arteries in mice – Relationship between coronary flow velocity reserve and coronary flow reserve in vivo using transthoracic echocardiography. Ultrasound Med Biol 34:1053–1062

20. Iskandrian AS, Verani MS, Heo J (1994) Pharmacologic stress testing: mechanism of action, hemodynamic responses, and results in detection of coronary artery disease. J Nucl Cardiol 1:94–111

21. Picano E (1992) Stress echocardiography. From pathophysiological toy to diagnostic tool. Circulation 85:1604–1612

22. Martin TW, Seaworth JF, Johns JP, et al (1992) Comparison of adenosine, dipyridamole, and dobutamine in stress echocardiography. Ann Intern Med 116:190–196

23. Rossen JD, Quillen JE, Lopez AG, et al (1990) Comparison of coronary vasodilation with intravenous dipyridamole and adenosine. J Am Coll Cardiol 15:373–377

24. Dimitrow PP (2003) Transthoracic Doppler echocardiography – noninvasive diagnostic window for coronary flow reserve assessment. Cardiovasc Ultrasound 1:4

25. Dimitrow PP, Galderisi M, Rigo F (2005) The non-invasive documentation of coronary microcirculation impairment: role of transthoracic echocardiography. Cardiovasc Ultrasound 3:18

26. Rigo F (2005) Coronary flow reserve in stress-echo lab. From pathophysiologic toy to diagnostic tool. Cardiovasc Ultrasound 3:8

27. Rigo F, Murer B, Ossena G et al (2008)Transthoracic echocardiographic imaging of coronary arteries: tips, traps, and pitfalls. Cardiovasc Ultrasound 6:7

28. Rigo F, Richieri M, Pasanisi E, et al (2003) Usefulness of coronary flow reserve over regional wall motion when added to dual-imaging dipyridamole echocardiography. Am J Cardiol 91:269–273

29. Nohtomi Y, Takeuchi M, Nagasawa K, et al (2003) Simultaneous assessment of wall motion and coronary flow velocity in the left anterior descending coronary artery during dipyridamole stress echocardiography. J Am Soc Echo 17:457–463

30. Lowenstein J, Tiano C, Marquez G, et al (2003) Simultaneous analysis of wall motion and coronary flow reserve of the left anterior descending coronary artery by transthoracic Doppler echocardiography during dipyridamole stress. J Am Soc Echo 17:735–744

31. Chirillo F, Bruni A, De Leo A, et al (2004) Usefulness of dipyridamole stress echocardiography for predicting graft patency after coronary artery bypass grafting. Am J Cardiol 93:24–30

32. Ascione L, De Michele M, Accadia M, et al (2006) Incremental diagnostic value of ultrasonographic assessment of coronary flow reserve with high-dose dipyridamole in patients with acute coronary syndrome. Int J Cardiol. 106:313–318

33. Lattanzi F, Picano E, Bolognese L, et al (1991) Inhibition of dipyridamole-induced ischemia by antianginal therapy in humans. Correlation with exercise electrocardiography. Circulation 83:1256–1262

34. Sicari R, Cortigiani L, Bigi R, et al; Echo-Persantine International Cooperative (EPIC) Study Group; Echo-Dobutamine International Cooperative (EDIC) Study Group (2004) Prognostic value of pharmacological stress echocardiography is affected by concomitant antiischemic therapy at the time of testing. Circulation 109:2428–2431

35. Voci P, Pizzuto F, Mariano E et al (2002) Measurement of coronary flow reserve in the anterior and posterior descending coronary arteries by transthoracic Doppler ultrasound. Am J Cardiol 90:988–991

36. Ueno Y, Nakamura Y, Takashima H et al (2002) Noninvasive assessment of coronary flow velocity and coronary flow velocity reserve in the right coronary artery by transthoracic Doppler echocardiography: comparison with intracoronary Doppler guidewire. J Am Soc Echocardiogr 15:1074–1079

37. Neglia D, Michelassi C, Trivieri MG, et al (2002) Prognostic role of myocardial blood flow impairment in idiopathic left ventricular dysfunction. Circulation 105:186–193

38. Cecchi F, Olivotto I, Gistri R et al (2003) Coronary microvascular dysfunction and prognosis in hypertrophic cardiomyopathy. N Engl J Med 349:1027–1035

39. Schächinger V, Britten M, Zeiher A (2000) Prognostic impact of coronary vasodilator dysfunction on adverse long-term outcome of coronary heart disease. Circulation 101:1899–1906

40. Albertal M, Voskuil M, Piek JJ, et al; The Doppler Endpoints Balloon Angioplasty Trial Europe (DEBATE) II Study Group (2002) Coronary flow velocity reserve after percutaneous interventions is predictive of periprocedural outcome. Circulation 105:1573–1578

41. Rigo F, Cortigiani L, Pasanisi E, et al (2006) The additional prognostic value of coronary flow reserve on left anterior descending artery in patients with negative stress echo by wall motion criteria. A Transthoracic Vasodilator Stress Echocardiography Study. Am Heart J 151:124–130

42. Rigo F, Sicari R, Gherardi S, et al (2008) The additive prognostic value of wall motion abnormalities and coronary flow reserve during dipyridamole stress echo. Eur Heart J 29:79–88

43. Rigo F, Sicari R, Gherardi S, et al (2007) Prognostic value of coronary flow reserve in medically treated patients with left anterior descending coronary disease with stenosis 51% to 75% in diameter. Am J Cardiol 100:1527–31

44. Meimoun P, Benali T, Elmkies F, et al (2008) Prognostic value of transthoracic coronary flow reserve in medically treated patients with proximal left anterior descending artery stenosis of intermediate severity. Eur J Echocardiogr 10:127–32

45. Cortigiani L, Bigi R, Sicari R, et al (2007) Comparison of prognostic value of pharmacologic stress echocardiography in chest pain patients with versus without diabetes mellitus and positive exercise electrocardiography. Am J Cardiol 100:1744–1749

46. Sicari R, Rigo F, Gherardi D, et al (2008) The prognostic value of Doppler echocardiographic-derived coronary flow reserve is not affected by concomitant antiischemic therapy at the time of testing. Am Heart J 155:1110–1117

47. Rigo F, Gherardi S, Galderisi M, et al (2006) The prognostic impact of coronary flow-reserve assessed by Doppler echocardiography in non-ischaemic dilated cardiomyopathy. Eur Heart J 27:1319–1323

48. Sicari R, Rigo F, Gherardi S et al (2008) Prognostic implications of coronary flow reserve on left anterior descending coronary artery in hypertrophic cardiomyopathy. Am J Cardiol 102:1634–1646

49. Tona F, Caforio AL, Montisci R, et al (2006) Coronary flow velocity pattern and coronary flow reserve by contrast-enhanced transthoracic echocardiography predict long-term outcome in heart transplantation. Circulation 114:I49–I55

50. De Bono DP, Samani NJ, Spyt TJ, et al (1992) Transcutaneous ultrasound measurements of blood flow in internal mammary artery to coronary artery graft. Lancet 339:379–381

51. Fusejima K, Takahara Y, Sudo Y, et al (1990) Comparison of coronary hemodynamics in patients with internal mammary artery and saphenous vein coronary artery bypass grafts: a noninvasive approach using combined two-dimensional and Doppler echocardiography. J Am Coll Cardiol 15:131–139

52. De Simone L, Caso P, Severino S, et al (1999) Noninvasive assessment of left and right internal mammary artery graft patency with high-frequency transthoracic echocardiography. J Am Soc Echocardiogr 12:841–849

53. Chirillo F, Bruni A, Balestra G, et al (2001) Assessment of internal mammary artery and saphenous vein graft patency and flow reserve using transthoracic Doppler echocardiography. Heart 86:424–431

54. Sicari R, Nihoyannopoulos P, Evangelista A, et al; European Association of Echocardiography (2009) Stress echocardiography expert consensus statement: European Association of Echocardiography (EAE) (a registered branch of the ESC). Eur J Echocardiogr 9:415–437

55. Shiina Y, Funabashi N, Lee K, et al (2007) Acute effect of oral flavonoid-rich dark chocolate intake on coronary circulation, as compared with non-flavonoid white chocolate, by transthoracic Doppler echocardiography in healthy adults. Int J Cardiol 131:424–9

56. Kiviniemi TO, Saraste A, Toikka JO, et al (2007) A moderate dose of red wine, but not de-alcoholized red wine increases coronary flow reserve. Atherosclerosis 195:e176–e181

57. Galderisi M, de Simone G, D'Errico A, et al (2008) Independent association of coronary flow reserve with left ventricular relaxation and filling pressure in arterial hypertension. Am J Hypertens 21:1060–6

58. Erdogan D, Yildirim I, Ciftci O, et al (2007) Effects of normal blood pressure, prehypertension, and hypertension on coronary microvascular function. Circulation 115:593–599

59. Kiviniemi TO, Saraste A, Toikka JO, et al (2008) Effects of cognac on coronary flow reserve and plasma antioxidant status in healthy young men. Cardiovasc Ultrasound 6:25

60. Galderisi M, Capaldo B, Sidiropulos M, et al (2007) Determinants of reduction of coronary flow reserve in patients with type 2 diabetes mellitus or arterial hypertension without angiographically determined epicardial coronary stenosis. Am J Hypertens 20:1283–1290

Technology and Training Requirements

10

Eugenio Picano

Stress echocardiography is relatively simple and widely available [1]. However, its easy access can become a problem in the clinical arena. Skill in interpretation cannot be acquired in a few days or weeks. With a handheld echocardiographic machine and an inexpensive drug or an ergometer, any sonographer can become a stress echocardiographer [2]. Ordering patterns might be distorted by financial incentives because the test can be performed in a physician's office. In the absence of a strict system of credentialing and quality control, we may soon experience a backlash of distrust regarding the technique [2]. Interpretation of stress echocardiography requires extensive experience in echocardiography and should be performed only by physicians with specific training in the technique [3, 4].

10.1
General Test Protocol

The patient lies in a decubitus position, the position required to achieve an optimal echocardiographic view. Electrocardiographic leads are placed at standard limb and precordial sites, slightly displacing (upward and downward) any leads that may interfere with the chosen acoustic window. A 12-lead electrocardiogram (ECG) is recorded in resting condition and each minute throughout the examination. An ECG lead is also continuously displayed on the echocardiography monitor to provide the operator with a reference for ST-segment changes and arrhythmias (Fig. 10.1). Cuff blood pressure is measured in resting condition and each minute thereafter with an automatic device. Echocardiographic monitoring is usually performed from the apical (both 4- and 2-chamber view) and parasternal (both long- and short-axis) approaches. In some cases the subxiphoidal view is employed. Images are recorded in resting condition from all views. The echocardiogram is continuously monitored and intermittently recorded. In the presence of obvious or suspected dyssynergy, a complete echocardiography examination is performed and recorded from all employed approaches to allow optimal

E. Picano, *Stress Echocardiography*,
© Springer-Verlag Berlin Heidelberg 2009

10

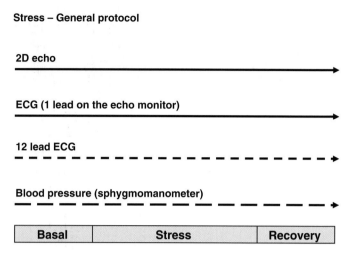

Stress – General protocol

2D echo

ECG (1 lead on the echo monitor)

12 lead ECG

Blood pressure (sphygmomanometer)

| Basal | Stress | Recovery |

Fig. 10.1 General protocol of stress echocardiography test

Table 10.1 Diagnostic end points of stress echocardiographic testing

Maximal dose/workload
Target heart rate
Obvious echocardiographic positivity
Severe chest pain
Obvious ECG changes (>2mm ST segment shift)

documentation of the presence and extent of myocardial ischemia. The same projections are obtained and recorded in the recovery phase, after cessation of the stress (exercise or pacing) or administration of the antidote (aminophylline for dipyridamole, beta-blockers for dobutamine). The segmental function can be evaluated by means of a triple comparison: stress vs. resting state; stress vs. recovery phase; and at peak stress, with the neighboring normally contracting segments. A clear standardization of the procedures allows the workplan to be optimized, thus improving the overall quality of diagnostic performance in the stress echocardiography laboratory. The nurse explains the procedure and the aims of testing to the patient, marks the acoustic approaches, and, in the case of pharmacological stresses, prepares the doses of drugs, including the antidote. A 12-lead ECG is recorded, and blood pressure is measured. After placement of the intravenous line (in the case of pharmacological stress) the sonographer records the resting echocardiogram and the stress starts. Throughout the study, the nurse keeps a written protocol of the study (clinical events, drugs injected, ECG and echocardiographic changes noted by the physician), infuses drugs or varies the workload, measures blood pressure, and evaluates the 12-lead ECG each minute. Diagnostic and nondiagnostic end points of stress echocardiography testing are reported in Tables 10.1 and 10.2, respectively.

Table 10.2 Submaximal nondiagnostic end points of stress echocardiography testing

Intolerance symptoms
Limiting asymptomatic side effects:
Hypertension: SAP>220mmHg; DAP>120mmHg
Hypotension (relative or absolute): >30mmHg drop in blood pressure
Supraventricular arrhythmias: supraventricular tachycardia, atrial fibrillation
Ventricular arrhythmias: ventricular tachycardia, frequent and polymorphic
premature ventricular beats

SAP, systolic arterial pressure; DAP, diastolic arterial pressure.

10.2
Imaging Equipment and Techniques

Digital acquisition of images has evolved from the days of stand-alone computers that digitized analog video signals, to the current era in which ultrasound systems have direct digital output [5]. By digitizing two-dimensional echocardiographic images, it is possible to put a single cardiac cycle into a continuous loop so that the cycle can be viewed whenever necessary for an indefinite period of time. This technique carries valuable advantages, especially for exercise echocardiography. Even in the exercising individual who is breathing rapidly and deeply, one can still see a technically good cardiac cycle between inspirations; therefore it reduces the respiratory artifact. Another advantage of using the computer to record the two-dimensional echocardiogram digitally is that it is possible to place the resting and stress cardiac cycles side-by-side in a split-screen or quad-screen format. This reduces the time and difficulty of analyzing the examination and may also simplify the recognition of subtle changes in wall motion. Although there is no evidence showing that it improves diagnostic accuracy when compared with videotape reading [6, 7], digital acquisition certainly makes storage, retrieval, analysis, and communication of stress echocardiography data faster and easier. Videotape recordings are recommended as a back-up.

Tissue harmonic imaging improves image quality over conventional imaging. This is obtained mainly through the elimination of ultrasound artifacts (namely the side-lobe, near-field, and reverberation artifacts) with consequent increase in lateral resolution and signal-to-noise ratio. The increased image quality is mirrored in a better visualization of the left ventricular endocardium and epicardium, and this has a favorable impact on evaluation of both global and regional left ventricular function at rest.

In the setting of stress echocardiography, tissue harmonic imaging reduces the number of uninterpretable segments, deflates observer variability, and increases diagnostic accuracy [8, 9]. The increase in interpretable myocardium is particularly valuable for the apical, lateral, and anterior wall segments (Fig. 10.2) imaged in the apical views at higher heart rates. Tissue harmonic imaging should be used for stress echocardiography imaging [3, 4]. When used in conjunction with harmonic imaging, contrast agents increase the number of interpretable left ventricular wall segments, enhance diagnostic confidence, and reduce the need for additional noninvasive tests due to equivocal noncontrast stress examination [10]. Contrast agents should be used when two or more segments are not well visualized [11].

10

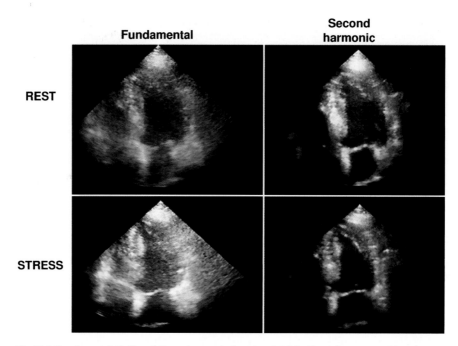

Fig. 10.2 Fundamental (*left*) and tissue harmonic imaging (*right*) of rest (*upper panels*) and stress (*lower panels*) end-systolic still frames of an apical four-chamber view. Basal and apical segments of the lateral wall are more sharply delineated with tissue harmonic imaging mode. (From [10])

10.3
Training Requirements

It is not reasonable to begin using stress echocardiography without thorough training in transthoracic echocardiography (level 2, American Society of Echocardiography). The basic skills required for imaging the heart under resting conditions are not substantially different from those required for imaging the same heart from the same projections during stress. Furthermore, the echocardiographic signs of ischemia are basically the same as those during myocardial infarction. In both cases, the assessment is based on a comparison between the "suspected" zone and the neighboring normal regions; in induced ischemia, however, the operator can use the suspected region as its own control, considering both resting conditions and the recovery phase. The use of stresses is associated with the possibility of life-threatening complications, both ischemia-related and ischemia-independent. Therefore, as happens with a simple exercise test, the cardiologist–sonographer (and the attendant nurse) should be certified in Basic and Advanced Life Support, as also required by the American Heart Association guidelines for stress testing [12].

The diagnostic accuracy of an experienced echocardiographer who is an absolute beginner in stress echocardiography is more or less equivalent to that achieved by tossing a coin (Fig. 10.3). However, 100 stress echocardiography studies are sufficient to build the individual learning curve and reach the plateau of diagnostic accuracy [13]. With Doppler,

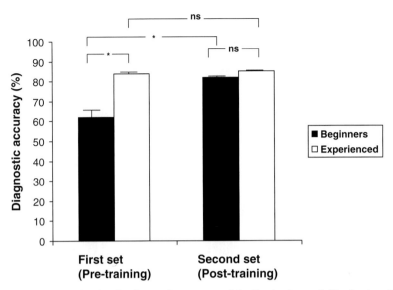

Fig. 10.3 Histograms showing the diagnostic accuracy of the five beginners (*white bars*) and five experts (*black bars*) who reviewed two sets of 50 videotapes before and after a 6-month training period (100 stress echocardiography studies with a supervisor); *$p< 0.001$. (From [2])

it is wise to assess one's own learning curve in cases where a recent catheterization provides a standard against which the presence and severity of regurgitation and gradients can be estimated; instead, with stress echocardiography it is wise to test one's initial performance in patients who have recently undergone coronary angiography, and possibly with other imaging techniques using the same stress.

After 15–30 days of exposure to a high-volume stress echocardiography laboratory, the physician should begin to accumulate his or her own experience with a stepwise approach, starting from more innocuous and simple stresses such as low-level supine exercise echocardiography and moving up to more technically demanding ones.

The interpretation of stress echocardiography is necessarily qualitative and subjective. In our laboratory, the cardiologist–echocardiographer performing the test evaluates the study on-line. Rarely is a "blind" reading by two independent observers made for diagnostic or clinical purposes. Quantitative analysis of regional wall motion is never performed for purely diagnostic reasons; quantitative methods are time consuming, require extra equipment and images of better quality than those interpretable with a qualitative assessment, and they certainly do not clarify uncertain readings; they simply measure and make the obvious "certain" without reducing the number of questionable studies. Diagnostic accuracy is not increased by quantitative methods, since the human eye naturally integrates space and time, and its discriminatory power is very difficult to equal and virtually impossible to surpass. It is also true, however, that different individuals have different eyes, and the degree of interinstitutional variability tested on identical images can be substantial, even among laboratories of unquestionable reputation (Fig. 10.4) [14]. Diagnostic accuracy is not only a function of experience; for a given diagnostic accuracy every observer

10

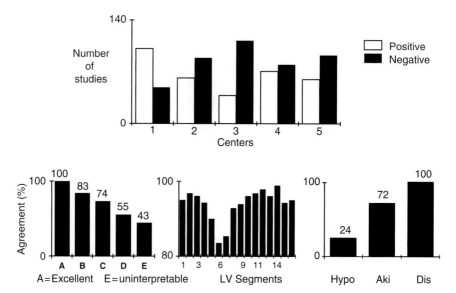

Fig. 10.4 Histogram showing interinstitutional variability in the reading of 150 dobutamine stress echocardiograms from five different centers with longstanding experience in stress echocardiography (Aachen, Cleveland, Essen, Pisa, Rotterdam). Positivity reading ranges from 102 of 150 (center 1) to 32 of 150 (center 3). Obviously, center 1 will have an outstanding sensitivity and poor specificity, whereas center 3, on the very same images, will have a low sensitivity and an outstanding specificity. Probably, both are right. Diagnostic accuracy compared with angiographically assessed coronary artery disease will be higher for center 1 in a population with a high prevalence of disease, and higher for center 3 in a population with a low prevalence of disease. This stunning interinstitutional reading variability is not without method, however. In the *bottom panel* the factors modulating variability are shown: image quality (*left*), location of the wall motion abnormality (*middle*), and severity of dysfunction (*right*). Variability is substantially higher for poor-quality images (*left*), for tricky segments such as the posterobasal segment or basal inferior septum (numbers *6* and *7* in *middle panel*), which may be "physiologically hypokinetic" even at baseline, and for a mild degree of dysfunction such as hypokinesia (*right*)

has his/her own sensitivity–specificity curve: there are "over-readers" (high sensitivity, low specificity) and "under-readers" (low sensitivity; high specificity), depending on whether images are aggressively or conservatively interpreted as abnormal. Many studies yield unquestionably negative or positive findings; still, there is a "gray zone" of interpretable tests in which the visualization of some regions can be suboptimal and the cardiologist's level of experience in interpreting the test is critical for a correct reading.

Interobserver variability is certainly a common problem in medicine, and in cardiology variability can be substantial with almost all diagnostic methods, including resting electrocardiography [15], exercise electrocardiography [16], perfusion scintigraphy [17], and coronary angiography [18]. For thallium perfusion images, the interobserver agreement for a majority of observers was found to be 75% for an abnormal and 68% for a normal interpretation [19]. In only 65% of coronary angiograms did all four experienced coronary angiographers (from the same institution) agree on the significance of a stenosis, defined as 50% narrowing of lumen diameter [18]. However, a perception of the diffuse nature of the problem does not reduce interobserver variability in stress echocardiography. There are several ways to minimize this variability, representing the key factor which may ultimately determine the real impact of stress echocardiography in modern cardiology. Again, experience with nuclear medicine has taught us that agreement can be doubled by moving from an interpretation without standardization to an interpretation with standardization of display and quantification [19]. Similarly, there are many precautions that may minimize variability, providing not only high accuracy but also better reproducibility.

These parameters are related to the physician interpreting the study, the technology used, the stress employed, and the patient under study (Table 10.3). Variability will be substantially reduced if one agrees in advance not to consider minor degrees of hypokinesia, since mild hypokinesia is a normal variant under most stresses and there is a wide overlap between normal and diseased populations [20, 21]. Also, the inclusion of isolated asynergy of posterobasal or basoinferoseptal segments among positivity criteria will inflate variability. Obviously, the inclusion of patients with resting images of borderline quality, or the use of stresses degrading image quality, will also dilate variability, which is closely linked to the quality of the images. The single most important factor deflating variability is dedicated training in a large-volume stress echocardiography laboratory with exposure to joint reading [22] and "a priori" development of standardized [23] and conservative [24] reading criteria (Fig. 10.5).

Table 10.3 Stress echocardiography and the human factor

	Increases variability	Reduces variability
Physician related:		
1. Previous training in stress echocardiography	No	Yes
2. Exposure to joint reading	No	Yes
3. Development of "a priori" reading criteria	No	Yes
4. Basal inferior septum	Yes	No
5. Positivity for "lack of hyperkinesis"	Yes	No
6. Positivity for "severe hypokinesis"	No	Yes
Technology related:		
7. Videotape instead of digital	Yes	No
8. Native tissue harmonic	No	Yes
Stress related:		
9. Use of stressor polluting image quality	Yes	No
Patient related:		
10. Resting images of borderline quality	Yes	No

10

VARIABILITY

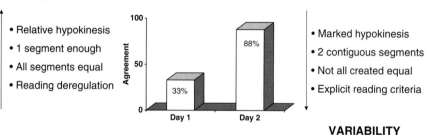

- Relative hypokinesis
- 1 segment enough
- All segments equal
- Reading deregulation

- Marked hypokinesis
- 2 contiguous segments
- Not all created equal
- Explicit reading criteria

VARIABILITY

Fig. 10.5 Madness and method in stress echocardiography reading. The wild variety of reading occurs when there is no a priori agreement in reading criteria. With strict characterization of conservative reading criteria (ignore mild hypokinesia, ignore relative hypokinesia, ignore isolated inferolateral hypokinesia, etc.) and a limited experience in joint reading, interobserver agreement rises spectacularly (*right panel*)

10.4
The Most Frequent Mistakes

The checklist for starting and keeping alive a stress echocardiography activity is reported in Table 10.4 (training requirements recommended by the American Society of Echocardiography) and in Table 10.5 (equally important cultural requirements suggested by the Task Force of the American College of Cardiology/American Heart Association) [12, 25]. However, regardless of the number of stress echocardiography studies performed and intensity of training, some readers still do not reach a satisfactory degree of accuracy [24]. This is true with all activities involving development of cognitive skills. The five most frequent mistakes in stress echocardiography training can be summarized as follows:

1. *Self-made stress echocardiography:* it is far better to perform and/or review 100 stress echocardiography studies with an expert supervisor than 1,000 stress echocardiography studies done all by yourself without a diagnostic reference standard (Fig. 10.5).
2. *Starting your learning curve at university level:* posttreadmill exercise is the most familiar stress for the cardiologist and the patient, but by far the most technically demanding. The best "technology" available today to improve image quality, diagnostic accuracy, and interobserver reproducibility is to use semisupine exercise as a physical stress and a vasodilator as a pharmacological stress.
3. *Underestimating ischemic risk:* the technicalities of pharmacological stress echocardiography can be surprisingly simple, but one has to know how to treat ischemia and its unforeseeable and potentially catastrophic complications. A stress echocardiography laboratory run by technicians and sonographers without an attending experienced cardiologist can be a deadly trap for the patient. For instance, the early stop of a pharmacological stress for a very initial asynergy developed after very low dose of a drug (dipyridamole or dobutamine) can make the difference between a patient's life and

Table 10.4 Summary of recommendations for training in stress echocardiography

	Fellows in training	Postfellowship training	Maintenance of skills
Qualifications for training	• Level 2 training + ability to interpret resting wall motion	• Level 2 training or equivalent • Current active practice of echocardiography*	Not applicable
Conditions for training	• Laboratory performing 40 stress echocardiography studies per month • Supervisor with level 3 training and experience with more than 200 stress echocardiography studies	• Laboratory performing 40 stress echocardiography studies per month • Supervisor with level 3 training and experience with more than 200 stress echocardiography studies	Not applicable
Number of cases recommended	• Participation in performance of at least 50 exercise echocardiography and/or pharmacologic stress echocardiography studies • Interpretation of at least 100 stress echocardiography studies with supervision as above	• Participation in performance of at least 50 exercise echocardiography and/or pharmacologic stress echocardiography studies • Interpretation of at least 100 stress echocardiography studies with supervision as above	Interpretation of 15 stress echocardiography studies per month

Table 10.5 Additive skills necessary to perform, interpret, and report pharmacological stress echocardiography

1. Knowledge of advantages and disadvantages of the different agents
2. Knowledge of the pharmacokinetics and the physiological response to the different agents
3. Knowledge of the contraindications to the different agents
4. Knowledge of the side effects and complications of the different agents and how to manage them
5. Competence in cardiopulmonary resuscitation
6. Knowledge of the end points of pharmacological stress and indications for termination the test

death. Not all patients were created equal during stress, and a fixed, inflexible approach can be dangerous. Similarly, the recognition of a vasospastic mechanism after adenosine or dobutamine completely changes the therapeutic approach: beta-blockers are the therapy of choice for antidote-resistant ischemia, and the ischemia trigger in vasospasm.

4. *Skills in resting echocardiography are not enough:* pediatric, transesophageal, transthoracic, and vascular echocardiography speak a different ultrasound idiom than does stress echocardiography. You have to learn stress echocardiography during dedicated training, or your experience will be disappointing and your results inconsistent.

5. *Technology without cardiology:* it is better to have the best eyes with a suboptimal technology than the worst eyes with the best technology. Usually, there is economic interest

in selling technology, not in improving culture. Unfortunately, to date no method for
quantitative analysis has increased the clinical impact of stress echocardiography. In the
future quantitative methods may serve as an adjunct to expert visual assessment of wall
motion. The widespread use of quantitative methods will require further validation and
simplification of analysis techniques [3, 4]. Stress echocardiography – and in particular
pharmacological stress echocardiography – requires a tight integration of echocardiographic knowledge and cardiological experience. If this happens, clinical rewards will
be outstanding, and stress echocardiography is now an integral part of the core curricu-
lum of the clinical cardiologist according to the European Society of Cardiology.

References

1. Picano E (1992) Stress echocardiography: from pathophysiological toy to diagnostic tool.
   Point of view. Circulation 85:1604–1612
2. Picano E (2003) Stress echocardiography: a historical perspective. Special article. Am J Med
   114:126–130
3. Pellikka PA, Nagueh SF, Elhendy AA, et al; American Society of Echocardiography (2007)
   American Society of Echocardiography recommendations for performance, interpretation,
   and application of stress echocardiography. J Am Soc Echocardiogr 20:1021–1024
4. Sicari R, Nihoyannopoulos P, Evangelista A, et al; European Association of Echocardiography
   (2008) Stress echocardiography expert consensus statement: European Association of
   Echocardiography (EAE) (a registered branch of the ESC). Eur J Echocardiogr. 9:415–437
5. Feigenbaum H (1988) Digital recording, display, and storage of echocardiograms. J Am Soc
   Echocardiogr 1:378–383
6. Castini D, Gentile F, Ornaghi M, Montani E, Lippolis A, Mangiarotti E, Esposti D, Cirino D,
   Maggi GC (1995) Dobutamine echocardiography: usefulness of digital image processing. Eur
   Heart J 16:1420–1424
7. Attenhofer CH, Pellikka PA, Oh JK, et al (1997) Is review of videotape necessary after review
   of digitized cine-loop images in stress echocardiography? A prospective study in 306 patients.
   J Am Soc Echocardiogr 10:179–184
8. Rodriguez O, Varga A, Dal Porto R, et al (1999) The impact of second harmonic imaging on
   stress echocardiography reading. Cardiologia 44:451–454
9. Franke A, Hoffmann R, Kuhl HP, et al (2000) Non-contrast second harmonic imaging improves
   interobserver agreement and accuracy of dobutamine stress echocardiography in patients with
   impaired image quality. Heart 83:133–140
10. Thanigaraj S, Nease RF Jr, Schechtman KB, et al (2001) Use of contrast for image enhance-
    ment during stress echocardiography is cost-effective and reduces additional diagnostic test-
    ing. Am J Cardiol 287:1430–1432
11. Douglas PS, Khandheria B, Stainback RF, et al; American College of Cardiology Foundation;
    American Society of Echocardiography; American College of Emergency Physicians; Ameri-
    can Heart Association; American Society of Nuclear Cardiology; Society for Cardiovascular
    Angiography and Interventions; Society of Cardiovascular Computed Tomography; Society
    for Cardiovascular Magnetic Resonance. (2008) ACCF/ASE/ACEP/AHA/ASNC/SCAI/
    SCCT/SCMR 2008 appropriateness criteria for stress echocardiography: a report of the
    American College of Cardiology Foundation Appropriateness Criteria Task Force, American
    Society of Echocardiography, American College of Emergency Physicians, American Heart
    Association, American Society of Nuclear Cardiology, Society for Cardiovascular Angiog-

raphy and Interventions, Society of Cardiovascular Computed Tomography, and Society for Cardiovascular Magnetic Resonance endorsed by the Heart Rhythm Society and the Society of Critical Care Medicine. J Am Coll Cardiol 51:1127–1147

12. Popp R, Agatston A, Armstrong W, et al (1998) Recommendations for training in performance and interpretation of stress echocardiography. Committee on Physician Training and Education of the American Society of Echocardiography. J Am Soc Echocardiogr 11:95–96

13. Picano E, Lattanzi F, Orlandini A, et al (1991) Stress echocardiography and the human factor: the importance of being expert. J Am Coll Cardiol 17:666–669

14. Hoffmann R, Lethen H, Marwick T, et al (1996) Analysis of interinstitutional observer agreement in interpretation of dobutamine stress echocardiograms. J Am Coll Cardiol 27:330–336

15. Segall HN (1960) The electrocardiogram and its interpretation: a study of reports by 20 physicians on a set of 100 electrocardiograms. Can Med Assoc 82:2–6

16. Blackburn H (1968) The exercise electrocardiogram: differences in interpretation. Am J Cardiol 21:871–880

17. Altwood JE, Jensen D, Froelicher V et al. (1981) Agreement in human interpretation of analog thallium myocardial perfusion images. Circulation 64:601–609

18. Zir LM, Miller SW, Dinsmore RE, et al (1976) Interobserver variability in coronary angiography. Circulation 53:627–632

19. Wackers FJT, Bodenheimer M, Fleiss JL, et al (1993) Factors affecting uniformity in interpretation of planar thallium-201 imaging in a multicenter trial. J Am Coll Cardiol 21:1064–1074

20. Borges AC, Pingitore A, Cordovil A, et al (1995) Heterogeneity of left ventricular regional wall thickening following dobutamine infusion in normal human subjects. Eur Heart J 16:1726–1730

21. Carstensen S, Ali SM, Stensgaard-Hansen FV, et al (1995) Dobutamine-atropine stress echocardiography in asymptomatic healthy individuals. The relativity of stress-induced hyperkinesia. Circulation 92:3453–3463

22. Varga A, Picano E, Dodi C, et al (1999) Madness and method in stress echo reading. Eur Heart J 20:1271–1275

23. Hoffmann R, Lethen H, Marwick T, et al (1998) Standardized guidelines for the interpretation of dobutamine echocardiography reduce interinstitutional variance in interpretation. Am J Cardiol 82:1520–1524

24. Imran M, Palinkas A, Pasanisi E, et al (2002) Optimal reading criteria in stress echocardiography. Am J Cardiol 90:444

25. Rodgers GP, Ayanian JZ, Balady G, et al (2000) American College of Cardiology/American Heart Association Clinical Competence statement on stress testing: a report of the American College of Cardiology/American Heart Association/American College of Physicians–American Society of Internal Medicine Task Force on Clinical Competence. J Am Coll Cardiol 36:1441–1453

Section 2

Stresses: How, When and Why

Exercise Echocardiography

11

Luc A. Piérard and Eugenio Picano

11.1
Historical Background

Many tests have been proposed in combination with echocardiography, but only a few have a role in clinical practice. For the diagnosis of organic coronary artery disease, exercise remains the paradigm of all stress tests and the first which was combined with stress echocardiography. In the early 1970s, *M*-mode recordings of the left ventricle were used in normal subjects [1] and in patients with coronary artery disease [2]. Subsequently, two-dimensional (2D) echocardiography was used to document ischemic regional wall motion abnormality during exercise [3]. The technique was at that time so challenging [4], that with the introduction of dipyridamole [5] and dobutamine [6] as pharmacological stressors many laboratories used pharmacological stress even in patients who were able to exercise. Large-scale, multicenter, effectiveness studies providing outcome data are in fact available only with pharmacological [7, 8] not with exercise echocardiography, offering a more robust evidence-based platform for their use in clinical practice. Exercise echocardiography was only really applied as a clinical tool in the early 1990s [4] and it is now increasingly used for the diagnosis of coronary artery disease, the functional assessment of intermediate stenosis, and risk stratification. A series of successive improvements led to a progressively widespread acceptance: digital echocardiographic techniques, allowing capture and synchronized display of the same view at different stages [9], improved endocardial border detection by harmonic imaging [10], and ultrasound contrast agents that opacify the left ventricle [11] (Fig. 11.1). In the USA, most laboratories use the posttreadmill approach with imaging at rest and as soon as possible during the recovery period [12, 13]. In Europe, a number of centers have implemented their stress echocardiography laboratory with a dedicated bed or table allowing bicycle exercise in a semisupine position and real-time continuous imaging throughout exercise [14, 15]. The diffusion of semisupine exercise

E. Picano, *Stress Echocardiography*,
© Springer-Verlag Berlin Heidelberg 2009

11

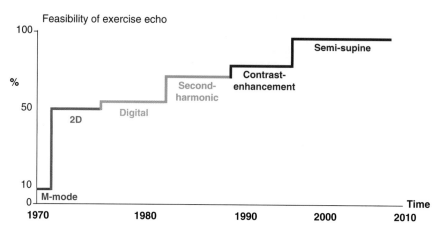

Fig. 11.1 The timeline of innovation in exercise echocardiography. The progressive increase in feasibility was linked to minor (digital acquisition) and major (2D, second-harmonic, contrast enhancement for border detection) technical improvements. Interestingly, the most important methodological improvement, i.e., the shift from posttreadmill to semisupine bicycle stress, is the most obvious, already clearly documented in the mid-1980s, and is still remarkably absent from US practice and the latest recommendations

imaging – much more user-friendly for the sonographer than the treadmill test – made image acquisition easier and interpretation faster [16–18]. Semisupine exercise gained its well-deserved role in the stress echocardiography laboratory for coronary artery disease diagnosis and, with growing frequency outside coronary artery disease, in the assessment of pulmonary hypertension, valve disease, cardiomyopathy, and heart failure [19, 20].

11.2
Pathophysiology

Exercise protocols are variable and include treadmill as well as upright and supine bicycle ergometry. All these forms of stress increase myocardial oxygen consumption and induce ischemia in the presence of a fixed reduction in coronary flow reserve [21] (Fig. 11.2). Of the determinants of myocardial oxygen demand, heart rate increases two- to three-fold, contractility three- to fourfold, and systolic blood pressure by 50% (Fig. 11.2) [21]. End-diastolic volume initially increases to sustain the increase in stroke volume through the Frank–Starling mechanism, and later falls at high heart rates (Fig. 11.3). Coronary blood flow increases three- to fourfold in normal subjects, but the reduction in diastolic time (much greater than shortening in systolic time) limits mostly the perfusion in the subendocardial layer – whose perfusion is mainly diastolic, whereas the perfusion in the subepicardial layer is also systolic [22]. In the presence of a reduction in coronary flow reserve, the regional myocardial oxygen demand and supply mismatch determines myocardial ischemia and regional dysfunction. When exercise is terminated, myocardial oxygen demand gradually declines, although the time course of resolution of the wall

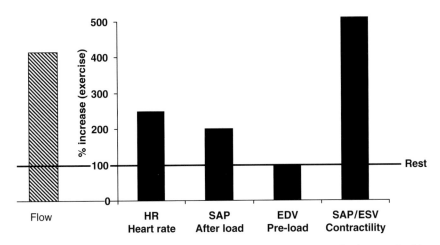

Fig. 11.2 The increase of main determinants of myocardial oxygen consumption in normal subjects referred for semi-supine exercise stress echo. Panel A: Heart rate (HR) increases two to threefold, the systolic arterial pressure (SAP) increases 1.5 to 2.5 fold, end-diastolic volume (EDV) 1.2 fold, and myocardial contractility (the most important determinant of myocardial oxygen consumption, measured as variation in elastance, i.e., the increase in end-systolic pressure divided for end-systolic volume) increases 4 to 8 fold versus baseline

motion abnormality is quite variable [23]. Some induced abnormalities may persist for several minutes, permitting their detection on postexercise imaging. However, wall motion usually recovers very rapidly, and postexercise imaging can easily miss wall motion abnormalities. Regional and global function, although closely linked, may behave differently during stress. For example, if a small wall motion abnormality develops as a result of limited ischemia, the remainder of the left ventricle may become hyperdynamic, and the ejection fraction will increase despite the presence of an ischemic wall motion abnormality. In such a case, a regional abnormality will be present in the absence of global dysfunction. Alternatively, severe exercise-induced hypertension in the absence of coronary artery disease may lead to an abnormal ejection fraction response without an associated wall motion abnormality. There are distinct advantages and disadvantages to exercise versus pharmacological stress, which are outlined in Table 11.1. The most important advantages of exercise are that it is a stress familiar to both patient and doctor; it adds echocardiography information on top of well-established and validated electro-cardiographic and hemodynamic information, and it is probably the safest stress procedure. The disadvantages are the limited ability to perform physical exercise in many individuals, who are either generally deconditioned or physically impeded by neurologic or orthopedic limitations. In addition, stress echocardiography during physical exercise is certainly more technically demanding than pharmacologic stress because of its greater difficulty and tighter time pressure [23].

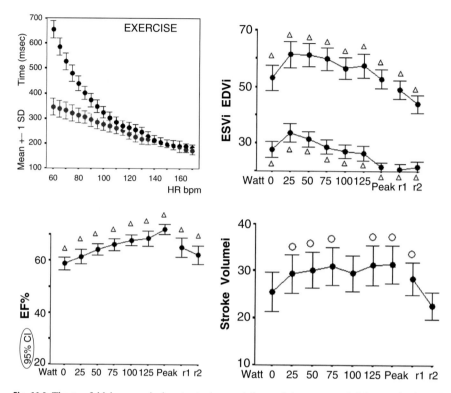

Fig. 11.3 The twofold increase in heart rate (*upper left panel*) is accompanied by a reduction of diastolic time, critical for subendocardial perfusion. The shortening of cardiological diastole is much more pronounced than shortening of cardiological systole, but the former is much more critical for subendocardial perfusion, even in the absence of coronary artery disease. (From [22])

Table 11.1 Exercise versus pharmacological stress

Parameter	Exercise	Pharmacological
Intravenous line required	No	Yes
Diagnostic utility of heart rate and blood pressure response	Yes	No
Use in deconditioned patients	No	Yes
Use in physically limited patients	No	Yes
Level of echocardiography imaging difficulty	High	Low
Safety profile	High	Moderate
Clinical role in valvular disease	Yes	No
Clinical role in pulmonary hypertension	Yes	No
Fatigue and dyspnea evaluation	Yes	No

11.3
Exercise Techniques

As a general rule, any patient capable of physical exercise should be tested with an exercise modality, as this preserves the integrity of the electrocardiogram (ECG) response and provides valuable information regarding functional status. Performing echocardiography at the time of physical stress also allows links to be drawn among symptoms, cardiovascular workload, and wall motion abnormalities. Exercise echocardiography can be performed using either a treadmill or bicycle protocol (Table 11.2). When treadmill exercise is performed, scanning during exercise is not feasible, and therefore most protocols rely on postexercise imaging [13]. It is imperative to complete postexercise imaging as soon as possible. To accomplish this, the patient is moved immediately from the treadmill to an imaging table and placed in the left lateral decubitus position so that imaging may be completed within 1–2 min. This technique assumes that regional wall motion abnormalities will persist long enough to be detected in the recovery phase. When abnormalities recover rapidly, false-negative results occur. The advantages of treadmill exercise echocardiography are the widespread availability of the treadmill system and the wealth of clinical experience that has accumulated with this form of stress testing. Information on exercise capacity, heart rate response, rhythm, and blood pressure changes are analyzed and, together with wall motion analysis, becomes part of the final interpretation. Bicycle exercise echocardiography is done with the patient either upright or recumbent (Fig. 11.4). The patient pedals against an increasing workload at a constant cadence (usually 60 rpm). The workload is escalated in a stepwise fashion while imaging is performed. Successful bicycle stress testing requires the patient's cooperation (to maintain the correct cadence) and coordination (to perform the pedaling action). The most important advantage of bicycle exercise is the chance to obtain images during the various levels of exercise (rather than relying on postexercise imaging). With the patient in the supine posture, it is relatively easy to record images from multiple views during graded exercise. With the development

Table 11.2 Exercise methods

Parameter	Treadmill	Upright bicycle	Supine bicycle
Ease of study for patients	Moderate	High	High
Ease of study for sonographer	Low	Moderate	High
Stage of onset of ischemia	No	Yes	Yes
Peak rate pressure product	High	High	High
Systolic blood pressure	Lower	Higher	Higher
Heart rate	Higher	Lower	Lower
Induction of coronary spasm	Higher	Lower	Lower
Preload increase	Lower	Lower	Higher
Ischemic strength	++ (+)	++ (+)	+++
Preferred modality in	USA	Europe	Echocardiography laboratory

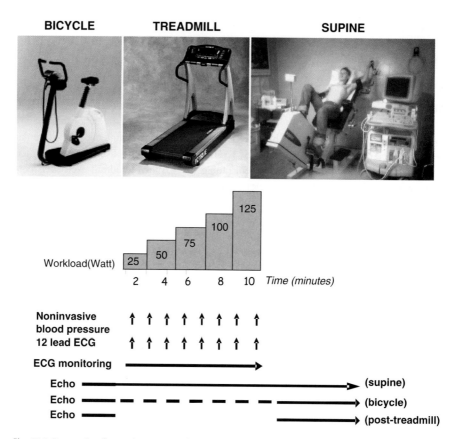

Fig. 11.4 Protocols of exercise stress echocardiography: upright bicycle (*left*); treadmill (*middle*); semisupine bicycle (*right*). Postexercise imaging is performed with treadmill only; at peak and postexercise with upright; and during, at peak, and after exercise with semisupine

of ergometers that permit leftward tilting of the patient, the ease of image acquisition has been further improved. In the upright posture, imaging is generally limited to either apical or subcostal views. By leaning the patient forward over the handlebars and extending the arms, apical images can be obtained in the majority of cases. To record subcostal views, a more lordotic position is necessary and care must be taken to avoid foreshortening of the apex. When considering the various forms of exercise, it is important to appreciate certain fundamental differences. For most patients, both duration of exercise and maximum achieved heart rate are slightly lower in the supine position [24, 25], due primarily to the development of leg fatigue at an earlier stage of exercise. The limitation is overcome in part by the occurrence of ischemia at a lower workload with supine exercise. The earlier development of ischemia is the result of both a higher end-diastolic volume and higher mean arterial blood pressure for a given level of stress in the supine position [25, 26]. These differences contribute to a higher wall stress and an associated increase in myocardial oxygen demand compared with an upright bicycle. Coronary spasms are provoked more frequently during treadmill than during bicycle exercise [27].

11.4 Safety and Feasibility

The safety of exercise stress is witnessed by decades of experience with ECG testing and stress imaging [28]. Also in exercise echocardiography registries collecting over 85,000 studies (25,000 in the international and 60,000 in the German registry), exercise echocardiography was the safest stress echocardiography test [29, 30]. Death occurs on average in 1 in 10,000 tests, according to the American Heart Association statements on exercise testing based on a review of more than 1,000 studies on millions of patients [28]. Major life-threatening effects (including myocardial infarction, ventricular fibrillation, sustained ventricular tachycardia, stroke) were reported in about 1 in 6,000 patients with exercise in the international stress echocardiography registry – fivefold less than with dipyridamole echocardiography, and tenfold less than with dobutamine echocardiography (Fig. 11.5). Although it is possible that patients referred for pharmacological stress are in general "sicker" than patients without contraindication to exercise, the available evidence suggests that while stress echocardiography is a safe method in the real world, exercise is safer than pharmacological stress [29], and dipyridamole [30] safer than dobutamine [31]. These conclusions are also in agreement with the preliminary results of the German Stress Echocardiography Registry, published only in abstract form, which recruited more than

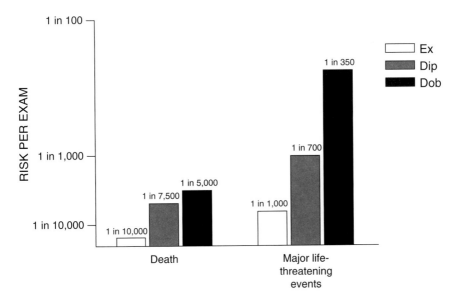

Fig. 11.5 Safety of stress echocardiography: highest for exercise, intermediate for dipyridamole, lowest for dobutamine stress. (Original data from [29–32], summarized in [15])

60,000 tests and reported a rate of complication of 0.6% with exercise, 3.6% with dobutamine, and 1.5% with dipyridamole [32].

The feasibility of obtaining interpretable studies of good quality – relatively unchanged versus baseline images – is sufficient with posttreadmill, good for upright, and almost excellent with semisupine testing which should be the test of choice for exercise stress echocardiography. From the perspective of the stress echocardiography laboratory, there is little question that semisupine exercise is easier, more feasible, and more informative than other forms of exercise stress. It is also undisputed that even semisupine exercise is more technically demanding than dobutamine and much more technically demanding than vasodilator stress.

11.5
Diagnostic Results for Detection of Coronary Artery Disease and Myocardial Viability

For the detection of angiographically significant coronary disease repeatedly assessed in a series of continuously updated meta-analyses [33–37], the overall sensitivity and specificity of exercise echocardiography has been reported to be 83 and 85%, respectively, according to the most updated meta-analysis of 55 studies with 3,714 patients (Table 11.3) [33–37]. The specificity of exercise echocardiography is similar to dobutamine echocardiography, lower than dipyridamole echocardiography, and higher for all forms of stress echocardiography compared to stress single-photon emission computed tomography (SPECT) [37]. The diagnostic accuracy is similar to other forms of stress imaging (dobutamine or dipyridamole stress echocardiography or stress SPECT) (Fig. 11.6). Although the available

Table 11.3 Sensitivity and specificity of exercise echocardiography (*echo*) according to meta-analysis of 55 studies with 3,714 patients (adapted from [37])

Test	No. of studies	Sensitivity % (95% CI)	Specificity % (95% CI)	lnDOR (95% CI)
Exercise echo	55	82.7 (80.2–85.2)	84.0 (80.4–87.6)[a]	3.0 (2.7–3.3)
Adenosine echo	11	79.2 (72.1–86.3)	91.5 (87.3–95.7)	3.0 (2.5–3.5)
Dipyridamole echo	58	71.9 (68.6–75.2)	94.6 (92.9–96.3)[a]	3.0 (2.8–3.2)
State of the art dipyridamole echo	5	81 (79–83)	91 (88–94)	3.1 (1.9–3.3)
Dobutamine echo	102	81.0 (79.1–82.9)	84.1 (82.0–86.1)[a]	2.9 (2.7–3.0)
Combined echo	226	79.1 (77.6–80.5)	87.1 (85.7–88.5)[a]	2.9 (2.8–3.0)
Combined SPECT	103	88.1 (86.6–89.6)[b]	73.0 (69.1–76.9)	2.8 (2.6–3.0)

CI confidence interval, *lnDOR* natural logarithm of the diagnostic odds ratio

[a] Nonoverlapping confidence intervals indicating a statistically higher specificity than the corresponding SPECT test

[b] Nonoverlapping confidence intervals indicating a statistically higher sensitivity than all other tests, except for adenosine and dipyridamole SPECT and a statistically lower specificity than all other tests except for exercise SPECT

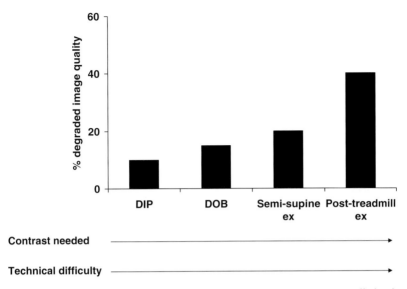

Fig. 11.6 The technical echocardiographic difficulty of different stresses. Factors polluting image quality are more frequent with posttreadmill, and least frequent with pharmacological stresses

information is only limited, exercise echocardiography can also be useful for detecting myocardial viability. Endogenous catecholamines produced during a low-level exercise test can also serve as a myocardial stressor to elicit contractile reserve in viable myocardium, with an accuracy comparable to low-dose dobutamine echocardiography [38, 39].

11.6
Prognostic Value

The presence, site, extent, and severity of exercise-induced wall motion abnormalities have a clearly proven prognostic impact, as shown by over 20 studies on 5,000 patients – ranging from patients with normal baseline function [40–43] to those evaluated early after an acute myocardial infarction [44–47], women [48], or hypertensive subjects [49]. The prognostic value of exercise stress echocardiography is high, comparable to other forms of pharmacological (dobutamine or dipyridamole) stress echocardiography and stress SPECT [49, 50] (Fig. 11.7).

Among patients who have a normal exercise echocardiogram, prognosis is favorable and the coronary event rate is quite low [40]. An abnormal stress echocardiogram, defined as a new or worsening wall motion abnormality, substantially increases the likelihood of a coronary event during the follow-up period. This finding, coupled with the presence or absence of resting left ventricular dysfunction and the exercise capacity of the patient, provides a great deal of prognostic information in an individual patient. The prognostic value is incremental over clinical and exercise electrocardiography variables [42, 50] (Fig. 11.8).

11

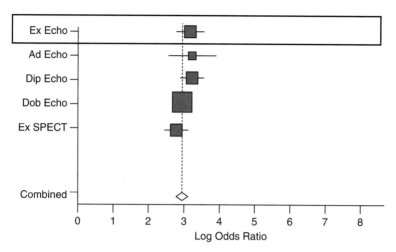

Fig. 11.7 The diagnostic accuracy of exercise echocardiography (*squared line*) versus other stress imaging test. The value of the log odds ratio is a measure of overall diagnostic accuracy. The size of the box is smaller for smaller sizes, with higher confidence intervals. (Modified from [37])

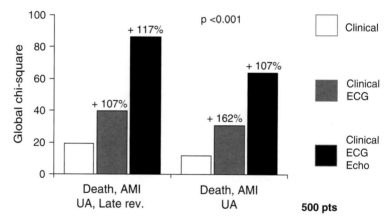

Fig. 11.8 The prognostic value of exercise echocardiography. (Modified from [42])

In patients evaluated for coronary artery disease, exercise echocardiography and exercise scintigraphy combined with the ECG variable provide comparable prognostic information and can be used interchangeably for risk stratification [50]. Other ancillary markers, beyond regional wall motion, can further stratify the prognosis during exercise echocardiography. In patients with a positive test result the prognosis is more malignant, and in patients with a negative test result the prognosis is less benign, with exercise-induced left ventricular cavity dilation [51] or severe mitral insufficiency [52, 53]. However, the systematic search of these ancillary markers of ischemia is unfeasible and technically challenging during exercise stress echocardiography, and may shift the focus of imaging away from wall motion, which remains the cornerstone of diagnosis. Their greatest clinical value is outside coronary artery disease, in patients with heart failure [20] or valvular heart disease [19].

11.7
Indications and Contraindications to Exercise Stress Echocardiography

Exercise is the most physiologic stressor of all and thus is preferable in patients who are capable of exercising (Table 11.4). For coronary artery disease diagnosis, exercise echocardiography is the appropriate first-line test, skipping the exercise electrocardiography test, in patients with conditions making the ECG uninterpretable, such as left bundle branch block or Wolf–Parkinson–White syndrome or ST-segment abnormalities on baseline resting ECG [54, 55, 56]. Exercise echocardiography is also the most suitable second-line stress test, when exercise ECG, performed as a first-line test reproduced ST-segment depression and/or angina or when the positive predictive value of these findings remains low (e.g., in women and/or hypertensive subjects) (Fig. 11.8). Exercise stress echocardiography is frequently performed inappropriately, as with all other stress imaging testing, as a first-line test in patients with low pretest probability of disease and in whom ECG is interpretable [57, 58]. There are contraindications to exercise echocardiography, such as the classical contraindications to exercise stress, including unstable hemodynamic conditions or severe, uncontrolled hypertension. Additional relative contraindications to exercise stress is the inability to exercise adequately, and – specifically for exercise echocardiography – a difficult resting echocardiogram. These conditions are not infrequent, especially in an elderly population, since out of five patients referred for testing, one is unable to exercise, one exercises submaximally [14], and one has an interpretable but challenging echocardiogram, which makes pharmacological stress echocardiography a more practical option. Exercise stress echocardiography has similar indications and contraindications to exercise SPECT, and similar diagnostic and prognostic accuracy as recognized by general cardiology guidelines [54, 55]. In a cost-conscious and radiation risk-conscious environment, this implies that stress echocardiography should be the obligatory choice [59, 60], even from a legal standpoint [61, 62], to avoid the environmental

Table 11.4 Indications to exercise stress echocardiography for diagnosis of coronary artery disease (adapted from [56])

	Appropriate	Uncertain	Inappropriate
Intermediate pretest probability of coronary artery disease	√		
ECG uninterpretable			
Prior stress ECG uninterpretable or equivocal	√		
Repeat stress echocardiography after 2 years, in asymptomatic stable symptoms		√	
Repeat stress echocardiography annually, in asymptomatic or stable symptoms		√	
Symptomatic, low pretest probability, interpretable ECG			√
Asymptomatic, low risk			√
Asymptomatic less than 1 year after percutaneous coronary intervention, with prior symptoms			√

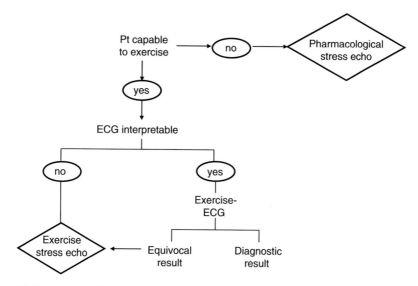

Fig. 11.9 The proposed algorithm for the use of exercise echocardiography

burden, radiological dose exposure (corresponding to 500–1,500 chest X-rays), and long-term risk (1 cancer in 500 exposed subsets) of stress scintigraphy [63, 64]. A unique advantage of exercise echocardiography over the other forms of stress is that it may offer helpful and tremendously versatile evaluation of valve function, of pulmonary hemodynamics, and of special subsets of patients, such as patients with heart failure, pulmonary hypertension, or valve disease (Table 11.4). In all these patients, the physiologic nature of exercise stress and the staggering versatility of the echocardiography technique allow one to tailor the most appropriate test to the individual patient in the stress echocardiography laboratory (Fig. 11.9).

References

1. Kraunz RF, Kennedy JW (1970) An ultrasonic determination of left ventricular wall motion in normal man. Studies at rest and after exercise. Am Heart J 79:36–43
2. Mason SJ, Weiss JL, Weisfeldt ML, et al (1979) Exercise echocardiography in detection of wall motion abnormalities during ischemia. Circulation 59:50–54
3. Wann LS, Faris JV, Childress RH, et al (1979) Exercise cross sectional echocardiography inischemic heart disease. Circulation 60:1300–1308
4. Bairey CN, Rozanski A, Berman DS (1988) Exercise echocardiography: ready or not? J Am Coll Cardiol 11:1355–1358
5. Picano E, Distante A, Masini M, et al (1985) Dipyridamole-echocardiography test in effort angina pectoris. Am J Cardiol 56:452–456
6. Berthe C, Pierard LA, Hiernaux M, et al (1986) Predicting the extent and location of coronary artery disease in acute myocardial infarction by echocardiography during dobutamine infusion. Am J Cardiol 58:1167–1172

7. Picano E, Landi P, Bolognese L, et al (1993) Prognostic value of dipyridamole echocardiography early after uncomplicated myocardial infarction: a large-scale, multicenter trial. The EPIC Study Group. Am J Med 95:608–618

8. Picano E, Sicari R, Landi P, et al (1998) Prognostic value of myocardial viability in medically treated patients with global left ventricular dysfunction early after an acute uncomplicated myocardial infarction: a dobutamine stress echocardiographic study. Circulation. 98:1078–84

9. Feigenbaum H (1994) A digital echocardiographic laboratory. J Am Soc Echocardiogr 7:105–106

10. Caidahl K, Kazzam E, Lidberg J, et al (1998) New concept in echocardiography: harmonic imaging of tissue without use of contrast agent. Lancet 352:1264–1270

11. Laskar R, Grayburn PA (2000) Assessment of myocardial perfusion with contrast echocardiography at rest and with stress: an emerging technology. Prog Cardiovasc Dis 43:245–258

12. Armstrong WF, Ryan T (2008) Stress echocardiography from 1979 to present. J Am Soc Echocardiogr 21:22–28

13. Pellikka PA, Nagueh SF, Elhendy AA, et al; American Society of Echocardiography (2007) American Society of Echocardiography recommendations for performance, interpretation, and application of stress echocardiography. J Am Soc Echocardiogr 20:1021–1041

14. Pierard LA (2007) Echocardiographic monitoring throughout exercise better than the post-treadmill approach? J Am Coll Cardiol 50:1864–1866

15. Sicari R, Nihoyannopoulos P., Evangelista A, et al (2008) Stress echocardiography consensus statement of the European Association of Echocardiography. Eur J Echocardiogr 9:415–437

16. Picano E, Lattanzi F,Masini M, et al (1987) Comparison of high-dose dipyridamole-echocardiography test and exercise 2-D echocardiography for diagnosis of coronary artery disease. Am J Cardiol 59:539–542

17. Hecht HS, DeBord L, Sho WR, et al (1993) Digital supine bicycle stress echocardiography: a new technique for evaluating coronary artery disease. J Am Coll Cardiol 21:950–956

18. Park TH, Tayan N, Takeda K, et al (2007) Supine bicycle echocardiography improved diagnostic accuracy and physiologic assessment of coronary artery disease with the incorporation of intermediate stages of exercise. J Am Coll Cardiol 50:1857–1863

19. Piérard LA, Lancellotti P (2007) Stress testing in valve disease. Heart 93:766–772

20. Tumminello G, Lancellotti P, Lempereur M, et al (2007) Determinants of pulmonary artery hypertension at rest and during exercise in patients with heart failure. Eur Heart J 28:569–574

21. Bombardini T, Gemignani V, Bianchini E, et al (2007) Cardiac reflections and natural vibrations: force-frequency relation recording system in the stress echo lab. Cardiovasc Ultrasound 5:42

22. Bombardini T, Nevola E, Giorgetti A, et al (2008) Prognostic value of left-ventricular and peripheral vascular performance in patients with dilated cardiomyopathy. J Nucl Cardiol 15:353–362

23. Beleslin BD,Ostojic M, Stepanovic J, et al (1994) Stress echocardiography in the detection of myocardial ischemia.Head-to-head comparison of exercise, dobutamine, and dipyridamole tests. Circulation 90:1168–1176

24. Thadani U,West RO,Mathew TM, et al (1977) Hemodynamics at rest and during supine and sitting bicycle exercise in patients with coronary artery disease.Am J Cardiol 39:776–783

25. Poliner LR, Dehmer GJ, Lewis SE, et al (1980) Left ventricular performance in normal subjects: a comparison of the responses to exercise in the upright and supine positions. Circulation. 62:528–534

26. Currie PJ, Kelly MJ, Pitt A (1983) Comparison of supine and erect bicycle exercise eletrocardiography in coronary artery disease: accentuation of exercise-induced ischemic ST segment depression by supine posture. Am J Cardiol 52:1167–1173

27. Yamakado T, Kasai A, Masuda T, et al (1996) Exercise-induced coronary spasm: comparison of treadmill and bicycle exercise in patients with vasospastic angina. Coron Artery Dis 7:819–822

28. Fletcher GF, Balady GJ, Amsterdam EA, et al (2001) Exercise standards for testing and training: a statement for healthcare professionals from the American Heart Association. Circulation 104:1694–740

29. Varga A, Garcia MA, Picano E; International Stress Echo Complication Registry (2006) Safety of stress echocardiography (from the International Stress Echo Complication Registry). Am J Cardiol 98:541–543

30. Picano E, Marini C, Pirelli S, et al (1992) Safety of intravenous high-dose dipyridamole echocardiography. The Echo-Persantine International Cooperative Study Group. Am J Cardiol 70:252–258

31. Picano E, Mathias W Jr, Pingitore A, et al (1994) Safety and tolerability of dobutamine-atropine stress echocardiography: a prospective, multicentre study. Echo Dobutamine International Cooperative Study Group. Lancet. 344:1190–1192

32. Beckmann S, Haug G (1999) National registry 1995–1998 on 150,000 stress echo examinations side effects and complications in 60,448 examinations of the registry 1997–1998, Circulation 100(suppl):3401A

33. Fleischmann KE, Hunink MG, Kuntz KM, et al (1998) Exercise echocardiography or exercise SPECT imaging? A meta analysis of diagnostic test performance. JAMA 280:913–920

34. Albuquerque de Fonseca L, Picano E (2001) Comparison of dipyridamole and exercise stress echocardiography for detection of coronary artery disease (a meta-analysis). Am J Cardiol 87:1193–1196

35. Kim C, Kwok YS, Heagerty P, et al (2001) Pharmacologic stress testing for coronary disease diagnosis: a meta-analysis. Am Heart J 142:934–944

36. Noguchi Y, Nagata-Kobayashi S, Stahl JE, et al (2005) A meta-analytic comparison of echocardiographic stressors. Int J Cardiovasc Imaging 21:189–207

37. Heijenbrok-Kal MH, Fleischmann KE, Hunink MG (2007) Stress echocardiography, stress single-photon-emission computed tomography and electron beam computed tomography for the assessment of coronary artery disease: a meta-analysis of diagnostic performance. Am Heart J 154:415–423

38. Hoffer EP, Dewe W, Celentano C, et al (1999) Low-level exercise echocardiography detects contractile reserve and predicts reversible dysfunction after acute myocardial infarction: comparison with low-dose dobutamine echocardiography. J Am Coll Cardiol 34:989–997

39. Lancellotti P, Hoffer EP, Piérard LA (2003) Detection and clinical usefulness of a biphasic response during exercise echocardiography early after myocardial infarction. J Am Coll Cardiol 41:1142–1147

40. Sawada SG, Ryan T, Conley M, et al (1990) Prognostic value of a normal exercise echocardiogram. Am Heart J 120:49–55

41. Olmos LI, Dakik H, Gordon R, et al (1998) Long-term prognostic value of exercise echocardiography compared with exercise 201Tl,ECG,and clinical variables in patients evaluated for coronary artery disease. Circulation 98:2679–2686

42. Marwick TH, Case C,Vasey C, et al (2001) Prediction of mortality by exercise echocardiography: a strategy for combination with the Duke treadmill score. Circulation 103:2566–2571

43. Arruda-Olson AM, Juracan EM, Mahoney DW, et al (2002) Prognostic value of exercise echocardiography in 5,798 patients: is there a gender difference? J Am Coll Cardiol 39:625–631

44. Jaarsma W, Visser C, Funke Kupper A (1986) Usefulness of two-dimensional exercise echocardiography shortly after myocardial infarction. Am J Cardiol 57:86–90

45. Applegate RJ, Dell'Italia LJ,Crawford MH (1987) Usefulness of two-dimensional echocardiography during low level exercise-testing early after uncomplicated myocardial infarction. Am J Cardiol 60:10–14

46. Ryan T, Armstrong WF, O'Donnel JA, et al (1987) Risk stratification following acute myocardial infarction during exercise two-dimensional echocardiography.Am Heart J 114:1305–1316

47. Quintana M, Lindvall K, Ryden L, et al (1995) Prognostic value of predischarge exercise stress echocardiography after acute myocardial infarction. Am J Cardiol 76:1115–1121

48. Heupler S, Mehta R, Lobo A, et al (1997) Prognostic implications of exercise echocardiography in women with known or suspected coronary artery disease. J Am Coll Cardiol 30:414–420

49. Marwick TH, Case C, Sawada S, et al (2002) Prediction of outcomes in hypertensive patients with suspected coronary disease. Hypertension 39:1113–1138

50. Shaw LJ, Marwick TH, Berman DS, et al (2006) Incremental cost-effectiveness of exercise echocardiography vs. SPECT imaging for the evaluation of stable chest pain. Eur Heart J 27:2448–2458

51. Yao SS, Shah A, Bangalore S, et al (2007) Transient ischemic left ventricular cavity dilation is a significant predictor of severe and extensive coronary artery disease and adverse outcome in patients undergoing stress echocardiography. J Am Soc Echocardiogr 20:352–358

52. Lancellotti P, Gérard PL, Piérard LA (2006) Long-term outcome of patients with heart failure and dynamic functional mitral regurgitation. Eur Heart J 27:187–192

53. Peteiro JC, Monserrat L, Bouzas A, et al (2006) Risk stratification by treadmill exercise echocardiography. J Am Soc Echocardiogr 19:894–901

54. Gibbons RJ, Abrams J, Chatterjee K, et al; American College of Cardiology; American Heart Association Task Force on practice guidelines (Committee on the Management of Patients With Chronic Stable Angina) (2003) ACC/AHA 2002 guideline update for the management of patients with chronic stable angina–summary article: a report of the American College of Cardiology/American Heart Association Task Force on practice guidelines (Committee on the Management of Patients With Chronic Stable Angina). J Am Coll Cardiol 41:159–168

55. Fox K, Garcia MA, Ardissino D, et al; Task Force on the Management of Stable Angina Pectoris of the European Society of Cardiology; ESC Committee for Practice Guidelines (CPG) (2006) Guidelines on the management of stable angina pectoris: executive summary: the Task Force on the Management of Stable Angina Pectoris of the European Society of Cardiology. Eur Heart J 27:1341–1381

56. Douglas PS, Khandheria B, Raymond F. et al. ACCF/ASE/ACEP/AHA/ASNC/SCAI/SCCT/ SCMR 2008 Appropriateness Criteria for Stress Echocardiography: A Report of the American College of Cardiology Foundation Appropriateness Criteria Task Force, American Society of Echocardiography, American College of Emergency Physicians, American Heart Association, American Society of Nuclear Cardiology, Society for Cardiovascular Angiography and Interventions, Society of Cardiovascular Computed Tomography, and Society for Cardiovascular Magnetic Resonance Endorsed by the Heart Rhythm Society and the Society of Critical Care Medicine. J Am Coll Cardiol 51: 1127–1147

57. Picano E, Pasanisi E, Brown J, et al (2007) A gatekeeper for the gatekeeper: inappropriate referrals to stress echocardiography. Am Heart J 154:285–290

58. Gibbons RJ, Miller TD, Hodge D, et al (2008) Application of appropriateness criteria to stress single-photon emission computed tomography sestamibi studies and stress echocardiograms in an academic medical center. J Am Coll Cardiol. 51:1283–1289

59. European Commission. Radiation protection 118: referral guidelines for imaging. http:/ /europa.eu.int/comm/environment/radprot/118/rp-118-en.pdf (accessed 10 January 2006)

60. Picano E (2003) Stress echocardiography: a historical perspective. Special article. Am J Med 114:126–130

61. Council Directive 97/43/EURATOM of 30 June 1997 on health protection of individuals against the dangers of ionizing radiation in relation to medical exposure and repealing Directive 84/466/Euratom
62. Picano E (2004) Sustainability of medical imaging. Education and debate. BMJ. 328:578–580
63. Picano E (2004) Informed consent and communication of risk from radiological and nuclear medicine examinations: how to escape from a communication inferno. Education and debate. BMJ 329:849–851
64. Amis S, Butler P, Applegate KE, et al (2007) American College of Radiology White Paper on Radiation Dose in Medicine. J Am Coll Radiol 4:272–284

Dobutamine Stress Echocardiography

12

Eugenio Picano

12.1
Historical Background

Among exercise-independent stresses, the most popular are dobutamine and dipyridamole. Dobutamine is the prototype of pharmacological adrenergic or inotropic stress. It was initially proposed for the diagnosis of coronary artery disease in combination with perfusion imaging [1] and later with two-dimensional (2D) echocardiography by the Liège group [2]. Other sympathomimetic agents have been proposed for stress echocardiography, including isoproterenol [3] and epinephrine [4], but these drugs often bring more pronounced arrhythmogenic side effects. Following the demonstration of low-dose dobutamine as a test of myocardial viability by Luc Pierard and his group [5], in the past decade dobutamine has been extensively adopted in pharmacological stress echocardiography. The evolution of dobutamine stress paralleled that of other pharmacological stresses. With echocardiography, it began at relatively "low" doses ($20\,\mu g\ kg^{-1}\ min^{-1}$), which gave low sensitivity values [6]; later, more aggressive doses were adopted (up to $40\,\mu g\ kg^{-1}\ min^{-1}$) [7, 8], and finally it was coadministered with atropine [9], which overcame the limitation of less than ideal sensitivity to minor forms of coronary artery disease.

12.2
Pharmacology and Pathophysiology

Dobutamine is a synthetic catecholamine resulting from the modification of the chemical structure of isoproterenol. It acts directly and mainly on beta-1 adrenergic receptors of the myocardium, producing an increase in heart rate, enhancement of atrioventricular conduction, and increased contractility (Fig. 12.1). In fact, alpha-adrenergic activity can mediate systemic vasoconstriction and an increase in blood pressure and – at the coronary level – increased constriction up to coronary vasospasm, especially when the alpha-mediated vasoconstriction is enhanced by chronic or acute beta-blockade. Stimulation of

E. Picano, *Stress Echocardiography*,
© Springer-Verlag Berlin Heidelberg 2009

12

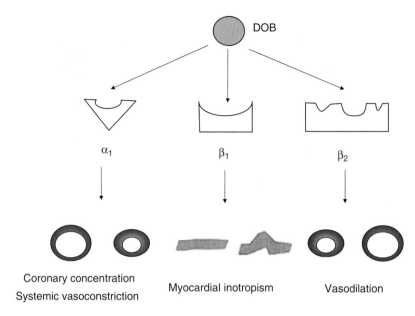

Fig. 12.1 The main cardiovascular receptor targets and physiologic effects of dobutamine

beta-2 receptors on coronary arterioles may induce coronary arteriolar vasodilation. However, endothelial dysfunction and enhanced alpha-adrenergic tone contribute to the loss of dobutamine-induced vasodilation in coronary atherosclerosis [10]. The short half-life (2 min) of dobutamine allows rapid resolution of its effects once the intravenous infusion is discontinued. However, the alpha-mediated coronaro-constrictive and platelet-aggregating effects are not reversed, and may be potentiated, by beta-blockers and peak at 30–45 min after the end of infusion.

Dobutamine provokes ischemia mainly through the inotropic and chronotropic response to stimulation of myocardial beta-1 receptors determining an increase in myocardial oxygen demand (Fig. 12.2). Other proischemic mechanisms are the flow maldistribution mediated by beta-2 receptors of coronary arterioles [11] and coronary vasospasm mediated by alpha-adrenoreceptors present on smooth muscle cells of epicardial arteries. The dobutamine dose usually employed for stress echocardiography testing causes a two- to threefold increase in coronary blood flow [12].

12.3
Methodology

The protocol displayed in Fig. 12.3 is the most widely used, the only one validated in a large-scale multicenter prospective trial [13], and it has been recently proposed as the state-of-the art protocol by both the American [14] and European [15] recommendations.

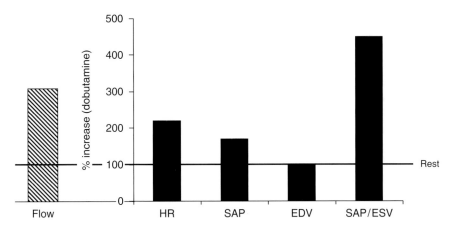

Fig. 12.2 The increase of main determinants of myocardial oxygen consumption in normal subjects referred for dobutamine stress echocardiography. Heart rate increases two- to threefold, end-diastolic volume (an index of preload) 1.2-fold, systolic arterial pressure 1.5- to twofold, and myocardial contractility (measured as elastance) increases four- to eightfold versus baseline

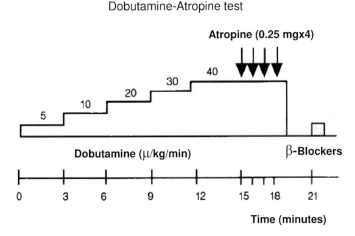

Fig. 12.3 Protocol of the dobutamine–atropine stress test. For viability detection in patients off beta-blockers, a 5-min step from 5 to 10 mcg is suggested

Doses lower than those shown in Fig. 12.3 are associated with insufficient sensitivity, while higher doses are associated with an unacceptable high rate of side effects. For viability assessment, steps of 5 min are used, starting from 5 up to 10 mcg [5]. However, to fully recruit the inotropic reserve in patients with heart failure and usually with beta-blocker therapy, high doses (without atropine) are required [16].

12

12.4
Feasibility and Safety

Minor but limiting side effects preclude the achievement of maximal pharmacological stress in about 10% of patients [13, 17]. In order of frequency, these side effects are: complex ventricular tachyarrhythmias (frequent, polymorphic, premature ventricular beats, couplets and triplets, nonsustained ventricular tachycardia); nausea and/or headache; hypotension (>30 mmHg drop in blood pressure) and or bradycardia; supraventricular tachyarrhythmias (supraventricular tachycardia or atrial fibrillation); hypertension. Limiting side effects are more often asymptomatic with dobutamine, and more often symptomatic with dipyridamole [17]. Side effects usually disappear upon interruption of drug infusion, since the half-life is 2–3 min. When symptoms or ischemia persist, IV beta-blockers – usually the short-acting drug esmolol – are given.

Both the patient and the physician should be aware of the rate of major complications that may occur during dobutamine stress. As concordantly shown by meta-analysis [18], single-center experiences [19–24], prospective multicenter studies [13], and retrospective registries [25–27] major life-threatening side effects occur in 1 of 300–350 cases (Table 12.1). The proliferating anecdotal reports of catastrophes also contribute in assessing the safety of the test. Cardiac rupture [28–31], ventricular fibrillation [32, 33], refractory

Table 12.1 Life-threatening complications in single-center experience (>1,000 patients), multicenter studies (EDIC), and multicenter registries for dobutamine stress echocardiography

Author, year	Patients	Complications (s)
Single institution experience		
Mertes et al.	1,118	None[a]
Pellikka et al.	1,000	1 AMI, 4 VT, 1 prol ischemia
Zahn et al.	1,000	1 VF, 1 LVF, 1 seizure
Ling et al.	1,968	None[a]
Seknus and Marwick	3,011	5 VT, 1 AMI, 1 prol ischamia, 1 hypo
Elhendy et al.	1,164	7 VT
Bremer et al.	1,035	1 VF, 1 VT
Poldermans et al.	1,734	3 VF, 13 VT, 6 hypo
Mathias et al.	4,033	1 VFm 8 VT, 1 MI; 5 atropine intoxications
Multicenter registry		
Picano et al. (EDIC), 1994	2,949	2 VF, 2 VT, 2 AMI, 1 prol ischemia, 1 hypo
Pezzano et al. (RITED) 1994	3,041	2 VF, 1 asystole
Beckmann, 1999	9,354	324 (2 VF)
Varga, 2001	35,103	63 (5 deaths)
Total	66,510	461

AMI acute myocardial infarction, *VT* ventricular tachyarrhythmia, *VF* ventricular fibrillation, *LVF*, *VFm*, *MI* myocardial infarction, prol prolonged, hypo hypotension
[a] No life-threatening complications reported; however, minor and self-limiting adverse effects were documented

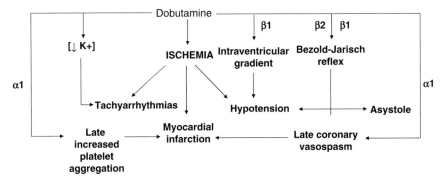

Fig. 12.4 Ischemia-dependent and ischemia-independent pathways of complications during dobutamine stress

coronary vasospasm [34, 35], myocardial infarction [36, 37], cardiac asystole [38, 39], and acute Tako Tsubo syndrome [40] have all been described during dobutamine testing. Tachyarrhythmias are the most frequent complication occurring during dobutamine stress echocardiography. In some cases they are subsequent to pharmacologically induced myocardial ischemia during the test, and therefore are associated with a transient wall motion abnormality. However, in many cases they are independent of ischemia and can also develop at low dobutamine doses. The mechanism of their onset can be attributed to the direct adrenergic arrhythmogenic effect of dobutamine, through myocardial β-receptor stimulation, which is particularly evident in patients with ischemic heart disease. Dobutamine infusion can also lower the blood potassium level, thereby contributing to the genesis of ventricular ectopy through a depolarizing effect on the cell membrane [41] (Fig. 12.4). Significant hypotension, sometimes associated with bradyarrhythmias, including asystole, is another frequent adverse reaction during dobutamine echocardiography. In some cases this finding has been attributed to dynamic interventricular obstruction provoked by inotropic action of dobutamine, especially in hypertrophic hearts [42]. A vasodepressor reflex triggered by left ventricular mechanoreceptor stimulation (Bezold–Jarish reflex) due to excessive inotropic stimulation may be an alternative mechanism [43]. Late and long-lasting transmural myocardial ischemia, with persistent ST-segment elevation, is probably due to the coronary vasoconstrictive effect of dobutamine, through α-receptor stimulation, sometimes involving multiple coronary segments. Moreover, dobutamine can induce increased platelet aggregation, possibly provoking coronary occlusion, prolonged myocardial ischemia, and acute myocardial infarction on the anatomic substrate of a vulnerable, possibly noncritical, plaque unable to induce ischemia during the stress [44, 13].

12.5
Diagnostic Results for Detection of Coronary Artery Disease

The accuracy in detecting angiographically assessed coronary artery disease has been consistently reported to be high, with sensitivity and specificity of 81 and 84%, respectively, in a meta-analysis of 102 studies with over 7,900 patients [45]. The diagnostic accuracy is

12

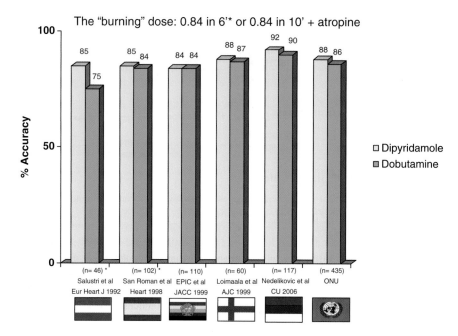

Fig. 12.5 The diagnostic accuracy (sensitivity on the *y*-axis, and specificity on the *x*-axis) for noninvasive detection of coronary artery disease of dobutamine echocardiography vs. dipyridamole echocardiography (all protocols) and state-of-the-art (high dose with atropine or fast high dose) dipyridamole echocardiography. (From meta-analysis of [45] and [47])

similar to other forms of stress testing, such as exercise echocardiography [45, 46], dipyridamole echocardiography [45, 46], or stress SPECT [45]. In particular, the sensitivity is identical to dipyridamole stress echocardiography when state-of-the-art protocols are used for both stresses (Fig. 12.5), as shown by a recent metaanalysis including 5 studies on 435 patients [47].

12.6
Identification of Myocardial Viability

Low-dose dobutamine recognizes myocardial viability with high specificity and good sensitivity, with excellent diagnostic [48] and prognostic [49] value. In patients with preserved global left ventricular function, myocardial viability identifies a greater risk to subsequent development of ischemia and nonfatal reinfarction early after acute myocardial infarction [50]. In patients with severe resting left ventricular dysfunction, a large amount of myocardial viability identified by low-dose dobutamine echocardiography is associated with a better survival [51]. This finding has been consistently described both in medically treated patients studied early after acute myocardial infarction [51]

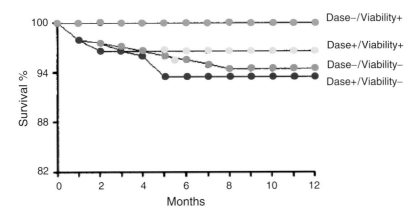

Fig. 12.6 Kaplan–Meier survival curves (considering only death as an end point) in patients stratified according to presence or absence of echocardiographically assessed viability and ischemia at
low and high doses of dobutamine, respectively. Best survival is observed in patients with low-dose
viability and no inducible ischemia; worst survival, in patients without viability and with inducible
ischemia. *Viability+* and *viability–* indicate presence or absence of myocardial viability at low-dose
dobutamine, respectively; *Dase+* and *Dase–*, presence or absence of myocardial ischemia at high-
dose dobutamine, respectively. (From [69])

(a model of stunned myocardium) (Fig. 12.6) and in revascularized patients studied after
chronic myocardial infarction (a model of hibernating myocardium) [52–54]. A contractile reserve identified by high-dose dobutamine (up to 40 mcg) identifies patients with
dilated cardiomyopathy and better response to medical therapy [55] and cardiac resynchronization therapy [56].

12.7
Prognostic Value

The presence, site, timing, extent, and severity of dobutamine-induced wall motion
abnormalities have a clear prognostic impact, as shown by over 50 studies on over 10,000
patients, including patients with or suspected coronary artery disease [57–66], evaluated
early after acute myocardial infarction [67–71], and patients undergoing major noncardiac vascular surgery [72–79]. These studies concordantly show that dobutamine stress
echocardiography results predict subsequent death, on the basis of coexistent fixed
resting wall motion abnormalities, dobutamine dose required to induce ischemia (Fig.
12.7), and peak wall motion score index (Fig. 12.8). The prognostic value of dobutamine
stress echocardiography is independent and additive to resting echocardiography and
exercise electrocardiography, and comparable to dipyridamole echocardiography [80,
81, 62] and stress SPECT [76, 82].

12

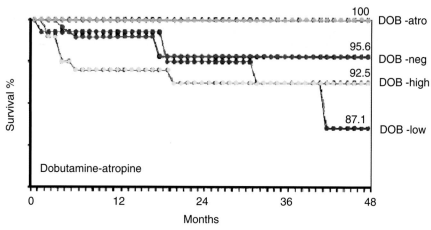

Fig. 12.7 Kaplan–Meier survival curves event-free of cardiac death in patients with negative and positive dobutamine echocardiography test results (*DOB*). Survival is worse in patients with positive DOB. In patients with positive DOB, a progressively worse survival is identified with positivity after atropine, high and low dose (*upper panel*). (From [62])

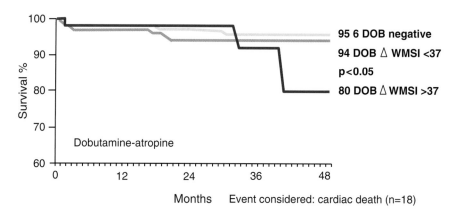

Fig. 12.8 Kaplan–Meier survival curves event-free of cardiac death in patients with negative and positive dobutamine echocardiography test results (*DOB*). In patients with positive DOB, a progressively worse survival is identified for patients with higher changes in peak wall motion score index (*WMSI, lower panel*). (From [62])

12.8
Indications and Contraindications

High-dose dobutamine is an appropriate choice for pharmacological stress echocardiography used for the detection of coronary artery disease, especially in patients with inability to exercise or contraindications to exercise [83] or with resting images of borderline

Table 12.2 Appropriate and inappropriate indications to dobutamine stress echocardiography

	Appropriate	Uncertain	Inappropriate
Diagnosis of CAD in patient unable to exercise	√		
Diagnosis of viability in ejection fraction <35%	√		
High-risk noncardiac surgery in inter-mediate-risk patient	√		
Low-flow, low-gradient aortic stenosis	√		
Need to evaluate antianginal therapy efficacy		√	
Intermediate risk noncardiac surgery in intermediate-risk patient		√	
Prediction of CRT efficacy		√	
First-line test in patients able to exercise			√
Severe hypertension, malignant ectopy, inferior wall aneurysm early after AMI			√
Low-risk noncardiac surgery in low-risk patient			√

AMI acute myocardial infarction, *CAD* coronary artery disease, *CRT* cardiac resynchronization therapy

quality which may make the more technically difficult exercise stress echocardiography a challenging task [84] (Table 12.2). It is also appropriate in intermediate-risk patients undergoing elective high-risk noncardiac surgery. Low-dose dobutamine is the first choice for identification of myocardial viability in patients with severe left ventricular dysfunction. It is also appropriate in low-flow, low-gradient aortic stenosis to separate true from pseudosevere aortic stenosis. Appropriateness is uncertain in intermediate-risk patients undergoing intermediate-risk noncardiac surgery. Patients with a history of complex atrial (paroxysmal atrial fibrillation, paroxysmal supraventricular tachycardia) or ventricular arrhythmias (sustained ventricular tachycardia or ventricular fibrillation) or with moderate to severe hypertension should probably not undergo dobutamine stress testing and be referred for safer vasodilator stress [85].

References

1. Mason JR, Palac RT, Freeman ML, et al (1984) Thallium scintigraphy during dobutamine infusion: nonexercise-dependent screening test for coronary disease. Am Heart J 107:481–485
2. Berthe CN, Pierard LA, Hienaux M, et al (1986) Predicting the extent and location of coronary artery disease in acute myocardial infarction by echocardiography during dobutamine infusion. Am J Cardiol 58:1167–1172
3. Fujita T, Ajisaka R, Matsumoto R, et al (1986) Isoproterenol infusion stress two-dimensional echocardiography in diagnosis of coronary artery disease in elderly patients: comparison with the other stress testing methods. Jpn Heart J 27:287–297
4. Ferrara N, Leosco D, Longobardi G, et al. (1986) Use of epinephrine test in diagnosis of coronary artery disease. Am J Cardiol 158:256–260

5. Pierard LA, De Landsheere CM, Berthe C, et al (1990) Identification of viable myocardium by echocardiography during dobutamine infusion in patients with myocardial infarction after thrombolytic therapy: comparison with positron emission tomography. J Am Coll Cardiol 15:1021–1031
6. Mannering D, Cripps T, Leech G, et al. (1988) The dobutamine stress test as an alternative to exercise testing after acute myocardial infarction. Br Heart J 59:521–526
7. Previtali M, Lanzarini L, Ferrario M, et al (1991) Dobutamine versus dipyridamole echocardiography in coronary artery disease. Circulation 83(Suppl 3):27–31
8. Cohen JL, Greene TO, Ottenwel!er J, et al (1991) Dobutamine digital echocardiography for detecting coronary artery disease. Am J Cardiol 67:1311–1318
9. McNeill AJ, Fioretti PM, EI-Said EM, et al (1992) Enhanced sensitivity for detection of coronary artery disease by addition of atropine to dobutamine stress echocardiography. Am J Cardiol 170:41–46
10. Barbato E, Bartunek J, Wyffels E, et al (2003) Effects of intravenous dobutamine on coronary vasomotion in humans. J Am Coll Cardiol 42:1596–601
11. Warltier DC, Zyvoloski M, Gross GJ, et al (1981) Redistribution of myocardial blood flow distal to a dynamic coronary arterial stenosis by sympathomimetic amines: comparison of dopamine, dobutamine and isoproterenol. Am J Cardiol 48:269–279
12. Severi S, Underwood R, Mohiaddin RH, et al (1995) Dobutamine stress: effects on regional myocardial blood flow and wall motion. J Am Coll Cardiol 26: 1187–1195
13. Picano E, Mathias W jr, Pingitore A, et al, on behalf of the EDIC study group (1994) Safety and tolerability of dobutamine-atropine stress echocardiography: a prospective, large-scale, multicenter trial. Lancet 344:1190–1192
14. Pellikka PA, Nagueh SF, Elhendy AA, et al; American Society of Echocardiography (2007) American Society of Echocardiography recommendations for performance, interpretation, and application of stress echocardiography. J Am Soc Echocardiogr 20:1021–1041
15. Sicari R, Nihoyannopoulos P, Evangelista A, et al; European Association of Echocardiography (2008). Stress echocardiography expert consensus statement: European Association of Echocardiography (EAE) (a registered branch of the ESC). Eur J Echocardiogr 9:415–437
16. Pratali L, Picano E, Otasevic P, et al (2001) Prognostic significance of the dobutamine echocardiography test in idiopathic dilated cardiomyopathy. Am J Cardiol 88:1374–1378
17. Pingitore A, Picano E, Colosso MQ, et al (1996) The atropine factor in pharmacologic stress echocardiography. Echo Persantine (EPIC) and Echo Dobutamine International Cooperative (EDIC) Study Groups. J Am Coll Cardiol 27:1164–1170
18. Lattanzi F, Picano E, Adamo E, et al (2000) Dobutamine stress echocardiography: safety in diagnosing coronary artery disease. Drug Safety 22:251–262
19. Mertes H, Sawada S, Ryan T, et al (1993) Symptoms, adverse effects, and complications associated with dobutamine stress echocardiography. Experience in 1118 patients. Circulation 88:15
20. Zahn R, Lotter R, Nohl H, et al (1996) Feasibility and safety of dobutamine stress echocardiography: experiences with 1,000 studies. Z Kardiol 85:28–34
21. Secknus MA, Marwick TH (1997) Evolution of dobutamine echocardiograpby protocols and indications: safety and side effects in 3,011 studies over 5 years. J Am Coll Cardiol 29:1234–1240
22. Pellikka PA, Roger VL, Oh JK, et al (1995) Stress echocardiography. Part II. Dobutamine stress echocardiography: techniques, implementation, clinical applications, and correlations. Mayo Clin Proc 70:16–27
23. Mathias W Jr, Arruda A, Santos FC, et al (1999) Safety of dobutamine-atropine stress echocardiography: a prospective experience of 4,033 consecutive studies. J Am Soc Echocardiogr 12:785–791

24. Poldermans D, Fioretti PM, Boersma E, et al (1994) Safety of dobutamine-atropine stress echocardiography in patients with suspected or proven coronary artery disease: experience in 650 consecutive examinations. Am J Cardiol 73:456–459

25. Pezzano A, Gentile F, Mantero A, et al (1998) RITED (Registro Italiano Test Eco-Dobutamina): side effects and complications of echo-dobutamine stress test in 3041 examinations. G Ital Cardiol 28:102–111

26. Beckmann SH, Haug G (1999) National registry 1995–1998 on 150,000 stress echo examinations: side effects and complications in 60,448 examinations of the registry 1997–1998. Circulation 100(suppl):3401

27. Varga A, Garcia MA, Picano E; International Stress Echo Complication Registry (2006). Safety of stress echocardiography (from the International Stress Echo Complication Registry). Am J Cardiol 98:541–543

28. Reisenhofer B, Squarcini G, Picano E (1998) Cardiac rupture during dobutamine stress test. Ann Intern Med 128:605

29. Orlandini AD, Tuero EI, Diaz R, et al (2000) Acute cardiac rupture during dobutamine-atropine echocardiography stress test. J Am Soc Echocardiogr 13:152–153

30. Daniels CJ, Orsinelli DA (1997) Cardiac rupture with dobutamine stress echocardiography. J Am Soc Echocardiogr 10:979–981

31. Zamorano J, Moreno R, Almeria C, et al (2002) Left ventricular free wall rupture during dobutamine stress echocardiography. Rev Esp Cardiol 55:312–314

32. Varga A, Picano E, Lakatos F (2000) Fatal ventricular fibrillation during a low-dose dobutamine stress test. Am J Med 108:352–353

33. Shaheen J, Mendzelevski B, Tzivoni D (1996) Dobutamine-induced ST segment elevation and ventricular fibrillation with nonsignificant coronary artery disease. Am Heart J 132:1058–60

34. Yamagishi H, Watanabe H, Toda I, et al (1998) A case of dobutamine-induced coronary arterial spasm with ST-segment elevation. Jpn Circ J 62:150–151

35. Alvarez L, Zamorano J, Mataix L, et al (2002) Coronary Spasm after Administration of Propranolol during Dobutamine Stress Echocardiography. Rev Esp Cardiol 55:778–781

36. Weidmann B, Lepique CU, Jansen W, et al (1997) Myocardial infarction as a complication of dobutamine stress echocardiography. J Am Soc Echocardiogr 10:768–771

37. Takeuchi M, Sonoda S, Hanada H, et al (1997) Acute myocardial infarction in a patient during dobutamine stress echocardiography. Cathet Cardiovasc Diagn 41:404–406

38. Lanzarini L, Previtali M, Diotallevi P (1996) Syncope caused by cardiac asystole during dobutamine stress echocardiography. Heart 75:320–321

39. Salustri A, Biferali F, Palamara A (1997) Cardiac arrest during dobutamine stress echocardiography. G Ital Cardiol 27:69–71

40. Merli E, Sutcliffe S, Gori M, Sutherland GG (2006) Tako-Tsubo cardiomyopathy: new insights into the possible underlying pathophysiology. Eur J Echocardiogr 7:53–61

41. Coma-Canella I (1991) Changes in plasma potassium during the dobutamine stress test. Int J Cardiol 33:55–59

42. Tanimoto M, Pai RG, Jintapakorn W, Shah PM (1995) Mechanisms of hypotension during dobutamine stress echocardiography in patients with coronary artery disease. Am J Cardiol 76:26–30

43. Heinle SK, Tice FD, Kisslo J (1995) Hypotension during dobutamine stress echocardiography: is it related to dynamic intraventricular obstruction? Am Heart J 130:314–317

44. Galloway MT, Paglieroni TG, Wun T et al (1995) Platelet activation during dobutamine stress echocardiography. Am Heart J 135:888–900

45. Heijenbrok-Kal MH, Fleischmann KE, Hunink MG (2007) Stress echocardiography, stress single-photon-emission computed tomography and electron beam computed tomography for

the assessment of coronary artery disease: a meta-analysis of diagnostic performance. Am Heart J 154:415–423

46. Noguchi Y, Nagata-Kobayashi S, Stahl JE, et al (2005) meta-analytic comparison of echocardiographic stressors. Int J Cardiovasc Imag 21:189–207

47. Picano E Molinaro S, Pasanisi E (2008). The diagnostic accuracy of pharmacological stress echocardiography for the detection of coronary artery disease: a meta-analysis. Cardiovasc Ultrasound 6:30

48. Bax JJ, Poldermans D, Elhendy A, Boersma E, Rahimtoola SH (2001) Sensitivity, specificity, and predictive accuracies of various noninvasive techniques for detecting hibernating myocardium. Curr Probl Cardiol 26:141–186

49. Allman KC, Shaw LJ, Hachamovitch R, Udelson JE (2002) Myocardial viability testing and impact of revascularization on prognosis in patients with coronary artery disease and left ventricular dysfunction: a meta-analysis. J Am Coll Cardiol 39:1151–1158

50. Sicari R, Picano E, Landi P, Pingitore A, Bigi R, Coletta C, Heyman J, Casazza F, Previtali M, Mathias W Jr, Dodi C, Minardi G, Lowenstein J, Garyfallidis X, Cortigiani L, Morales MA, Raciti M (1997) Prognostic value of dobutamine-atropine stress echocardiography early after acute myocardial infarction. Echo Dobutamine International Cooperative (EDIC) Study. J Am Coll Cardiol 29:254–260

51. Picano E, Sicari R, Landi P, Cortigiani L, Bigi R, Coletta C, Galati A, Heyman J, Mattioli R, Previtali M, Mathias W Jr, Dodi C, Minardi G, Lowenstein J, Seveso G, Pingitore A, Salustri A, Raciti M (1998) Prognostic value of myocardial viability in medically treated patients with global left ventricular dysfunction early after an acute uncomplicated myocardial infarction: a dobutamine stress echocardiographic study. Circulation 15:1078–1084

52. Meluzin J, Cerny J, Frelich M, Stetka F, Spinarova L, Popelova J, Stipal R (1998) Prognostic value of the amount of dysfunctional but viable myocardium in revascularized patients with coronary artery disease and left ventricular dysfunction. Investigators of this Multicenter Study. J Am Coll Cardiol 32:912–920

53. Senior R, Kaul S, Lahiri A (1999) Myocardial viability on echocardiography predicts long-term survival after revascularization in patients with ischemic congestive heart failure. J Am Coll Cardiol 33:1848–1854

54. Sicari R, Picano E, Cortigiani L, Borges AC, Varga A, Palagi C, Bigi R, Rossini R, Pasanisi E; VIDA (Viability Identification with Dobutamine Administration) Study Group (2003).Prognostic value of myocardial viability recognized by low-dose dobutamine echocardiography in chronic ischemic left ventricular dysfunction. Am J Cardiol 92:1263–1266

55. Eichhorn J, Fink C, Bock M, Delorme S, Brockmeier K, Ulmer HE (2002). Images in cardiovascular medicine. Time-resolved three-dimensional magnetic resonance angiography for assessing a pulmonary artery sling in a pediatric patient. Circulation 106:e61–e62

56. Ciampi Q, Villari B (2007) Role of echocardiography in diagnosis and risk stratification in heart failure with left ventricular systolic dysfunction. Cardiovasc Ultrasound 5:34

57. Afridi I, Quinones MA, Zoghbi WA, Cheirif J (1994) Dobutamine stress echocardiography: sensitivity, specificity and predictive value for future cardiac events. Am Heart J 127:1510

58. Poldermans D, Fioretti PM, Boersma E, Cornel JH, Borst F, Vermeulen EG, Arnese M, el-Hendy A, Roelandt JR (1994) Dobutamine-atropine stress echocardiography and clinical data for predicting late cardiac events in patients with suspected coronary artery disease. Am J Med 97:119–125

59. Marcovitz PA, Shayna V, Horn RA, Hepner A, Armstrong WF (1996) Value of dobutamine stress echocardiography in determining the prognosis in patients with known or suspected coronary artery disease. Am J Cardiol 78:404–408

60. Steinberg EH, Madmon L, Patel CP, Sedlis SP, Kronzon I, Cohen JL (1997) Long-term prognostic significance of dobutamine echocardiography in patients with suspected coronary artery disease: results of a 5-Year follow-up study. J Am Coll Cardiol 29:269–273

61. Chuah SC, Pellikka PA, Roger VL, McCully RB, Seward JB (1998) Role of dobutamine stress echocardiography in predicting outcome in 860 patients with known or suspected coronary artery disease. Circulation 1998 97:1474–1480

62. Pingitore A, Picano E, Varga A, Gigli G, Cortigiani L, Previtali M, Minardi G, Colosso MQ, Lowenstein J, Mathias W Jr, Landi P (1999) Prognostic value of pharmacological stress echocardiography in patients with known or suspected coronary artery disease: a prospective, large-scale, multicenter, head-to-head comparison between dipyridamole and dobutamine test. Echo-Persantine International Cooperative (EPIC) and Echo-Dobutamine International Cooperative (EDIC) Study Groups. J Am Coll Cardiol 34:1769–1777

63. Krivokapich J, Child JS, Walter DO, Garfinkel A (1999) Prognostic value of dobutamine stress echocardiography in predicting cardiac events in patients with known or suspected coronary artery disease. J Am Coll Cardiol 33:708–716

64. Poldermans D, Fioretti PM, Boersma E, Bax JJ, Thomson IR, Roelandt JR, Simoons ML (1999) Long-term prognostic value of dobutamine-atropine stress echocardiography in 1737 patients with known or suspected coronary artery disease: a single-center experience. Circulation 99:757–762

65. Marwick TH, Case C, Sawada S, Rimmerman C, Brenneman P, Kovacs R, Short L, Lauer M (2001) Prediction of mortality using dobutamine echocardiography. J Am Coll Cardiol 37:754–760

66. Sicari R, Pasanisi E, Venneri L, Landi P, Cortigiani L, Picano E; Echo Persantine International Cooperative (EPIC) Study Group; Echo Dobutamine International Cooperative (EDIC) Study Group. (2003) Stress Echo Results Predict Mortality: a Large Scale Multicenter Prospective International Study. J Am Coll Cardiol 41:589–595

67. Carlos ME, Smart SC, Wynsen JC, Sagar KB (1997) Dobutamine stress echocardiography for risk stratification after myocardial infarction. Circulation 18:1402–1410

68. Greco CA, Salustri A, Seccareccia F, Ciavatti M, Biferali F, Valtorta C, Guzzardi G, Falcone M, Palamara A (1997) Prognostic value of dobutamine echocardiography early after uncomplicated acute myocardial infarction: a comparison with exercise electrocardiography. J Am Coll Cardiol 29:261–267

69. Picano E, Sicari R, Landi P, Cortigiani L, Bigi R, Coletta C, Galati A, Heyman J, Mattioli R, Previtali M, Mathias W Jr, Dodi C, Minardi G, Lowenstein J, Seveso G, Pingitore A, Salustri A, Raciti M (1998) Prognostic value of myocardial viability in medically treated patients with global left ventricular dysfunction early after an acute uncomplicated myocardial infarction: a dobutamine stress echocardiographic study. Circulation 98:1078–1084

70. Previtali M, Fetiveau R, Lanzarini L, Cavalotti C, Klersy C (1998) Prognostic value of myocardial viability and ischemia detected by dobutamine stress echocardiography early after acute myocardial infarction treated with thrombolysis. J Am Coll Cardiol 32:380–386

71. Sicari R, Landi P, Picano E, Pirelli S, Chiaranda G, Previtali M, Seveso G, Gandolfo N, Margaria F, Magaia O, Minardi G, Mathias W (2002) Exercise-electrocardiography and/ or pharmacological stress echocardiography for non-invasive risk stratification early after uncomplicated myocardial infarction. A prospective international large scale multicentre study. Eur Heart J 23:1030–1037

72. Eichelberger JP, Schwarz KQ, Black ER, Green RM, Ouriel K (1993) Predictive value of dobutamine echocardiography just before noncardiac vascular surgery. Am J Cardiol 72:602–607

73. Davila-Roman VG, Waggoner AD, Sicard GA, Geltman EM, Schechtman KB, Perez JE (1993) Dobutamine stress echocardiography predicts surgical outcome in patients with an aortic aneurysm and peripheral vascular disease. J Am Coll Cardiol 21:957–963

74. Poldermans D, Arnese M, Fioretti PM, Salustri A, Boersma E, Thomson IR, Roelandt JR, van Urk H (1995) Improved cardiac risk stratification in major vascular surgery with dobutamine-atropine stress echocardiography. J Am Coll Cardiol 26:648–653

75. Poldermans D, Arnese M, Fioretti PM, Boersma E, Thomson IR, Rambaldi R, van Urk H (1997) Sustained prognostic value of dobutamine stress echocardiography for late cardiac events after major noncardiac vascular surgery. Circulation 195:53–58

76. Shaw LJ, Peterson ED, Kesler K, Hasselblad V, Califf RM (1996) Meta-analysis of intravenous dipyridamole-thallium-201 imaging (1985 to 1994) and dobutamine echocardiography (1991 to 1994) for risk stratification before vascular surgery. Am J Cardiol 78:1327–1337

77. Kertai MD, Boersma E, Bax JJ, Heijenbrok-Kal MH, Hunink MG, L'talien GJ, Roelandt JR, van Urk H, Poldermans D (2003). A meta-analysis comparing the prognostic accuracy of six diagnostic tests for predicting perioperative cardiac risk in patients undergoing major vascular surgery. Heart 89:1327–1334

78. Beattie WS, Abdelnaem E, Wijeysundera DN (2006) A meta-analytic comparison of preoperative stress echocardiography and nuclear scintigraphy imaging. Anesth Analg 102:8–16

79. Vahanian A, Alfieri O, Al-Attar N, et al; European Association of Cardio-Thoracic Surgery; European Society of Cardiology; European Association of Percutaneous Cardiovascular Interventions. (2008) Transcatheter valve implantation for patients with aortic stenosis: a position statement from the European Association of Cardio-Thoracic Surgery (EACTS) and the European Society of Cardiology (ESC), in collaboration with the European Association of Percutaneous Cardiovascular Interventions (EAPCI). Eur Heart J 29:1463–1470

80. Minardi G, Di Segni M, Manzara CC, et al (1997) Diagnostic and prognostic value of dipyridamole and dobutamine stress echocardiography in patients with Q-wave acute myocardial infarction. Am J Cardiol 80:847–851

81. Schröder K, Wieckhorst A, Völler H (1997) Comparison of the prognostic value of dipyridamole and dobutamine stress echocardiography in patients with known or suspected coronary artery disease. Am J Cardiol 79:1516–1518

82. Schinkel AF, Bax JJ, Elhendy A, van Domburg RT, et al (2004)-term prognostic value of dobutamine stress echocardiography compared with myocardial perfusion scanning in patients unable to perform exercise tests. Am J Med 117:1–9

83. Douglas PS, Khandheria B, Raymond F. et al (2008) ACCF/ASE/ACEP/AHA/ASNC/SCAI/SCCT/SCMR 2008 Appropriateness criteria for stress echocardiography: a report of the American College of Cardiology Foundation Appropriateness Criteria Task Force, American Society of Echocardiography, American College of Emergency Physicians, American Heart Association, American Society of Nuclear Cardiology, Society for Cardiovascular Angiography and Interventions, Society of Cardiovascular Computed Tomography, and Society for Cardiovascular Magnetic Resonance Endorsed by the Heart Rhythm Society and the Society of Critical Care Medicine. J Am Coll Cardiol 51:1127–1147

84. Beleslin BD, Ostojic M, Stepanovic J, et al (1994). Stress echocardiography in the detection of myocardial ischemia. Head-to-head comparison of exercise, dobutamine, and dipyridamole tests. Circulation 90:1168–1176

85. Cortigiani L, Bigi R, Rigo F, et al; Echo Persantine International Cooperative Study Group (2003). Diagnostic value of exercise electrocardiography and dipyridamole stress echocardiography in hypertensive and normotensive chest pain patients with right bundle branch block. J Hypertens 21:2189–2194

Dipyridamole Stress Echocardiography 13

Eugenio Picano

13.1
Historical Background

Dipyridamole was the first pharmacological stress agent used for the diagnosis of coronary artery disease, with a pioneering indicator proposed in Europe for the identification of ischemia during stress echocardiography [1] and later in the USA by Lance Gould as hyperemic stress perfusion imaging [2]. Its main cardiac imaging applications stem from two fundamental properties, which are the two imaging sides of the same pathophysiological coin of coronary arteriolar vasodilation: the hyperemic effect and the proischemic effect [3]. The hyperemic is the conceptual basis for myocardial perfusion imaging, usually with radionuclide scintigraphy but today also with cardiovascular magnetic resonance (CMR) [4]. The ischemic effect is the requisite for functional imaging, usually with two-dimensional (2D) echocardiography (Fig. 13.1), but today also performed with CMR [5]. The two entities – hyperemic stress and ischemic stress – are closely linked and can be considered as two different aspects of the same phenomenon, which requires endogenous adenosine accumulation as the common biochemical pathway (Table 13.1). The predominance of the hyperemic over the ischemic manifestation will depend on the dose of dipyridamole (determining the amount of adenosine accumulation) and on the underlying coronary anatomy. With relatively low intravenous dipyridamole doses, in the presence of absent to moderate coronary artery disease, the hyperemic effect will prevail. With relatively high doses, in the presence of moderate to severe coronary artery disease, the ischemic effect will dominate. With echocardiography imaging that requires ischemia as a mandatory end point, testing began with relatively low doses (0.56 mg kg^{-1} over 4 min), which gave low sensitivity values [6]. Later, more aggressive doses were adopted (up to 0.84 mg kg^{-1} over 10 min) [7]. Finally it was coadministered with atropine [8]) or – more simply – with a high dose but a shorter infusion time (the accelerated protocol) [9], which overcame the limitation of less than ideal sensitivity to minor forms of coronary artery disease, especially in patients receiving antianginal therapy (Fig. 13.2). The two lines of functional (wall motion) and hyperemic (coronary flow reserve) imaging are destined to converge conceptually and clinically with the diffusion of new-generation imaging technologies such as myocar-

E. Picano, *Stress Echocardiography*,
© Springer-Verlag Berlin Heidelberg 2009

DIPYRIDAMOLE PEDIGREE

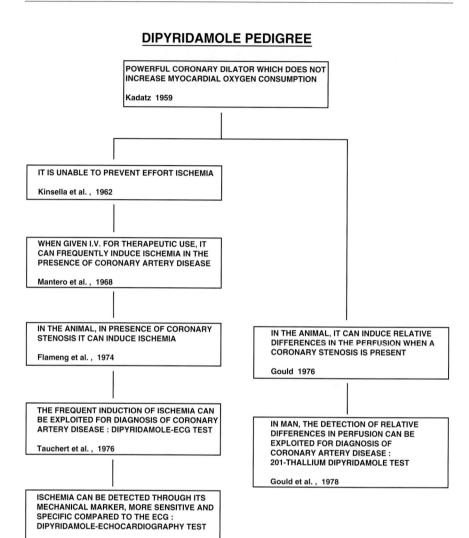

Fig. 13.1 Dipyridamole stress pedigree. On the *left*, the ischemic arm and on the right the hyperemic arm. The pioneer of dipyridamole as an exercise-independent stress test was Martin Tauchert, a German cardiologist who proposed dipyridamole ECG. Only years later did Lance Gould introduce the concept of vasodilator stress imaging, which did not conceptually require myocardial ischemia for test positivity. In recent years, it became clear that wall motion information can be ideally added to perfusion imaging, during contrast echocardiography or coronary flow imaging of the left anterior descending artery. The two arms (hyperemic and ischemic) of dipyridamole stress are destined to merge with last-generation dual imaging stress echocardiography or stress cardiovascular magnetic resonance imaging. (Modified from [3])

Table 13.1 The dual nature of dipyridamole stress

Parameter	Hyperemic imaging	Ischemic imaging
End point	Flow heterogeneity	Wall motion abnormality
Ischemia required	No	Yes
Dominant imaging technique	Radionuclide scintigraphy	Two-dimensional echocardiography
Dose–effect response	Flat over 0.56 mg/kg	Steep up to 0.84 mg/kg
Optimal use	0.56 mg/kg	0.84 mg/kg

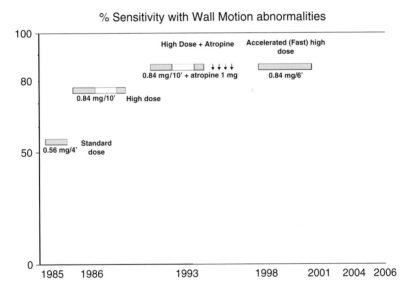

Fig. 13.2 Evolving dipyridamole stress echocardiography protocols over the years. The most sensitive and accurate protocols proposed over the last 15 years are the high dose (0.84 mg kg^{-1} in 10 min) with atropine up to 1 mg (recommended by the American Society of Echocardiography guidelines in 1998 and 2007) or the fast (or accelerated) high dose (0.84 mg kg^{-1} in 6 min). The latter is currently endorsed as the state-of-the-art protocol by the European Association of Echocardiography 2008 recommendations, and is usually preferred since the imaging time is shorter and no multiple drug administration is needed. (Modified from [83], with permission)

dial contrast echocardiography [10] and coronary flow velocity imaging [11], which will allow simultaneous assessment of flow and function at the same high, fast infusion protocol, which is currently recommended as state of the art by the European Association of Echocardiography (EAE) [12]. The fast high-dose dipyridamole protocol is the best choice to kill "two birds with one stone", i.e., to image function and perfusion (two birds) in one

13

sitting with a single stress (one stone). This approach is obviously simpler than the "two birds, two stones" approach (with separate testing of perfusion with low-dose adenosine or dipyridamole and function with dobutamine). It is, however, imperative that your "stone" (stress) is of sufficient weight (high cumulative dose) and thrown with sufficient speed (fast infusion rate) to kill the two diagnostic birds.

13.2
Pharmacology and Pathophysiology

Dipyridamole is a vasodilator test that reduces myocardial oxygen supply through flow maldistribution (steal) phenomena by stimulating $A2_A$ adenosinergic receptors present on the endothelial and smooth muscle cells of coronary arterioles. Acting indirectly, dipyridamole increases endogenous adenosine levels by reduction of cellular reuptake and metabolism. It acts as a prodrug, increasing the interstitial levels of adenosine by the combined effect of inhibition of cellular uptake of adenosine and inhibition of its breakdown by adenosine deaminase. The peak vasodilatory effect is obtained 4–8 min after the end of infusion, and the half-life is 6 h [3], which suggests that the antidote aminophylline that blocks adenosine receptors should be routinely given at the end of the stress, even in negative cases. The dipyridamole dose usually employed for stress echocardiography testing (0.84 mg kg^{-1}) causes a three- to fourfold increase in coronary blood flow in normals [13] over resting values and a threefold increase in adenosine concentration in systemic venous blood [14].

Dipyridamole provokes ischemia mainly through steal phenomena [3], although the coadministration of atropine may also increase myocardial oxygen demand to a significant extent. Coronary collateral circulation represents a steal-prone coronary anatomy, probably providing the morphological background facilitating horizontal steal phenomena [15]. In the absence of collateral circulation, the most likely mechanism of dipyridamole-induced ischemia is the vertical steal [3]. The regional coronary flow in the ischemia-producing vessel remains unchanged when dipyridamole doses are increased from subischemic to ischemic [16], suggesting that an ischemic dysfunction develops for a transmural flow redistribution, causing hypoperfusion of the subendocardial layer. The flow increase is also considered to be important for the inotropic response of viable myocardium. In fact, the increased coronary flow reserve of hibernating myocardium is mirrored by the myocardial inotropic reserve in segments with resting dysfunction [17]. The cardioprotective effect on viable myocardium can also be evoked by very low, subhyperemic doses [18]. The three effects – viability, hyperemia, and ischemia – are elicited with different, increasing doses [19] observed one after the other during a single stress with dose titration [19]: Fig. 13.3. The exposure of vulnerable myocardium to the sunlight of coronary blood flow leads to three separate or sometimes overlapping effects: the "cold light" of the viability effect, the "warning" of regular-dose hyperemia, and the "burning" with high-dose ischemia.

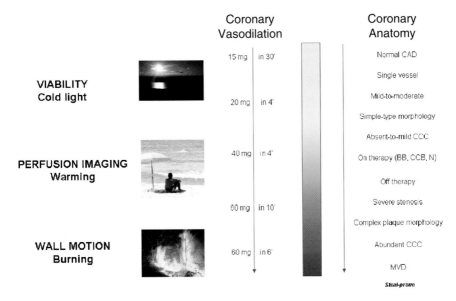

Fig. 13.3 The pathophysiological effects of dipyridamole at different dose windows and as a function of the underlying coronary anatomy in the individual patient. The proischemic, myocardial burning effects dominate at the higher doses; the cardioprotective, cold light effect at very low doses, and the warming hyperemic effect at intermediate doses. (From [37])

13.3
Methodology

The standard or regular dipyridamole protocol consists of an intravenous infusion of $0.84\,mg\ kg^{-1}$ over 10 min, in two separate infusions: $0.56\,mg\ kg^{-1}$ over 4 min (standard dose), followed by 4 min of no dose and, if still negative, and additional $0.28\,mg\ kg^{-1}$ over 2 min. If no end point is reached, atropine (doses of 0.25 mg up to a maximum of 1 mg) is added, as recommended by the guidelines of the American Society of Echocardiography for a decade [20, 21]. The same overall dose of $0.84\,mg\ kg^{-1}$ can also be given over 6 min, as currently suggested by the 2008 recommendations of the European Association of Echocardiography [12]. Aminophylline (240 mg IV) should be available for immediate use in case an adverse dipyridamole-related event occurs and routinely infused at the end of the test, regardless of the result.

For a selective assessment of myocardial viability, a very low dose of dipyridamole ($0.28\,mg\ kg^{-1}$) has the same diagnostic accuracy as low-dose dobutamine [18, 22]. In special subsets of patients in whom a very high sensitivity for the diagnosis of coronary artery disease is required, high-dose dipyridamole ($0.84\,mg\ kg^{-1}$) can be followed by maximal exercise [23, 10] or – less safely – by high-dose dobutamine [24]. Whenever suitable technology and dedicated expertise are available, it is recommended to perform dual imaging vasodilator stress echocardiography with combined wall motion and coronary flow reserve assessment with pulsed Doppler velocity imaging on the left anterior descending coronary artery [11, 12] (Fig. 13.4).

All caffeine-containing foods (coffee, tea, chocolate, bananas, and cola drinks) should be avoided for 12 h before testing, and all theophylline-containing drugs (aminophylline) should be discontinued for at least 24 h.

13.4
Feasibility and Safety

Minor but limiting side effects preclude the achievement of maximal pharmacological stress in less than 5% of patients [25]. In order of frequency, they are hypotension and/or bradycardia, headache, dizziness, and/or nausea. Roughly two-thirds of patients studied with the high-dose dipyridamole protocol experience minor side effects such as flushing and headache, which reflect the systemic vasodilatory effect of the drug. These side effects usually disappear following administration of aminophylline at the end of testing. On rare occasions, dipyridamole-induced ischemia becomes resistant to aminophylline [26]. In these cases, the marked late rise in the rate–pressure product during the test, which is due to sympathetic excitatory reflexes triggered by ischemia, exceeds the ischemic threshold on effort, maintaining ischemia when the flow maldistribution has been reversed by administration of aminophylline. In these cases, the administration of nitrates is necessary to reverse ischemia. Aminophylline is routinely given at the end of testing, also in negative cases, but on rare occasions it may trigger coronary vasospasm in about one-third of patients with variant angina: transient ST-segment elevation is the usual pattern, and nitrates (not further aminophylline or beta-blockers!) should be given immediately to relieve spasm [27]. Major life-threatening complications – i.e., myocardial infarction, third-degree atrioventricular block, cardiac asystole, sustained ventricular tachycardia, or pulmonary edema – occur in about 1 in 1,000 cases, as shown by series encompassing over 35,000 patients with high-dose stress echocardiography techniques [26, 28, 29]. The test induces major complications three times less frequently than dobutamine [28–30] (Table 13.2).

13.5
Diagnostic Results for Detection of Coronary Artery Disease

The accuracy in detecting angiographically assessed coronary artery disease has been consistently shown to be high, with sensitivity and specificity 72% and 95%, respectively, in a meta-analysis of 58 studies (all generations of protocols included) [31]. The diagnostic accuracy is similar to other forms of stress testing, such as exercise echocardiography or stress SPECT [31]. When state-of-the-art protocols are used for both stresses [32–36], the sensitivity, specificity, and accuracy of fast (or atropine-potentiated) high-dose dipyridamole is identical to dobutamine stress echocardiography, as shown by a meta-analysis including five studies with 435 patients [37]: Fig. 13.5.

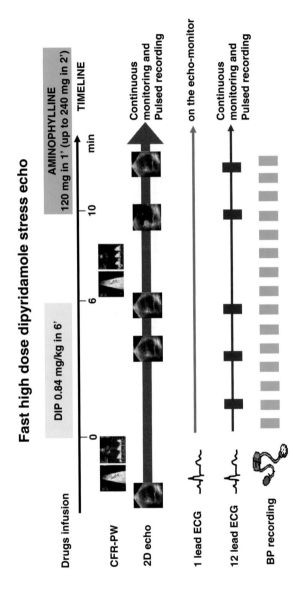

Fig. 13.4 The state-of-the-art protocol of high-dose, fast dipyridamole echocardiography test with dual imaging (wall motion and coronary flow reserve on the left anterior descending coronary artery)

Table 13.2 Safety profile of pharmacologic stress echocardiography

	Dobutamine	Dipyridamole
% Submaximal tests	10%	5%
Side effects	1/300 exams	1/1,000
VT, VF	++	+
High-grade AV block	+	++
Death	1/5,000	1/10,000

VT ventricular tachycardia, *VF* ventricular fibrillation

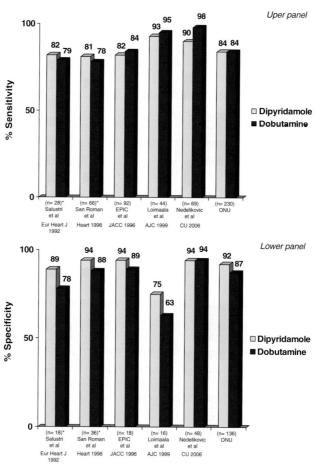

Fig. 13.5 Sensitivity (*upper panel*) and specificity (*lower panel*) for 5 individual studies and cumulative analysis of dipyridamole vs dobutamine stress echocardiography. Asterisk indicates fast dipyridamole protocol; no asterisk is the high dose plus atropine protocol

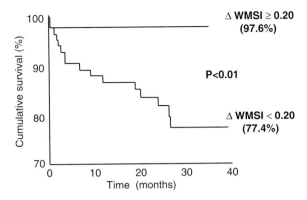

Fig. 13.6 Kaplan–Meier survival curves (with the end point as death only) in patients undergoing coronary revascularization. Myocardial viability could be distinguished by the number of segments which had improved, using as a cut-off value the difference between the resting wall motion score index and the low-dose dipyridamole wall motion score index (delta WMSI) set at 0.20. A small amount of viable myocardium is associated with a greater incidence of cardiac death ($p<0.01$). (From [38])

13.6
Viability

Very-low-dose (0.28 mg kg^{-1}) dipyridamole recognizes myocardial viability with high specificity (higher than dobutamine) [18], good sensitivity (lower than dobutamine) [22], and excellent prognostic value (comparable to dobutamine) [38] (Fig. 13.6).

13.7
Prognostic Value

The prognostic value of dipyridamole stress echocardiography based on wall motion abnormalities has been extensively proven, confirmed, and reconfirmed in different subsets of patients with chronic coronary artery disease [39–42], recent myocardial infarction [43–49], or major noncardiac vascular surgery [50–55]. The prognostic value has been extensively demonstrated in special patient subsets, including hypertensives [56, 57], elderly patients [58], women [59], patients with left bundle branch block [60], with right bundle branch block and/or left anterior hemiblock [61], outpatients [62], patients with single-vessel disease [63], and in a chest pain unit [64, 65]. Dipyridamole stress results can predict subsequent cardiac death, mainly on the basis of two parameters: dipyridamole time (i.e., the interval between test onset and appearance of obvious dyssynergies) and peak wall motion score index (Fig. 13.7). The prognostic value of dipyridamole stress echocardiography is independent of and additive to simpler clinical and laboratory variables such as resting echocardiography and exercise electrocardiography testing, and it has also been confirmed by prospective large-scale multicenter studies [45, 49] (Table 13.3).

13

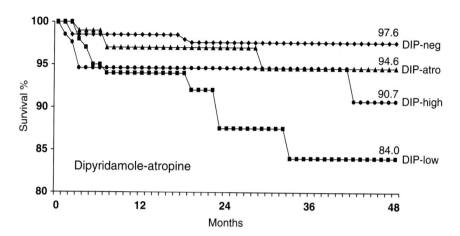

Fig. 13.7 Kaplan–Meier survival curves free of cardiac death in patients with negative and positive dipyridamole echocardiography tests (*DIP*). Survival is worse in patients with positive DIP. In patients with positive DIP, progressively worse survival is identified with positivity after atropine of high and low dose. DIP + low dose vs. DIP negative, $p<0.0001$. Cardiac death ($n = 18$); follow-up 38 $\pm$ 21 months. (Modified from [75])

Table 13.3 Life-threatening complications in multicenter studies (EPIC) and multicenter registries for dipyridamole stress (scintigraphy or echocardiography)

Author, year	Patients	Complications
Multicenter registry		
Picano et al. 1992	10,451	1 cardiac death, 1 asystole, 2 acute myocardial infarctions, 1 pulmonary edema, 1 sustained ventricular tachycardia
Varga et al. 2006	24,599	19 (1 death)
Total	108,856	60

Ongoing ischemic therapy at the time of testing not only lowers the diagnostic sensitivity in a way somewhat symmetrical to the effects on exercise testing [66], but also heavily modulates the prognostic value of pharmacological stress echocardiography. In the presence of concomitant anti-ischemic therapy, a positive test is more prognostically malignant, and a negative test less prognostically benign [67]. The prognostic value of dipyridamole stress echocardiography has also been evaluated in direct head-to-head comparisons with other forms of stress testing, and it was shown to be similar to dobutamine echocardiography [55, 68–70] and probably better than perfusion scintigraphy [47, 53].

The prognostic information supplied by vasodilator stress echocardiography based on wall motion (functional) imaging has been recently expanded with the systematic use of dual imaging and with combined wall motion and coronary flow reserve imaging [11, 71–74]. The use of coronary flow reserve as a stand-alone diagnostic criterion suffers from many structural limitations that render it little more than an academic toy: firstly, only the

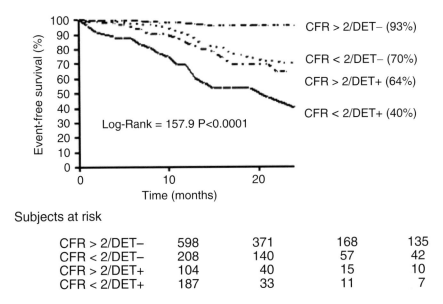

Fig. 13.8 The additive prognostic value of wall motion and coronary flow reserve. (Modified from [77])

left anterior descending (LAD) artery is sampled, and secondly, the coronary flow reserve cannot distinguish between microvascular and macrovascular coronary disease [75, 13]. Therefore, it is more interesting (and clinically plausible) to evaluate the additive value over conventional wall motion for prognostic stratification. From the pathophysiologic viewpoint, wall motion positivity requires ischemia and epicardial artery stenosis as a necessary prerequisite, whereas coronary flow reserve can be normal only if microvascular integrity is also preserved. The combination of conventional wall motion analysis with 2D echocardiography and coronary flow reserve with pulsed Doppler flowmetry of the mid-distal left anterior descending (LAD) artery has been shown to provide an added and complementary power of prognostication in patients with known or suspected coronary artery disease [76–78], normal coronary arteries [79, 80], diabetes [81, 82], and idiopathic dilated cardiomyopathy [83, 84]. A reduced coronary flow reserve is an additional parameter of severity in the risk stratification of the stress echocardiographic response, whereas patients with a negative test for wall motion criteria and normal coronary flow reserve have a favorable outcome during dipyridamole stress echocardiography (Fig. 13.8).

13.8
Indications and Contraindications

Fast, high-dose dipyridamole stress echocardiography is an appropriate choice for pharmacological stress echocardiography used for the detection of coronary artery disease, especially in patients with inability to exercise or contraindications to exercise, or with

Table 13.4 Indications to dipyridamole stress echocardiography

	Appropriate	Uncertain	Inappropriate
Diagnosis of CAD in patients unable to exercise	√		
Diagnosis of CAD in patients with sufficient image quality	√		
High-risk noncardiac surgery in intermediate risk patients	√		
Need to evaluate therapy efficacy in patients unable to exercise		√	
Intermediate-risk noncardiac surgery in intermediate-risk patients		√	
Diagnosis of viability in EF<35% and intolerant to dobutamine		√	
First-line test in patients capable to exercise and good acoustic window			√
Asthma, theophylline therapy			√
Chronic dipyridamole therapy, recent (<12 h) coffee, tea, chocolate ingestion			√

EF ejection fraction, *CAD* coroany artery disease

resting images of borderline quality, making exercise echocardiography especially challenging. It is technically easier than exercise or dobutamine, since the image quality is less degraded by tachycardia, hyperventilation, and hypercontractility [85, 86]: "from the technical viewpoint, dipyridamole is the elementary school, dobutamine the secondary school, and exercise the university in the stress echo cursus studiorum" [86]. It is equally accurate, and technically easier [85, 86] and safer, than dobutamine stress echocardiography: as clearly stated by the 2008 EAE recommendations, "exercise is safer than pharmacological stress. Among pharmacological stresses, dipyridamole is safer than dobutamine" [12]. It is subjectively better tolerated by the patients than adenosine [87]. Dipyridamole stress echocardiography is also appropriate in intermediate-risk patients undergoing elective high-risk noncardiac surgery. Appropriateness is uncertain in intermediate-risk patients undergoing intermediate-risk noncardiac surgery (Table 13.4). For the identification of myocardial viability in patients in whom low-dose dobutamine is unsafe or not tolerated, low-dose dipyridamole can be an effective alternative, although the appropriateness of the specific indication is restricted by limited experience. Patients with second- or third-degree atrioventricular block or with sick sinus syndrome should not receive dipyridamole (unless they have a functioning pacemaker). Also, patients with bronchial asthma or a tendency to bronchospasm are not indicated for dipyridamole testing. Patients using dipyridamole chronically should not undergo adenosine testing for at least 24 h after withdrawal of therapy, because their blood levels of adenosine could be unpredictably high. Withdrawal of long-term theophylline or caffeine for at least 24 h is also required in order to have adenosine receptors free. The main differences between dipyridamole and dobutamine stress

Table 13.5 Pharmacological test for detection of coronary stenosis

	Vasodilator	Dobutamine
Receptor target	A2A adenosine	Alpha-1; beta-1; beta-2 adrenergic
Hemodynamics	Reduces supply	Increases demand
Physiological targets	Coronary arterioles	Myocardium
Cellular target	Smooth muscle cells	Myocytes
Antidote	Aminophylline	β-Blockers
Stress	Dipyridamole (adenosine)	Dobutamine
Contraindications	Asthmatic disease, bradyarrhythmias	Tachyarrhythmias, uncontrolled hypertension

echocardiography are reported in Table 13.5. Inotropic and vasodilator stresses should both be used in a stress echocardiography laboratory, for several reasons. Basically, each test has different limitations and specific advantages: a versatile use of both makes it possible to tailor the stress to the individual patient. Whatever type of stress is the laboratory's first choice, in the case of submaximal results due to limiting side effects, the second choice should be used, to avoid the inaccuracies of nondiagnostic submaximal testing.

References

1. Tauchert M, Behrenbeck DW, Hotzel J, et al (1976) A new pharmacological test for diagnosing coronary artery disease. Dtsch Med Wochenschr 101:35–37
2. Gould KL, Westcott RJ, Albro PC, et al (1978) Noninvasive assessment of coronary stenoses by myocardial imaging during pharmacologic coronary vasodilatation. II. Clinical methodology and feasibility. Am J Cardiol 41:279–287
3. Picano E (1989) Dipyridamole-echocardiography test: historical background and physiologic basis. Eur Heart J 10:365–376
4. Bodi V, Sanchis J, Lopez-Lereu MP, et al (2007) Prognostic value of dipyridamole stress cardiovascular magnetic resonance imaging in patients with known or suspected coronary artery disease. J Am Coll Cardiol 50:1174–1179
5. Pingitore A, Lombardi M, Scattini B, et al (2008) Head to head comparison between perfusion and function during accelerated high-dose dipyridamole magnetic resonance stress for the detection of coronary artery disease. Am J Cardiol 101:8–14
6. Picano E, Distante A, Masini M, et al (1985) Dipyridamole-echocardiography test in effort angina pectoris. Am J Cardiol 56:452–456
7. Picano E, Lattanzi F, Masini M, et al (1986) High dose dipyridamole echocardiography test in effort angina pectoris. J Am Coll Cardiol 8:848–854
8. Picano E, Pingitore A, Conti U, et al (1993) Enhanced sensitivity for detection of coronary artery disease by addition of atropine to dipyridamole echocardiography. Eur Heart J 14:1216–1222
9. Dal Porto R, Faletra F, Picano E, et al (2001) Safety, feasibility, and diagnostic accuracy of accelerated high-dose dipyridamole stress echocardiography. Am J Cardiol 87:520–524

10. Moir S, Haluska BA, Jenkins C, et al (2004) Incremental benefit of myocardial contrast to combined dipyridamole-exercise stress echocardiography for the assessment of coronary artery disease. Circulation 110:1108–1113

11. Rigo F, Richieri M, Pasanisi E, et al (2003) Usefulness of coronary flow reserve over regional wall motion when added to dual-imaging dipyridamole echocardiography. Am J Cardiol 91:269–273

12. Sicari R, Nihoyannopoulos P, Evangelista A, et al; European Association of Echocardiography (2008) Stress echocardiography expert consensus statement: European Association of Echocardiography (EAE) (a registered branch of the ESC). Eur J Echocardiogr 9:415–437

13. Rigo F (2005) Coronary flow reserve in stress-echo lab. From pathophysiologic toy to diagnostic tool. Cardiovasc Ultrasound 3:8

14. Laghi-Pasini F, Guideri F, Petersen C, et al (2003) Blunted increase in plasma adenosine levels following dipyridamole stress in dilated cardiomyopathy patients. J Intern Med 254:591–596

15. Gliozheni E, Picano E, Bernardino L, et al (1996) Angiographically assessed coronary collateral circulation increases vulnerability to myocardial ischemia during vasodilator stress testing. Am J Cardiol 78:1419–1424

16. Hutchinson SJ, Shen A, Soldo S, et al (1996) Transesophageal assessment of coronary flow velocity reserve during "regular" and "high"-dose dipyridamole stress testing. Am J Cardiol 77:1164–1168

17. Torres MA, Picano E, Parodi G, et al (1997) Flow-function relation in patients with chronic coronary artery disease and reduced regional function. A positron emission tomographic and two-dimensional echocardiographic study with coronary vasodilator stress. J Am Coll Cardiol 30:65–70

18. Varga A, Ostojic M, Djordjevic-Dikic A, et al (1996) Infra-low dose dipyridamole test. A novel dose regimen for selective assessment of myocardial viability by vasodilator stress echocardiography. Eur Heart J 17:629–634

19. Picano E (2002) Dipyridamole in myocardial ischemia: Good Samaritan or Terminator? Int J Cardiol 83:215–216

20. Armstrong WF, Pellikka PA, Ryan T, et al (1998) Stress echocardiography: recommendations for performance and interpretation of stress echocardiography. Stress Echocardiography Task Force of the Nomenclature and Standards Committee of the American Society of Echocardiography. J Am Soc Echocardiogr 11:97–104

21. Pellikka PA, Nagueh SF, Elhendy AA, et al; American Society of Echocardiography (2007) American Society of Echocardiography recommendations for performance, interpretation, and application of stress echocardiography. J Am Soc Echocardiogr 20:1021–1041

22. Picano E, Ostojic M, Varga A, et al (1996) Combined low-dose dipyridamole-dobutamine stress echocardiography to identify myocardial viability. J Am Coll Cardiol 27:1422–1428

23. Picano E, Lattanzi F, Masini M, et al (1988) Usefulness of the dipyridamole-exercise echocardiography test for diagnosis of coronary artery disease. Am J Cardiol 62:67–70

24. Ostojic M, Picano E, Beleslin B, et al (1994) Dipyridamole-dobutamine echocardiography: a novel test for the detection of milder forms of coronary artery disease. J Am Coll Cardiol 23:1115–1122

25. Picano E, Marini C, Pirelli S, et al (1992) Safety of intravenous high-dose dipyridamole echocardiography. The Echo-Persantine International Cooperative Study Group. Am J Cardiol 70:252–8

26. Picano E, Lattanzi F, Distante A, et al (1989) Role of myocardial oxygen consumption in dipyridamole-induced ischemia. Am Heart J 118:314–319

27. Picano E, Lattanzi F, Masini M, et al (1988) Aminophylline termination of dipyridamole stress as a trigger of coronary vasospasm in variant angina. Am J Cardiol 62:694–697

28. Varga A, Garcia MA, Picano E; International Stress Echo Complication Registry (2006) Safety of stress echocardiography (from the International Stress Echo Complication Registry). Am J Cardiol 98:541–54

29. Beckmann S, Haug G (1999) National registry 1995–1998 on 150.000 stress echo examinations side effects and complications in 60,448 examinations of the registry 1997–1998. Circulation 100(suppl):3401A

30. Picano E, Mathias W Jr, Pingitore A, Bigi R, Previtali M (1994) Safety and tolerability of dobutamine-atropine stress echocardiography: a prospective, multicentre study. Echo Dobutamine International Cooperative Study Group. Lancet 344:1190–1192

31. Heijenbrok-Kal MH, Fleischmann KE, Hunink MG (2007) Stress echocardiography, stress single-photon-emission computed tomography and electron beam computed tomography for the assessment of coronary artery disease: a meta-analysis of diagnostic performance. Am Heart J 154:415–423

32. Salustri A, Fioretti PM,McNeill AJ, et al (1992) Pharmacological stress echocardiography in the diagnosis of coronary artery disease and myocardial ischaemia: a comparison between dobutamine and dipyridamole. Eur Heart J 13:1356–1362

33. Pingitore A, Picano E, Quarta Colosso M, et al (1996) The atropine factor in pharmacologic stress echocardiography. Echo Persantine (EPIC) and Echo Dobutamine International Cooperative (EDIC) Study Groups. J Am Coll Cardiol 27:1164–1170

34. San Román JA, Vilacosta I, Castillo JA, et al (1998) Selection of the optimal stress test for the diagnosis of coronary artery disease. Heart 80:370–376

35. Loimaala A,Groundstroem K, Pasanen M, et al (1999) Comparison of bicycle, heavy isometric, dipyridamole-atropine and dobutamine stress echocardiography for diagnosis of myocardial ischemia. Am J Cardiol 84:1396–1400

36. Nedeljkovic I, Ostojic M, Beleslin B, et al (2006) Comparison of exercise, dobutamine-atropine and dipyridamole-atropine stress echocardiography in detecting coronary artery disease. Cardiovasc Ultrasound 4:22

37. Picano E, Molinaro S, Pasanisi E (2008) The diagnostic accuracy of pharmacological stress echocardiography for the assessment of coronary artery disease: a meta-analysis. Cardiovasc Ultrasound 6:30

38. Sicari R, Ripoli A, Picano E, et al; VIDA (Viability Identification with Dipyridamole Administration) Study Group (2001) The prognostic value of myocardial viability recognized by low dose dipyridamole echocardiography in patients with chronic ischaemic left ventricular dysfunction. Eur Heart J 22:837–844

39. Picano E, Severi S, Michelassi C, et al (1989) Prognostic importance of dipyridamole echocardiography test in coronary artery disease. Circulation 80:450–457

40. Severi S, Picano E, Michelassi C, et al (1994) Diagnostic and prognostic value of dipyridamole echocardiography in patients with suspected coronary artery disease. Comparison with exercise electrocardiography. Circulation 89:1160–1173

41. Coletta C, Galati A, Greco G, et al (1995) Prognostic value of high-dose dipyridamole echocardiography in patients with chronic coronary artery disease and preserved left ventricular function. J Am Coll Cardiol 26:887–894

42. Sicari R, Pasanisi E,Venneri L, et al on behalf of the Echo-Persantine International Cooperative (EPIC) and Echo-Dobutamine International Cooperative (EDIC) Study Groups (2003) Stress echo results predict mortality: a large-scale multicenter prospective international study. J Am Coll Cardiol 19:589–595

43. Bolognese L, Rossi L, Sarasso G, et al (1992) Silent versus symptomatic dipyridamole induced ischemia after myocardial infarction: clinical and prognostic significance. J Am Coll Cardiol 19:953–959

44. Sclavo MG, Noussan P, Pallisco O, et al (1992) Usefulness of dipyridamole-echocardiographic test to identify jeopardized myocardium after thrombolysis. Limited clinical predictivity of dipyridamole-echocardiographic test in convalescing acute myocardial infarction: correlation with coronary angiography. Eur Heart J 13:1348–1355

45. Picano E, Landi P, Bolognese L, et al (1993) Prognostic value of dipyridamole echocardiography early after uncomplicated myocardial infarction: a large-scale, multicenter trial. The EPIC Study Group. Am J Med 95:608–618

46. Chiarella F, Domenicucci S, Bellotti P, et al (1994) Dipyridamole echocardiographic test performed 3 days after an acute myocardial infarction: feasibility, tolerability, safety and in-hospital prognostic value. Eur Heart J 15:842–850

47. Van Daele ME, McNeill AJ, Fioretti PM, et al (1994) Prognostic value of dipyridamole sestamibi single-photon emission computed tomography and dipyridamole stress echocardiography for new cardiac events after an uncomplicated myocardial infarction. J Am Soc Echocardiogr 7:370–380

48. Neskovic AN, Popovic AD, Babic R, et al (1995) Positive high-dose dipyridamole echocardiography test after acute myocardial infarction is an excellent predictor of cardiac events. Am Heart J 129:31–39

49. Sicari R, Landi P, Picano E, et al; EPIC (Echo Persantine International Cooperative); EDIC (Echo Dobutamine International Cooperative) Study Group (2002) Exercise-electrocardiography and/or pharmacological stress echocardiography for non-invasive risk stratification early after uncomplicated myocardial infarction. A prospective international large scale multicentre study. Eur Heart J 23:1030–1037

50. Tischler MD, Lee TH, Hirsch AT, et al (1991) Prediction of major cardiac events after peripheral vascular surgery using dipyridamole echocardiography. Am J Cardiol 68:593–597

51. Sicari R, Picano E, Lusa AM, et al (1995) The value of dipyridamole echocardiography in risk stratification before vascular surgery. A multicenter study. The EPIC (Echo Persantine International Study) Group-Subproject: risk stratification before major vascular surgery. Eur Heart J 16:842–847

52. Rossi E, Citterio F, Vescio MF, et al (1998) Risk stratification of patients undergoing peripheral vascular revascularization by combined resting and dipyridamole echocardiography. Am J Cardiol 82:306–310

53. Pasquet A, D'Hondt AM, Verhelst R, et al (1998) Comparison of dipyridamole stress echocardiography and perfusion scintigraphy for cardiac risk stratification in vascular surgery patients. Am J Cardiol 82:1468–1470

54. Sicari R, Ripoli A, Picano E, et al on behalf of the EPIC study group (1999) Perioperative prognostic value of dipyridamole echocardiography in vascular surgery: a large-scale multi-center study on 509 patients. Circulation 100(19 Suppl):II269–II274

55. Zamorano J, Duque A, Baquero M, et al (2002) Stress echocardiography in the pre-operative evaluation of patients undergoing major vascular surgery. Are results comparable with dipyridamole versus dobutamine stress echo? Rev Esp Cardiol 55:121–126

56. Cortigiani L, Paolini EA, Nannini E (1998) Dipyridamole stress echocardiography for risk stratification in hypertensive patients with chest pain. Circulation 98:2855–2859

57. Mondillo S, Agricola E, Ammaturo T, et al (2001) Prognostic value of dipyridamole stress echocardiography in hypertensive patients with left ventricular hypertrophy, chest pain and resting electrocardiographic repolarization abnormalities. Can J Cardiol 17:571–577

58. Camerieri A, Picano E, Landi P, et al (1993) Prognostic value of dipyridamole echocardiography early after myocardial infarction in elderly patients. Echo Persantine Italian Cooperative (EPIC) Study Group. J Am Coll Cardiol 22:1809–1815

59. Cortigiani L, Dodi C, Paolini EA, et al (1998) Prognostic value of pharmacological stress echocardiography in women with chest pain and unknown coronary artery disease. J Am Coll Cardiol 32:1975–1981

60. Cortigiani L, Picano E, Vigna C, et al on behalf of the EPIC and EDIC study groups (2001) Prognostic value of pharmacologic stress echocardiography in patients with left bundle branch block. Am J Med 110:361–369

61. Cortigiani L, Bigi R, Gigli G et al (2003) Prognostic significance of intraventricular conduction defects in patients undergoing stress echocardiography for suspected coronary artery disease. Am J Med 15:126–132

62. Cortigiani L, Picano E, Coletta C, et al on behalf of the EPIC (Echo Persantine International Cooperative) and EDIC (Echo Dobutamine International Cooperative) Study Groups (2002) Safety, feasibility and prognostic implication of pharmacologic stress echocardiography in 1482 patients evaluated in an ambulatory setting. Am Heart J 141:621–629

63. Cortigiani L, Picano E, Landi P, et al (1998) Value of pharmacologic stress echocardiography in risk stratification of patients with single-vessel disease: a report from the Echo-Persantine and Echo-Dobutamine International Cooperative Studies. J Am Coll Cardiol 32:69–74

64. Orlandini A, Tuero E, Paolasso E, et al (2000) Usefulness of pharmacologic stress echocardiography in a chest pain center. Am J Cardiol 86:1247–1250, A6

65. Bedetti G, Pasanisi EM, Tintori G, et al (2005) Stress echo in chest pain unit: the SPEED trial. Int J Cardiol 102:461–467

66. Lattanzi F, Picano E, Bolognese L, et al (1991) Inhibition of dipyridamole-induced ischemia by antianginal therapy in humans. Correlation with exercise electrocardiography. Circulation 83:1256–1262

67. Sicari R, Cortigiani L, Bigi R, et al; Echo-Persantine International Cooperative (EPIC) Study Group; Echo-Dobutamine International Cooperative (EDIC) Study Group (2004) Prognostic value of pharmacological stress echocardiography is affected by concomitant antiischemic therapy at the time of testing. Circulation 109:2428–2431

68. Schröder K, Wieckhorst A, Völler H (1997) Comparison of the prognostic value of dipyridamole and dobutamine stress echocardiography in patients with known or suspected coronary artery disease. Am J Cardiol 79:1516–1518

69. Minardi G, Di Segni M, Manzara CC, et al (1997) Diagnostic and prognostic value of dipyridamole and dobutamine stress echocardiography in patients with Q-wave acute myocardial infarction. Am J Cardiol 80:847–851

70. Pingitore A, Picano E, Varga A, et al (1999) Prognostic value of pharmacological stress echocardiography in patients with known or suspected coronary artery disease: a prospective, large-scale, multicenter, head-to-head comparison between dipyridamole and dobutamine test. Echo-Persantine International Cooperative (EPIC) and Echo-Dobutamine International Cooperative (EDIC) Study Groups. J Am Coll Cardiol 34:1769–1777

71. Nohtomi Y, Takeuchi M, Nagasawa K, et al (2003) Simultaneous assessment of wall motion and coronary flow velocity in the left anterior descending coronary artery during dipyridamole stress echocardiography. J Am Soc Echocardiogr 16:457–463

72. Lowenstein J, Tiano C, Marquez G, et al (2003) Simultaneous analysis of wall motion and coronary flow reserve of the left anterior descending coronary artery by transthoracic doppler echocardiography during dipyridamole stress echocardiography. J Am Soc Echocardiogr 16:607–613

73. Chirillo F, Bruni A, De Leo A, et al (2004) Usefulness of dipyridamole stress echocardiography for predicting graft patency after coronary artery bypass grafting. Am J Cardiol 93:24–30

74. Ascione L, De Michele M, Accadia M, et al (2006) Incremental diagnostic value of ultrasonographic assessment of coronary flow reserve with high-dose dipyridamole in patients with acute coronary syndrome. Int J Cardiol 106:313–318

75. Picano E, Pálinkás A, Amyot R (2001) Diagnosis of myocardial ischemia in hypertensive patients. J Hypertens 19:1177–1183

76. Rigo F, Cortigiani L, Pasanisi E, et al (2006) The additional prognostic value of coronary flow reserve on left anterior descending artery in patients with negative stress echo by wall motion

13

criteria. A Transthoracic Vasodilator Stress Echocardiography Study. Am Heart J 151:124–130

77. Rigo F, Sicari R, Gherardi S, et al (2008) The additive prognostic value of wall motion abnormalities and coronary flow reserve during dipyridamole stress echo. Eur Heart J 29:79–88

78. Sicari R, Rigo F, Gherardi S, et al (2008) The prognostic value of doppler echocardiographic derived coronary flow reserve is not affected by concomitant anti-ischemic therapy at the time of testing. Am Heart J 156:573–579

79. Sicari R, Palinkas A, Pasanisi EG, et al (2005) Long-term survival of patients with chest pain syndrome and angiographically normal or near-normal coronary arteries: the additional prognostic value of dipyridamole echocardiography test (DET). Eur Heart J 26:2136–2141

80. Sicari R, Rigo F, Gherardi S, et al (2008) Long-term survival of patients with chest pain syndrome and angiographically normal or near normal coronary arteries: the additional prognostic value of coronary flow reserve. Eur Heart J (abstract suppl)

81. Cortigiani L, Bigi R, Sicari R, et al (2006) Prognostic value of pharmacological stress echocardiography in diabetic and nondiabetic patients with known or suspected coronary artery disease. J Am Coll Cardiol 47:605–610

82. Cortigiani L, Rigo F, Gherardi S, et al (2007) Additional prognostic value of coronary flow reserve in diabetic and nondiabetic patients with negative dipyridamole stress echocardiography by wall motion criteria. J Am Coll Cardiol 50:1354–1361

83. Pratali L, Otasevic P, Rigo F, et al (2005) The additive prognostic value of restrictive pattern and dipyridamole-induced contractile reserve in idiopathic dilated cardiomyopathy. Eur J Heart Fail 7:844–851

84. Rigo F, Gherardi S, Galderisi M, et al (2006) The prognostic impact of coronary flow-reserve assessed by Doppler echocardiography in non-ischaemic dilated cardiomyopathy. Eur Heart J 27:1319–1323

85. Beleslin BD, Ostojic M, Stepanovic J, et al (1994) Stress echocardiography in the detection of myocardial ischemia. Head-to-head comparison of exercise, dobutamine, and dipyridamole tests. Circulation 90:1168–1176

86. Sochowski RA, Yvorchuk KJ, Yang Y, et al (1995) Dobutamine and dipyridamole stress echocardiography in patients with a low incidence of severe coronary artery disease. J Am Soc Echocardiogr 8:482–487

87. Martin TW, Seaworth JF, Johns JP, et al (1992) Comparison of adenosine, dipyridamole, and dobutamine in stress echocardiography. Ann Intern Med 116:190–196

Adenosine Stress Echocardiography

14

Eugenio Picano, Miodrag Ostojic, and Rodolfo Citro

14.1
Historical Background

Adenosine stress testing is a procedure in which patients are exposed to intravenous infusion of adenosine with simultaneous monitoring of symptoms, hemodynamic parameters, electrocardiogram, and imaging [1]. It is a second-generation vasodilator adenosinergic stress, evolving from the first-generation prototype dipyridamole stress, which acts through the accumulation of endogenous adenosine [2]: Table 14.1. Perfusion imaging with scintigraphy is the dominant application of adenosine stress. Of the 8.4 million myocardial perfusion studies conducted in the USA in 2006, pharmacological stress was used in 3.7 million tests, including infusion of adenosine in 63%, dipyridamole in 30%, and dobutamine in 7% [3]. Radionuclide scintigraphy [4], positron emission tomography [5], or magnetic resonance imaging [6] can be utilized for myocardial perfusion imaging. The conventional stress echocardiography approach is based on functional imaging, which recognizes regional wall motion abnormalities as a diagnostic criterion and ischemia as the necessary end point [7]. Similarly to what happens with dipyridamole [2], high doses of adenosine are required in this case to have high diagnostic sensitivity [8]. Perfusion imaging is also potentially applicable in the stress echocardiography laboratory with myocardial contrast echocardiography [9] and with greater feasibility with coronary flow velocity imaging [10], which is currently recommended in combination with wall motion during vasodilation stress echocardiography [11]. With adequate dosing, adenosine stress echocardiography therefore also has the potential "to kill two birds with one stone," i.e., to assess wall motion and coronary flow reserve simultaneously in one sitting, with a single stress [12], as it is the currently recognized state-of-the-art standard for dipyridamole stress echocardiography [13], also recommended by the European Association of Echocardiography [11]. The clinical appeal of adenosinergic stress may be further enhanced by third-generation

Table 14.1 Three generations of adenosinergic stress

	Prototype	First clinical application	Mediator	Stimulated receptors	Half-life
First generation	Dipyridamole	1980	Endogenous adenosine	A1, A2A, A2B, A3	Hours
Second generation	Adenosine	1990	Exogenous adenosine	A1, A2A, A2B, A3	Seconds
Third generation	Regadenoson	2000	Selective adenosine agonist	A2A (A1)	Minutes

adenosinergic stresses, i.e., selective A2A adenosine agonists, such as regadenoson [14]. Regadenoson (CVT-3146, Cardiovascular Therapeutics, Palo Alto, CA, USA) is a short-acting third-generation adenosinergic stress agent currently being evaluated in two phase-3 randomized, double-blind clinical trials enrolling more than 2,000 patients worldwide. The affinity of regadenoson for human adenosine A2A receptors exceeds that for adenosine A1 receptors by more than ninefold, and its affinity for A2B and A3 receptors is minimal. Given its selectivity, this A2A receptor agonist has the potential to increase the safety and tolerability of adenosine stress, especially in asthmatic patients. In fact, adenosine accumulates in inflamed bronchial mucosa under conditions of cell stress and hypoxia, and contributes as a mediator of bronchoconstriction in both acute and chronic asthma, mainly through stimulation of A2B receptors.

14.2
Pharmacology and Pathophysiology

Adenosine is a nucleoside, i.e., a purine-based adenine bound to sugar ribose [15] acting through its specific receptors located on the outer surface of the cell membrane. It is produced inside the cell, so it is diffused, driven by the concentration gradient, to extracellular space to activate its receptors, which can be divided into two major subtypes: (1) A1 inhibitory receptors and (2) A2 stimulatory receptors. The A1 receptors predominate in the myocardium, whereas the A2 receptors are found in the coronary arteries (endothelial and smooth muscle cells). Probably the chemistry signal that induces adenosine synthesis is the oxygen supply/demand ratio via the variation of the potential of phosphorylation. In fact, in case of insufficient oxygen supply, there is a reduction in the potential of phosphorylation and the consequent increment of free AMP in the cytoplasm that is available as a substrate of 5'-nucleotidase [16]. The increment of 5'-nucleotidase determines an increased production of adenosine. A2A receptors play a key role in mediating inappropriate arteriolar vasodilation leading to hyperemia and – in presence of critical coronary stenosis – to subendocardial ischemia for vertical and horizontal steal phenomena and regional wall motion abnormality [2]. The human adenosine A2A receptor gene has been localized on chromosome 22q and several genetic polymorphisms have been identified [17] as

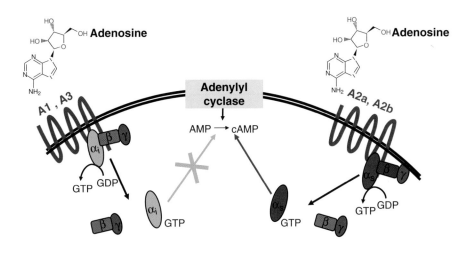

A1, A3 receptors inhibit Adenyl cyclase
A2a, A2b receptors activate Adenyl cyclase

Fig. 14.1 The molecular structure of adenosine receptors

potentially responsible, at least in part, for the heterogeneity in response to coronary flow during stress imaging [18] (Fig. 14.1).

When adenosine binds with phosphate it becomes a nucleotide, i.e., adenosine monophosphate, adenosine diphosphate, and adenosine triphosphate. Actually, one of the pathways of adenosine generation is degradation of those nucleotides, which under normal conditions contribute only up to 10% of the endogenous adenosine in the heart. Approximately 90% of adenosine in the heart is created by the *S*-adenosylhomocysteine hydrolase pathway [4]. A certain amount is also generated by degradation of extracellular AMP. Extracellular adenosine returns into the cell by reuptake through cell membrane by facilitated diffusion, where in a very short time it is degraded by enzyme adenosine deaminase to inosine, which is biologically inactive. It is the end stage of adenosine degradation in myocytes, but in the endothelial cells adenosine is broken down from inosine to hypoxanthine and uric acid. At physiological concentrations, adenosine is predominantly salvaged, i.e., metabolized to adenosine 5-monophosphate (AMP) by the enzyme adenosine kinase. At higher concentrations such as those following administration of diagnostic doses, adenosine is deaminated to inosine [4]. Dipyridamole blocks adenosine reuptake with a resultant increase of adenosine in extracellular space and greater activity on the receptor site. Theophylline and other methylxanthines (such as caffeine) block adenosine receptors in a dose-dependent manner [4] (Fig. 14.2). The main physiological effects of endogenous adenosine, classified according to involvement of A1, A2, or A3 receptors are presented in Table 14.2. When patients receiving adenosine ($140\,\mu g\,kg^{-1}$ per min) for controlled hypotension were pretreated with clinical doses of dipyridamole (to reduce the dose requirements of adenosine),

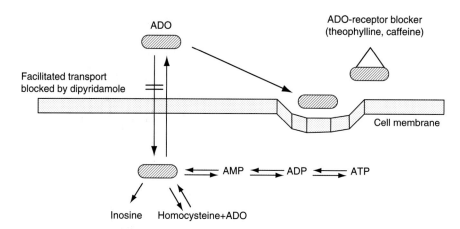

Fig. 14.2 Metabolism and mechanisms of action of adenosine in the coronary arteries. *ADO* adenosine, *AMP* adenosine monophosphate, *ADP* adenosine diphosphate, *ATP* adenosine triphosphate. (Modified from [4])

Table 14.2 Adenosine receptors: a view from the imaging laboratory

Receptor	Effect	Desired diagnostic end point
A1	Atrioventricular block Bradycardia Preconditioning	
A2A		Coronary vasodilation
A2B	Bronchoconstriction due to mast cell degranulation	
A3	Anti-inflammatory effects (peripheral blood mono-nuclear cells)	

Table 14.3 Cardiovascular effects of exogenous adenosine administered intravenously in humans

- Vagal inhibition (low doses), increase in heart rate
- Inhibition of the sinus node and AV conduction in high doses, bradycardia, AV block
- Antiadrenergic effect
- Vasodilatation in all arteriolar beds, except vasoconstriction in renal preglomerular arterioles; decrease in reperfusion injury
- Hyperventilation (explained by interaction with carotid chemoreceptors)

the arterial plasma concentration was 2.5 µM, a level ten times the normal level [19]. The adenosine effects listed in Table 14.3 substantiate the proposed potential clinical uses of adenosine listed in Table 14.4. Cardiac stress imaging is the most important diagnostic application of adenosine infusion. The intravenous infusion of adenosine induces a slight increase in heart rate and cardiac output, and a slight decrease in systemic pressure. The mild tachycardia occurs in spite of the direct, negative chronotropic and dromotropic effects of adenosine for stimulation of A1 myocardial receptors; it is a consequence of adrenergic activation, occurring either through direct stimulation of sympathic excitatory arterial chemoreceptors [20] or indirectly, through systemic vasodilation. In normal subjects, the coronary blood flow increases to four to five times the baseline flow following adenosine – an increase comparable to that caused by high-dose dipyridamole and substantially higher than that induced by exercise or dobutamine, during which coronary blood flow increases about three times the baseline value [21]. The maximal coronary dilatory effect is reached within 2 min of adenosine administration and wears off rapidly within 2.5 min after the infusion is stopped. Adenosine can induce elevation in pulmonary capillary wedge pressure and/or left ventricular end-diastolic pressure only in presence of myocardial ischemia [22]. The power and time course of the coronary vasodilator effect of adenosine and other newer synthetic adenosine-receptor agonists are shown in Fig. 14.3 [14].

Table 14.4 Potential clinical uses of adenosine

• Paroxysmal supraventricular tachycardia

• Exercise-induced ventricular tachycardia

• Controlled hypotension during intracranial vascular surgeries

• Afterload reduction in congestive heart failure

• Antiplatelet aggregation (cardiopulmonary bypass, hemodialysis)

• Reduction of reperfusion injury

• Diagnosis and prognosis of coronary artery disease (13)

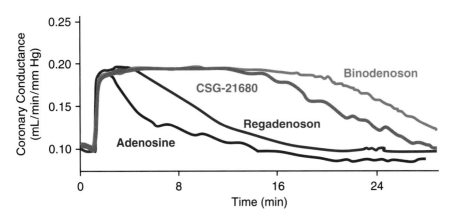

Fig. 14.3 The vasodilatory effect of adenosine and newer selective A2A receptor agonists. (Adapted from [33])

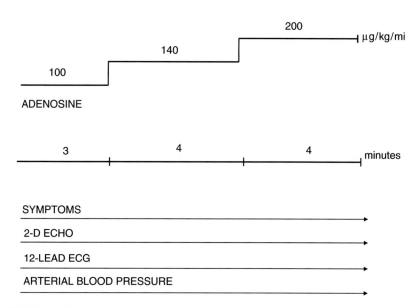

Fig. 14.4 Protocol of adenosine stress echocardiography

14.3
Methodology

For echocardiographic imaging, the dose is usually started at 100 μg kg^{-1} per minute and is increased gradually up to 200 μg kg^{-1} per minute [8] (Fig. 14.4). When side effects are intolerable, down-titration of the dose is also possible. Similar to dobutamine, administration of adenosine requires an infusion pump, whereas dipyridamole may be injected with a handheld syringe. As with dipyridamole, test sensitivity can be potentiated using a handgrip [23], which can be added to adenosine or to ATP infusion [24]. Some authors suggest infusing adenosine for no more than 90 s, taking into account that the maximal hyperemic effect is already reached at 30–60 s [25, 26]. The adenosine injection of 2.5 mg bolus produces an increment in coronary flow reserve similar to that obtained a by 3-min venous infusion and has no significant side effects [27]. The short adenosine infusion seems to be effective, safer, and better tolerated than the standard dosage, but it has the disadvantage that there is not enough time to assess contemporary left ventricular wall motion.

14.4
Tolerability and Safety

Side effects are very frequent and are limiting in a significant number of patients – up to 20% [28]. The most frequent limiting side effects include high-degree atrioventricular block, arterial hypotension, intolerable chest pain (sometimes unrelated to underlying ischemia,

Table 14.5 Side effects of pharmacological stress protocols

Stress protocol	Dipyridamole 0.56 mg kg^{-1}	Dipyridamole 0.84 mg kg^{-1}	Adenosine 140 mcg kg^{-1} per min	Dobutamine 40 mcg kg^{-1} per min ± atropine
Reference	Lette et al	Picano et al	Cerqueira et al	Picano et al
No. of patients	73,806 (9,066 with 0.75 or 0.84 mg kg^{-1})	10,451	9,256	2,949
Major side effects	0.04%	0.07%	<0.10%	0.4%
Fatal MI	0.01%	0.01%	0%	0%
Nonfatal MI	0.017%	0.02%	0.01%	0.07%
VT/VF	0.008%	0.01%	0%	0.05%

MI myocardial infarction, *VT* sustained ventricular tachycardia, *VF* ventricular fibrillation

possibly induced for direct stimulation of myocardial A1 adenosine receptors), shortness of breath, flushing, and headache. All side effects disappear upon termination of adenosine infusion. On very rare occasions, an infusion of aminophylline is required. The quality of side effects is similar to that experienced by the same patients during dipyridamole stress, but these effects are quantitatively more pronounced during adenosine stress. In one study [26], it was found that among adenosine, dipyridamole, and dobutamine, adenosine was the test most disliked by the patients. Although side effects are frequent, the incidence of major life-threatening complications (such as myocardial infarction, ventricular tachycardia, and shock) has been shown to be very low, with only one nonfatal myocardial infarction in approximately 10,000 cases. Among pharmacological stress tests [25–29], adenosine is probably the least well tolerated subjectively, but at the same time possibly the safest (see Table 14.5).

14.5
Diagnostic Accuracy for Detection of Coronary Artery Disease and Myocardial Viability

The full range of sensitivities has been reported [33–37, 7, 8, 26], with higher values coming from expert centers evaluating patients with previous myocardial infarction and multivessel disease (Table 14.6). Higher adenosine dose [8] and/or the combination with a handgrip [22] showed higher sensitivity without significant loss in specificity. On the basis of a recent meta-analysis on 11 studies, adenosine stress echocardiography, based on wall motion abnormalities, showed the same sensitivity (79%), specificity (91.5%), and accuracy as exercise echocardiography, dipyridamole echocardiography, and dobutamine echocardiography, with superior specificity when compared to SPECT stress imaging [38]. With last-generation (wall motion and coronary flow reserve, 11) three basic patterns can be identified during dual imaging adenosine stress echocardiography (Fig. 14.5): a normal response, with increased regional function and preserved coronary flow reserve (>2.0);

Table 14.6 Diagnostic accuracy of adenosine echocardiography

Authors	Reference	Year	Patients	Dose	Sensitivity (%)	Specificity (%)
Zoghbi et al.	33	1991	73	100–140	85	92
Edlund et al.	34	1991	54	60–200	89	Na
Martin et al.	35	1992	37	140	76	60
Marwick et al.	36	1993	97	180	86	71
Case et al.	37	1994	26	140	96	100
Takeishi et al.	38	1994	61	140	51	Na
Tawa et al.	39	1995	67	180	64	91
Djordievic al.	40	1996	58	200	92	88

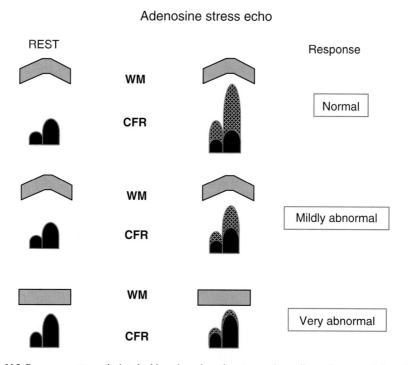

Fig. 14.5 Response patterns during dual imaging adenosine stress echocardiography: normal (hyperkinetic wall motion; greater than twofold increase in diastolic coronary flow velocity); mildly abnormal (normal wall motion but reduced hyperemic response); markedly abnormal (wall motion abnormalities that can be made even more malignant by concomitant reduction in coronary flow reserve in LAD territory)

an abnormal response, with reduction in coronary flow reserve (<2.0) but with normal wall motion response (indicative of microvascular disease or moderate epicardial coronary artery stenosis); and a markedly abnormal response with inducible wall motion abnormalities, suggestive of anatomically significant epicardial artery stenosis. Some initial data suggest that adenosine infusion may elicit an inotropic response in viable myocardium with resting dysfunction [39], thereby representing an alternative to dobutamine for the recognition of viability through pharmacological stimulation.

14.6
Prognostic Value

Data on the prognostic value of adenosine stress echocardiography findings are conspicuously lacking to date. By extrapolation from the wealth of data available with dipyridamole stress echocardiography [11, 40] and from more recent data with adenosine scintigraphy [40] and adenosine magnetic resonance imaging [41], it is reasonable to expect adenosine-induced wall motion abnormalities to identify troublemakers in the short run (within months), whereas isolate reduction in coronary flow reserve, without associated wall motion abnormalities, may identify troublemakers in the long run (years).

14.7
Indications and Contraindications

The merits and limitations of adenosine in comparison with the prototype vasodilator dipyridamole are shown in Table 14.7. The list of indications and contraindications to adenosine is identical to that for dipyridamole (Table 14.8). Exogenous adenosine has an even more pronounced negative chronotropic and dromotropic effect than endogenous adenosine [14], making the appearance of advanced atrioventricular blocks more frequent with adenosine than with dipyridamole for equivalent doses. Adenosine is a direct alternative to dipyridamole – the prototype of vasodilator adenosinergic stress. Like dipyridamole, antianginal drugs lower adenosine stress echocardiography sensitivity, whereas concomitant

Table 14.7 Adenosine versus dipyridamole for vasodilator stress testing

	Dipyridamole	Adenosine
Half-life	Hours	Seconds
Aminophylline requirement	Always	Almost never
Echocardiographic difficulty	Mild	Mild to moderate
Limiting side effects	5%	10–20%
Patient tolerance	Good	Beta-blockers
Prognostic value	Proven	Unknown

14

Table 14.8 Patients with indications to adenosine stress echocardiography

	Indicated	Uncertain	Contraindicated
Indication to dual imaging vasodilatory stress echocardiography	√		
Unstable carotid disease	√		
Elderly patients	√		
Viability detection in patients intolerant to dobutamine		√	
Theophylline use, COPD, asthma			√
Previously intubated because of respiratory failure			√
History of first-degree (or greater) AV block or sinus mode disease without functioning artificial pacemaker			√
Intake of caffeine or other methylxanthine-containing foods (chocolate, tea, banana) for 24 h before stress			√

therapy with oral dipyridamole potentiates the cardiovascular effects of adenosine. The safety record and short half-life make adenosine especially indicated in patients with severe aortic stenosis [42] or elderly patients [43], who may be especially vulnerable to complications during dipyridamole or dobutamine stress. In some countries, an additional limitation of adenosine is its exorbitant cost: in the USA, adenosine costs $ 179, dipyridamole $ 95, and dobutamine $ 1 per exam. In Europe, adenosine costs € 100, dipyridamole € 3, and dobutamine € 9. However, it is also possible to have a galenic formulation of adenosine from the hospital pharmacy at a very low cost of around € 1. Possibly, more expensive third-generation selective A2A agonists may find a selective indication in patients with moderate and severe chronic obstructive pulmonary disease [44], who have an indication to stress imaging and may want to avoid adenosine-induced bronchoconstriction and respiratory compromise, although in these patients the use of the bronchodilator dobutamine might be more reasonable.

References

1. Verani MS, Mahmarian JJ, Hixson JB, et al (1990) Diagnosis of coronary artery disease by controlled coronary vasodilation with adenosine and thallium-201 scintigraphy in patients unable to exercise. Circulation 82:80–87
2. Picano E (1989) Dipyridamole-echocardiography test: historical background and physiologic basis. Eur Heart J 10:365–376
3. Arlington Medical Resources (2006) The myocardial perfusion market guide (US and Europe). Arlington Medical Resources, Arlington, VA
4. Verani MS (1991) Adenosine thallium 201 myocardial perfusion scintigraphy. Am Heart J 122:269–278

5. Bateman TM (2004) Cardiac positron emission tomography and the role of adenosine pharmacologic stress. Am J Cardiol 94:19D–24D

6. Paetsch I, Jahnke C, Wahl A, et al (2004) Comparison of dobutamine stress magnetic resonance, adenosine stress magnetic resonance, and adenosine stress magnetic resonance perfusion. Circulation 110:835–842

7. Zoghbi WA (1991) Use of adenosine echocardiography for diagnosis of coronary artery disease. Am Heart J 122:285–292

8. Djordjevic-Dikic AD, Ostojic MC, Beleslin BD, et al (1996) High-dose adenosine stress echocardiography for noninvasive detection of coronary artery disease. J Am Coll Cardiol 28:1689–1695

9. Lafitte S, Masugata H, Peters B, et al (2001) Accuracy and reproducibility of coronary flow rate assessment by real-time contrast echocardiography: in vitro and in vivo studies. J Am Soc Echocardiogr 14:1010–1019

10. Caiati C, Zedda N, Montaldo C, et al (1999) Contrast-enhanced transthoracic second harmonic echo Doppler with adenosine: a noninvasive, rapid and effective method for coronary flow reserve assessment. J Am Coll Cardiol 34:122–130

11. Sicari R, Nihoyannopoulos P, Evangelista A, et al; European Association of Echocardiography (2008) Stress echocardiography consensus statement of the European Association of Echocardiography. Eur J Echocardiogr 9:415–437

12. Korosoglou G, Dubart AE, DaSilva KG Jr, et al (2006) Real-time myocardial perfusion imaging for pharmacologic stress testing: added value to single photon emission computed tomography. Am Heart J 151:131–138

13. Cerqueira MD (2004) The future of pharmacologic stress: selective A2A adenosine receptor agonists. Am J Cardiol 94:33D–40D

14. Iskandrian AE, Bateman TM, Belardinelli L, Blackburn B, Cerqueira MD, Hendel RC, Lieu H, Mahmarian JJ, Olmsted A, Underwood SR, Vitola J, Wang W; ADVANCE MPI Investigators. (2007) Adenosine versus regadenoson comparative evaluation in myocardial perfusion imaging: results of the ADVANCE phase 3 multicenter international trial. J Nucl Cardiol 14:645–658

15. Fredholm BB, Abbracchio MP, Burnstock G, et al (1994) Nomenclature and classification of purinoceptors. Pharmacol Rev 46:143–156

16. Drury AN, Szent-GyorgyA (1929) The physiological activity of adenine compounds with especial reference to their action upon the mammalian heart. J Physiol 68:213–237

17. MacCollin M, Peterfreund R, MacDonald M, et al (1994) Mapping of a human A2a adenosine receptor (ADORA2) to chromosome 22. Genomics 20:332–333

18. Andreassi MG, Foffa I, Gherardi S, et al (2008) Genetic polymorphism in the adenosine A2A receptor affects coronary flow reserve response in non-ischemic dilated cardiomyopathy. Eur Heart J 29, Suppl 1

19. Conradson T-BG, Dixon CMS, Clarke B, et al (1987) Cardiovascular effects of infused adenosine in man: potentiation by dipyridamole. Acta Physiol Scand 129:387–391

20. Biaggioni I, Olafsson B, Robertson RM, et al (1987) Cardiovascular and respiratory effects of adenosine in conscious man. Evidence for chemoreceptor activation. Circ Res 61:779–786

21. Iskandrian AS, Verani MS, Heo J (1994) Pharmacologic stress testing: mechanism of action, hemodynamic responses, and results in detection of coronary artery disease. J Nucl Cardiol 1:94–111

22. Beleslin BD, Ostojic M, Djordjevic-Dikic A, et al (1997) Coronary vasodilation without myocardial erection. Simultaneous haemodynamic, echocardiographic and arteriographic findings during adenosine and dipyridamole infusion. Eur Heart J 18:1166–1174

23. Tawa CB, Baker WB, Kleiman NS, et al (1996) Comparison of adenosine echocardiography, with and without isometric handgrip, to exercise echocardiography in the detection of ischemia in patients with coronary artery disease. J Am Soc Echocardiogr 9:33–43

24. Miyazono Y, Kisanuki A, Toyonaga K, et al (1998) Usefulness of adenosine triphosphate-atropine stress echocardiography for detecting coronary artery stenosis. Am J Cardiol 82:290–294

25. Pizzuto F, Voci P, Mariano E, et al (2001) Assessment of flow velocity reserve by transthoracic Doppler and venous adenosine infusion, before and after left anterior descending coronary stenting. J Am Coll Cardiol 38:155–162

26. Wilson RF, Wyche K, Christensen BV, et al (1990) Effects of adenosine on human coronary arterial circulation. Circulation 82:1595–1606

27. Kern M, Deligonul U, Tatineni S, et al (1991) Intravenous adenosine: continuous infusion and low dose bolus administration for determination of coronary vasodilator reserve in patients with and without coronary artery disease. J Am Coll Cardiol 18:718–729

28. Cerqueira MD, Verani MS, Schwaiger M, et al (1994) Safety profile of adenosine stress perfusion imaging: results from the Adenoscan Multicenter Trial Registry. J Am Coll Cardiol 23:384–389

29. Martin TW, Seaworth JF, Johns JP, et al (1992) Comparison of adenosine, dipyridamole, and dobutamine in stress echocardiography. Ann Intern Med 116:190–196

30. Lette J, Tatum JL, Fraser S, et al (1995) Safety of dipyridamole testing in 73,806 patients: the Multicenter Dipyridamole Safety Study. J Nucl Cardiol 2:3–17

31. Picano E, Marini C, Pirelli S, et al (1992) Safety of intravenous high-dose dipyridamole echocardiography. The Echo-Persantine International Cooperative Study Group. Am J Cardiol 70:252–258

32. Picano E, Mathias W Jr, Pingitore A, et al on behalf of the EDIC study group (1994) Safety and tolerability of dobutamine-atropine stress echocardiography: a prospective, large-scale, multicenter trial. Lancet 344:1190–1192

33. Zoghbi WA, Cheirif J, Kleiman NS, et al (1991) Diagnosis of ischemic heart disease with adenosine echocardiography. J Am Coll Cardiol 18:1271–1279

34. Edlund A, Albertsson P, Caidahl K, et al (1991) Adenosine infusion to patients with ischaemic heart disease may provoke left ventricular dysfunction detected by echocardiography. Clin Physiol 11:477–488

35. Marwick T, Willemart B, D'Hondt AM, et al (1993) Selection of the optimal nonexercise stress for the evaluation of ischemic regional myocardial dysfunction and malperfusion. Comparison of dobutamine and adenosine using echocardiography and 99mTc-MIBI single photon emission computed tomography. Circulation 87:345–354

36. Case RA, Buckmire R, McLaughlin DP, et al (1994) Physiological assessment of coronary artery disease and myocardial viability in ischemic syndromes using adenosine echocardiography. Echocardiography 11:133–143

37. Takeishi Y, Chiba J, Abe S, et al (1994) Adenosine-induced heterogeneous perfusion accompanies myocardial ischemia in the presence of advanced coronary artery disease. Am Heart J 127:1262–1268

38. Heijenbrok-Kal MH, Fleischmann KE, Hunink MG (2007) Stress echocardiography, stress single-photon-emission computed tomography and electron beam computed tomography for the assessment of coronary artery disease: a meta-analysis of diagnostic performance. Am Heart J 154:415–423

39. Djordjevic-Dikic A, Ostojic M, Beleslin B, et al (2003) Low-dose adenosine stress echocardiography: detection of myocardial viability. Cardiovasc Ultrasound 1:7

40. Hachamovitch R, Hayes SW, Friedman JD, et al (2005) A prognostic score for prediction of cardiac mortality risk after adenosine stress myocardial perfusion scintigraphy. J Am Coll Cardiol 45:722–729

41. Jahnke C, Nagel E, Gebker R, et al (2007) Prognostic value of cardiac magnetic resonance stress tests: adenosine stress perfusion and dobutamine stress wall motion imaging. Circulation 115:1769–1776

42. Patsilinakos SP, Kranidis AI, Antonelis IP, et al (1999) Detection of coronary artery disease in patients with severe aortic stenosis with noninvasive methods. Angiology 50:309–317

43. Anthopoulos LP, Bonou MS, Kardaras FG, et al (1996) Stress echocardiography in elderly patients with coronary artery disease: applicability, safety and prognostic value of dobutamine and adenosine echocardiography in elderly patients. J Am Coll Cardiol 28:52–59

44. Thomas GS, Tammelin BR, Schiffman GL, et al (2008) Safety of regadenoson, a selective adenosine A2A agonist, in patients with chronic obstructive pulmonary disease: a randomized, double-blind, placebo-controlled trial (RegCOPD trial). J Nucl Cardiol 15:319–328

Eugenio Picano

15.1
Historical Background

High-rate pacing is a valid stress test to be used in conjunction with echocardiography; it is independent of physical exercise and does not require drug administration. It has evolved over the last 20 years, starting from an invasive (intravenous) right atrial pacing modality, combined with an ionizing imaging technique such as radionuclide ventriculography [1], moving to a semi-invasive modality combined with two-dimensional (2D) echocardiography, using a transnasal [2] or transoral [3] catheter for transesophageal left atrial pacing, and finally evolving to a totally noninvasive modality with external programming in patients with a permanent pacemaker for right atrial or ventricular pacing [4].

15.2
Pathophysiology

Pacing can be atrial or ventricular (Table 15.1). The paced chamber is the left atrium in transesophageal pacing and the right atrium or the right ventricle in permanent pacemaker stimulation. The pathophysiological rationale of pacing stress is obvious, with the stress determined by a controlled increase in heart rate, which is a major determinant of myocardial oxygen demand, and thereby tachycardia may exceed a fixed coronary flow reserve in the presence of hemodynamically significant coronary artery disease. Cardiac volumes decrease [5] and blood pressure does not change significantly during pacing, whereas contractility increases only minimally, possibly due to the Bowditch-Treppe or staircase phenomenon [6], i.e., the increase in contractility due to the increase in heart rate [7, 8]. At increased heart rate, the coronary flow is decreased through reduction in diastolic duration in the presence of coronary stenosis [9]. Heart rate is a major factor influencing transmural blood flow distribution and regional function, because when coronary vasodilation is maximal there is an inverse relationship between the heart rate level and subendocardial perfusion [10]. The drop in the subendocardial-to-subepicardial flow ratio associated with rapid atrial pacing in the presence

Table 15.1 Pacing mode and contractile pattern in pacing stress echocardiography

	Paced chamber	Non-invasiveness	Septal movement	Simplicity of echocardiographic reading
Permanent PM atrial mode	Right atrium	++	Normal	++
Permanent PM ventricular mode	Right ventricle	++	Paradoxical (60%)	±
Permanent PM biventricular	Right and left ventricle	++	Normal	++
Transesophageal	Left atrium	±	Normal	++
Transvenous	Right atrium	–	Normal	++

++ excellent, + good, – poor

of a tight coronary stenosis [10] is critical to the development of regional dysfunction, because regional percent systolic thickening is linearly and tightly related to subendocardial, but not to transmural flow. In patients with permanent right ventricular pacing, perfusion defects can often be found in the inferior and apical wall, which are probably the earliest activated sites under right ventricular apical pacing [11, 12]. The regional coronary flow reserve can be impaired in the dominant coronary artery perfusing these regions, whereas it is usually normal in the left anterior descending coronary artery. This abnormality is at least partially responsible for the uncertain specificity of stress myocardial scintigraphy [13]. In patients with permanent pacemakers, chronic right ventricular pacing also induces asymmetric thickness of the left ventricular wall and redistribution of left ventricular mass [14]. In fact, asynchronous electric activation of the left ventricle decreases mechanical load in early vs. late activated regions of the ventricular wall. Accordingly, chronic right ventricular pacing induces redistribution of left ventricular mass, with thinning of early vs. late activated myocardium. Septal motion during right ventricular pacing can vary according to the site of stimulation and heart rate. Pre-ejection septal beaking is observed – similarly to what can be found in other patients with relatively delayed left ventricular activation, caused by left bundle branch block or type B Wolff–Parkinson–White syndrome (Fig. 4.4 in Chap. 4). The pre-ejection period septal beaking is not due to early activation and unopposed contraction of the interventricular septum, but rather it occurs in response to an altered transseptal pressure gradient. When pacing causes the right ventricle to be activated before the left, right ventricular pressure begins to increase in systole before left ventricular pressure, altering the normal left-to-right transseptal pressure gradient [15]. Coincident with the early unopposed increase in right ventricular pressure, the septum abruptly moves posteriorly toward the left ventricle. With the subsequent onset of left ventricular contraction, left ventricular pressure increases, the normal transseptal pressure gradient is restored, and the septum returns in the anterior direction toward its end-diastolic position. In the ejection phase, a ventricularly paced left ventricle can show a normal posterior motion and thickening (more frequent with pacing from the right ventricular apex) or a flat or paradoxical (anterior) motion (more frequent with pacing from right ventricular outflow or right ventricular inflow) [11]. The interpretation can be easier in the first case than in the second case, especially considering that in 30% of patients, a normal or flat motion can become paradoxical at high pacing rates over 120 per min.

15.3
Methodology

The main features of different pacing techniques are summarized in Table 15.1. All have good diagnostic results. However, intravenous atrial pacing [1] requires catheterization, which nullifies its utilization in the echocardiography laboratory. Utilization of the transesophageal approach as a stress test for ischemia has become possible thanks to recent improvements in this technique, enabling effective atrial capture at a relatively low threshold, which has reduced patient discomfort [2], and transoral stimulation with 10-French catheters [3]. The results reported have been good, but semi-invasiveness substantially limits the applicability of this approach. In a more clinically plausible approach, the presence of a permanent pacemaker can be exploited to conduct a pacing stress test in a totally noninvasive way by programming the pacemaker to increasing frequencies [4]. The paced chamber is the right atrium in atrial stimulation and the right ventricle in ventricular stimulation mode. The diffusion of biventricular pacing also expands the domain of application of pacing stress echocardiography, since this pacing mode induces a physiological contraction of the septum, making echocardiography interpretation easier. The interpretation must consider that regional wall motion in the septum is differently affected by the pacing mode (Fig. 15.1).

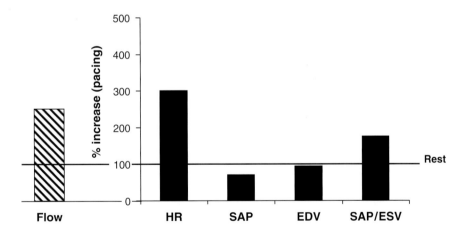

Fig. 15.1 Determinants of myocardial oxygen supply and demand in normal subjects referred for pacing stress echocardiography. The coronary flow reserve is normally around 250% (lower values than those obtained with dipyridamole or adenosine stress echocardiography). Heart rate (*HR*) increases two- to threefold, end-diastolic volume (*EDV*) remains stable or decreases slightly, systolic arterial pressure (*SAP*) does not change to any significant extent, and myocardial contractility (noninvasively measured as elastance, or systolic arterial pressure, end-systolic volume (*ESV*) ratio), increases by only 30%, probably as a result of Bowditch-Treppe or staircase phenomenon

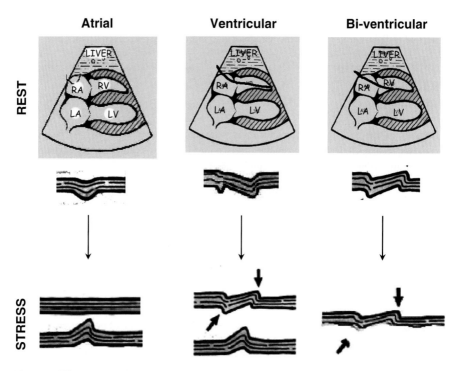

Fig. 15.2 Different types of baseline septal motion and stress-induced ischemia according to the pacing-mode (AAI vs. VVI) and (in VVI) according to the site of stimulation. *RV* right ventricle, *IVS* interventricular septum. LA=left atrium; LV=left ventricle; RA=right atrium; AAI=atrial stimulation mode; VVI=ventricular stimulation mode

In the atrial and biventricular stimulation mode, the normal, physiological electrical activation sequence is preserved; therefore the septal wall motion is normal and there are no special interpretation problems. Roughly two out of three patients with permanent pacemakers are studied in the right ventricular pacing mode. In approximately 30% of right ventricular-paced patients, the septal wall motion is normal [14, 15], but in the majority of them an anterior systolic interventricular septal motion (paradoxical motion) is present at baseline (Fig. 15.2). In this case, it is necessary to focus on wall thickening rather than endocardial excursion, and on nonseptal regions of the left anterior descending territory to identify left anterior descending stenosis, but this interpretation will always be a challenge, especially at high heart rates. Pacemaker stress echocardiography can only be used with patients with a permanent pacemaker, a large and expanding population in today's cardiology practice [4]. In addition, this test is especially useful in patients with a permanent pacemaker. In fact, the noninvasive diagnosis of coronary artery disease in patients with a permanent pacemaker is an extremely difficult task, since the induced rhythm by right ventricular pacing makes the electrocardiogram uninterpretable and stress scintigraphy is plagued by an exorbitant number of false-positive results [8].

With external programming of the pacemaker, pacing is started at 110 bpm and increased every 2 min by 10 bpm until 85% of the target heart rate (220 minus years of age for men; 200 minus years of age for women) is achieved (Fig. 15.3) or until other standard end points are

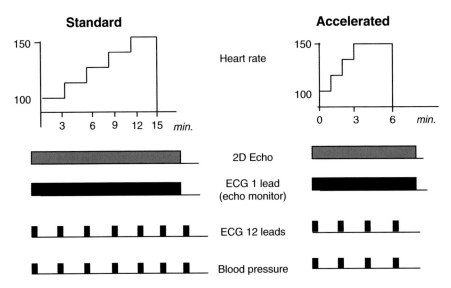

Fig. 15.3 Protocol of pacing stress echocardiography: standard (*left*) or accelerated (*right*)

reached. The same protocol can also be followed in an accelerated fashion, with faster steps (20–30 s each) up to the target heart rate. The examination is done with the patient supine or in left lateral decubitus position. 2D echocardiographic images are obtained before pacing and throughout the stress test, the last recording being obtained after 3 min pacing at the highest rate reached (usually 150 bpm) or the target heart rate. Blood pressure and the electrocardiogram are monitored throughout the examination. Left ventricular wall motion abnormalities are evaluated at rest, during pacing, and immediately after pacing interruption.

15.4
Clinical Results and Comparison with Other Stress Echocardiography Tests

Good diagnostic results have been obtained with invasive pacing stress echocardiography, with good sensitivity and specificity [16–19]. As with other stress echocardiography tests, the positivity can be effectively titrated in the time and space domain [4], and more severe degrees of underlying coronary artery disease are associated with a lower heart rate, necessary to induce ischemia and with more extensive wall motion abnormality (Fig. 15.4). Pacing-induced ischemia is also helpful in risk stratification of the patient with known or suspected coronary artery disease [20, 21].

15.5
Limitations and Indications

Myocardial oxygen consumption as high as that reached with exercise is not obtained by atrial pacing because cardiac volumes decrease and blood pressure does not change significantly, such that in some patients with mild coronary artery disease, wall motion

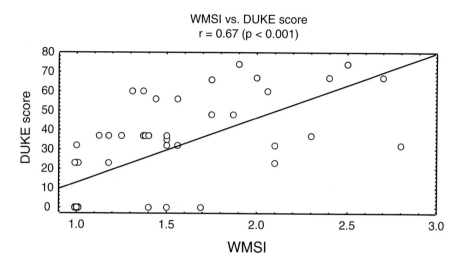

Fig. 15.4 Extent and severity of coronary artery disease (expressed by the prognostically validated Duke score) is predicted by peak Wall Motion Score Index (*WMSI*) during pacing stress echocardiography

Table 15.2 Pacing vs. pharmacologic stress echocardiography

	Pacemaker	Pharmacological
Patient tolerability	Very high	High
Stress imaging time	5–10 min	10–20 min
Safety	Very high	High
Intravenous line	Usually not required	Required
Clinical experience	Initial	Extensive
Applicability	Patients with permanent pacemaker	All patients

abnormalities may not develop. At a high rate, there are fewer video frames during the ejection period and less time to appreciate a regional wall motion abnormality. Only one-half of patients can be stressed in an atrial stimulation or biventricular mode that preserves the physiological sequence of contraction of the left ventricle [22]. In patients with ventricular stimulation of long duration, specificity can perhaps be lowered. The external programming of the permanent pacemaker is simple and fast, but it requires technology (external programmer) and expertise not readily available in the echocardiography laboratory – also requiring minimum cooperation and coordination with the pacemaker laboratory – which is usually, but not always and anywhere, easy to obtain. Noninvasive pacemaker stress echocardiography has several advantages in comparison to conventional diagnostic techniques. The relative merits and limitations of noninvasive pacemaker stress echocardiography vs. pharmacological stress echocardiography are reported in Table 15.2. The ability

Table 15.3 Indications to pacing stress in patients referred for stress echocardiography

	Appropriate	Uncertain	Inappropriate
Patients with implanted pacemaker (atrial- or biventricular mode)	√		
Patients with implanted pacemakers (ventricular mode)		√	
Patients without implanted pacemaker (transesophageal)			√

to instantly lower the rate and terminate stress results in high test safety. Pacemaker stress echocardiography is rapid and can be conducted at bedside and is therefore well tolerated by the patient and user-friendly for the physician. In contrast to physical stress, it does not require patient capability to exercise; contrary to pharmacological stress, it does not require an intravenous line and the additional cost (and risk) of drug administration. Imaging time is also shorter, because the median time of pacing is less than 10 min with the accelerated protocol, which compares favorably with the approximately 10 min of imaging time for dipyridamole and about 20 min for dobutamine–atropine. In patients with a permanent pacemaker, 2D echocardiography during pacing is a useful tool in the detection of coronary artery disease. Because of its safety and repeatability, noninvasive pacing stress echocardiography can be the first-line stress test in patients with permanent pacemakers (Table 15.3), especially if the stimulation can be performed in the most physiological and less technically challenging atrial or biventricular mode.

References

1. Tzivoni D, Weiss AT, Solomon J, et al (1981) Diagnosis of coronary artery disease by multigated radionuclide angiography during right atrial pacing. Chest 80:562–565
2. Chapman PD, Doyle TP, Troup PJ, et al (1984) Stress echocardiography with transesophageal atrial pacing: preliminary report of a new method for detection of ischemic wall motion abnormalities. Circulation 70:445–450
3. Atar S, Nagai T, Cercek B, et al (2000) Pacing stress echocardiography: an alternative to pharmacologic stress testing. J Am Coll Cardiol 36:1935–1941
4. Picano E, Alaimo A, Chubuchny V, et al (2002) Noninvasive pacemaker stress echocardiography for diagnosis of coronary artery disease: a multicenter study. J Am Coll Cardiol 40:1305–1310
5. Rozenman Y, Weiss AT, Atlan H, et al (1984) Left ventricular volumes and function during atrial pacing in coronary artery disease: a radionuclide angiographic study. Am J Cardiol 53:497–502
6. Bombardini T, Agrusta M, Natsvlishvili N, et al (2005) Noninvasive assessment of left ventricular contractility by pacemaker stress echocardiography. Eur J Heart Fail 7:173–181
7. Bombardini T, Gemignani V, Bianchini E, et al (2007) Cardiac reflections and natural vibrations: force-frequency relation recording system in the stress echo lab. Cardiovasc Ultrasound 5:42
8. Bombardini T (2005) Myocardial contractility in the echo lab: molecular, cellular and pathophysiological basis. Cardiovasc Ultrasound 3:27
9. Heusch G (2008) Heart rate in the pathophysiology of coronary blood flow and myocardial ischaemia: benefit from selective bradycardic agents. Br J Pharmacol 153:1589–601

10. Indolfi C, Ross J Jr (1993) The role of heart rate in myocardial ischemia and infarction: impli-
    cations of myocardial perfusion-contraction matching. Prog Cardiovasc Dis 36:61–74
11. Takeuchi M, Nohtomi Y, Kuroiwa A (1997) Effect of ventricular pacing on coronary blood
    flow in patients with normal coronary arteries. Pacing Clin Electrophysiol 20:2463–2469
12. Skalidis EI, Kochiadakis GE, Koukouraki SI, et al (2001) Myocardial perfusion in patients with
    permanent ventricular pacing and normal coronary arteries. J Am Coll Cardiol 37:124–129
13. Prinzen FW, Cheriex EC, Delhaas T, et al (1995) Asymmetric thickness of the left ventricular
    wall resulting from asynchronous electric activation: a study in dogs with ventricular pacing
    and in patients with left bundle branch block. Am Heart J 130:1045–1053
14. Little WC, Reeves RC, Arciniegas J, et al (1982) Mechanism of abnormal interventricular
    septal motion during delayed left ventricular activation. Circulation 65:1486–1492
15. Gomes JA, Damato AN, Akhtar M, et al (1977) Ventricular septal motion and left ventricular
    dimensions during abnormal ventricular activation. Am J Cardiol 39:641–650
16. Baldo V, Biscione F, Battista M, et al (1997) Right ventricular echo-pacing test in the diag-
    nosis of ischemic cardiopathy in patients with VVI pacemaker. Cardiovasc Imaging 8(Suppl
    2):342–346
17. Volkov GV, Osipov MA, Bashinskii, et al (1994) A new method for the diagnosis of myocar-
    dial ischemia in patients with an implanted programmable pacemaker. Ter Arkh 66:25–27
18. Benchimol D,Mazanof M, Dubroca B, et al (2000) Detection of coronary stenoses by stress
    echocardiography using a previously implanted pacemaker for ventricular pacing: preliminary
    report of a new method. Clin Cardiol 23:842–848
19. Płonska-Gosciniak E, Lancellotti P, Kleinrok A, et al (2008) Influence of gender on diag-
    nostic accuracy of rapid atrial and ventricular pacing stress echocardiography for the detec-
    tion of coronary artery disease: a multicenter study (Pol-RAPSE final results). J Am Soc
    Echocardiogr 21:1116–1120
20. Chubuchny V, Plonska E, Baldini U, et al (2002) Prognostic value of noninvasive pacemaker
    stress echocardiography in patients with permanent pacemakers: a multicenter study (abstract).
    Circulation 108(Suppl II):608
21. Biagini E, Schinkel AF, Elhendy A, et al (2005) Pacemaker stress echocardiography predicts
    cardiac events in patients with permanent pacemaker. Am J Med 118:1381–1386
22. Stojnic BB, Stojanov PL, Angelkov L, et al (1996) Evaluation of asynchronous left ventricu-
    lar relaxation by Doppler echocardiography during ventricular pacing with AV synchrony
    (VDD): comparison with atrial pacing (AAI). Pacing Clin Electrophysiol 19:940–944

Ergonovine Stress Echocardiography for the Diagnosis of Vasospastic Angina

16

Jae-Kwan Song and Eugenio Picano

Coronary artery spasm has been considered one of the major mechanisms causing *dynamic* stenosis of epicardial coronary arteries, which can evoke acute myocardial ischemia. Vasospastic angina caused by coronary artery spasm has a wide clinical spectrum: one of its typical clinical manifestations is variant angina. Coronary vasospasm has also been documented to contribute to the development of unstable angina or acute myocardial infarction [1]. Classically, coronary artery spasm is diagnosed by an invasive provocative procedure during diagnostic coronary angiography. Since various noninvasive diagnostic tests for fixed atherosclerotic stenosis of epicardial coronary arteries (exercise ECG, stress echocardiography, and nuclear tests) are being used in routine daily practice, it would be useful to establish a reliable, noninvasive, and safe diagnostic method to document coronary artery spasm in the management of patients with vasospastic angina.

The rare episodic nature of coronary artery spasm makes it extremely difficult to document spontaneous coronary vasospasm in clinical practice. The noninvasive stress tests currently used are ergonovine [2], acetylcholine [3], and systemic alkalosis by hyperventilation [4]. Of these, spasm-provocation testing using ergonovine is considered the gold standard for diagnosis of coronary artery spasm because of its high sensitivity and specificity. Acetylcholine seems to have comparable diagnostic validity for intracoronary administration, but its short half-life for the abundant pseudocholinesterase in human plasma makes intravenous injection inadequate for spasm provocation.

16.1
Basic Considerations

Ergonovine maleate is an important oxytocin alkaloid and a member of the ergobasine group, an amine alcohol derivative of lysergic acid. This drug can induce coronary vasoconstriction in patients who have undergone heart transplantation, which suggests that it does not act via the central nervous system. This drug is believed to stimulate α-adrenergic

E. Picano, *Stress Echocardiography*,
© Springer-Verlag Berlin Heidelberg 2009

and 5-hydroxytryptamine (serotonin) receptors [5]. After intravenous injection, the half-life of the distribution phase is between 1.8 and 3 min, and the half-life of the disappearance phase is between 32 and 116 min [6]. This rapid mode of action explains why coronary spasm most often occurs between 2 and 4 min after the injection. The use of ergonovine in incremental doses starting with an intravenous injection of 0.05–0.1 mg followed by small increments of 0.1–0.15 mg at 5-min intervals up to a maximum cumulative dosage of 0.35 or 0.4 mg is generally recommended [1]. This general guideline is based on the finding that the cumulative doses (0.1 + 0.2 + 0.3 + 0.4 mg) at 5-min intervals have the same effects as a single dose of 0.4 mg [1]. The provocative test with ergonovine performed in the cardiac catheterization laboratory has a high sensitivity (98%) and specificity (98.7%) [7].

16.2
Protocol

For a diagnosis of vasospastic angina, the possibility of significant fixed atherosclerotic stenosis of major epicardial coronary arteries is usually ruled out by means of the exercise stress test and/or pharmacological stress echocardiography. All cardioactive drugs (β-receptor blocker, calcium channel blocker, and nitrates) should be discontinued for at least five half-lives; however, nitroglycerin should be administered sublingually as necessary. Resting hypertension is usually controlled using angiotensin-converting enzyme inhibitors; uncontrolled hypertension is a contraindication of this test.

It should be remembered that some drugs, especially long-action calcium channel blockers, may have persistent effects on coronary vasomotor tone as long as 2–3 weeks after discontinuation [8, 9].

Figure 16.1 shows the classic protocol of ergonovine echocardiography. A bolus injection of ergonovine (50 µg) is administered intravenously at 5-min intervals until a positive

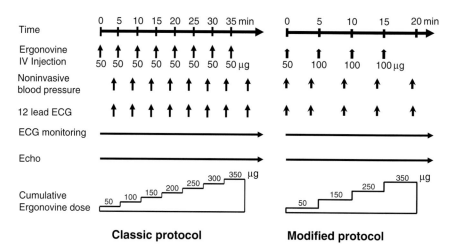

Fig. 16.1 Classic (*left*) and modified (*right*) protocols for ergonovine echocardiography

response is obtained or a total dose of 0.35 mg is reached. The 12-lead ECG is recorded after each ergonovine injection and left ventricular wall motion is monitored continuously. Positive criteria for the test include the appearance of transient ST-segment elevation or depression greater than 0.1 mV at 0.08 s after the J point (ECG criteria) or reversible wall motion abnormality by two-dimensional echocardiography (echocardiographic criteria). The criteria for terminating the test are as follows: positive response defined as ECG or echocardiographic criteria, total cumulative dose of 0.35 mg ergonovine, or development of significant arrhythmia or changes in vital signs (systolic blood pressure>200 mmHg or <90 mmHg). An intravenous bolus injection of nitroglycerin is administered as soon as an abnormal response is detected; sublingual nifedipine (10 mg) is also recommended to counter the possible delayed effects of ergonovine. These drugs can be administered as needed. The protocol can be modified just to decrease the test time (Fig. 16.1), with bolus doses of 50, 100, 100, and 100 μg every 5 min up to a cumulative dose of 350 μg.

16.3
Noninvasive Diagnosis of Coronary Artery Spasm: Clinical Data

Bedside ergonovine echocardiography has been reported to be accurate and safe [8–18] (Figs. 16.2, 16.3). The sensitivity of echocardiographic criteria (detection of reversible regional wall motion abnormalities) is higher than 90%,which is far greater than that of ECG criteria (ST-segment displacement, 40–50%). Characteristic ST-segment elevation during ergonovine testing occurred in about one-third of patients with variant angina [16]; the lower sensitivity with ECG criteria can be partially explained by an earlier development of regional wall asynergy during myocardial ischemia in the so-called pre-electrocardiographic phase rather than a true false-negative finding [10–13]. The earlier detection of ischemia with higher sensitivity is very important from the safety point of view, as the vicious cycle of the ischemic cascade can be terminated earlier and the risk associated with prolonged ischemia reduced. According to the recent report of ergonovine echocardiography performed on 1,372 patients [16], the test showed very high feasibility (99.1%); transient arrhythmias – including sinus bradycardia ($n = 10$), ventricular premature beats ($n = 10$), short-run ventricular tachycardia ($n = 2$), and atrioventricular block ($n = 4$) – developed in 1.9% (26/1,372) of the patients studied. All of these arrhythmias were transient and promptly reversed with the administration of nitroglycerin and nifedipine, as described earlier. Although intracoronary nitroglycerin could not be used to reverse coronary vasospasm in this protocol, there were no serious complications such as development of myocardial infarction or fatal arrhythmia during the test [8, 9].

Unlike other stress tests for fixed atherosclerotic stenosis of coronary artery, this test shows high sensitivity even in patients with single-vessel spasm [16]; the transmural nature of supply ischemia due to coronary artery spasm may explain this difference.

As this test also showed very high specificity (>90%) for the diagnosis of coronary artery spasm before coronary angiography, invasive coronary angiography and spasm-provocation testing can be avoided for the diagnosis of vasospastic angina [16, 18].

16

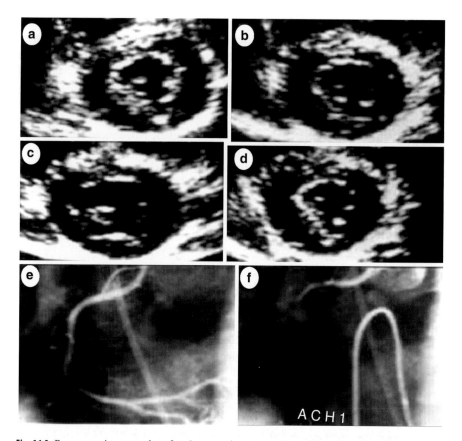

Fig. 16.2 Representative examples of **a–d** ergonovine stress echocardiography and **e, f** coronary angiography in a 53-year-old man with early-morning chest pain. Treadmill test results were negative up to stage 4 of the Bruce protocol, and ergonovine echocardiography was done. Left ventricular wall motion at end-systole recorded in the parasternal short-axis view was demonstrated in quad screen format. **a** Basal status. **b** Left ventricular wall motion after injection of 0.05 mg ergonovine. **c** Regional loss of systolic myocardial thickening in the mid-inferior segment with an ergonovine dose of 0.1 mg and **d** recovery of regional wall motion abnormality with nitroglycerin, a finding suggestive of myocardial ischemia in the region of the right coronary artery due to coronary vasospasm. **e** Coronary angiogram taken 2 days later revealed a normal right coronary artery. **f** Intracoronary injection of acetylcholine (ACH) provoked total occlusion of the proximal right coronary artery, which was compatible with coronary vasospasm. (From [9], with permission)

16.4
Special Safety Considerations

Issues regarding the safety of spasm-provocation testing are summarized in Table 16.1.

Ergonovine echocardiography testing, undertaken either in the catheterization laboratory or at the bedside, is a risky and challenging procedure, demanding a high degree of

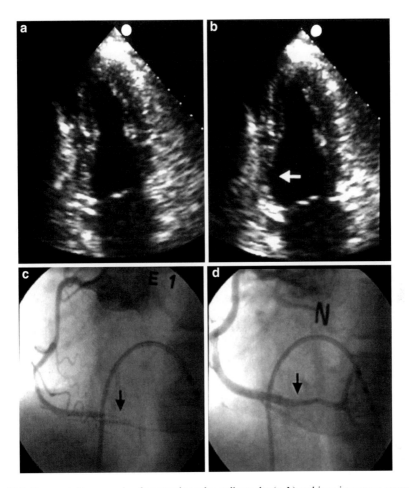

Fig. 16.3 Representative example of ergonovine echocardiography (**a**, **b**) and invasive spasm provocation testing during diagnostic coronary angiography (**c**, **d**) in a 47-year-old man. Left ventricular wall motion at end-systole recorded in the apical two-chamber view was demonstrated (**a**, **b**). Compared with the basal status (**a**), prominent loss of systolic thickening in the inferior wall developed with an ergonovine dose of 0.15 mg (**b**, *white arrow*), which was compatible with myocardial ischemia due to coronary artery spasm in the right coronary artery territory. Coronary angiogram taken 3 days later revealed no significant fixed disease. Intravenous injection of ergonovine (*E1*) provoked total occlusion of the distal right coronary artery (*C*), and the angiogram after injection of nitroglycerin (*N*) showed completely normal right coronary artery and relief of total occlusion (**d**). (Adapted from [16], with permission)

skill on the part of the operator [8]. Angiographic demonstration of reversible total occlusion of one of the major epicardial coronary arteries is in itself enough for a diagnosis of coronary vasospasm. If, however, angiography reveals only moderate vasoconstriction, as occurs more frequently in the daily clinical practice of provocation testing, other indexes of myocardial ischemia are necessary before a definite diagnosis of coronary vasospasm

16

Table 16.1 Potential advantages and disadvantages of spasm-provocation testing in the catheterization laboratory and at the bedside

	Advantages	Disadvantages
Provocation test during angiography	Angiographic demonstration of reversible vasoconstriction	Relatively late and insensitive ischemic markers (chest pain, electrocardiographic changes)
	Direct intracoronary injection of nitroglycerin	Invasive, perturbs vasomotor tone
	Temporary pacemaker backup	Injecting contrast agent into coronary circulation
		Continuous monitoring of whole ischemic process impossible
Bedside ergonovine echocardiography	Detection of regional wall motion abnormalities: sensitive and specific marker of myocardial ischemia, continuous monitoring, early detection and termination of ischemic cascade	Intracoronary injection of nitroglycerin impossible
	Noninvasive, does not perturb vasomotor tone	Temporary pacemaker backup impossible
	Repeat and follow-up studies	Dependent on acoustic window

can be made. In the catheterization laboratory, the development of chest pain and electrocardiographic changes, well known as relatively late events in ischemic cascade, are classic markers of myocardial ischemia. The usual 3- to 4-min wait after each injection of the drug before repeat angiography without sensitive monitoring of ischemic cascade in the catheterization laboratory may also contribute to the potential danger of the procedure. This is because the development of serious arrhythmia or myocardial infarction depends on the duration of the preceding myocardial ischemia during spasm provocation.

In addition to concerns about disturbing vasomotor tone with the catheter, injecting a contrast agent into the coronary circulation during a severe ischemic episode may increase the risk of the procedure. Myocardial imaging rather than angiography has been proposed as a more sensitive, more specific, and safer method of identifying coronary vasospasm by some physicians. The importance of intracoronary nitroglycerin for reversing an intractable vasospasm that is not responsive to sublingual and intravenous nitroglycerin has been reported [19, 20], but other published investigations indicate that intracoronary nitroglycerin is not a prerequisite for spasm-provocation testing [8–18].

The most important advantage of ergonovine echocardiography is its capacity for detecting regional wall motion abnormalities, which are sensitive and specific markers of myocardial ischemia, even before the appearance of chest pain or electrocardiographic changes. During ergonovine echocardiography, the wall of the left ventricle can be continuously monitored, with early termination of myocardial ischemia based on the detection of regional wall motion abnormality; this is a potential and theoretical advantage of the test. In our study [8, 16], less than half of the patients with definite wall motion abnormalities showed ECG changes suggestive of myocardial ischemia, which is compatible with the premise described above. Further multicenter investigation is needed to determine whether early detection and termination of myocardial ischemia based on regional wall motion abnormalities can completely obviate the need for temporary pacemaker backup.

16.5
Clinical Impact

Noninvasive ergonovine stress echocardiography is an effective and reasonably safe way of diagnosing coronary vasospasm in routine clinical practice for patients visiting the outpatient clinic [16] or for those admitted to the coronary care unit under the clinical impression of unstable angina pectoris [15]. Although clinical usage of spasm provocation testing has decreased significantly in Western countries and spasm provocation testing is no longer a routine diagnostic procedure, recent investigation [21] reveals significantly higher mortality and event rates with a positive result of ergonovine stress echocardiography (Fig. 16.4) in patients with near normal coronary angiogram or in those with negative stress test results for significant fixed stenosis. These results demonstrate the powerful prognostic implication of noninvasive ergonovine stress echocardiography in routine daily practice for differential diagnosis of chest pain syndrome. As this test provides an effective and powerful means of risk stratification on the basis

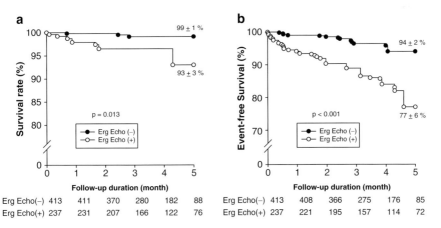

Fig. 16.4 Survival (**a**) and event-free survival rates (**b**) according to the results of ergonovine echocardiography (*Erg Echo*) in patients with near normal coronary angiogram or negative stress test results for significant fixed stenosis. (−), negative test; (+), positive test. (Adapted from [21])

16

of the presence of provocable ischemia in patients with no evidence of significant fixed coronary stenosis, either by direct invasive or noninvasive (by 64-slice computed tomography) coronary angiography or by noninvasive stress testing, consideration of ergonovine stress echocardiography for complete differential diagnosis of mechanisms of myocardial ischemia should be encouraged in various clinical scenarios involving patients with chest pain syndrome [22], such as patients with angiographically normal coronary arteries and a history of angina at rest, aborted sudden death [23], flash pulmonary edema [24], or suspected left ventricular apical ballooning syndrome [25]. The usefulness of the ergonovine test in monitoring the efficacy of antianginal therapy has been documented [26], but its clinical value remains uncertain. It is probably inappropriate to use the test in patients in whom the diagnosis is already established by clinical history or with concomitant ischemia in presence of angiographically documented coronary artery disease. The test can be less safe in patients with uncontrolled hypertension and previous stroke [27]. It is also important to consider vasospasm – and, if appropriate, vasospasm testing – in several clinical settings remote from the cardiology ward when ergometrine-containing or serotonin-agonist drugs are routinely given and may occasionally precipitate "out-of the-blue" cardiological catastrophes mediated by coronary vasospasm: ergometrine given in the obstetric clinic to reduce uterine blood loss in the puerperium phase [28–33] or bromocriptine given for milk suppression [34, 35], sumatriptan or ergometrine used in neurology for migraine headaches [36–39], 5-fluorouracil and capecitabine (an oral 5-fluorouracil prodrug) given as chemotherapy in (breast and colon-rectal) cancer [40–44], and, with increasing frequency, cocaine as a cause of chest pain in the ER [44–45]. In all these conditions, it is essential to think of vasospasm so as to recognize it (Table 16.2).

Table 16.2 Indications to ergometrine stress echocardiography

	Appropriate	Uncertain	Inappropriate
Patients with angina at rest and normal or near normal coronary arteries	√		
Patients with chest pain assuming cocaine, 5-FU, capecitabine, ergometrine, bromocriptine, sumatriptan	√		
Patients with suspected Tako-Tsubo syndrome	√		
Patients with unexplained flash pulmonary edema with normal coronary arteries	√		
Patients with known variant angina to test therapy efficacy		√	
Patients with known variant angina			√
Patients with uncontrolled hypertension or previous stroke			√

References

1. Maseri A (1987) Role of coronary artery spasm in symptomatic and silent myocardial ischemia. J Am Coll Cardiol 9:249–262
2. Heupler FA Jr, Proudfit WL, Razavi M, et al (1978) Ergonovine maleate provocative test for coronary arterial spasm. Am J Cardiol 41:631–640
3. Yasue H, Horio Y, Nakamura N, et al (1986) Induction of coronary artery spasm by acetylcholine in patients with variant angina: possible role of the parasympathetic nervous system in the pathogenesis of coronary artery spasm. Circulation 74:955–963
4. Yasue H, Nagao M, Omote S, et al (1978) Coronary arterial spasm and Prinzmetal's variant form of angina induced by hyperventilation and Tris-buffer infusion. Circulation 58:56–62
5. Muller-Schweinitzer E (1980) The mechanism of ergometrine-induced coronary arterial spasm. In vitro studies on canine arteries. J Cardiovasc Pharmacol 2:645–655
6. Mantyla R, Kanto J (1981) Clinical pharmacokinetic of methylergometrine (methylergonovine). Int J Clin Pharmacol Biopharm 19:386–391
7. Heupler FA (1980) Provocative testing for coronary arterial spasm. Risk, method and rationale. Am J Cardiol 46:335–337
8. Song JK, Park SW, Kim JJ, et al (1994) Values of intravenous ergonovine test with two-dimensional echocardiography for diagnosis of coronary artery spasm. J Am Soc Echocardiogr 7:607–615
9. Song JK, Lee SJK, Kang DH, et al (1996) Ergonovine echocardiography as a screening test for diagnosis of vasospastic angina before coronary angiography. J Am Coll Cardiol 27:1156–1161
10. Distante A, Rovai D, Picano E, et al (1984) Transient changes in left ventricular mechanics during attacks of Prinzmetal's angina: an *M*-mode echocardiographic study. Am Heart J 107:465–474
11. Distante A, Rovai D, Picano E, et al (1984) Transient changes in left ventricular mechanics during attacks of Prinzmetal's angina: a two-dimensional echocardiographic study. Am Heart J 108:440–446
12. Distante A, Picano E, Moscarelli E, et al (1985) Echocardiographic versus hemodynamic monitoring during attacks of variant angina pectoris. Am J Cardiol 55:1319–1322
13. Rovai D, Distante A, Moscarelli E, et al (1985) Transient myocardial ischemia with minimal electrocardiographic changes: an echocardiographic study in patients with Prinzmetal's angina. Am Heart J 109:78–83
14. Morales MA, Lombardi M, Distante A, et al (1985) Ergonovine-echo test assess the significance of chest pain at rest without ECG changes. Eur Heart J 16:1361–1366
15. Song JK, Park SW, Kang DH, et al (1998) Diagnosis of coronary vasospasm in patients with clinical presentation of unstable angina using ergonovine echocardiography. Am J Cardiol 82:1475–1478
16. Song JK, Park SW, Kang DH, et al (2000) Safety and clinical impact of ergonovine stress echocardiography for diagnosis of coronary vasospasm. J Am Coll Cardiol 35:1850–1856
17. Nedeljkovic MA, Ostojic M, Beleslin B, et al (2001) Efficiency of ergonovine echocardiography in detecting angiographically assessed coronary vasospasm. Am J Cardiol 88:1183–1187
18. Palinkas A, Picano E, Rodriguez O, et al (2002) Safety of ergot stress echocardiography for noninvasive detection of coronary vasospasm. Coron Artery Dis 12:649–654
19. Buxton A, Goldberg S, Hirshfeld JW, et al (1980) Refractory ergonovine-induced vasospasm: importance of intracoronary nitroglycerin. Am J Cardiol 46:329–334
20. Pepine CJ, Feldman RJ, Conti CR (1982) Action of intracoronary nitroglycerin in refractory coronary artery spasm. Circulation 65:411–414

21. Song JK, Park SW, Kang DH, et al (2002) Prognostic implication of ergonovine echocardiography in patients with near normal coronary angiogram or negative stress test for significant fixed stenosis. J Am Soc Echocardiogr 15:1346–1352

22. Hamilton KK, Pepine CJ (2000) A renaissance of provocative testing for coronary spasm? J Am Coll Cardiol 35:1857–1859

23. van der Burg AE, Bax JJ, Boersma E, et al (2004) Standardized screening and treatment of patients with life-threatening arrhythmias: the Leiden out-of-hospital cardiac arrest evaluation study. Heart Rhythm 1:51–57

24. Epureanu V, San Román JA, Vega JL, et al (2002) Acute pulmonary edema with normal coronary arteries: mechanism identification by ergonovine stress echocardiography. Rev Esp Cardiol 55:775–777

25. Previtali M, Repetto A, Panigada S, et al (2008) Left ventricular apical ballooning syndrome: prevalence, clinical characteristics and pathogenetic mechanisms in a European population. Int J Cardiol May 26

26. Lombardi M, Morales MA, Michelassi C, et al (1993) Efficacy of isosorbide-5-mononitrate versus nifedipine in preventing spontaneous and ergonovine-induced myocardial ischaemia. A double-blind, placebo-controlled study. Eur Heart J 14:845–851

27. Barinagarrementeria F, Cantú C, Balderrama J (1992) Postpartum cerebral angiopathy with cerebral infarction due to ergonovine use. Stroke 23:1364–1366

28. Salem DN, Isner JM, Hopkins P, et al (1984) Ergonovine provocation in postpartum myocardial infarction. Angiology 35:110–114

29. Nall KS, Feldman B (1998) Postpartum myocardial infarction induced by Methergine. Am J Emerg Med 16:502–504

30. Yaegashi N, Miura M, Okamura K (1999) Acute myocardial infarction associated with postpartum ergot alkaloid administration. Int J Gynaecol Obstet 64:67–68

31. Ribbing M, Reinecke H, Breithardt G et al (2001) Acute anterior wall infarct in a 31-year-old patient after administration of methylergometrine for peripartal vaginal hemorrhage. Herz 26:489–493

32. Hayashi Y, Ibe T, Kawato H, et al (2003) Postpartum acute myocardial infarction induced by ergonovine administration. Intern Med 42:983–986

33. Ichiba T, Nishie H, Fujinaka W, et al (2005) Acute myocardial infarction due to coronary artery spasm after caesarean section. Masui 54:54–56

34. Larrazet F, Spaulding C, Lobreau HJ, et al (1993) Possible bromocriptine-induced myocardial infarction. Ann Intern Med 118:199–200

35. Hopp L, Weisse AB, Iffy L (1996) Acute myocardial infarction in a healthy mother using bromocriptine for milk suppression. Can J Cardiol 12:415–418

36. Castle WM, Simmons VE (1992) Coronary vasospasm and sumatriptan. BMJ 305:117–118

37. Mueller L, Gallagher RM, Ciervo CA (1996) Vasospasm-induced myocardial infarction with sumatriptan. Headache 36:329–331

38. Wackenfors A, Jarvius M, Ingemansson R, et al (2005) Triptans induce vasoconstriction of human arteries and veins from the thoracic wall. J Cardiovasc Pharmacol 45:476–484

39. Bassi S, Amersey R, Henderson R et al (2004) Thyrotoxicosis, sumatriptan and coronary artery spasm. J R Soc Med 97:285–287

40. Kleiman NS, Lehane DE, Geyer CE Jr et al (1987) Prinzmetal's angina during 5-fluorouracil chemotherapy. Am J Med 82:566–568

41. Lestuzzi C, Viel E, Picano E, et al (2001) Coronary vasospasm as a cause of effort-related myocardial ischemia during low-dose chronic continuous infusion of 5-fluorouracil. Am J Med 111:316–318

42. Sestito A, Sgueglia GA, Pozzo C, et al (2006) Coronary artery spasm induced by capecitabine. J Cardiovasc Med 7:136–138
43. Papadopoulos CA, Wilson H (2008) Capecitabine-associated coronary vasospasm: a case report. Emerg Med J 25:307–309
44. Rezkalla SH, Kloner RA (2007) Cocaine-induced acute myocardial infarction. Clin Med Res 5:172–176
45. McCord J, Jneid H, Hollander JE et al (2008) American Heart Association Acute Cardiac Care Committee of the Council on Clinical Cardiology. Management of cocaine-associated chest pain and myocardial infarction: a scientific statement from the American Heart Association Acute Cardiac Care Committee of the Council on Clinical Cardiology. Circulation 117:1897–1907

Hyperventilation Test

17

Eugenio Picano

Hyperventilation tests have been mainly used in clinical practice as a provocative test for coronary artery vasospasm in patients with suspected or documented vasospastic angina [1–4]. The rationale for the use of hyperventilation testing for this purpose is based on the demonstration that, in susceptible patients, hyperventilation may trigger a vasospasm of a major epicardial coronary artery associated with chest pain and ischemic electrocardiographic changes similar to those observed during spontaneous anginal attacks [1].

17.1
Pathophysiology

Prolonged, vigorous overbreathing decreases plasma hydrogen ion concentration, leading to metabolic alkalosis, which can trigger coronary artery spasm [1]. The increase in arterial blood pH reaches the peak at the end of hyperventilation, while ST-segment elevation usually develops during the recovery phase early after the end of the test, when arterial pH is already decreasing toward baseline but is still significantly elevated compared to basal values [4].

Another mechanism of coronary spasm in this setting can ensue, with increases in intracellular concentration of calcium ions following a decrease in the concentration of hydrogen ions, which compete with calcium for active transmembrane transport [5] (Fig. 17.1). The increase in intracellular calcium concentration can in turn elicit a vasospastic constriction of smooth muscle cells in susceptible coronary epicardial arteries [5].

17.2
Protocol

The patient hyperventilates for 5 min, with increased frequency (30 per min) and depth of breathing (Fig. 17.2). The time window of positivity usually occurs 1–5 min after the end of hyperventilation, therefore without degrading the quality of echocardiographic imaging.

E. Picano, *Stress Echocardiography*,
© Springer-Verlag Berlin Heidelberg 2009

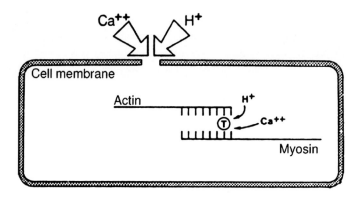

Fig. 17.1 The mechanism of contraction induced by alkalosis in smooth muscle cell. With a reduced concentration of hydrogen ions, more calcium enters the cell from the outside and more intracellular calcium reaches the regulatory troponin site, triggering contraction. (Modified from [5], with permission)

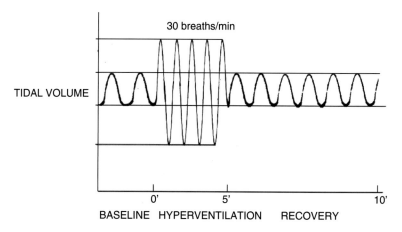

Fig. 17.2 Protocol of the hyperventilation stress echocardiography test

17.3
Diagnostic Value

The sensitivity of the test is markedly affected by the spontaneous activity of the disease; when spontaneous attacks occur frequently, a positive response to hyperventilation is observed in more than 80% of patients, while the sensitivity of the test decreases to 50% or less in patients with less active disease [1, 3, 4, 6–10]. Since hyperventilation may produce chest pain and pseudoischemic changes in vasospasm, echocardiographic monitoring during the test can be particularly useful to demonstrate normal regional wall motion and thickening and therefore rule out the diagnosis of vasospastic myocardial ischemia. In patients with variant angina, hyperventilation can also be used to predict the ability of antianginal drugs to prevent spontaneous attacks and to select an effective medical treatment [8]; moreover, if the test yields negative results during long-term follow-up, this may indicate a spontaneous remission of the disease [8].

17.4
Diagnostic Value and Clinical Guidelines

The hyperventilation test has shown excellent safety and satisfactory feasibility associated with good sensitivity (slightly lower than ergometrine) and specificity for the diagnosis of vasospastic angina (Table 17.1). It is considered slightly safer than the ergonovine test because the stimulus to vasospasm wanes as soon as the intracellular pH returns to normal; however, one should be aware that consequences of ischemia are largely independent of the form of provocation [11, 12]. Both total duration of the test and the imaging time are shorter with hyperventilation (about 10 min) than with ergonovine (approximately 20 min) (Table 17.1).

It can therefore be a useful test for the diagnosis of vasospastic angina in outpatients and in patients with contraindications to ergometrine such as arterial hypertension or previous stroke (Table 17.1). It may unmask the vasospastic origin of symptoms in patients with syncopal angina [13, 14]. However, hyperventilation is demanding for the patient who may not be able to complete it and is contraindicated in epilepsy. In patients with typical symptoms, a positive response to hyperventilation is diagnostic, thus avoiding the need to perform ergometrine testing. In patients with a negative or nondiagnostic response to hyperventilation but with symptoms suggesting vasospastic angina, ergonovine testing

Table 17.1 Tests for coronary vasospasm

	Hyperventilation	Ergometrine
Sensitivity	++	+++
Specificity	+++	+++
Safety	+++	++(+)
Imaging time	10 min	20 min
Arterial hypertension	Yes	No
Epilepsy	No	Yes
Previous stroke	Yes	No
Physically deconditioned	No	Yes

should be performed since the sensitivity of the hyperventilation test in patients with sporadic symptoms is suboptimal and a negative response cannot rule out the presence of vasospastic angina. Our policy is to perform ergometrine testing only in inpatients, whereas hyperventilation is also performed in outpatients.

Hyperventilation testing can also be used to assess the efficacy of medical therapy, such as endothelium-protective estradiol supplementation in variant angina [15] or atrial natriuretic peptide (ANP) [16] infusion. Novel, promising approaches combine mild hyperventilation followed by exercise [17] or the cold pressor test [18–21] to enhance the test sensitivity for vasospasm detection. Conceptually, this approach is similar to the combined stress approach for the diagnosis of minor forms of fixed coronary artery stenosis. In the latter case, a vasodilator stress reducing subendocardial flow supply through steal phenomenon (dipyridamole) is administered and, if the stress is negative, a second additive stressor (exercise or dobutamine), with a different mechanism of action, is administered on the shoulder of the first one to increase myocardial oxygen demand [22, 23]. In the diagnosis of coronary vasospasm, there is a hierarchy of testing for stressor potency with ergometrine being the most potent, hyperventilation the intermediate, and exercise and cold pressor the least potent stressor [9] (Fig. 17.3). Since hyperventilation acts in a different fashion than exercise and cold, the sensitivity for vasospasm critically increases with the combination of hyperventilation and either the cold pressor or exercise test (Fig. 17.3).

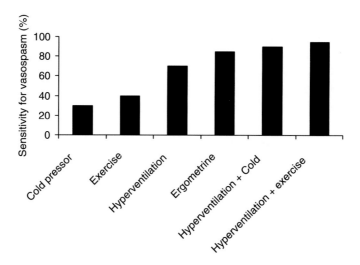

Fig. 17.3 The hierarchy of test sensitivity for the diagnosis of coronary artery disease. The continuous transverse line indicates the fixed ceiling of coronary flow reserve, which is not reduced in this ideal case of pure vasospastic angina. The *dashed lines* indicate the fluctuations of coronary tone. They occur spontaneously (*far left*, variant angina) or can be provoked by stress testing. The power of stress testing is indicated by the depth of the *dashed line*. Only tests arriving below the line of oxygen consumption at rest evoke ischemia. Cold and exercise are relatively weak stressors when used alone, but they can critically potentiate the sensitivity of hyperventilation

References

1. Yasue H, Nagao M, Omote S, et al (1978) Coronary arterial spasm and Prinzmetal's variant form of angina induced by hyperventilation and Tris-buffer infusion. Circulation 58:56–62
2. Mortensen SA, Vilhelmsen R, Sandoe E (1983) Non-pharmacological provocation of coronary vasospasm. Experience with prolonged hyperventilation in the coronary care unit. Eur Heart J 4:391–397
3. Rasmussen K, Bagger JP, Bottzauw J, et al (1984) Prevalence of vasospastic ischaemia induced by the cold pressor test or hyperventilation in patients with severe angina. Eur Heart J 5:354–361
4. Previtali M, Ardissino D, Barberis P, et al (1989) Hyperventilation and ergonovine tests in Prinzmetal's variant angina pectoris in men. Am J Cardiol 63:17–20
5. Weber S, Pasquier G, Guiomard A, et al (1981) Clinical application of the alkalosis induction test for coronary artery spasm. Arch Mal Coeur Vaiss 74:1389–1395
6. Ardissino D, De Servi S, Falcone C, et al (1987) Role of hypocapnic alkalosis in hyperventilation-induced coronary artery spasm in variant angina. Am J Cardiol 59:707–709
7. Morales MA, Reisenhofer B, Rovai D, et al (1993) Hyperventilation-echocardiography test for the diagnosis of myocardial ischaemia at rest. Eur Heart J 14:1088–1093
8. Girotti LA, Crosatto JR, Messuti H, et al (1982) The hyperventilation test as a method for developing successful therapy in Prinzmetal's angina. Am J Cardiol 49:834–841
9. Kaski JC, Crea F, Meran D, et al (1986) Local coronary supersensitivity to diverse vasoconstrictive stimuli in patients with variant angina. Circulation 74:1255–1265
10. Fujii H, Yasue H, Okumura K, et al (1988) Hyperventilation-induced simultaneous multivessel coronary spasm in patients with variant angina: an echocardiographic and arteriographic study. J Am Coll Cardiol 12:1184–1192
11. Maseri A (1996) Variant angina. In: Maseri A (ed) Ischemic heart disease. Churchill Livingston, London, pp 559–588
12. Nakao K, Ohgushi M, Yoshimura M, et al (1997) Hyperventilation as a specific test for diagnosis of coronary artery spasm. Am J Cardiol 80:545–549
13. Astarita C, Rumolo S, Liguori E (1999) Syncopal vasospastic angina in a patient with familial non-obstructive hypertrophic cardiomyopathy. G Ital Cardiol 29:159–162
14. Alcala Lopez JE, Azpitarte Almagro J, Alvarez Lopez M, et al (1995) Syncope and chest pain. Demonstration of the mechanism by the hyperventilation test. Rev Esp Cardiol 48:631–633
15. Kawano H, Motoyama T, Hirai N, et al (2001) Estradiol supplementation suppresses hyperventilation-induced attacks in postmenopausal women with variant angina. J Am Coll Cardiol 37:735–740
16. Tanaka H, Yasue H, Yoshimura M, et al (1993) Suppression of hyperventilation-induced attacks with infusion of atrial natriuretic peptide in patients with variant angina pectoris. Am J Cardiol 72:128–133
17. Sueda S, Fukuda H, Watanabe K, et al (2001) Usefulness of accelerated exercise following mild hyperventilation for the induction of coronary artery spasm: comparison with an acetylcholine test. Chest 119:155–162
18. Hirano Y, Ozasa Y, Yamamoto T, et al (2001) Hyperventilation and cold-pressor stress echocardiography for non-invasive diagnosis of coronary artery spasm. J Am Soc Echocardiogr 14:626–633
19. Hirano Y, Ozasa Y, Yamamoto T, et al (2002) Diagnosis of vasospastic angina by hyperventilation and cold-pressor stress echocardiography: comparison to I-MIBG myocardial scintigraphy. J Am Soc Echocardiogr 15:617–623

17

20. Hirano Y, Uehara H, Nakamura H, et al (2007) Diagnosis of vasospastic angina: comparison of hyperventilation and cold-pressor stress echocardiography, hyperventilation and cold-pressor stress coronary angiography, and coronary angiography with intracoronary injection of acetylcholine. Int J Cardiol 116:331–337

21. Yilmaz A, Mahrholdt H, Athanasiadis A, et al (2007) Non-invasive evaluation of coronary vasospasm using a combined hyperventilation and cold-pressure-test perfusion CMR protocol. J Cardiovasc Magn Reson 9:759–764

Grading of Ischemic Response

18

Eugenio Picano

The need for a dichotomy (yes/no) classification of the results of both provocative tests (positive or negative) and coronary angiography (disease present or absent) in conventional sensitivity/specificity analysis of test results has at least three important limitations [1]:

1. Coronary artery disease is not an all-or-nothing condition; a binary classification requires arbitrary threshold criteria and creates artificial distinctions in coronary artery disease, which in reality shows a continuous spectrum of severity.
2. Sensitivity and specificity values tend to be affected by the disease's distribution in the study population; a sample distribution with a high frequency of mild disease will be placed centrally near the threshold values, where scatter is more likely to lower sensitivity and specificity [2].
3. Percent diameter narrowing is not an adequate standard for quantifying stenosis severity in clinical studies [3]; in unselected populations, this anatomical parameter has a poor correlation with the coronary flow reserve. Thus coronary artery disease is a complex phenomenon that cannot be described adequately by means of a simple normality versus disease paradigm; there are in fact significant differences as regards the degree and the extent of disease that carry important implications for both therapy and prognosis. A stress test should not only predict the presence or absence of coronary disease, but should also stratify disease severity. The diagnosis of myocardial ischemia by stress echocardiography should be delimited by time and space coordinates of the circumferential (horizontal) extent of ischemia (x-axis), the transmural (vertical) depth of ischemia (y-axis), and the ischemia-free stress time (i.e., the time from the start of stress to the appearance of ischemia; z-axis) (Fig. 18.1).

The anatomical–functional degree of coronary artery disease is related to the area included in this three-axis system. From the theoretical point of view, poststress imaging (e.g., postexercise echocardiography) emphasizes the importance of the extent of asynergy. Time to ischemia is more informative in pharmacological tests in which continuous monitoring of images during stress is obtained and the appearance of asynergy is the absolute end point; this usually makes it impossible to observe the effect of coronary stenoses that are less severe than the one that first provoked ischemia. Both parameters – time and space – can

E. Picano, *Stress Echocardiography*,
© Springer-Verlag Berlin Heidelberg 2009

18

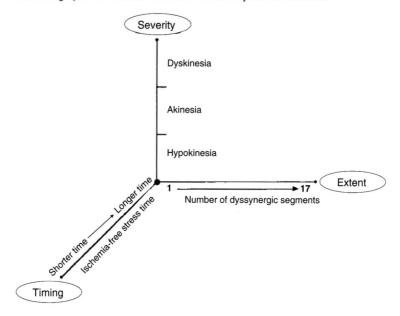

Fig. 18.1 Space and time coordinates of the ischemic response during stress echocardiography: *x-axis*, the number of segments in which the left ventricle is dyssynergic; *y-axis*, the severity of dyssynergy that is correlated to the degree of coronary flow impairment; *z-axis*, ischemia-free stress time

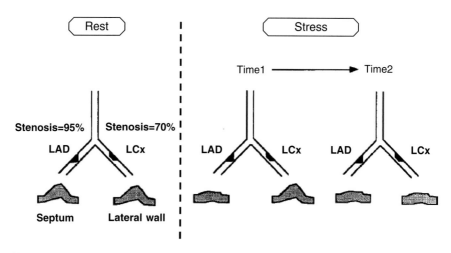

Fig. 18.2 Relationship between stress-induced asynergy and the extent of coronary artery disease. The extent of disease is best reflected by the extent of dyssynergy. A greater extent of coronary artery disease is mirrored by a greater extent of asynergy during stress. *LAD* left anterior descending artery, *LCx* left circumflex artery

be usefully combined to describe the test's degree of positivity: the extent of dyssynergy reflects the extent of coronary artery disease (Figs. 18.2 and 18.3), whereas the time to ischemia is better related to the degree of stenosis in the ischemia-producing vessel (Figs. 18.4 and 18.5). Another less common sign of disease severity is represented by slow and/ or incomplete recovery after interruption of the stress and by the appearance of stress-induced arrhythmias. Other signs of disease severity, apart from short stress time and slow recovery (antidote resistance), include dyskinesis, heterozonal positivity (multiple coronary regions), and left ventricular dilatation.

18.1
Degree of Asynergy

The degree of subendocardial hypoperfusion and the transmural effect of ischemia are reflected in the severity of regional dyssynergy and hypokinesis indicating a milder and transmurally less extensive ischemia in comparison to akinesis and dyskinesis [4].

18.2
Extent of Asynergy

The extension of the risk zone can be identified and quantified by evaluating the number of asynergic segments during stress. The wall motion score index in resting conditions and at peak stress represents an integrated estimation of spatial extent and of the severity of asyn-

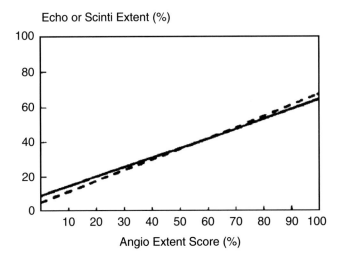

Fig. 18.3 Relationship between angiographically assessed coronary artery disease (*x-axis*) with dobutamine stress (*y axis*) and extent and severity of the perfusion defect during sestamibi scintigraphy or wall motion dysfunction during simultaneous echocardiographic imaging with dobutamine stress. *Solid line* scintigraphic score, *dashed line* echocardiographic score. (From [7], with permission)

18

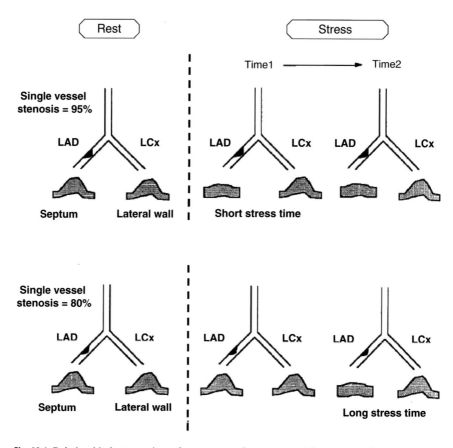

Fig. 18.4 Relationship between time of appearance of asynergy and the severity of coronary artery disease. The sensitivity of disease is best reflected by the timing of dyssynergy. Higher degrees of stenosis are mirrored by an earlier appearance of synergy during the test. *LAD* left anterior descending artery, *LCx* left circumflex artery

ergy. Also, it is linearly correlated to the extent and severity of angiographically assessed coronary artery disease (Fig. 18.2) and to the perfusion defect simultaneously assessed with radionuclide scintigraphy [5–7] (Fig. 18.3). In patients with previous myocardial infarction, the appearance of homozonal asynergy during stress (in the site of necrosis) suggests that a critical residual stenosis is present in the infarct-related vessel [8, 9], whereas the presence of heterozonal asynergy identifies multivessel coronary artery disease [10–12]. However, a low wall motion score index or homozonal positivity cannot rule out multivessel coronary artery disease. This may be due to the test protocol employed in stress echocardiography, since the development of a new wall motion abnormality is an absolute end point of the test, chosen in order to prevent potential complications from severe or prolonged ischemia.

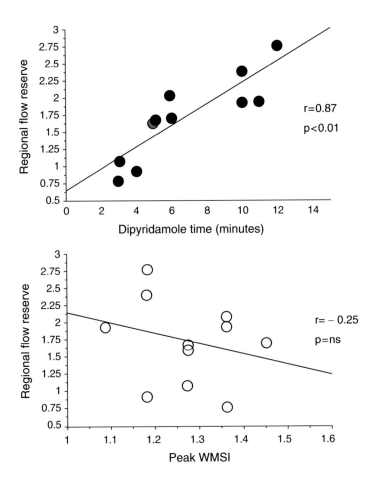

Fig. 18.5 Relationship between regional coronary flow reserve (*ordinates*) and either dipyridamole time (*abscissae, top*) or peak wall motion score index (*MWMSI; abscissae, bottom*) in patients with coronary artery disease and positive dipyridamole echocardiographic test. The relationship is significant only with dipyridamole time. (From [21], with permission)

18.3
Ischemia-Free Stress Time

The most important diagnostic information extracted from the exercise test is the cardiac workload capable of inducing electrocardiographically [13] or echocardiographically [14] assessed myocardial ischemia. For a given extent and severity of induced ischemia, patients with more severe coronary artery disease and worse prognosis are identified on the basis of exercise time, corresponding to the level of stress necessary to provoke ischemia.

The positive response on the basis of ischemia-free stress time (i.e., the time lag between the start of stress and the onset of echocardiographically detected ischemia) can also be stratified by exercise-independent tests. From the theoretical point of view, the step-by-step increase in heart rate induced by atrial pacing or the administration of scalar doses of a drug represent a graduated stress, similar to a multistage exercise test. The amount of stress capable of provoking myocardial ischemia (expressed as doses of drugs, heart rate, duration of exercise, or – for all stresses – ischemia-free stress time) is inversely related to the severity of coronary artery disease [15–22]. An early positivity with the lower dose of the drug indicates a more severe coronary artery disease from the anatomical [18, 19], functional [20–22], and prognostic points of view [23], as compared to late positivity with a higher dose. In single-vessel disease, severity of coronary stenosis and impairment in regional flow reserve are greater when the stress-induced dyssynergy appears earlier during the test (Fig. 18.4). In patients with a positive dipyridamole echocardiography study, regional coronary flow reserve (measured by dynamic positron emission tomography) correlated well with dipyridamole time, but not with the peak wall motion score index [21] (Fig. 18.5). For dobutamine and exercise or pacing, the shorter the ischemia-free stress time was, the more severe the underlying stenosis provoking ischemia was [17–20]. Patients with low-dose positivity are also at higher risk for subsequent cardiac events (Fig. 18.6). Clearly, for proper recognition of the ischemia-free stress time, continuous echocardiographic monitoring is needed in order to obtain a cinematographic representation of ischemic stress. Poststress imaging cannot provide any information on the timing of asynergy during stress; the representation of ischemia in this case is photographic rather than cinematographic. In fact, two images are compared, one in basal conditions and the other after stress. The lack of the time coordinate reduces the overall diagnostic information provided by the stress test.

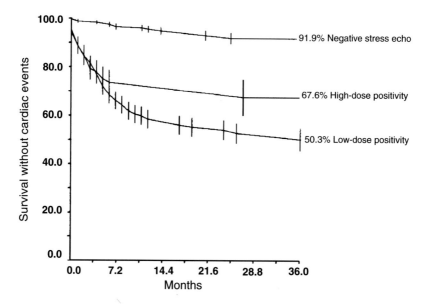

Fig. 18.6 Cumulative survival rates in patients free of cardiac events in group A (negative dipyridamole echocardiographic test), group B (positive high-dose echocardiographic test, i.e., with ischemia-free stress time longer than 8 min), and group C (positive low-dose dipyridamole echocardiographic test)

The stress time is also a useful parameter to assess the effects of both antianginal therapy and revascularization procedures. These therapeutic procedures might determine a full negativity of a previously positive test, but when the test remains positive after the intervention, the potential beneficial effects can be assessed on the basis of a reduction in the peak wall motion score index and an increase in ischemia-free stress time. During both exercise and pharmacological stress, the echocardiographic evaluation of the wall motion score index and particularly of ischemia-free stress time allows an objective evaluation of either pharmacological [24–28] or mechanical [29–32] therapy. In addition, serial assessment of stress echocardiographic response on repeated testing allows one to separate angiographic progressors and nonprogressors efficiently, simply by taking into account the presence, timing, extent, and severity of stress-induced abnormalities of wall motion [33]. The prediction of angiographic progression is substantially more accurate with stress echocardiography than with exercise electrocardiography [34].

18.4
Slow or Incomplete Recovery

In 5–10% of tests, the interruption of stress – cessation of exercise or, in the case of pharmacological tests, antidote administration – fails to reverse the induced ischemia. A longer recovery time (i.e., the time from the end of stress to the return to basal function) indicates more severe coronary artery disease. A possible explanation for a slow recovery may be the prolonged ischemia or greater severity of the coronary lesions underlying reperfusion. From the clinical point of view, this phenomenon is almost always associated with severe or extensive coronary artery disease [35].

18.5
False Friends of Stress-Induced Ischemia Severity:
Arrhythmias and Hypotension

The administration of stress may induce arrhythmias for the stress per se or secondary to the induced ischemia. For example, adenosine and dipyridamole, albeit rarely, can provoke atrial standstill up to asystolia for the depressor effect of adenosine on the impulse formation and conduction [36]. Other stresses, such as dobutamine, have significant arrhythmogenic effects independently of ischemia [37–39] and can induce transient atrioventricular block for a neurally mediated vagal reflex [40]. These primary arrhythmic phenomena have no diagnostic value in the assessment of coronary artery disease; however, they may be useful ancillary markers to identify arrhythmic tendencies, which should be confirmed by other diagnostic evidence (such as Holter monitoring or the head-up tilting test). For instance, in patients with transient atrioventricular block during a negative dobutamine stress, the head-up tilting test is frequently positive [40].

The significance of stress-induced hypotension is different for exercise and pharmacological stress: during exercise, a fall in blood pressure implies the presence of acute cardiac insufficiency and is very often associated with advanced forms of coronary artery disease [13, 14]. In contrast, during pharmacological stress, hypotension can be induced without implying pump failure and is not related to the presence and severity of coronary artery disease. During dipyridamole, hypotension is probably caused by hypersensitivity to negative chronotropic effects of adenosine (hypotension and bradycardia) and/or to peripheral vasodilatory effects of adenosine (isolated hypotension). During dobutamine, the two main hypothesized ischemia-independent mechanisms are vasodepressor reflex triggered by left ventricular mechanoreceptor stimulation due to excessive inotropic stimulation [41] and the development of dynamic intraventricular pressure gradient mirrored by the increased left ventricular outflow tract velocity [42–44]. While mild (20 mmHg) hypotension during dobutamine is frequent (20%) and probably prognostically benign, profound (drop in systolic pressure >50 mmHg) hypotension during dobutamine is rare (3% of cases) and has been associated with a worse prognosis for subsequent cardiac events [45, 46].

18.6
The Fourth Coordinate: Perfusion and/or Coronary Flow Reserve

The classic model of stratification on the basis of three spatial and temporal coordinates shown in Fig. 18.1 has been expanded in recent years by the ability to include a further severity stratification on the basis of the type of positivity: reduction of coronary flow reserve (or perfusion changes) or wall motion abnormality. In the last 5 years, coronary flow reserve on the left anterior descending artery has become routine added information in the clinical setting of vasodilatory stress echocardiography [47]. In this way, the stress echocardiography response can be stratified on the basis of ischemic cascade, as occurs with other imaging techniques such as cardiovascular magnetic resonance [48]. In the absence of regional wall motion abnormalities, a reduced coronary flow reserve makes the wall motion negativity less prognostically benign [49, 50]. In presence of wall motion positivity, a reduced coronary flow reserve makes the wall motion positivity more prognostically malignant [51]. This introduces a further, fourth dimension (type of positivity) in the coordinates of stress echocardiographic stratification.

18.7
Conclusion

The presence (or absence) of inducible wall motion abnormalities separates patients with different prognosis. A normal stress echocardiogram yields an annual risk of 0.4–0.9%. Thus in patients with suspected coronary artery disease, a normal stress echocardiography implies excellent prognosis and coronary angiography can safely be avoided. The positive and negative responses can be further stratified with interaction with clinical parameters (diabetics, renal dysfunction, and therapy at test time), resting echocardiography (global LV and additive stress echocardiography parameters, especially coronary flow reserve on the left anterior descending artery during vasodilation stress testing) [52]. A positive stress echocardiography result is more prognostically malignant (Table 18.1), and a negative stress echocardiography result less prognostically benign (Table 18.2), if one considers

Table 18.1 Stress echocardiographic risk titration of a positive test result

1-year risk (hard events)	Intermediate (1–3% year)	High (>10% year)
Dose/workload	High	Low
Resting EF	>50%	<40%
Antiischemic therapy	Off	On
Coronary territory	LCx/RCA	LAD
Peak WMSI	Low	High
Recovery	Fast	Slow
Positivity or baseline dyssynergy	Homozonal	Heterozonal
CFR	>2.0	>2.0

EF ejection fraction, *LAD* left anterior descending artery, *LCX* left circumflex, *RCA* right coronary artery, *WMSI* wall motion score index

Table 18.2 Stress echocardiographic risk titration of a negative test result

1-year risk (hard events)	Very low (<0.5% year)	Low (1–3%year)
Stress	Maximal	Submaximal
Resting EF	>50%	<40%
Antiischemic therapy	Off	On
CFR	>2.0	<2.0

EF ejection fraction, *CFR* coronary flow reserve

simple variables in addition to regional wall motion. In patients with positive stress echocardiography results, the timing and extent of wall motion abnormalities powerfully stratify the prognostic risk. In patients with a negative stress echocardiography result, a reduced coronary flow reserve helps to identify the "wolf in sheep's clothes," in whom prognosis is less good, in spite of the falsely reassuring negativity of wall motion.

References

1. Demer LL, Gould KL, Goldstein RA, et al (1989) Assessment of coronary artery disease severity by positron emission tomography. Comparison with quantitative arteriography in 193 patients. Circulation 79:825–835
2. Hlatky MA, Mark DB, Harrell FE Jr, et al (1987) Rethinking sensitivity and specificity. Am J Cardiol 59:1195–1198
3. Marcus ML, Skorton DJ, Johnson MR, et al (1988) Visual estimates of percent diameter coronary stenosis: "a battered gold standard." J Am Coll Cardiol 11:882–885
4. Ross J Jr (1991) Myocardial perfusion-contraction matching. Implications for coronary heart disease and hibernation. Circulation. 83:1076–1083
5. Sawada SG, Segar DS, Ryan T, et al (1991) Echocardiographic detection of coronary artery disease during dobutamine infusion. Circulation 83:1605–1614

18

6. Picano E, Alaimo A, Chubuchny V, et al (2002) Noninvasive pacemaker stress echocardiography for diagnosis of coronary artery disease: a multicenter study. J Am Coll Cardiol 40:1305–1310

7. Marwick T, D'Hondt AM, Baudhuin T, et al (1993) Optimal use of dobutamine stress for the detection and evaluation of coronary artery disease: combination with echocardiography or scintigraphy, or both? J Am Coll Cardiol 22:159–167

8. Armstrong WF, O'Donnell J, Ryan T, et al (1987) Effect of prior myocardial infarction and extent and location of coronary disease on accuracy of exercise echocardiography. J Am Coll Cardiol 10:531–538

9. Bolognese L, Sarasso G, Bongo AS, et al (1991) Dipyridamole echocardiography test. A new tool for detecting jeopardized myocardium after thrombolytic therapy. Circulation 84:1100–1106

10. Berthe C, Pierard LA, Hiernaux M, et al (1986) Predicting the extent and location of coronary artery disease in acute myocardial infarction by echocardiography during dobutamine infusion. Am J Cardiol 58:1167–1172

11. Jaarsma W, Visser CA, Kupper AJ, et al (1986) Usefulness of two-dimensional exercise echocardiography shortly after myocardial infarction. Am J Cardiol 57:86–90

12. Bolognese L, Sarasso G, Aralda D, et al (1989) High-dose dipyridamole echocardiography early after uncomplicated acute myocardial infarction: correlation with exercise testing and coronary angiography. J Am Coll Cardiol 14:357–363

13. Chaitman BR (1996) Exercise stress testing. In: Braunwald E (ed) Heart disease. A textbook of cardiovascular medicine, 5th edn. Saunders, Philadelphia, pp153–176

14. Armstrong WF (1988) Exercise echocardiography: ready, willing and able. J Am Coll Cardiol 11:1359–1361

15. Crouse LJ, Harbrecht JJ, Vacek JL, et al (1991) Exercise echocardiography as a screening test for coronary artery disease and correlation with coronary arteriography. Am J Cardiol 67:1213–1218

16. Ryan T, Segar DS, Sawada SG, et al (1993) Detection of coronary artery disease with upright bicycle exercise echocardiography. J Am Soc Echocardiogr 6:186–197

17. Sheikh KH, Bengtson JR, Helmy S, et al (1990) Relation of quantitative coronary lesion measurements to the development of exercise-induced ischemia assessed by exercise echocardiography. J Am Coll Cardiol 15:1043–1051

18. Segar DS, Brown SE, Sawada SG, et al (1992) Dobutamine stress echocardiography: correlation with coronary lesion severity as determined by quantitative angiography. J Am Coll Cardiol 19:1197–1202

19. Baptista J, Arnese M, Roelandt JR, et al (1994) Quantitative coronary angiography in the estimation of the functional significance of coronary stenosis: correlations with dobutamine atropine stress test. J Am Coll Cardiol 23:1434–1439

20. Amico A, Iliceto S, D'Ambrosio G, et al (1987) Evaluation of timing of occurrence of wall motion abnormalities during incremental atrial pacing aids in the prediction of the severity of coronary artery disease. Eur Heart J 8:190–194

21. Picano E, Parodi O, Lattanzi F, et al (1994) Assessment of anatomic and physiological severity of single-vessel coronary artery lesions by dipyridamole echocardiography. Comparison with positron emission tomography and quantitative arteriography. Circulation 89:753–761

22. Picano E, Lattanzi F, Masini M, et al (1987) Different degrees for ischemic threshold stratified by the dipyridamole-echocardiography test. Am J Cardiol 59:71–73

23. Picano E, Severi S, Michelassi C, et al (1989) Prognostic importance of dipyridamole echocardiography test in coronary artery disease. Circulation 80:450–457

24. Lattanzi F, Picano E, Bolognese L, et al (1991) Inhibition of dipyridamole-induced ischemia by antianginal therapy in humans. Correlation with exercise electrocardiography. Circulation 83:1256–1262

25. Ferrara N, Longobardi G, Nicolino A, et al (1992) Effect of beta-adrenoceptor blockade on dipyridamole-induced myocardial asynergies in coronary artery disease. Am J Cardiol 70:724–727
26. Fioretti PM, Poldermans D, Salustri A, et al (1994) Atropine increases the accuracy of dobutamine stress echocardiography in patients taking beta-blockers. Eur Heart J 15:355–360
27. Dodi C, Pingitore A, Sicari R, et al (1997) Effects of antianginal therapy with a calcium antagonist and nitrates on dobutamine-atropine stress echocardiography. Comparison with exercise electrocardiography. Eur Heart J 18:242–247
28. Lombardi M, Morales MA, Michelassi C, et al (1993) Efficacy of isosorbide-5-mononitrate versus nifedipine in preventing spontaneous and ergonovine-induced myocardial ischaemia. A double-blind, placebo-controlled study. Eur Heart J 14:845–851
29. Picano E, Pirelli S, Marzilli M, et al (1989) Usefulness of high-dose dipyridamole echocardiography test in coronary angioplasty. Circulation 80:807–815
30. Mertes H, Erbel R, Nixdorff U, et al (1993) Exercise echocardiography for the evaluation of patients after nonsurgical coronary artery revascularization. J Am Coll Cardiol 21:1087–1093
31. Sawada SG, Judson WE, Ryan T, et al (1989) Upright bicycle exercise echocardiography after coronary artery bypass grafting. Am J Cardiol 64:1123–1129
32. Crouse LJ, Vacek JL, Beauchamp GD, et al (1992) Exercise echocardiography after coronary artery bypass grafting. Am J Cardiol 70:572–576
33. Rodriguez O, Picano E, Fedele S, et al (2001) Non-invasive prediction of angiographic progression of coronary artery disease by dipyridamole-stress echocardiography. Coron Artery Dis 12:197–204
34. Rodriguez O, Picano E, Fedele S, et al (2002) Noninvasive prediction of coronary artery disease progression by comparison of serial exercise electrocardiography and dipyridamole stress echocardiography. Int J Cardiovasc Imaging 18:93–99
35. Picano E, Lattanzi F, Distante A, et al (1989) Role of myocardial oxygen consumption in dipyridamole-induced ischemia. Am Heart J 118:314–319
36. Picano E, Marini C, Pirelli S, et al (1992) Safety of intravenous high-dose dipyridamole echocardiography. The Echo-Persantine International Cooperative Study Group. Am J Cardiol 70:252–258
37. Picano E, Mathias W Jr, Pingitore A, et al (1994) Safety and tolerability of dobutamine atropine stress echocardiography: a prospective, multicentre study. Echo Dobutamine International Cooperative Study Group. Lancet 344:1190–1192
38. Bigi R, Partesana N, Verzoni A et al (1995) Incidence and correlates of complex ventricular arrhythmias during dobutamine stress echocardiography after acute myocardial infarction. Eur Heart J 16:1819–1824
39. De Sutter J, Poldermans D, Vourvouri E et al (2003) Long-term prognostic significance of complex ventricular arrhythmias induced during dobutamine stress echocardiography. Am J Cardiol 91:242–244
40. Hung KC, Lin FC, Chern MS et al (1999) Mechanisms and clinical significance of transient atrioventricular block during dobutamine stress echocardiography. J Am Coll Cardiol 34:998–1004
41. Rosamond TL, Vacek JL, Hurwitz A, et al (1992) Hypotension during dobutamine stress echocardiography: initial description and clinical relevance. Am Heart J 123:403–407
42. Pellikka PA, Oh JK, Bailey KR, et al (1992) Dynamic intraventricular obstruction during dobutamine stress echocardiography. A new observation. Circulation 86:1429–1432
43. Heinle SK, Tice FD, Kisslo J (1995) Hypotension during dobutamine stress echocardiography: is it related to dynamic intraventricular obstruction? Am Heart J 130:314–317

18

44. Lieberman EB, Heinle SK, Wildermann N, et al (1995) Does hypotension during dobutamine stress echocardiography correlate with anatomic or functional cardiac impairment? Am Heart J 129:1121–1126
45. Dhond MR, Whitley TB, Singh S et al (2000) Incidence and significance of profound hypotension during dobutamine stress echocardiography. Clin Cardiol 23:47–50
46. Day SM, Younger JG, Karavite D et al (2000) Usefulness of hypotension during dobutamine echocardiography in predicting perioperative cardiac events. Am J Cardiol 85:478–483
47. Rigo F, Richieri M, Pasanisi E, et al (2003) Usefulness of coronary flow reserve over regional wall motion when added to dual-imaging dipyridamole echocardiography. Am J Cardiol 91:269–273
48. Bodi V, Sanchis J, Lopez-Lereu MP et al (2007) Prognostic value of dipyridamole stress cardiovascular magnetic resonance imaging in patients with known or suspected coronary artery disease. J Am Coll Cardiol 50:1174–1179
49. Rigo F, Cortigiani L, Pasanisi E, et al (2006) The additional prognostic value of coronary flow reserve on left anterior descending artery in patients with negative stress echo by wall motion criteria. A Transthoracic Vasodilator Stress Echocardiography Study. Am Heart J 151:124–130
50. Cortigiani L, Bigi R, Sicari R, et al (2007) Comparison of prognostic value of pharmacologic stress echocardiography in chest pain patients with versus without diabetes mellitus and positive exercise electrocardiography. Am J Cardiol 100:1744–1749
51. Rigo F, Sicari R, Gherardi S, et al (2008) The additive prognostic value of wall motion abnormalities and coronary flow reserve during dipyridamole stress echo. Eur Heart J 29:79–88
52. Sicari R, Nihoyannopoulos P, Evangelista A, et al. European Association of Echocardiography (2008) Stress echocardiography expert consensus statement: European Association of Echocardiography (EAE) (a registered branch of the ESC). Eur J Echocardiogr 9:415–437

Diagnostic Results and Indications

19

Eugenio Picano

The relationship between the data obtained from provocative tests and angiographically assessed coronary artery disease is usually expressed in terms of sensitivity and specificity, where sensitivity is the frequency of a positive test result in a population of patients with coronary artery disease and specificity is the frequency of a negative test result in a population of patients without disease. In a given population, sensitivity and specificity values are affected by a constellation of factors (some of which – more relevant to stress echocardiography – are summarized in Tables 19.1 and 19.2) related to the angiographic standard, patient population, stress methodology, and interpretation criteria. In the presence of more severe and extensive coronary artery disease, any stress echocardiography test will give higher sensitivity values [1]. For any given level of stenosis, angiographic coronary lesions of the complex type (i.e., with intraluminal filling defects and/or irregular margins suggestive of thrombus and/or ulcers) will give higher sensitivity values for vasodilator stresses [2], but not inotropic stresses [3]. Abundant coronary collateral circulation makes the myocardium more vulnerable to ischemia during vasodilator stresses [4], whereas exercise or inotropic stress results are independent of angiographically assessed collateral circulation [5]. All stresses yield better sensitivity results in populations with previous myocardial infarction and in patients studied while off antianginal therapy, which lowers the sensitivity of both physical and pharmacological stresses [6, 7]. The evaluation of patients with variant angina inflates sensitivity since stresses such as exercise or dobutamine may elicit vasospasm – and therefore ischemia – independently of the underlying organic stenosis. Stress-related factors are also important. Submaximal stresses sharply lower test sensitivity (to a greater extent than perfusion imaging sensitivity) [6]. During exercise, a peak stress acquisition yields better sensitivity than poststress imaging such as the one performed after treadmill exercise. The use of more aggressive test protocols leads to higher sensitivities; however, the user-friendliness of the test declines. For pharmacological tests, the best trade-off between accuracy and feasibility for primary diagnostic purposes is probably a high dose with atropine for dobutamine and an accelerated high dose for dipyridamole (Fig. 19.1).

E. Picano, *Stress Echocardiography*,
© Springer-Verlag Berlin Heidelberg 2009

Table 19.1 Factors affecting stress echocardiography sensitivity

	Increases sensitivity	Decreases sensitivity
Previous myocardial infarction	Present	Absent
Antianginal therapy	Absent	Present
Stenosis severity	>75%	50–75%
Stenosis extent	Multivessel disease	Single-vessel disease
Stenosis morphology	Complex	Simple
Stenosis location	LAD	LCx
Stress intensity	Maximal	Submaximal
Variant (vasospastic) angina	Yes	No
Echocardiography interpretation criteria	Lack of hyperkinesia	Marked hypokinesia
Echocardiography reader	Expert	Beginner

LAD left anterior descending artery, *LCx* left circumflex artery

Table 19.2 Factors affecting stress echocardiography specificity

	Increases sensitivity	Decreases sensitivity
Resting wall motion abnormalities	Absent	Present
Left ventricular hypertrophy, left bundle branch block	Absent	Present
Stress intensity	Submaximal	Maximal
Variant (vasospastic) angina	No	Yes
Echocardiography interpretation criteria	Marked hypokinesia	Lack of hyperkinesia
Interpreting the basal third of the inferior wall	No	Yes
Echocardiography reader	Expert	Beginner

LAD left anterior descending artery, *LCx* left circumflex artery

The interpretation criteria also affect sensitivity. The lack of hyperkinesis will provide a higher sensitivity when compared with the more specific criterion of transient regional dyssynergy. An expert reading and high-quality two-dimensional (2D) imaging using a top-quality instrument will obviously improve the diagnostic accuracy. Digital acquisition capabilities do not increase accuracy compared to videotape recordings, but they probably do make the reading more reproducible. Specificity is also affected by many factors, some of which – not surprisingly – are the same as those affecting specificity. As a rule, several factors increasing sensitivity symmetrically lower specificity.

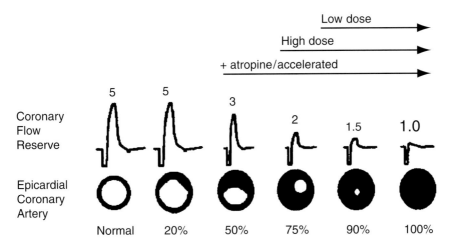

Fig. 19.1 Pharmacological test protocols for the detection of coronary artery disease (CAD). The various protocols can be ranked according to their different abilities to pick up different levels of CAD severity, the high-dose test protocol with atropine coadministration being the most sensitive, high-dose protocols (up to 40 µg kg^{-1} per min for dobutamine, up to 0.84 mg kg^{-1} for dipyridamole) of intermediate sensitivity, and low-dose protocols (up to 20 µg kg^{-1} per min for dobutamine, up to 0.56 mg kg^{-1} for dipyridamole) being the least sensitive

19.1
Stress Echocardiography Versus Other Diagnostic Tests

Given the many factors affecting the values of diagnostic accuracy, reliable information on the relative value of different tests can only be gained by studying an adequate number of patients in head-to-head comparisons under the same conditions. On the basis of these studies and meta-analyses, some conclusions on the relative value of various stress tests can be drawn.

When compared to standard exercise electrocardiography testing, stress echocardiography has an advantage in terms of sensitivity and a particularly impressive advantage in terms of specificity [7]. Compared to nuclear perfusion imaging, stress echocardiography at least has similar accuracy, with a moderate sensitivity gap, especially in patients with single-vessel disease of mild severity (50–80% stenosis) evaluated under antianginal therapy with submaximal stresses [6]; this sensitivity gap is virtually filled by state-of-the-art protocols (with atropine coadministration) and is more than balanced by a marked specificity gap in favor of stress echocardiography, which is particularly striking in populations with left ventricular hypertrophy, syndrome X, hypertension, and hypertrophic cardiomyopathy [8]. The sensitivity gap in favor of nuclear vs. echocardiography is slightly more pronounced with adenosine (often stopped at a submaximal level in order to limit side effects [8]) since it is less well tolerated subjectively than dipyridamole [9]. The extent and severity of the perfusion deficit by nuclear imaging is paralleled by the extent and severity of the wall motion dyssynergy

19

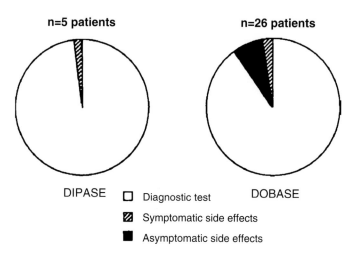

Fig. 19.2 Feasibility of dobutamine–atropine test (DOBASE, *right*) vs. dipyridamole–atropine (DIPASE, *left*). EPIC–EDIC study group. (From [22], with permission)

during stress [8–10], and both perfusion and functional defects are correlated to the extent and severity of angiographically assessed coronary artery disease. Exercise, dipyridamole, and dobutamine stress echocardiography have similar overall accuracy [11, 12] comparable to stress perfusion scintigraphy [13]. Dipyridamole has a higher feasibility than dobutamine (Fig. 19.2). With dobutamine, the most frequent side effects are tachyarrhythmias and hypertension, whereas during dipyridamole infusion bradyarrhythmias and hypotension are frequent. Dipyridamole has more often symptomatic, and dobutamine asymptomatic limiting side effects. Dipyridamole–atropine and dobutamine–atropine stress echocardiography have similar sensitivity and specificity (Fig. 19.3) and a similar capability to stratify the ischemic response according to ischemia-free stress time and peak wall motion score index (Fig. 19.4) [14]. Dipyridamole and dobutamine stress echocardiography also have a comparable prognostic value [15] and similar accuracy for identification of myocardial viability [16]. As far as subjective tolerance is concerned, dipyridamole and dobutamine are similarly well tolerated and both are significantly better tolerated than adenosine [17]. Some data are also available concerning the direct assessment of the relative intrinsic echocardiographic difficulty of the two tests. It has been said that "from the technical viewpoint, dipyridamole represents the primary school, dobutamine the secondary school, and exercise the university in the stress echo cursus studiorum" [18]. Another report semiquantitatively addressed the issue of image degradation during stress and described that image quality worsened significantly more frequently during dobutamine stress than with dipyridamole stress [19]. Also, for the recognition of myocardial viability, both tests in principle have a comparable diagnostic accuracy for predicting spontaneous or revascularization induced functional recovery, with dipyridamole being slightly more specific and dobutamine slightly more sensitive. Dobutamine is the only one extensively validated and accepted by guidelines with this indication [20–22]. From the practical viewpoint, both tests should be used to optimize the diagnostic performance of

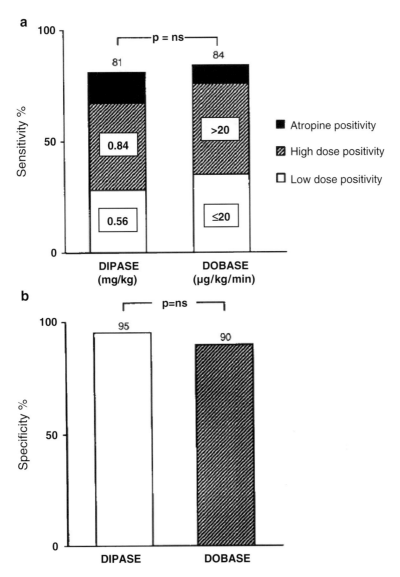

Fig. 19.3 (**a**) Sensitivity and (**b**) specificity of the dobutamine–atropine test (*DOBASE*) vs. dipyridamole–atropine (*DIPASE*). EPIC-EDIC study group. *ns* Not significant. (From [22], with permission)

the stress echocardiography laboratory – a policy that is justified for several reasons. Each patient referred for stress evaluation might suffer from relative or absolute contraindications to either stress modality. For instance, a patient with severe hypertension and/or a history of significant atrial or ventricular arrhythmias is more reasonably subjected to the dipyridamole stress test, which, unlike dobutamine, has no arrhythmogenic or hypertensive effect.

19

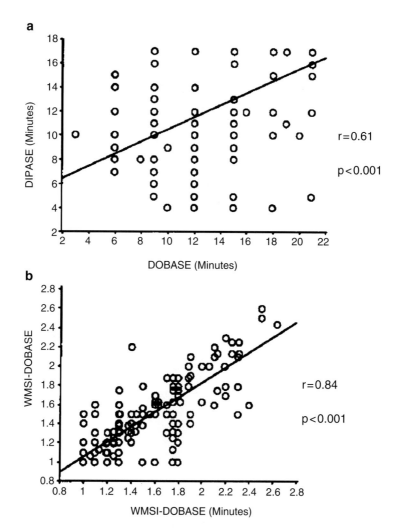

Fig. 19.4 Stratification of the stress echocardiography response in (**a**) the time domain and (**b**) the space domain. EPIC–EDIC study group. *DOBASE* dobutamine atropine test, *DIPASE* dipyridamole–atropine test, *WMSI* wall motion score index. (From [22], with permission)

In contrast, a patient with severe conduction disturbances or advanced asthmatic disease should undergo the dobutamine stress test, since adenosine has a negative chronotropic and dromotropic effect, as well as a documented bronchoconstrictor activity. Patients either taking xanthine medication or under the effect of caffeine contained in drinks (tea, coffee, cola) should undergo the dobutamine test. Both dipyridamole and dobutamine have excellent overall tolerability and feasibility [21]. Nevertheless, submaximal nondiagnostic tests do occur in some patients because of side effects: less than 5% of patients with dipyridamole infusion and about 10% (20% of normal patients) of patients with dobutamine infusion [14, 21].

Obviously, the negative predictive value for both diagnostic and prognostic standards is much lower when the peak dose is not achieved, as with a submaximal exercise stress test. Patients with a submaximal pharmacological stress should be switched over to the other stress. In addition, for the detection of minor, less extensive forms of coronary artery disease or of minor forms of myocardial viability, a combined pharmacological stress procedure may be needed. Dipyridamole and dobutamine are good options for the diagnosis of coronary artery disease, with dipyridamole having better feasibility and a more reassuring safety record [21]. The choice of one test over the other depends on patient characteristics, clinical issues, local drug cost, and the physician's preference. It is important for all stress echocardiography laboratories to become familiar with both stresses to achieve a flexible and versatile diagnostic approach that allows the best stress to be tailored to individual patient needs.

19.2
Stress Echocardiography and the Effects of Medical Therapy

Patients may be undergoing various forms of antianginal therapy at the time of testing, both an advantage and a disadvantage for stress echocardiography testing. The disadvantage is that antianginal therapy reduces sensitivity, since stress-induced wall motion abnormalities are caused by the development of obligatory myocardial ischemia. The advantage is that the effect of therapy can be assessed using an objective, primary ischemic end point such as changes in stress-induced wall motion abnormalities. The presence of ischemia can be titrated on the basis of the ischemic-free stress time and the extent and severity of the induced dyssynergy. The various forms of stress are differently affected by various forms of therapy (Table 19.3). Antianginal therapy lowers the sensitivity of exercise echocardiography, as it does with vasodilator stress testing [20, 21]. The beneficial effect of therapy on dipyridamole time parallels variations in exercise time, providing the possibility of an exercise-independent assessment of efficacy of medical therapy (Fig. 19.5). Interestingly, the positive effects of β-blockers on dipyridamole stress are largely independent of the effect on heart rate, possibly involving a direct antisteal effect [22, 23]. Monotherapy with a calcium antagonist and nitrates also protects the patient from dipyridamole-induced ischemia [22, 24]. Angiotensin-converting enzyme inhibitors have no effect on dipyridamole stress echocardiography results [25]. Aminophylline obviously blunts dipyridamole-induced

Table 19.3 Effects of oral therapy on stress testing sensitivity

	Stress exercise	Dipyridamole	Dobutamine
β-Blockers	↓	↓	↓↓
Calcium channel blockers	↓	↓	↓↔
Nitrates	↓	↓	↓↔
ACE inhibitors	↔	↔	↔
Aminophylline	↓↔	↓↓	↔

ACE angiotensin-converting enzyme, ↓ decreased sensitivity, ↓↓ markedly decreased sensitivity, ↔ no effect on sensitivity, ↓ ↔ mild decrease in sensitivity

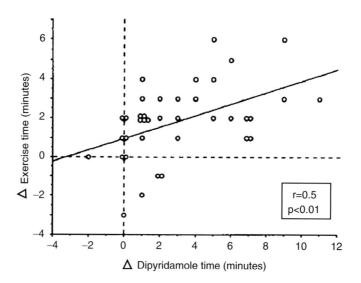

Fig. 19.5 Correlation between therapy-induced variations in dipyridamole time (i.e., the time from onset of dipyridamole infusion to obvious dyssynergy) and exercise time (i.e., the time from onset of exercise to 0.1 mV of ST-segment depression) in the 38 patients with positivity on both tests when off treatment. Δ variations. (From [40], with permission)

ischemia, whereas concomitant oral dipyridamole therapy might potentiate it. The sensitivity of dobutamine is heavily affected by concomitant β-blocker therapy. Beta-blockers effect a rightward shift in the dose–response curve to dobutamine and sharply lower test sensitivity, unless atropine is used [26]. Calcium antagonists and/or nitrates only mildly reduce dobutamine stress sensitivity [21, 27] and they do so in a manner unrelated to changes induced in exercise tolerance [27]. Concomitant antiischemic therapy at the time of testing heavily modulates the prognostic value of pharmacological stress echocardiography. In presence of concomitant antiischemic therapy, a positive test is prognostically more malignant, and a negative test prognostically less benign. However, the decision to remove a patient from β-blocker therapy for stress testing should be made on an individual basis and should be done carefully to avoid a potential hemodynamic rebound effect, which can lead to accelerated angina or hypertension [28].

19.3
Contraindications to Stress Testing

The absolute and relative contraindications to stress testing are summarized in Table 19.4. Obviously, a poor acoustic window makes any form of stress echocardiography unfeasible. However, a difficult resting echocardiography greatly increases the probability of obtaining no interpretable study results during exercise and should be an indication for the less technically demanding pharmacological stress echocardiography to be used (Table 19.5). Specific contraindications to dipyridamole (or adenosine) echocardiography include the presence

Table 19.4 Absolute and relative contraindications to stress testing

	To all forms of stress testing		To stress echocardiography	To exercise stress	Dob	Dip	Atro
	Absolute	Relative					
Acute myocardial infarction (<2 days)	√						
Unstable angina not stabilized	√						
Uncontrolled cardiac arrhythmias	√						
Severe aortic stenosis	√						
Uncontrolled symptomatic heart failure	√						
Acute pulmonary embolism	√						
Acute myocarditis or pericarditis	√						
Acute aortic dissection	√						
Left main coronary stenosis		√					
Moderate aortic stenosis		√					
Electrolyte abnormalities		√					
Severe arterial hypertension (SAP>200; DAP 110 mmHg)		√					
Tachyarrhythmias or bradyarrhythmias		√					
High degree of atrioventricular block		√					
Poor acoustic window (obesity)			√				
Inability to exercise adequately				√			
Moderate hypertension, ventricular ectopy					√		
2nd–3rd degree A-V block						√	
Relative hypotension					√	√	
Unstable carotid disease					√	√	√
Glaucoma, severe prostatic disease							√

SAP systolic arterial pressure, *DAP* diastolic arterial pressure

of severe conduction disturbances, since adenosine can cause transient block at the AV node, and severe bronchopneumopathic disease requiring chronic xanthine therapy, since adenosine is a powerful bronchoconstrictor. Patients with resting systolic blood pressure

Table 19.5 Pretest probability of coronary artery disease by age, gender, and symptoms (adapted from [31])

Age (years)	Gender	Typical/ definite angina pectoris	Atypical/ probable angina pectoris	Nonanginal chest pain	Asymptomatic
30–39	Men	Intermediate	Intermediate	Low	Very low
	Women	Intermediate	Very low	Very low	Very low
40–49	Men	High	Intermediate	Intermediate	Low
	Women	Intermediate	Low	Very low	Very low
50–59	Men	Intermediate	Intermediate	Intermediate	Low
	Women	Intermediate	Intermediate	Low	Very low
60–69	Men	Intermediate	Intermediate	Intermediate	Low
	Women	Intermediate	Intermediate	Intermediate	Low

Typical or definite angina pectoris can be defined as (1) substernal chest pain or discomfort that is (2) provoked by exertion or emotional stress and (3) relieved by rest and/or nitroglycerin. Atypical or probable angina can be defined as chest pain or discomfort that lacks one of the three characteristics of definite or typical angina pectoris

under 100 mmHg generally should not receive dobutamine or dipyridamole. Dobutamine causes an increase in systolic blood pressure in the majority of patients but can also cause a significant decrease in systolic blood pressure in a substantial minority of patients. Dipyridamole usually causes a modest decrease in systolic blood pressure of 10–20 mmHg, but occasionally causes a more severe decrease. Adenosine is the preferred option because of its rapid half-life (<10 s) in patients with unstable carotid artery disease. Significant hypertension and prolonged hypotension should be avoided in these patients, making adenosine the agent of choice. Patients who do not achieve the target heart rate with dobutamine alone or inducible ischemia with dipyridamole alone, are commonly administered atropine. Atropine use in this setting is a risk only for closed-angle glaucoma patients, a minority of patients with glaucoma. If eye pain occurs the patient should call an ophthalmologist within the day [2]. Severe prostatic disease is also a contraindication to atropine use.

19.4
Indications for Stress Testing

Indications for stress echocardiography can also be grouped in very broad categories, which eventually could encompass the overwhelming majority of patients: diagnosis of coronary artery disease; prognosis and risk stratification in patients with established diagnosis, for instance, after myocardial infarction; assessment of preoperative risk; evaluation for cardiac etiology of exertional dyspnea; evaluation after revascularization; and localization of ischemia [20–22]. As a rule, the less informative the exercise ECG test is, the stricter the indication to stress echocardiography is. Out of five patients, one is unable to exercise, one exercises submaximally, and one exercises maximally but the ECG is uninterpretable [21]. The three main specific indications for pharmacological stress echocardiography can be summarized as follows [21]:

1. Patients in whom the exercise stress test is contraindicated (e.g., patients with severe arterial hypertension)
2. Patients in whom the exercise stress test is not feasible (e.g., those with intermittent claudication)
3. Patients in whom the exercise stress test was nondiagnostic or gave ambiguous results: inability to achieve the target heart rate response; presence of chest pain in the absence of significant electrocardiographic changes; a concomitance of conditions lowering the reliability of the ECG marker of ischemia (female sex, arterial hypertension, repolarization abnormalities on ECG under resting conditions or after hyperventilation, and the need to continue drugs such as digitalis or antiarrhythmics that potentially induce ST-T changes)

The published evidence in this field is rapidly growing and may possibly change some of the present indications in the near future. In more general terms, evaluation of the clinical utility of a diagnostic test is far more difficult than assessment of the efficacy of a therapeutic intervention, because the diagnostic test cannot have the same direct effect on patient survival or recovery. Furthermore, there are no double-blind, randomized studies to prove the usefulness of the technique in a given situation [21]. As always, the appropriateness of the indication should be found in the point of balance between published evidence, personal experience, available resources, and common sense.

19.5
Inappropriate Use of Stress Testing

Whatever the stress test used, some common rules in stress test indication and/or interpretation should be considered [21, 29].

1. All available information (clinical, stress, and imaging data) should be considered when interpreting the test. In the Bayesian analysis, the probability of the patient having the disease before the test is considered the a priori (pretest) likelihood, since it can be estimated by retrospective observations (Table 19.5). The Bayes theorem states that the probability of a patient having the disease after the test is performed will be the product of the disease probability before the test and the probability that the test provided a true result. After the test, the new value of the probability of the patient having the disease will be the posttest likelihood. For instance, a positive exercise electrocardiography test indicates a probability of coronary artery disease of 90% in a patient with typical angina, 80% in a patient with atypical chest pain, and 35% in an asymptomatic subject. The clinician often makes this calculation intuitively, for instance, when he or she suspects a false result when a 30-year-old woman with atypical angina has an abnormal exercise test result (low pretest probability).

The same abnormal response would be intuitively considered a true-positive result in a 60-year-old man with typical angina pectoris (high pretest probability) [29].

2. Most patients with a normal or near normal resting ECG who are able to exercise adequately should undergo standard exercise treadmill testing rather than exercise or pharmacological imaging. Standard exercise ECG tests are currently underutilized in favor of more expensive imaging tests. However, in patients with normal ECG, the negative predictive value of exercise ECG is almost as good as that of a stress imaging test. Exercise ECG should be the first-line test in these patients.

All forms of stress echocardiography (or stress imaging) testing are inappropriately applied as a first-line test in lieu of exercise ECG testing, for instance when screening asymptomatic patients with low pretest likelihood of disease and/or when doing routine assessment of asymptomatic patients after revascularization [21].

3. The prescribing physician should decide which stress imaging study to order. Expertise with the various imaging modalities should be the most important factor determining selection of a specific modality in an individual patient [21]. If more than one technique is available in a given practice or institution, the technique that has been found to be most accurate should generally be the modality of choice [29].

4. Useless testing should be avoided. Every test has a cost and a risk. If the physician's decision will be the same whatever the result of the test, the test should not be ordered. If the physician will in any case go to angiography in view of an anatomy-guided revascularization, the imaging test is useless. Compared with the treadmill exercise test, the cost of stress echocardiography is at least 2.1 times higher, stress single-photon emission computed tomography myocardial imaging is 5.7 times higher, and coronary angiography is 21.7 times higher [28].

References

1. Philbrick JT, Horwitz RI, Feinstein AR (1980) Methodologic problems of exercise testing for coronary artery disease: groups, analysis and bias. Am J Cardiol 46:807–812
2. Lu C, Picano E, Pingitore A,et al (1995) Complex coronary artery lesion morphology influences results of stress echocardiography. Circulation 91:1669–1675
3. Heyman J, Salvade P, Picano E,et al (1997) The elusive link between coronary lesion morphology and dobutamine stress echocardiography results. The EDIC (Echo Dobutamine International Cooperative) Study Group. Int J Card Imaging 13:395–401
4. Gliozheni E, Picano E, Bernardino L, et al (1996) Angiographically assessed coronary collateral circulation increases vulnerability to myocardial ischemia during vasodilator stress testing. Am J Cardiol 78:1419–1424
5. Beleslin BD, Ostojic M, Djordjevic-Dikic A, et al (1999) Integrated evaluation of relation between coronary lesion features and stress echocardiography results: the importance of coronary lesion morphology. J Am Coll Cardiol 33:717–726
6. Marwick T, Willemart B, D'Hondt AM, et al (1993) Selection of the optimal nonexercise stress for the evaluation of ischemic regional myocardial dysfunction and malperfusion. Comparison of dobutamine and adenosine using echocardiography and 99mTc-MIBI single photon emission computed tomography. Circulation 87:345–354

7. Severi S, Picano E, Michelassi C, et al (1994) Diagnostic and prognostic value of dipyrida-mole echocardiography in patients with suspected coronary artery disease. Comparison with exercise electrocardiography. Circulation 89:1160–1173

8. Marwick T, D'Hondt AM, Baudhuin T, et al (1993) Optimal use of dobutamine stress for the detection and evaluation of coronary artery disease: combination with echocardiography or scintigraphy, or both? J Am Coll Cardiol 22:159–167

9. Parodi G, Picano E, Marcassa C, et al (1999) High dose dipyridamole stress imaging: simul-taneous sestamibi scintigraphy and two-dimensional echocardiography for the detection and evaluation of coronary artery disease. Coron Artery Dis 10:177–184

10. Quinones MA, Verani MS, Haichin RM, et al (1992) Exercise echocardiography versus 201Tl single-photon emission computed tomography in evaluation of coronary artery disease. Anal-ysis of 292 patients. Circulation 85:1026–1031

11. De Albuquerque Fonseca L, Picano E (2001) Comparison of dipyridamole and exercise stress echocardiography for detection of coronary artery disease (a meta-analysis). Am J Cardiol 87:1193–1196

12. Picano E, Molinaro S, Pasanisi E (2008) The diagnostic accuracy of pharmacological stress echocardiography for the assessment of coronary artery disease: a meta-analysis. Cardiovasc Ultrasound 6:30

13. Imran MB, Palinkas A, Picano E (2002) Head to head comparison of dipyridamole echocar-diography and stress perfusion scintigraphy for the detection of coronary artery disease: a metaanalysis. Int J Cardiovasc Imaging 19:23–28

14. Pingitore A, Picano E, Colosso MQ, et al (1996) The atropine factor in pharmacologic stress echocardiography. Echo Persantine (EPIC) and Echo Dobutamine International Cooperative (EDIC) Study Groups. J Am Coll Cardiol 27:1164–1170

15. Pingitore A, Picano E, Varga A, et al (1999) Prognostic value of pharmacological stress echocardiography in patients with known or suspected coronary artery disease: a prospective, large-scale, multicenter, head-to-head comparison between dipyridamole and dobutamine test. Echo-Persantine International Cooperative (EPIC) and Echo-Dobutamine International Cooperative (EDIC) Study Groups. J Am Coll Cardiol 34:1769–1777

16. Picano E, Ostojic M, Varga A, et al (1996) Combined low dose dipyridamole-dobutamine stress echocardiography to identify myocardial viability. J Am Coll Cardiol 27:1422–1428

17. Martin TW, Seaworth JF, Johns JP, et al (1992) Comparison of adenosine, dipyridamole, and dobutamine in stress echocardiography. Ann Intern Med 116:190–196

18. Beleslin BD, Ostojic M, Stepanovic J, et al (1994) Stress echocardiography in the detection of myocardial ischemia. Head-to-head comparison of exercise, dobutamine, and dipyridamole tests. Circulation 90:1168–1176

19. Sochowski RA, Yvorchuk KJ, Yang Y, et al (1995) Dobutamine and dipyridamole stress echocardiography in patients with a low incidence of severe coronary artery disease. J Am Soc Echocardiogr 8:482–487

20. Pellikka PA, McCully RB (2007) Stress echocardiography: so much to do, so little time. J Am Coll Cardiol 50:1990–1991

21. Sicari R, Nihoyannopoulos P, Evangelista A, et al; European Association of Echocardiogra-phy (2008) Stress echocardiography expert consensus statement: European Association of Echocardiography (EAE) (a registered branch of the ESC). Eur J Echocardiogr 9:415–437

22. Douglas PS, Khandheria B, Stainback RF, et al; American College of Cardiology Founda-tion; American Society of Echocardiography; American College of Emergency Physicians; American Heart Association; American Society of Nuclear Cardiology; Society for Cardio-vascular Angiography and Interventions; Society of Cardiovascular Computed Tomography; Society for Cardiovascular Magnetic Resonance (2008) ACCF/ASE/ACEP/AHA/ASNC/ SCAI/SCCT/SCMR 2008 appropriateness criteria for stress echocardiography: a report of the

American College of Cardiology Foundation Appropriateness Criteria Task Force, American Society of Echocardiography, American College of Emergency Physicians, American Heart Association, American Society of Nuclear Cardiology, Society for Cardiovascular Angiography and Interventions, Society of Cardiovascular Computed Tomography, and Society for Cardiovascular Magnetic Resonance endorsed by the Heart Rhythm Society and the Society of Critical Care Medicine. J Am Coll Cardiol 51:1127–1147

23. Ferrara N, Coltorti F, Leosco D, et al (1995) Protective effect of beta-blockade on dipyridamole- induced myocardial ischaemia. Role of heart rate. Eur Heart J 16:903–908

24. Ferrara N, Longobardi G, Nicolino A, et al (1992) Effect of beta-adrenoceptor blockade on dipyridamole-induced myocardial asynergies in coronary artery disease. Am J Cardiol 70:724–727

25. Longobardi G, Ferrara N, Leosco D, et al (1995) Failure of protective effect of captopril and enalapril on exercise and dipyridamole-induced myocardial ischemia. Am J Cardiol 76:255–258

26. Fioretti PM, Poldermans D, Salustri A, et al (1994) Atropine increases the accuracy of dobutamine stress echocardiography in patients taking beta-blockers. Eur Heart J 15:355–360

27. Dodi C, Pingitore A, Sicari R, et al (1997) Effects of antianginal therapy with a calcium antagonist and nitrates on dobutamine-atropine stress echocardiography. Comparison with exercise electrocardiography. Eur Heart J 18:242–247

28. Gibbons RJ, Balady GJ, Timothy Bricker J, et al (2002) ACC/AHA 2002 guideline update for exercise testing: summary article. A report of the American College of Cardiology/American Heart Association Task Force on Practice Guidelines (Committee to Update the 1997 Exercise Testing Guidelines). J Am Coll Cardiol 40:1531–1540

29. Fox K, Garcia MA, Ardissino D, et al; Task Force on the Management of Stable Angina Pectoris of the European Society of Cardiology; ESC Committee for Practice Guidelines (CPG) (2006) Guidelines on the management of stable angina pectoris: executive summary: the Task Force on the Management of Stable Angina Pectoris of the European Society of Cardiology. Eur Heart J 27:1341–1381

Myocardial Viability

20

Luc Piérard and Eugenio Picano

20.1
Historical Background

When facing dangerous environmental situations, most animal species react with a sympathoadrenergic fight or flight activation; others, such as the opossum, react with a vagal sympathoinhibitory discharge, or the play dead reaction, which discourages possible predators. The myocardium reacts to dangerous situations with opossum-like behavior. In several altered myocardial states (ischemia, hibernation, stunning), when the local supply–demand balance of the cell is critically endangered, the cell minimizes expenditure of energy used for development of contractile force, accounting at rest for about 60% of the high-energy phosphates produced by cell metabolism, and utilizes whatever is left for the maintenance of cellular integrity. The echocardiographic counterpart of this cellular strategic choice is the regional asynergy of viable segments [1]. Both viable and necrotic segments show a depressed resting function [2], but the segmental dysfunction of viable regions can be transiently normalized by proper inotropic stimulus. From the pathophysiological and experimental viewpoint, stunning and hibernation are sharply separated entities (Table 20.1). Between fully reversible ischemia and ischemia lasting more than 15–20 min, invariably associated with necrotic phenomena, there is a blurred transition zone. Within this gray zone, ischemia is too short to cause myocardial necrosis but long enough to induce myocardial stunning: a persistent contractile dysfunction lasting for hours, days, and even weeks after the restoration of flow [1].

The stunned myocardium differs from the "hibernated" myocardium (Table 20.1). In the hibernating myocardium, myocardial perfusion is chronically reduced (for months or years), but remains beyond the critical threshold indispensable to keep the tissue viable, albeit with depressed performance. While in the stunned myocardium a metabolic alteration causes an imbalance between energy supply and work produced [3], the hibernating myocardial cell adapts itself to a chronically reduced energy supply, and its survival is

E. Picano, *Stress Echocardiography*,
© Springer-Verlag Berlin Heidelberg 2009

Table 20.1 Altered myocardial states

	Stunned	Hibernated
Resting function	Depressed	Depressed
Flow	Normal/increased	Decreased/normal
Coronary anatomy	Any	Severe stenosis or occlusion
Duration	Hours to days	Days to months
Recovery	Spontaneous	After revascularization
Clinical significance	Prognostic	Therapeutic
Clinical models	Acute myocardial infarction	Ischemic cardiomyopathy

guaranteed by a reduced or abolished contractile function [4, 5]. Rahimtoola referred to the hibernating heart as a "smart heart" [6], appropriately downregulating its biochemical and physiological activity as an act of self-preservation aimed at ensuring the long-term survival of the anatomical and physiological integrity of its constituent cardiac cells. Currently hibernation is not viewed as a simple consequence of an oxygen deficit, but as an adaptive response to maintain cardiomyocyte viability in the setting of reduced blood flow. Reduced calcium responsiveness and alterations in adrenergic receptor density have been proposed as mechanisms for decreased contractility. Morphologically, hibernating myocardium displays features of dedifferentiation, with loss of cardiomyocytes and myofibrils, and of degeneration with increased interstitial fibrosis [6].

Persistent but reversible postischemic dysfunction was initially an experimental observation described by Heyndrickx [1], later popularized with the successful term "myocardial stunning" by Braunwald in 1982 [2]. Conversely, myocardial hibernation was a clinical impression – copyrighted by a cardiac surgeon, Rahimtoola – describing hearts with severely depressed resting preoperative function that spectacularly recover following revascularization [4]. While myocardial stunning might be referred to as a laboratory phenomenon [1] in search of a clinical manifestation, hibernation would seem to be a clinical condition in search of a good laboratory model [3]. Although their separation is clear-cut from the conceptual and pathophysiological viewpoint, stunning and hibernation are sometimes indistinguishable in the clinical setting. They can coexist in the same patient in space (with islands of hibernated and stunned tissue interspersed with necrotic and/or normal cells) and in time (with early phenomena of acute stunning progressively leading to chronic hibernation, as may occur after an acute myocardial infarction with critical residual stenosis of the infarct-related artery). What is clinically important is the distinction between asynergic viable and asynergic but necrotic segments (Table 20.2).

20.2
Pathophysiology Behind Viability Imaging

The clinical cardiologist can address the viability issue with a variety of imaging techniques, including nuclear, magnetic resonance, and echocardiographic methods. The markedly hypokinetic or akinetic regions, which are the target of our diagnostic efforts to

Table 20.2 Differentiation between viable and necrotic myocardium

	Viable	Necrotic
Myocyte	Normal to altered	Absent
Fibrosis	Normal	Increased
Coronary flow reserve	Usually present	Absent
Inotropic response	Usually present	Absent
Recovery	Usually present	Absent
Th, MIBI, FDG uptake	Yes	No
End-diastolic thickness	Normal	Normal to reduced
Microvascular integrity	Present	Absent

Th thallium scintigraphy, *MIBI* Tc 99m-sestamibi, *FDG* fluorodeoxyglucose

Table 20.3 Viability cascade

Levels of damage	DOB	Thallium, FDG	DE-CMR	Chance of recovery	% Viable myocytes
Mild	+	+	25%	High	>75%
Moderate	–	+	25–75%	Moderate	25–75%
Severe	–	–	>75%	Low	<25%

DE-CMR delayed enhancement cardiovascular magnetic resonance, *DOB* dobutamine, *FDG* fluorodeoxyglucose

recognize myocardial viability, can have a continuous spectrum of damage, from mild to irreversible (Table 20.3). The different diagnostic probes sample different markers of the viability cascade. If a function is strictly essential to cell survival, e.g., cell membrane integrity, it will be lost only for advanced, close to irreversible degrees of damage (Fig. 20.1). Conversely, other functions such as functional response to low-level inotropic stimulation indicate that the damage is limited and the segment is highly likely to recover. Hibernation has different depths similar to sleep stages that correspond to increasing levels of myocardial damage and decreasing chances of functional recovery upon revascularization (Table 20.3). The initial stages of dysfunction are probably caused by chronic stunning. These stages are characterized by normal resting perfusion but reduced flow reserve, mild myocyte alterations, maintained membrane integrity (allowing the transport of both thallium and glucose), preserved capacity to respond to an inotropic stimulus, and little or no tissue fibrosis. After revascularization, functional recovery will probably be rapid and complete. On the other hand, the more advanced stages of dysfunction are likely to correspond to chronic hibernation. They usually are associated with reduced rest perfusion, increased tissue fibrosis, more severe myocyte alterations (degeneration, apoptosis), and a decreased ability to respond to inotropic stimuli. Nonetheless, membrane function and glucose metabolism may remain preserved for a long period of time. After revascularization,

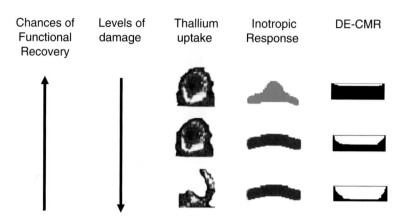

Chances of Functional Recovery	Levels of damage	Thallium uptake	Inotropic Response	DE-CMR

Fig. 20.1 The viability cascade. Higher degrees of cellular damage correspond to progressive loss of cellular functions. Mild damage is associated with preserved inotropic response and thallium uptake. Moderate damage can be identified as a loss of contractile response with preserved thallium uptake. Severe preterminal damage is expressed by loss of contractile response, no thallium uptake, and transmural scar

functional recovery, if there is any, will probably be quite delayed and mostly incomplete. The possibility of recruiting the inotropic reserve might appear paradoxical in the presence of hibernation. The traditional concept is that a decrease in resting coronary blood flow indicates that coronary vasodilating reserve was exhausted. However, hibernating segments have some vasodilatory reserve, which is mirrored by contractile reserve [7]. The hibernating myocardium acts like King Lear, the Shakespearean character: once rich and now poor in coronary supply for the presence of a severe flow-limiting coronary stenosis, precluding a normal myocardial function even at rest. However, even the most stunned or hibernating myocardium has some superfluous flow reserve, which can be recruited by the appropriate pharmacological stimulus: "Oh! Reason not the need: our basest beggars are in the poorest thing superfluous" (Shakespeare, King Lear, II, IV, 262–263). The increase in flow will lead to increased function [8], since the physiology of myocardium is that an "erectile" organ [9], and the augmentation of flow is paralleled – in the low flow range – by a parallel increase not only in stiffness, but also in function, both in experimental animals and in humans [10]. As stated by Salisbury in the original description in 1960, quoting Webster's unabridged dictionary, "erection in physiology indicates a becoming or being hard and swollen by filling with blood," and myocardium fills these requirements. In a physiologic sense, vasodilation (primarily achieved with adenosine, or secondarily with dobutamine) is a "Viagra test" of the viable but hibernating heart.

20.3
Nuclear and Magnetic Resonance Techniques for the Identification of Myocardial Viability

Nuclear medicine long had a monopoly on the diagnosis of myocardial viability. The viable myocardial cell does not move, but still maintains a series of biochemical and metabolic activities that are critical for cell survival and are highly useful markers for the clinical

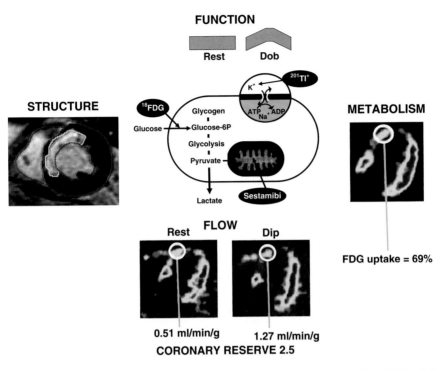

FUNCTION

Rest   Dob

STRUCTURE   METABOLISM

^{18}FDG ^{201}Tl$^+$

Glycogen

Glucose → Glucose-6P

Glycolysis

Pyruvate

Lactate   Sestamibi

FLOW

Rest   Dip

FDG uptake = 69%

0.51 ml/min/g   1.27 ml/min/g

CORONARY RESERVE 2.5

Fig. 20.2 Echocardiographic, nuclear, and magnetic resonance markers of myocardial viability. Cell viability can be identified by 201-thallium, a potassium analog requiring integrity of ionic pumps, by technetium sestamibi, which is trapped intracellularly, or by fluorodeoxyglucose (*FDG*) uptake, which images the glycolytic pathway (*central panel*). With echocardiography (*upper panel*), viability is imaged through its functional fruit of contractile reserve. With magnetic resonance (*left panel*), myocardial structure is imaged through the roots of the transmural extent of the scar, visualized with the delayed enhancement technique: scar tissue is *bright*

identification of viability using nuclear techniques [11] (Fig. 20.2). The viable cells have a residual coronary flow, which can be visualized with a flow tracer such as technetium sestamibi (gamma-emitting and therefore detectable by a gamma camera) or rubidium (positron-emitting and therefore detectable by positron emission tomography). The viable cell has membrane integrity and intact function of ionic pumps and is therefore capable of taking up 201-thallium, a potassium analog, and storing it intracellularly. The viable cell can also metabolize glucose, which can be traced with fluorodeoxyglucose, a positron-emitting glucose analog. It competes intracellularly for phosphorylation by means of cellular exokinase. Phosphorylated fluorodeoxyglucose cannot be further metabolized and remains trapped with the cell as a viability marker. With a completely different approach, cardiovascular magnetic resonance (CMR) with a delayed gadolinium enhancement (DE) technique [12] directly visualizes myocardial scar as hyperenhanced areas in T1-weighted images. The imaging study is performed at rest (no stress required) and after several minutes from contrast medium injection, since the redistribution phase of the tissue (and not the first pass effect of the vessels) is the diagnostic target [12]. Summarizing the versatility of diagnostic markers of viability, we might say that of the viability plant, DE-CMR evaluates the structural roots, contrast echocardiography (or scintigraphy) the lymph, and stress echocardiography the fruit (functional response). If the fruit is present, the roots (normal structure) and the lymph (microcirculatory integrity) must be present. If roots are destroyed (wall thickness<6 mm or delayed enhancement>50% of wall thickness) the lymph and the fruit will generally be absent.

20.4
Resting Echocardiography

Echocardiography can provide a reasonably accurate detection of myocardial viability with several parameters derived from different techniques, i.e., resting echocardiography, contrast echocardiography, tissue characterization and myocardial velocity imaging, and pharmacological stress echocardiography (Table 20.4). Each of these techniques detects a separate variable of the myocardial segments with resting dysfunction, i.e., connective tissue increase, microvascular integrity, intramural function, and contractile reserve. The echocardiographic appearance of a markedly thinned myocardial wall, with an end-diastolic thickness of less than 6 mm and obviously increased echocardiographic reflectivity [13], possibly with a thrombus adhering to the asynergic wall, is a poorly sensitive but highly specific marker of necrosis, because of the extensive replacement of myocytes with fibrous tissue determining thinning and increased wall brightness (Fig. 20.3) [14].

Table 20.4 Ultrasonic assessment of viable myocardium

	Rest 2D echocardiography	Pharmacological stress echocardiography	Contrast echocardiography	Myocardial velocity
Sign	Dyskinetic, thinned, hyperechoic region	Functional improvement	Contrast opacification	Preserved subendocardial strain
Physiological variable	Transmural extent of necrosis	Contractile reserve	Microvascular integrity	Sarcomere shortening
Advantages	Simple	Fast	Simultaneous flow–function assessment	No intervention needed
Limitations	Insensitive	Stress echocardiography know-how	Catheter for intracoronary injection, inadequate evidence for intravenous	Inadequate/ unsatisfactory evidence for clinical use
Clinical value	Mild	Excellent	Unsatisfactory	Unsatisfactory

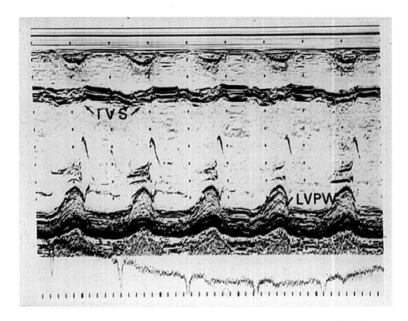

Fig. 20.3 *M*-mode resting echocardiogram of a previous old anteroseptal myocardial infarction, suggesting no residual viability. The posterior wall shows normal thickness, texture, motion, and thickening, whereas the necrotic septum is thinned and hyperechoic, with no active systolic thickening. There is a slight passive systolic movement due to tethering from adjacent normally contracting myocardium. *IVS* interventricular septum, *LVPW* posterior (inferolateral) wall of left ventricle

20.5
Myocardial Contrast Echocardiography

Microvascular integrity is a prerequisite for myocardial viability detection by contrast echocardiography. Viability is associated with the presence of collateral blood flow within the infarct bed, and this preserved flow can be detected with intracoronary [15–18] and – less accurately – with intravenous contrast echocardiography [19–21]. Echocontrast negativity is invariably associated with no response to dobutamine and no functional recovery, whereas echocontrast positivity can be found with and without dobutamine-induced response [18]. The combination of inotropic response and echocontrast information may be useful to titrate the sensitivity of damage, with mild degrees of damage (echocontrast with dobutamine response) associated with prompt recovery, moderate degrees (echocontrast with no dobutamine response) associated with possible, but unlikely recovery, and severe degrees (no echocontrast and no dobutamine response) virtually never associated with recovery, the specific marker of irreversible microvascular and myocyte damage. In the viability cascade (Table 20.3), the loss of microvascular integrity corresponds to levels of damage very close to irreversibility. If there is no lymph in the plant of viability, it is useless to look for the fruit of inotropic reserve. It is also true that lymph (microcirculatory integrity) can be present, without the fruit of functional integrity: the myocardial region may show contrast echocardiography positivity, with no improvement after revascularization.

20.6
Tissue Characterization and Myocardial Velocity Imaging

The myocardial wall has an echoreflectivity that is not stable during the cardiac cycle, showing a physiological systolic-to-diastolic cyclic variation. Myocardial echodensity decreases with contraction. This quantitative parameter can be translated into the more familiar gray-level codification: the image of a normal wall is darker during end-systole and brighter during end-diastole. The systodiastolic excursion of echodensity is due, in a very complex way, to wall thickening and intramural function. After a few minutes of ischemia, systodiastolic variation is abolished, but is promptly restored in the case of effective reperfusion for the preserved intramural function, when regional wall motion is still compromised. The usefulness of this index has been demonstrated in the research and clinical settings [23]. Necrotic regions do not show cyclic gray-level variation, which is preserved in asynergic but viable segments. With a conceptually similar approach, in myocardial infarction, transmural extension of scar distribution in the infarct zone is proportionally related to the reduction in systolic function measured by the radial transmural velocity gradient or strainrate imaging or peak radial strain using the speckle tracking technique [24–26].

20.7
Dobutamine Stress Echocardiography

Ten years before the description by Rahimtoola of hibernated myocardium [4], several clinical and experimental studies had recognized the inotropic reserve as a marker of reversible myocardial dysfunction after revascularization during cardiac catheterization (ante litteram hibernation). Regional wall motion was evaluated at ventriculography and the inotropic stimulus was either postextrasystolic beat or adrenaline [27–29]. After many years, the same mechanism was employed for the recognition of myocardial viability through pharmacological stress echocardiography. Asynergic, but viable myocardium preserves a contractile reserve, which may be evoked by an appropriate stimulus (Prince Charming's kiss) awakening the seemingly dead myocardium. The recovery of function may take place either through a primary inotropic stimulus (determining a secondary increase in flow to meet the augmented metabolic demands) or through a primary vasodilatory stimulus (determining the increment of regional function) [10]. The prototype of an inotropic stress for viability assessment is low-dose dobutamine [30], originally proposed by Luc Pierard in 1990 and today the reference standard for the recognition of viability by stress echocardiography. Dobutamine is usually employed as an ischemic stress at a dosage of 5–40 µg kg^{-1} per min. The viability assessment is usually performed at a dose of 5–10 µg kg^{-1} per min. In fact, the effects on myocardial receptors can be obtained at a very low dose of dobutamine, which does not elicit major increases in either heart rate or blood pressure, with the consequent modification of regional function by extrinsic mechanisms.

Following the pioneering observation by Pierard [30], several groups have confirmed that low-dose dobutamine can identify viable myocardium both early after an acute myocardial infarction (stunning) [31–35] and in chronic coronary artery disease (hibernation) [36–45]. Dobutamine-induced functional recovery correlates well with other, more complex imaging techniques, including fluorodeoxyglucose uptake with positron emission tomography (PET) and thallium scintigraphy. In a population of asynergic segments, thallium uptake occurs more frequently than a dobutamine-induced response [40–42]. Thallium demonstrates the ability of the myocardium to take up a cation by an active process that takes place at the cell membrane level. Stress echocardiography assesses the ability of the cardiac muscle to increase its contraction in response to an inotropic stimulus, which requires the functional integrity of the cell's contractile machinery. These different cellular functions are not all simultaneously and equally present in the viable myocardium, but are hierarchically ranked according to a sequence outlining a viability cascade (Fig. 20.1), conceptually similar to the well-known ischemic cascade. In the viability cascade, a preserved inotropic response to dobutamine expresses a mild level of damage, which will usually allow prompt restoration of function following revascularization (Table 20.3). For presumably more severe levels of damage, a segment can be unresponsive to inotropic stress and still be capable of taking up a significant amount of thallium [36]. This is likely to correspond to a more advanced form of cellular damage, in which only those cellular functions that are strictly essential to cell survival (such as membrane integrity) are preserved. From the pooled analysis of available studies using functional recovery following revascularization as a gold standard [42], thallium has a sensitivity superior to stress echocardiography, but a lower specificity, with similar overall accuracy [11, 39–43] (Fig. 20.4). Thus a significant number of myocardial segments with baseline systolic dysfunction will lack

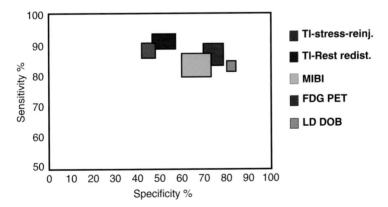

Fig. 20.4 Sensitivity and specificity of nuclear techniques and dobutamine echocardiography in predicting functional recovery. (From a meta-analysis conducted by Bax et al [42].) Low-dose dobutamine echocardiography has a clearly better specificity and a slightly lower sensitivity than nuclear techniques

inotropic reserve during dobutamine administration in spite of preserved thallium uptake. Only a minority of these dobutamine-nonresponsive and thallium-uptaker segments are destined to recover following revascularization [11, 39].

In general, there is an excellent correlation between PET and dobutamine echocardiography results [47, 48]. The increased sensitivity of PET compared with dobutamine echocardiography occurs at the expense of lower specificity regarding the recovery of function. In quantitative terms, contractile reserve evidenced by a positive dobutamine response requires at least 50% viable myocytes in a given segment, whereas scintigraphic methods also identify segments with less viable myocytes [47]. Minor levels of viability, characterized by scintigraphic positivity and dobutamine echocardiography negativity, are often unable to translate into functional recovery, but may contribute to an improvement in exercise capacity after revascularization, which is better correlated to the extent of viability by PET than to the extent of viability by dobutamine echocardiography [48].

When compared to DE-CMR, dobutamine stress echocardiography has similar overall accuracy, although for regions with less than 25% scar, it is possible that dobutamine may provide a higher positive predictive value than DE-CMR [49–51]. Both dobutamine echocardiography and DE-CMR require intravenous access, but the latter does not require infusion of pharmacological stress agent. Thus, DE-CMR is safer, requires less intensive monitoring, and is also somewhat easier to interpret. However, it is more expensive, less widely available, and cannot be performed at bedside [52]. In poorly echogenic patients, the dobutamine test can be coupled with CMR [49]. An advantage of dobutamine echocardiography is its ability to distinguish between presumably stunned myocardium and presumably hibernating myocardium using both low and high doses of dobutamine. Sustained improvement corresponds in the setting of acute coronary syndrome to stunned myocardium – improvement of contractility in dyssynergic segments until peak dose without deterioration – than can recover its function progressively without revascularization. In the setting of chronic coronary artery disease, sustained improvement implies the presence of nontransmural necrosis and preserved coronary flow reserve. A biphasic response – initial improvement of contractility at low-dose dobutamine followed by subsequent worsening at high-dose dobutamine – implies viable but jeopardized myocardium with blunted flow reserve. Timely revascularization is required in this condition. Too early follow-up echocardiography may result in underestimation of the extent of possible functional improvement which can continue to progress.

20.8
Alternative Stress Echocardiography Methods

Dobutamine is widely used to assess myocardial viability in both acute and chronic postinfarction patients. However, it does have limitations:

1. In a certain number of patients, even at low doses, it induces myocardial ischemia, which obscures the recognition of viability. Such percentages have been reported to be especially consistent in patients with chronic coronary artery disease evaluated before bypass surgery [37]. For some patients, a more selective stress is needed for viability that will not induce ischemia.

2. Concomitant β-blocker therapy blunts the inotropic response to low-dose dobutamine. Although good results have been reported in populations largely on β-blocker therapy [21], β-blockers may conceivably alter the ability to detect contractile reserve at low-dose testing [35]. This problem becomes clinically relevant since patients with acute myocardial infarction or chronic coronary artery disease are largely on chronic β-blocker therapy, and withdrawal may be impractical and possibly dangerous.
3. Even in the ideal conditions of selected patients without inducible ischemia and off therapy, dobutamine has a suboptimal sensitivity for predicting recovery. If a segment shows improved wall motion with dobutamine, it is likely to be viable and move better with revascularization but viability is still possible even if wall motion does not improve with dobutamine.

These limitations have led to the identification of alternative stresses to evoke an inotropic response in viable segments. Enoximone is a phosphodiesterase inhibitor increasing cyclic adenosine monophosphate (cAMP) concentration independently of β-receptor activation [53]. Dipyridamole evokes a vasodilation through A2-adenosine receptor stimulation, although a flow-independent effect due to direct stimulation of A1-myocyte adenosine receptors has also been suggested [54]. These stresses have a lower ischemic potential than low-dose dobutamine and are unaffected by β-blocker therapy. Low-dose dipyridamole stress ($0.28\,mg\ kg^{-1}$ over 4 min) for viability has a diagnostic accuracy comparable to that of dobutamine for predicting spontaneous and revascularization-induced functional recovery [55]. In addition, low-dose dipyridamole can be used in combination with low-dose dobutamine for recruiting inotropic reserve [56] in segments which are thallium-uptakers, nonresponders to dobutamine, and destined to recover following revascularization [57]. It has an impressive prognostic value in identifying patients with severe left ventricular dysfunction who can benefit more from revascularization [58]. Also, low-level exercise can recruit a contractile reserve in viable myocardium through production of endogenous catecholamines and with an accuracy comparable to low-dose dobutamine [59]. An exercise test with continuous monitoring of regional function can also identify a biphasic response [60].

20.9
The Clinical Value of Myocardial Viability: Critical or Luxury Information?

The recognition of myocardial viability is associated with a higher incidence of unstable angina in patients evaluated early after an acute myocardial infarction [54].

If patients with severe resting dysfunction are considered, myocardial viability is associated with a better survival rate, both in medically treated patients after acute myocardial infarction (Fig. 20.5) [60–63] and in patients with chronic coronary artery disease submitted to revascularization procedures [64–67] (Fig. 20.6). The quest for myocardial viability is per se prognostically and therapeutically critical in patients with ischemic cardiomyopathy (Table 20.5), with the clinical picture dominated by heart failure symptoms (Fig. 20.7), the coronary anatomy suitable for revascularization, and no spontaneous or inducible ischemia. The indication for revascularization is stronger in those patients with severe left ventricular dysfunction, but with preserved myocardial viability and suitable coronary anatomy. When viability is restricted to

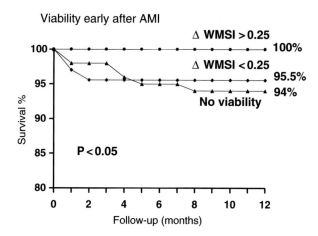

Fig. 20.5 Kaplan–Meier survival curves (considering only death as an end point) in patients with absence (no viability) and presence (viability) of myocardial viability. Patients with myocardial viability are separated on the basis of the number of segments showing improvement by use of an arbitrary cutoff value for the difference between rest *WMSI* (wall motion score index) and low-dose dobutamine WMSI (ΔWMSI) set at 0.25. Absence of myocardial viability is associated with greater incidence of cardiac death ($p<0.05$). Survival in patients with little myocardial viability is comparable to patients without myocardial viability. (Adapted from [63])

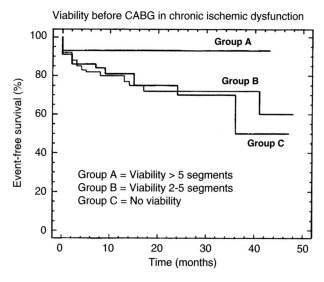

Fig. 20.6 Kaplan–Meier curves showing survival free of cardiac events (including death, nonfatal MI, unstable AP requiring hospitalization, and hospitalization for heart failure) in groups A (viability in more than five segments), B (viability in fewer than five segments), and C (no viability) patients. Event-free survival was significantly better in group A than in group B or group C, both being $p<0.05$. (Adapted from [64])

Table 20.5 Clinical relevance of myocardial viability

	Luxury information	Critical information
Global left ventricular function	Preserved	Impaired
Typical history	Single recent infarction	Multiple previous infarctions
Prognostic significance of viability	Predicts angina	Predicts death
Prevailing pathophysiological substrate	Stunned	Hibernated
Method of choice	Stress for ischemia and viability (high-dose pharmacological stress echocardiography)	Selective assessment of viability (low-dose pharmacological stress echocardiography)

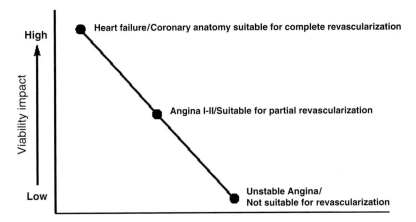

Fig. 20.7 Clinical and angiographic variables modulating the clinical impact of viability testing, which is higher in patients with heart failure symptoms, little or no anginal symptoms, and with coronary anatomy suitable for complete revascularization

only certain coronary areas, selective revascularization (usually with angioplasty) can be performed, targeted at stenotic coronary arteries feeding asynergic, yet viable regions. In patients with markedly reduced resting function (ejection fraction<35%) and chronic coronary artery disease, the stress echocardiography documentation of myocardial viability is associated with a much lower mortality rate in revascularized patients than in medically treated patients [68]. The absence of viable myocardium downstream from a critical coronary artery stenosis in the absence of inducible ischemia substantially weakens the indication for revascularization and directs the clinical decision toward medical therapy or, if possible, cardiac transplantation.

These conclusions apply to the recognition of myocardial viability by virtually all methods, including thallium-perfusion imaging, fluorodeoxyglucose metabolic imaging,

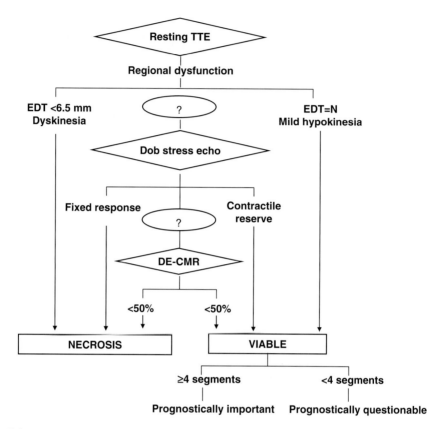

Fig. 20.8 Algorithm for the diagnosis of myocardial viability. A sequential application of resting echocardiography, dobutamine echocardiography, and delayed enhancement-cardiac magnetic resonance provides a very accurate diagnosis of myocardial viability at very reasonable cost and without the long-term risks due to radiation burden of scintigraphy and positron emission tomography. EDT=end-diastolic thickness; DE-CMR=delayed enhancement cardiac magnetic resonance; TTE=transthoracic echocardiography

or dobutamine echocardiography, with no measurable performance difference for predicting revascularization benefit between the three testing techniques [68]. In patients with viability, there is a direct relationship between severity of left ventricular dysfunction and magnitude of benefit with revascularization [68]. In patients with viability, revascularization was associated with 80% reduction in annual mortality (16% vs. 3.2%) compared to medical treatment (Fig. 20.8).

20.10
The Prognostic Value of Myocardial Viability: A Moonlight Serenade

Viability information is like a moon in the sky of prognosis: in the daytime of a preserved global left ventricular function (ejection fraction>35%) the sun shines, and the moon – even if present in the sky – gives no additional prognostic light. The prognosis is linked to the clouds of ischemia, which obscure the sun of preserved resting function. In these good ventricles, with ejection fraction greater than 35%, the documentation of ischemia should dictate a revascularization oriented by the results of physiological testing. In the prognostic night light of a reduced left ventricular function (ejection fraction<35%), the adverse prognostic effects of ischemia are magnified and ischemia, per se, warrants revascularization. For any given level of inducible ischemia, the prognosis worsens with the worsening of the left ventricular function. The documentation of a large amount of viable myocardium reduces the risk of revascularization and viability-oriented revascularization determines a survival advantage in comparison to medically treated patients. It is important, however, that the "viability moonlight" can direct the cardiologist only when a "full moon" is present, i.e., a considerable amount of viable myocardium. Similar to ischemia, viability response should also be titrated. Viability is not a binary, dichotomous response, but it is a continuous response that should be stratified in different shades of gray. The prognostic protection conferred by viability is only detected when it exceeds a critical threshold of at least four segments or 20% of the total left ventricle [11, 68]. The beneficial impact of viability on survival is observed only in revascularized patients.

20.11
Myocardial Viability in Context

At present various problems increase the difficulty of clinical assessment of myocardial viability and clinical decision making based on the recognition of myocardial viability. We evaluate diagnostic tests in terms of their capacity to predict functional recovery, and this is the best available gold standard. However, we now know that not all segments destined to recover do so early after revascularization. Moreover, some partially viable segments do not recover at all. In addition, functional improvement can occur during inotropic stimulation in the absence of salvageable myocardium.

– *Not all segments destined to recover do so in days or weeks.* Functional recovery is frequently used for comparison in studies evaluating different techniques to assess myocardial viability. It is the gold standard against which the sensitivity and specificity of the various techniques are assessed. In fact, recovery of ventricular function depends on many factors, including quality of the revascularization procedure, perioperative ischemia, and recurrence of obstruction in native or graft vessels. The time course of recovery can be extremely variable, since recovery of ventricular function depends on the quality and completeness of the revascularization procedure and the severity of histological abnormalities: the higher the dedifferentiation of myocytes, the longer the time needed for recovery. In the later stages of hibernation, intracellular glycogen accumulates and myofibrillar units drop out, offering a morphological substrate to the reduced or absent inotropic response to low-dose dobutamine infusion. Therefore, the time course of recovery can be highly variable; assessment too early may underestimate the prevalence and degree of functional improvement.
– *Viability can be present without late functional improvement.* Even if tissue is viable preoperatively, the revascularization is complete, and the follow-up is appropriately

long, the myocardium can remain asynergic and still the restoration of flow can produce beneficial clinical effects [69]. In fact, systolic thickening occurs largely as a result of subendocardial thickening. The presence of viable myocardium in the outer layers of the ventricular wall may induce greater thickening during inotropic stimulation for transmural tethering. Perfusion may actually improve in a large amount of viable myocardium, outside the subendocardial layer, and this may not necessarily translate into an improved resting function. However, the beneficial effects may extend above and beyond functional recovery [70]; viable, well-perfused tissue may exert an antiremodeling effect, contributing to maintaining left ventricular shape and size by preventing infarct expansion and subsequent heart failure. In patients with acute myocardial infarction and ischemic cardiomyopathy, a substantial amount of viable myocardium prevents ongoing left ventricular remodeling after revascularization and is associated with persistent improvement of symptoms and better outcome [71, 72, 73]. Exercise capacity may improve, and substrate for arrhythmias may change with a possible antiarrhythmic effect of improved perfusion, without functional recovery.

– *Functional improvement can occur during inotropic stress without viability.* An inotropic stress can induce improvement in an asynergic region even in the absence of significant viability; this occurs because of transmural or horizontal tethering in nontransmural infarctions [63]. This effect is more prominent when the inotropic stimulus is also exerted in normal myocardium and when it is of a moderate to marked degree. This may explain the declining specificity associated with increasing doses of dobutamine. In spite of these theoretical, pathophysiological, and clinical limitations, pharmacological stress echocardiography can now be considered the technique of choice for the recognition of myocardial viability. Its major advantage is the simultaneous insight it provides into resting function, which determines the overall clinical relevance of the viability issue, and into myocardial ischemia, which integrates the prognostic impact of viability and can be assessed at high doses of the drug. The accuracy is high and comparable to scintigraphy and CMR techniques (Table 20.5), but the cost is lower [74] and, similarly to CMR, there is no radiation dose and biological burden increasing long-term cancer risk [75–77]. This is especially important in patients with heart disease who undergo multiple imaging tests with high and cumulative radiation exposure [78] of which neither the cardiologist [79] nor the patient [80] are fully aware. No new technologies (including contrast echocardiography or myocardial velocity imaging) can be proposed for a clinically oriented use today [81, 82] (Table 20.6).

Despite the absence of published randomized trials (the results of the STICH study are not yet available), extensive myocardial viability can be considered a factor strongly supporting coronary revascularization in itself only in patients with severe resting left ventricular dysfunction, absence of spontaneous or induced ischemia, chronic coronary artery disease, and suitable coronary anatomy. The currently accepted appropriate (and less appropriate) indications for clinically driven testing of myocardial viability [83] are summarized in Table 20.7.

Table 20.6 Methods to assess myocardial viability

	Relative cost	Radiation dose (CXr)	Cancer risk per exam	Accuracy
Stress echocardiography	1	0	0	++
DE-CMR	5.5	0	0	++
MIBI scintigraphy	3.5	500	1 in 1,000	++
Thallium scintigraphy	3.5	>1,000	>1 in 500	++
PET-FDG	14	500	1 in 1,000	++

CXr chest radiograph, *DE-CMR* delayed enhancement, *MIBI* Tc 99m-sestamibi, *PET-FDG* positron emission tomography fluorodeoxyglucose

Table 20.7 Most frequent appropriate/uncertain/inappropriate indications in CAD detection and/or risk stratification (adapted from [83])

	Appropriate	Uncertain	Inappropriate
Ischemic cardiomyopathy, known CAD, patient eligible for revascularization	√		
Equivocal aortic stenosis, low cardiac output	√		
Risk stratification in nonischemic cardiomyopathy		√	
EF>40% and/or patient eligible for revascularization			√

CAD coronary artery disease, *EF* ejection fraction

References

1. Heyndrickx GR, Millard RW, McRitchie RJ, et al (1975) Regional myocardial functional and electrophysiological alterations after brief coronary artery occlusion in conscious dogs. J Clin Invest 56:978–985
2. Braunwald E, Kloner RA (1982) The stunned myocardium: prolonged, postischemic ventricular dysfunction. Circulation 66:1146–1149
3. Rahimtoola SH (1985) A perspective on the three large multivessel randomized clinical trials of coronary bypass surgery for chronic stable angina. Circulation 72(Suppl V): V123–V135
4. Braunwald E, Rutherford JD (1986) Reversible ischemic left ventricular dysfunction: evidence for "hibernating myocardium". J Am Coll Cardiol 56:978–985
5. Rahimtoola SH (1989) The hibernating myocardium. Am Heart J 117:211–220
6. Flameng W, Suy R, Schwartz F et al (1981) Ultrastructural correlates of left ventricular contraction abnormalities in patients with chronic ischemic heart disease: determinants of reversible segmental asynergy post-revascularization surgery. Am Heart J 102:846–857

7. Torres MA, Picano E, Parodi G, et al (1997) Residual coronary reserve identifies segmental viability in patients with wall motion abnormalities. J Am Coll Cardiol 30:65–70

8. Gregg DE (1963) Effect of coronary perfusion pressure or coronary flow on oxygen usage of the myocardium. Circ Res 13:497–500

9. Salisbury PF, Cross CE, Rieben PA (1960) Influence of coronary artery pressure upon myocardial elasticity. Circ Res 8:794–800

10. Stahl LD, Aversano TR, Becker LC (1986) Selective enhancement of function of stunned myocardium by increased flow. Circulation 74:843–851

11. Bonow RO (2002) Myocardial viability and prognosis in patients with ischemic left ventricular dysfunction. J Am Coll Cardiol 39:1159–1162

12. Wagner A, Mahrholdt H, Holly TA, et al (2003) Contrast-enhanced MRI and routine single photon emission computed tomography (SPECT) perfusion imaging for detection of subendocardial myocardial infarcts: an imaging study. Lancet 361:374–379

13. Faletra F, Crivellaro W, Pirelli S, et al (1995) Value of transthoracic two-dimensional echocardiography in predicting viability in patients with healed Q-wave anterior wall myocardial infarction. Am J Cardiol 76:1002–1006

14. Cwajg JM, Cwajg E, Nagueh SF, et al (2000) End-diastolic wall thickness as a predictor of recovery of function in myocardial hibernation: relation to rest-redistribution Tl-201 tomography and dobutamine stress echocardiography. J Am Coll Cardiol 35:1152–1161

15. Sabia PJ, Powers ER, Ragosta M, et al (1992) An association between collateral blood flow and myocardial viability in patients with recent myocardial infarction. N Engl J Med 327:1825–1831

16. Ragosta M, Camarano G, Kaul S, et al (1994) Microvascular integrity indicates myocellular viability in patients with recent myocardial infarction. New insights using myocardial contrast echocardiography. Circulation 89:2562–2569

17. Ito H, Iwakura K, Oh H, et al (1995) Temporal changes in myocardial perfusion patterns in patients with reperfused anterior wall myocardial infarction. Their relation to myocardial viability. Circulation 91:656–662

18. Bolognese L, Antoniucci D, Rovai D, et al (1996) Myocardial contrast echocardiography versus dobutamine echocardiography for predicting functional recovery after acute myocardial infarction treated with primary coronary angioplasty. J Am Coll Cardiol 28:1677–1683

19. deFilippi CR, Willett DL, Irani WN, et al (1995) Comparison of myocardial contrast echocardiography and low-dose dobutamine stress echocardiography in predicting recovery of left ventricular function after coronary revascularization in chronic ischemic heart disease. Circulation 92:2863–2868

20. Meza MF, Ramee S, Collins T, et al (1997) Knowledge of perfusion and contractile reserve improves the predictive value of recovery of regional myocardial function postrevascularization: a study using the combination of myocardial contrast echocardiography and dobutamine echocardiography. Circulation 96:3459–3465

21. Balcells E, Powers ER, Lepper W, et al (2003) Detection of myocardial viability by contrast echocardiography in acute infarction predicts recovery of resting function and contractile reserve. J Am Coll Cardiol 41:827–833

22. Milunski MR, Mohr GA, Perez JE, et al (1989) Ultrasonic tissue characterization with integrated backscatter. Acute myocardial ischemia, reperfusion, and stunned myocardium in patients. Circulation 80:491–503

23. Marini C, Picano E, Varga A, et al (1996) Cyclic variation in myocardial gray level as a marker of viability in man. A videodensitometric study. Eur Heart J 17:472–479

24. Thibault H, Derumeaux G (2008) Assessment of myocardial ischemia and viability using tissue Doppler and deformation imaging: the lessons from the experimental studies. Arch Cardiovasc Dis 101:61–68

25. Zhang Y, Chan AK, Yu CM, et al (2005) Strain rate imaging differentiates transmural from non-transmural myocardial infarction: a validation study using delayed-enhancement magnetic resonance imaging. J Am Coll Cardiol 46:864–871

26. Becker M, Lenzen A, Ocklenburg C, et al (2008) Myocardial deformation imaging based on ultrasonic pixel tracking to identify reversible myocardial dysfunction. J Am Coll Cardiol 51:1473–1481

27. Dyke SH, Cohn PF, Gorlin R, et al (1974) Detection of residual myocardial function in coronary artery disease using post-extra systolic potentiation. Circulation 50:694–699

28. Horn HR, Teichholz LE, Cohn PF, et al (1974) Augmentation of left ventricular contraction pattern in coronary artery disease by an inotropic catecholamine. The epinephrine ventriculogram. Circulation 49:1063–1071

29. Dyke SH, Urschel CW, Sonnenblick EH, et al (1975) Detection of latent function in acutely ischemic myocardium in the dog: comparison of pharmacologic inotropic stimulation and postextrasystolic potentiation. Circ Res 36:490–497

30. Pierard LA, De Landsheere CM, Berthe C, et al (1990) Identification of viable myocardium by echocardiography during dobutamine infusion in patients with myocardial infarction after thrombolytic therapy: comparison with positron emission tomography. J Am Coll Cardiol 15:1021–1031

31. Smart SC, Sawada S, Ryan T, et al (1993) Low-dose dobutamine echocardiography detects reversible dysfunction after thrombolytic therapy of acute myocardial infarction. Circulation 88:405–415

32. Watada H, Ito H, Oh H, et al (1994) Dobutamine stress echocardiography predicts reversible dysfunction and quantitates the extent of irreversibly damaged myocardium after reperfusion of anterior myocardial infarction. J Am Coll Cardiol 24:624–630

33. Poli A, Previtali M, Lanzarini L, et al (1996) Comparison of dobutamine stress echocardiography with dipyridamole stress echocardiography for detection of viable myocardium after myocardial infarction treated with thrombolysis. Heart 75:240–246

34. Barilla F, Gheorghiade KP, Alam M, et al (1993) Low-dose dobutamine in patients with acute myocardial infarction identifies viable but not contractile myocardium and predicts the magnitude of improvement in wall motion abnormalities in response to coronary revascularization. Am Heart J 51:1312–1316

35. Zaglavara T, Haaverstad R, Cumberledge B, et al (2002) Dobutamine stress echocardiography for the detection of myocardial viability in patients with left ventricular dysfunction taking beta blockers: accuracy and optimal dose. Heart 87:329–335

36. Cigarroa CG, deFilippi CR, Brickner ME, et al (1993) Dobutamine stress echocardiography identifies hibernating myocardium and predicts recovery of left ventricular function after coronary revascularization. Circulation 88:430–436

37. La Canna G, Alfieri O, Giubbini R, et al (1994) Echocardiography during infusion of dobutamine for identification of reversibly dysfunction in patients with chronic coronary artery disease. J Am Coll Cardiol 23:617–626

38. Afridi I, Kleiman NS, Raizner AE, et al (1995) Dobutamine echocardiography in myocardial hibernation. Optimal dose and accuracy in predicting recovery of ventricular function after coronary angioplasty. Circulation 91:663–670

39. Arnese M, Cornel JH, Salustri A, et al (1995) Prediction of improvement of regional left ventricular function after surgical revascularization. A comparison of low-dose dobutamine echocardiography with 201Tl single-photon emission computed tomography. Circulation 91:2748–2752

40. Perrone-Filardi P, Pace L, Prastaro M, et al (1995) Dobutamine echocardiography predicts improvement of hypoperfused dysfunctional myocardium after revascularization in patients with coronary artery disease. Circulation 91:2556–2565

41. Haque T, Furukawa T, Takahashi M, et al (1995) Identification of hibernating myocardium by dobutamine stress echocardiography: comparison with thallium-201 reinjection imaging. Am Heart J 130:553–563

42. Bax JJ, Wijns W, Cornel JH, et al (1997) Accuracy of currently available techniques for prediction of functional recovery after revascularization in patients with left ventricular dysfunction due to chronic coronary artery disease: comparison of pooled data. J Am Coll Cardiol 30:1451–1460

43. Charney R, Schwinger ME, Chun J, et al (1994) Dobutamine echocardiography and resting redistribution thallium-201 scintigraphy predicts recovery of hibernating myocardium after coronary revascularization. Am Heart J 128:864–869

44. Marzullo P, Parodi O, Reisenhofer B, et al (1993) Value of rest thallium-201/technetium-99m sestamibi scans and dobutamine echocardiography for detecting myocardial viability. Am J Cardiol 71:166–172

45. Perrone-Filardi P, Pace L, Prastaro M, et al (1996) Assessment of myocardial viability in patients with chronic coronary artery disease. Rest-4-hour-24-hour 201Tl tomography versus dobutamine echocardiography. Circulation 94:2712–2719

46. Panza JA, Dilsizian V, Laurienzo JM, et al (1995) Relation between thallium uptake and contractile response to dobutamine. Implications regarding myocardial viability in patients with chronic coronary artery disease and left ventricular dysfunction. Circulation 91:990–998

47. Baumgartner H, Porenta G, Lau YK, et al (1998) Assessment of myocardial viability by dobutamine echocardiography, positron emission tomography and thallium-201 SPECT: correlation with histopathology in explanted hearts. J Am Coll Cardiol 32:1701–1708

48. Pagano D, Bonser RS, Townend JN, et al (1998) Predictive value of dobutamine echocardiography and positron emission tomography in identifying hibernating myocardium in patients with post ischaemic heart failure. Heart 79:281–288

49. Wellnhofer E, Olariu A, Klein C, et al (2004) Magnetic resonance low-dose dobutamine test is superior to SCAR quantification for the prediction of functional recovery. Circulation 109:2172–2174

50. Bove CM, DiMaria JM, Voros S, et al (2006) Dobutamine response and myocardial infarct transmurality: functional improvement after coronary artery bypass grafting – initial experience. Radiology 240:835–841

51. Ramani K, Judd RM, Holly TA, et al (1998) Contrast magnetic resonance imaging in the assessment of myocardial viability in patients with stable coronary artery disease and left ventricular dysfunction. Circulation 98:2687–2694

52. Kim RJ, Manning WJ (2004) Viability assessment by delayed enhancement cardiovascular magnetic resonance: will low-dose dobutamine dull the shine? Circulation 109:2476–2479

53. Lu C, Carlino M, Fragasso G, et al (2000) Enoximone echocardiography for predicting recovery of left ventricular dysfunction after revascularization: a novel test for detecting myocardial viability. Circulation 101:1255–1260

54. Picano E, Marzullo P, Gigli G, et al (1992) Identification of viable myocardium by dipyridamole- induced improvement in regional left ventricular function assessed by echocardiography in myocardial infarction and comparison with thallium scintigraphy at rest. Am J Cardiol 70:703–710

55. Varga A, Sicari R, Picano E, et al (1996) Infra-low dose dipyridamole test. A novel dose regimen for selective assessment of myocardial viability by vasodilator stress echocardiography. Eur Heart J 17:629–634

56. Picano E, Ostojic M, Varga A, et al (1996) Combined low dose dipyridamole-dobutamine stress echocardiography to identify myocardial viability. J Am Coll Cardiol 27:1422–1428

57. Sicari R, Varga A, Picano E, et al (1999) Comparison of combination of dipyridamole and dobutamine during echocardiography with thallium scintigraphy with thallium scintigraphy to improve viability detection. Am J Cardiol 83:6–10

58. Sicari R, Ripoli A, Picano E, et al, VIDA (Viability Identification with Dipyridamole Administration) Study Group (2001) The prognostic value of myocardial viability recognized by low dose dipyridamole echocardiography in patients with chronic ischaemic left ventricular dysfunction. Eur Heart J 22:837–844

59. Hoffer EP, Dewe W, Celentano C, et al (1999) Low-level exercise echocardiography detects contractile reserve and predicts reversible dysfunction after acute myocardial infarction: comparison with low-dose dobutamine echocardiography. J Am Coll Cardiol 34:989–997

60. Lancellotti P, Hoffer EP, Piérard LA (2003) Detection and clinical usefulness of a biphasic response during exercise echocardiography early after myocardial infarction. J Am Coll Cardiol 41:1142–1147

61. Sicari R, Picano E, Landi P, et al (1997) Prognostic value of dobutamine-atropine stress echocardiography early after acute myocardial infarction. Echo Dobutamine International Cooperative (EDIC) Stud y. J Am Coll Cardiol 29:254–260

62. Carlos ME, Smart SC, Wynsen JC, et al (1997) Dobutamine stress echocardiography for risk stratification after myocardial infarction. Circulation 95:1402–1410

63. Lee KS, Marwick T, Cook SA, et al (1995) Prognosis of patients with left ventricular dysfunction with and without viable myocardium after myocardial infarction: relative efficacy of medical therapy and revascularization. Circulation 90:2687–2694

64. Picano E, Sicari R, Landi P, et al (1998) Prognostic value of myocardial viability in medically treated patients with global left ventricular dysfunction early after an acute uncomplicated myocardial infarction: a dobutamine stress echocardiographic study. Circulation 98:1078–1084

65. Meluzin J, Cerny J, Frelich M, et al (1998) Prognostic value of the amount of dysfunctional but viable myocardium in revascularized patients with coronary artery disease and left ventricular dysfunction. Investigators of this Multicenter Study. J Am Coll Cardiol 32:912–920

66. Senior R, Kaul S, Lahiri A (1999) Myocardial viability on echocardiography predicts long-term survival after revascularization in patients with ischemic congestive heart failure. J Am Coll Cardiol 33:1848–1854

67. Cortigiani L, Sicari R, Picano E, et al (2007) VIDA (Viability Identification with Dobutamine Administration) Study Group. Dobutamine stress echocardiography and the effect of revascularization on outcome in diabetic and non-diabetic patients with chronic ischaemic left ventricular dysfunction. Eur J Heart Fail 9:1038–1043

68. Sicari R, Picano E, Cortigiani L, et al (2003) VIDA (Viability Identification with Dobutamine Administration) Study Group. Prognostic value of myocardial viability recognized by low-dose dobutamine echocardiography in chronic ischemic left ventricular dysfunction. Am J Cardiol 92:1263–1266

69. Allman KC, Shaw LJ, Hachamovitch R, et al (2002) Myocardial viability testing and impact of revascularization on prognosis in patients with coronary artery disease and left ventricular dysfunction: a meta-analysis. J Am Coll Cardiol 39:1151–1158

70. Kaul S (1995) There may be more to myocardial viability than meets the eye. Circulation 92:2790–2793

71. Armstrong WF (1996) "Hibernating" myocardium: asleep or part dead? J Am Coll Cardiol 28:530–535

72. Bolognese L, Cerisano G, Buonamici P, et al (1997) Influence of infarct-zone viability on left ventricular remodeling after acute myocardial infarction. Circulation 96:3353–3359

73. Rizzello V, Poldermans D, Boersma E, et al (2004) Opposite patterns of left ventricular remodeling after coronary revascularization in patients with ischemic cardiomyopathy: role of myocardial viability. Circulation 110:2383–2388
74. Chan J, Khafagi F, Young AA, et al (2008) Impact of coronary revascularization and transmural extent of scar on regional left ventricular remodelling. Eur Heart J 29:1608–1617
75. Pennell DJ, Sechtem UP, Higgins CB, et al (2004) Society for Cardiovascular Magnetic Resonance; Working Group on Cardiovascular Magnetic Resonance of the European Society of Cardiology: clinical indications for cardiovascular magnetic resonance [CMR]: Consensus Panel report. Eur Heart J 25:1940–1965
76. Picano E (2004) Sustainability of medical imaging. Educational and Debate. BMJ 328:578–80
77. Picano E (2004) Informed consent and communication of risk from radiological and nuclear medicine examinations: how to escape from a communication inferno. BMJ Educational and Debate. BMJ 329:849–851
78. Picano E (2003) Stress echocardiography: a historical perspective. Am J Med 114:126–130
79. Bedetti G, Botto N, Picano E, et al (2008) Cumulative patient effective dose in cardiology. BJR 81:805–813
80. Correia MJ, Hellies A, Picano E, et al (2005) Lack of radiological awareness among physicians working in a tertiary-care cardiological centre. Int J Cardiol 105:307–311
81. Bedetti G, Pizzi C, Picano E, et al (2008) Suboptimal awareness of radiologic dose among patients undergoing cardiac stress scintigraphy. J Am Coll Radiol 5:126–131
82. Pellikka PA, Nagueh SF, Elhendy AA, et al, American Society of Echocardiography (2007). American Society of Echocardiography recommendations for performance, interpretation, and application of stress echocardiography. J Am Soc Echocardiogr 20:1021–1041
83. Sicari R, Nihoyannopoulos P, Evangelista A, et al, European Association of Echocardiography (2008) Stress echocardiography expert consensus statement: European Association of Echocardiography (EAE) (a registered branch of the ESC). Eur J Echocardiogr 9:415–437
84. Douglas PS, Khandheria B, Stainback RF, et al, American College of Cardiology Foundation; American Society of Echocardiography; American College of Emergency Physicians; American Heart Association; American Society of Nuclear Cardiology, Society for Cardiovascular Angiography and Interventions; Society of Cardiovascular Computed Tomography, Society for Cardiovascular Magnetic Resonance (2008) ACCF/ASE/ACEP/AHA/ASNC/SCAI/SCCT/SCMR 2008 appropriateness criteria for stress echocardiography: a report of the American College of Cardiology Foundation Appropriateness Criteria Task Force, American Society of Echocardiography, American College of Emergency Physicians, American Heart Association, American Society of Nuclear Cardiology, Society for Cardiovascular Angiography and Interventions, Society of Cardiovascular Computed Tomography, and Society for Cardiovascular Magnetic Resonance endorsed by the Heart Rhythm Society and the Society of Critical Care Medicine. J Am Coll Cardiol 51:1127–1147

Diagnostic Flowcharts

21

Eugenio Picano

In patients with known or suspected coronary artery disease, diagnosis and risk stratification can be aided by noninvasive tests for myocardial ischemia. Guidelines for choosing among the different stress testing approaches have been published [1–5], but the use of these tests by physicians varies widely according to diagnostic yields, cost, and convenience. Some general principles should be considered. First, no single test or strategy has been proven to be overall superior [5]. Second, all published research consistently demonstrates that stress testing with radionuclide scintigraphy and echocardiography provides more information than exercise electrocardiography alone [1–4].

However, the fact that a test provides more information does not mean that it is the most appropriate test. Other important issues are whether the additional information is sufficient to change patient care in ways that would be expected to improve outcomes [5]. Third, regardless of which test is used, a normal test result should never be considered a guarantee that the patient does not have coronary artery disease or has no risk of cardiovascular events [3]. The rational diagnostic approach can be divided into four successive steps, progressing from the clinical picture to exercise electrocardiography, then to the imaging stress test. In highly selected cases, testing for coronary vasospasm can be considered.

21.1
Step 1: Clinical Picture

Simple ECG and resting echocardiography can integrate the clinical picture sufficiently to identify patients with a higher probability of severe disease, warranting coronary angiography. In such patients, the good cardiologist needs hardly any help to place the patient on the fast-track of coronary angiography. Early after myocardial infarction associated with ischemic, mechanical, or arrhythmic complications, patients with unstable angina that is not alleviated by maximal therapy, or patients with malignant arrhythmias associated with spontaneous episodes, should be referred directly for coronary angiography (Table 21.1). The guidelines from the American College of Cardiology and of the American Heart Association consistently indicate exercise electrocardiography as the appropriate first test

E. Picano, *Stress Echocardiography*,
© Springer-Verlag Berlin Heidelberg 2009

21

Table 21.1 Indications for the use of stress imaging rather than exercise electrocardiography[a]

Coronary angiography first	EET first	Stress imaging first (rather than exercise electrocardiography)
Complicated myocardial infarction	After uncomplicated myocardial infarction	Complete LBBB
Unstable coronary syndromes after maximal therapy	Stable chest pain syndrome	Electronically paced ventricular rhythm
Aborted sudden death, etc.	Capability to exercise	More than 1 mm ST-segment depression on resting ECG
	No contraindications to exercise testing	Unable to exercise
	Interpretable ECG	Poor left ventricular function if viability is critical

EET exercise electrocardiography, *ECG* electrocardiography, *LBBB* left bundle branch block
[a] Modified and adapted from the guidelines developed by the American College of Cardiology, the American Heart Association, the American College of Physicians, and the American Society of Internal Medicine [1–5]

[1–4] in the initial assessment of a patient with known or suspected stable coronary artery disease, who is capable of exercising and has an interpretable baseline ECG. Exercise electrocardiography is of little diagnostic value in patients with particular electrocardiographic abnormalities at rest, including left bundle branch block, electronically paced ventricular rhythm, and ST-segment depression greater than 1 mm (Table 21.1). In such patients, and in patients who are unable to exercise, and/or with poor left ventricular function if viability is critical, noninvasive testing with some forms of imaging is indicated by default [5].

21.2
Step 2: Exercise Electrocardiography Stress Test

The high feasibility, excellent safety record, ease of application, and low cost make exercise electrocardiography a first-line tool for screening patients with known or suspected coronary artery disease. The rate of acute myocardial infarction or death for this test is about 1 in 2,500 [6]. Compared to stress echocardiography and stress single photon emission computed tomography, the cost of exercise electrocardiography is at least two to five times lower, respectively. In addition, the exercise test provides information not only on the coronary reserve, but also on cardiovascular efficiency (i.e., the way in which coronary reserve can be translated into external work). Both these variables (coronary reserve and cardiovascular efficiency) concur in determining exercise tolerance and, therefore, quality of life in the individual patient [7, 8]. A negative exercise electrocardiography test result is associated with 99.3% survival at 5-year follow-up in patients with normal resting function [9]. Survival is only slightly lower in patients with previous myocardial infarction. It is hard to believe that one can improve on this extraordinarily good prognosis with any form of intervention. Therefore, in a patient capable of adequate physical effort and with

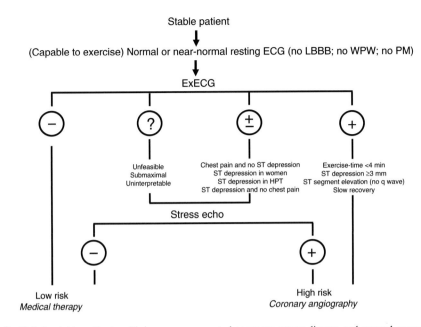

Fig. 21.1 In stable patients with known or suspected coronary artery disease and normal or near-normal resting ECG, the diagnostic algorithm should start with the exercise electrocardiography test. This remains the first noninvasive test to be done and often the last one: a maximal negative test result is associated with an extremely good prognosis; at the other end of the spectrum, a response of severe ischemia warrants coronary angiography without further investigations. In patients with ambiguous or uninterpretable results during exercise electrocardiography or patients in whom exercise is submaximal or contraindicated, stress echocardiography is an excellent choice. A normal stress echocardiogram identifies a low-risk group. A positive finding on a stress echocardiogram warrants a more aggressive therapeutic approach. HPT, hypertensives; LBBB, left bundle branch block; PM, pacemaker; WPW, Wolff-Parkinson-White

interpretable ECG, exercise electrocardiography should be the first step in the diagnostic sequence and, in case of negativity for both electrocardiographic criteria and chest pain at a maximal load, should also be the last (Fig. 21.1). The exercise electrocardiography test can also show a high-risk response (Fig. 21.1), including at least one of the following signs [10]:

1. Early positivity (with an exercise time of less than 4 min)
2. Prolonged positivity with slow recovery (>8 min)
3. Marked positivity (>3 mm of ST-segment depression or ST-segment elevation in the absence of resting Q waves)
4. Global ST-segment changes
5. Associated hypotension, which may indicate either left main or advanced triple-vessel coronary artery disease over underlying left ventricular dysfunction
6. Reproducible malignant arrhythmias

In patients with these or other markers of adverse prognosis, angiography is warranted without any further imaging testing (Fig. 21.1).

21

21.3
Step 3: Stress Imaging Testing

Exercise electrocardiography positivity at an intermediate to high load, as well as negativity at a submaximal workload, or negativity in the presence of chest pain, warrants a stress echocardiography test. The latter should establish the diagnosis of ischemia with a higher reliability and should define its extent and severity. Stress echocardiography test negativity makes the presence of a prognostically important organic coronary disease unlikely. The excellent outcome associated with this response does not support the decision to proceed with coronary angiography.

Stress echocardiography test positivity identifies a group of patients at higher risk in whom coronary angiography is warranted (Fig. 21.1). However, as discussed in Chap. 17, stress echocardiography positivity should be titrated, since the associated risk may range anywhere between 2 and 20% mortality per year, depending on the time, space, extent, severity, recovery of inducible wall motion abnormalities, and concomitant therapy at the time of testing (Table 21.2).

In the choice of an imaging technique (as detailed elsewhere; see Chaps. 1 and 36) stress echocardiography has to be preferred for logistic and economic reasons. However, nuclear perfusion imaging can still be a viable alternative in four basic situations, which can be related to the institution, the patient, or the stress used. These situations can be minimized, but not totally abolished, and therefore access to a high-quality nuclear laboratory remains an important resource for the clinical cardiologist. The situations in which nuclear perfusion imaging can be performed are the following: no stress echocardiography activity, stress echocardiography activities but semi-random results, patients with a poor acoustic window, and ambiguous stress echocardiography results, which can occur even in technically satisfactory studies (Chap. 36). In all these conditions, perfusion imaging can help considerably in patient work-up. In institutions with cardiac magnetic resonance facilities, this is the imaging test of choice as an alternative to stress echocardiography (Chap. 35).

Table 21.2 Stress echocardiography risk titration

Risk	Low (2% year)	High (20% year)
Dose/workload	High	Low
Resting EF	>50%	<40%
Antiischemic therapy	Off	On
Coronary territory	LCx/RCA	LAD
Peak WMSI	Low	High
Recovery	Fast	Slow
Positivity on baseline dyssynergy	Homozonal	Heterozonal
ESV increase at peak stress	No	Yes

EF ejection fraction, *WMSI* wall motion score index, *ESV* end-systolic volume, *LCx* left circumflex, *RCA* right coronary artery, *LAD* left anterior descending

Table 21.3 Stress echocardiography: which test for which patient

Patient characteristics	Exercise	Dipyridamole	Dobutamine
Inability to exercise	3	1	1
Contraindication to exercise	3	1	1
Positive EET at ≤6 min of exercise in hypertensives, women, baselne ECG changes	1	2	2
Asthmatic patient	2	3	1
Under theophylline therapy	1	3	1
Severe hypertension	3	1	3
Well-controlled hypertension	2	1	2
Relative hypotension	1	3	3
Malignant ventricular ectopy	1	1	3
2nd- to 3rd-degree AV block	1	3	2
Suboptimal acoustic window	3	1	2
Evaluation of antiischemic therapy efficacy	1	1	2
Unstable carotid disease	2	2	2
Permanent pacemaker	Pacemaker stress echocardiography		

1, Especially indicated; 2, relatively contraindicated; 3, contraindicated
EET exercise electrocardiography, *ECG* electrocardiography, *AV* atrioventricular

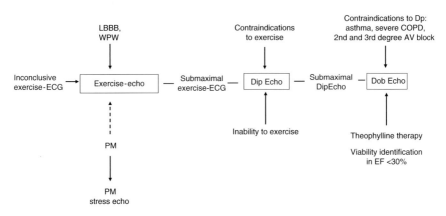

Fig. 21.2 The right type of stress echocardiography (exercise, dipyridamole, dobutamine, or pacemaker stress echocardiography) can be chosen according to several clinical, resting electrocardiography, resting echocardiography, and exercise electrocardiography test variables

It is important to choose the right stress echocardiography test for the right patient. Table 21.3 and Fig. 21.2 summarize the relative indications and contraindications to each of the major stresses according to the evidence more extensively discussed on Chap. 18.

21

Exercise echocardiography can, and should, be the first-line test, skipping the exercise electrocardiography test in patients with conditions making ECG uninterpretable, such as left bundle branch block or Wolff-Parkinson-White syndrome or baseline ST-segment abnormalities [1–4] (Fig. 21.2). Instead of pharmacological stress echocardiography, it may also be wise to choose exercise echocardiography in patients with an ambiguous positive result during an exercise electrocardiographic test at a workload of 6 min or less. This kind of patient (typically, a middle-aged hypertensive woman with ST-segment depression at a peak rate pressure product below 20,000) can have either angiographically normal or severely diseased coronary arteries. Exercise has the advantage of being the safest test and also being highly feasible and less technically demanding for low levels of exercise.

21.4
Step 4: Testing for Vasospasm

The possibility of testing for coronary vasospasm should be considered after complete negativity of maximal exercise stress testing or imaging stress at the end of the diagnostic evaluation (Fig. 15.4 in Chap. 15). Vasospasm testing is the last resort if chest pain is present and a coronary origin is sought. Before angiography, coronary vasospasm can be suspected in patients with angina at rest, particularly at night or in the early morning, and good or extremely variable effort tolerance. After angiography, the suspicion of spasm should be raised if coronary arteries are normal or mildly diseased, paradoxically in conflict with severe ischemia (Fig. 21.3). Clinically, the suspicion of vasospasm is also high

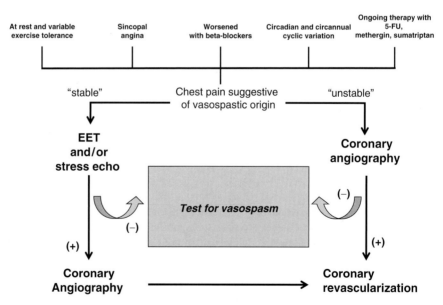

Fig. 21.3 The indication for coronary vasospasm testing in Pisa echocardiography laboratory. EET, exercise-electrocardiography testing; 5-FU, 5-fluorouracil

in patients with syncopal angina [11–14] or aborted sudden death [15, 16]. In susceptible patients, coronary vasospasm can be triggered by noncardiological medications such as the chemotherapeutic agent 5-fluorouracil in patients with cancer [17–19], sumatriptan in migraine sufferers [20, 21], or ergometrine given to young mothers in the puerperium phase [22–24] to reduce uterine blood loss through arterial vasoconstriction [23, 24], or bromocriptine, which is also given in obstetric clinics for milk suppression [25, 26]. In all these conditions, the diagnosis and treatment are easy and potentially life-saving only if one thinks of it in clinical scenarios far from the classic cardiological stage.

In properly selected patients, vasospasm testing (either with ergometrine or hyperventilation) can be performed safely and practically outside the cardiac catheterization laboratory. Testing for vasospasm is the only way to make a diagnosis that can be missed by conventional testing, imaging stress, and even coronary angiography. After all, according to Maseri [20], the single most important factor affecting the frequency with which variant angina is recognized depends on the physician's awareness of its existence.

References

1. Gibbons RJ, Balady GJ, Beasley JW, et al (1997) ACC/AHA Guidelines for exercise testing. A report of the American College of Cardiology/American Heart Association Task Force on Practice Guidelines (Committee on Exercise Testing). J Am Coll Cardiol 30:260–311
2. Ritchie JL, Bateman TM, Bonow RO, et al (1995) Guidelines for clinical use of cardiac radionuclide imaging. Report of the American College of Cardiology/American Heart Association Task Force on Assessment of Diagnostic and Therapeutic Cardiovascular Procedures (Committee on Radionuclide Imaging), developed in collaboration with the American Society of Nuclear Cardiology. J Am Coll Cardiol 25:521–547
3. Gibbons RJ, Chatterjee K, Daley J, et al (1999) ACC/AHA/ACP-ASIM guidelines for the management of patients with chronic stable angina: a report of the American College of Cardiology/American Heart Association Task Force on Practice Guidelines (Committee on Management of Patients With Chronic Stable Angina). J Am Coll Cardiol 33:2092–2197
4. Cheitlin MD, Alpert JS, Armstrong WF, et al (1997) ACC/AHA Guidelines for the clinical application of echocardiography. A report of the American College of Cardiology/American Heart Association Task Force on Practice Guidelines (Committee on Clinical Application of Echocardiography). Developed in collaboration with the American Society of Echocardiography. Circulation 95:1686–1744
5. Lee TH, Boucher CA (2001) Clinical practice. Noninvasive tests in patients with stable coronary artery disease. N Engl J Med 344:1840–1845
6. Stuart RJ Jr, Ellestad MH (1980) National survey of exercise stress testing facilities. Chest 77:94–97
7. L'Abbate A (1991) Pathophysiological basis for noninvasive functional evaluation of coronary stenosis. Circulation 83(Suppl III) 83:2–7
8. Lauer MS (2002) The "exercise" part of exercise echocardiography. J Am Coll Cardiol 39:1353–1355
9. Severi S, Picano E, Michelassi C, et al (1994) Diagnostic and prognostic value of dipyridamole echocardiography in patients with suspected coronary artery disease. Comparison with exercise electrocardiography. Circulation 89:1160–1173
10. Mark DB, Shaw L, Harrell FE Jr, et al (1991) Prognostic value of a treadmill exercise score in outpatients with suspected coronary artery disease. N Engl J Med 325:849–853

11. MacAlpin RN (1993) Cardiac arrest and sudden unexpected death in variant angina: complications of coronary spasm that can occur in the absence of severe organic coronary stenosis. Am Heart J 125:1011–1017
12. Unverdorben M, Haag M, Fuerste T, et al (1997) Vasospasm in smooth coronary arteries as a cause of asystole and syncope. Cathet Cardiovasc Diagn 41:430–434
13. Astarita C, Rumolo S, Liguori E (1999) Syncopal vasospastic angina in a patient with familial nonobstructive hypertrophic cardiomyopathy. G Ital Cardiol 29:159–162
14. Drakos SG, Anastasiou-Nana MI, Nanas JN (2002) Exacerbation of variant angina by metoprolol resulting in syncope due to transient atrioventricular block. Int J Cardiol 82:83–85
15. Lacroix D, Kacet S, Lekieffre J (1994) Vasospastic angina without flow-limiting coronary lesions as a cause for aborted sudden death. Int J Cardiol 43:247–249
16. Meisel SR, Mazur A, Chetboun I, et al (2002) Usefulness of implantable cardioverter defibrillators in refractory variant angina pectoris complicated by ventricular fibrillation in patients with angiographically normal coronary arteries. Am J Cardiol 89:1114–1116
17. Kleiman NS, Lehane DE, Geyer CE Jr, et al (1987) Prinzmetal's angina during 5-fluorouracil chemotherapy. Am J Med 82:566–568
18. Lestuzzi C, Viel E, Picano E, et al (2001) Coronary vasospasm as a cause of effort-related myocardial ischemia during low-dose chronic continuous infusion of 5-fluorouracil. Am J Med 111:316–318
19. Maseri A, Lanza G (2001) Fluorouracil-induced coronary artery spasm. Am J Med 111:326–327
20. Castle WM, Simmons VE (1992) Coronary vasospasm and sumatriptan. BMJ 305:117–118
21. Mueller L, Gallagher RM, Ciervo CA (1996) Vasospasm-induced myocardial infarction with sumatriptan. Headache 36:329–331
22. Nall KS, Feldman B (1998) Postpartum myocardial infarction induced by Methergine. Am J Emerg Med 16:502–504
23. Yaegashi N, Miura M, Okamura K (1999) Acute myocardial infarction associated with postpartum ergot alkaloid administration. Int J Gynaecol Obstet 64:67–68
24. Ribbing M, Reinecke H, Breithardt G, et al (2001) Acute anterior wall infarct in a 31-year-old patient after administration of methylergometrine for peripartal vaginal hemorrhage. Herz 26:489–493
25. Larrazet F, Spaulding C, Lobreau HJ, et al (1993) Possible bromocriptine-induced myocardial infarction. Ann Intern Med 118:199–200
26. Hopp L, Weisse AB, Iffy L (1996) Acute myocardial infarction in a healthy mother using bromocriptine for milk suppression. Can J Cardiol 12:415–418

Prognosis

22

Eugenio Picano

According to Maseri, "Identification of patients with known ischemic heart disease who are at low risk is important, first, because it is reassuring for the patient; second, because in such a group the prognostic accuracy of any diagnostic test becomes very low; third, because it is difficult to demonstrate that even the most aggressive treatments can increase life expectancy when the latter is not reduced appreciably" [1]

Echocardiography is most useful for the identification of these patients. In fact resting left ventricular function, myocardial viability and stress-induced ischemia showed their prognostic impact in the preechocardiographic era, when evaluated by different tools, i.e., radioisotopic techniques for ventricular function [2], fluorodeoxyglucose uptake for viability [3], and exercise electrocardiography [4] and myocardial scintigraphy [5] for inducible ischemia. Only echocardiography allowed all these pieces of information – previously scattered among several diagnostic techniques – to be put together in a synoptic way.

22.1
Left Ventricular Function

The risk increases hyperbolically with the reduction in ventricular function [2], with relatively moderate increments of mortality for values of ejection fraction between 50 and 30% and with marked increments below 30% [6] (Fig. 22.1). In the steep segment of the curve, a reduction of 10% of ejection fraction (from 30 to 20%) results in an 8–16% increase in mortality at 6 months; in the flat part of the curve, the same reduction in ejection fraction (from 60 to 50%) leads to an undetectable, nonsignificant increase in mortality, from 1 to 1.5%.

The asynergic regions might be viable and therefore may potentially recover to normal function. The more dysfunctional myocardium there is, the more important the search for viability will be (see Chap. 20).

E. Picano, *Stress Echocardiography*,
© Springer-Verlag Berlin Heidelberg 2009

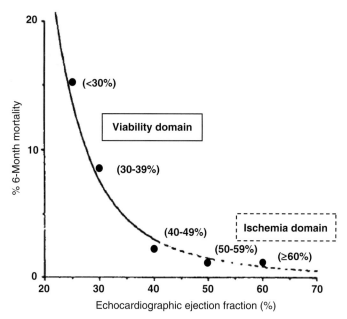

Fig. 22.1 Hyperbolic curve relating 6-month mortality and values of ejection fraction in patients recovering from an acute myocardial infarction. Beyond 40%, even large increases in ejection fraction determine only a mild increase in mortality; this is the "flat" arm of the curve, where the impact of viability is probably minimal. Below 40%, even small changes in ejection fraction determine marked changes in mortality; this is the "steep" arm of the curve, where the impact of viability is probably critical to survival. (Redrawn and modified from [6], with permission)

22.2
Myocardial Viability

In patients with good ventricles (dashed line in Fig. 22.1), viability is basically neutral for survival, and cardiac death can be predicted only on the basis of the extent and severity of induced ischemia [7]. However, myocardial viability detected with low-dose dobutamine tends to be associated with unstable angina and nonfatal reinfarction (Fig. 22.2). In patients with severe chronic left ventricular dysfunction (solid line in Fig. 22.1), the presence of myocardial viability is associated with a better survival rate in revascularized patients [8–13] (Fig. 22.3) (see also Fig. 22.4 of Chap. 11 and Fig. 22.7 of Chap. 12). These data may be considered consistent with the finding of the Coronary Artery Surgery Study, which 20 years ago – well before myocardial viability entered the clinical scene – showed improved survival after bypass grafting (vs patients randomized to medical therapy) in the subgroup of patients with three-vessel disease and low ejection fraction [14]. A likely explanation is that a proportion of patients had hibernating myocardium with preserved viability and functional recovery after surgery. Also, in patients with severe left ventricular dysfunction evaluated early after an acute myocardial infarction, myocardial viability is associated with better survival both in revascularized and in medically treated patients [15, 16].

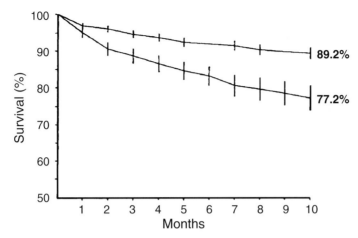

Fig. 22.2 Cumulative survival rates free of spontaneously occurring events (including death, reinfarction, and unstable angina) in patients with absence (*top curve*) and presence (*bottom curve*) of myocardial viability, recognized as functional improvement in a segment with rest wall motion abnormalities after low-dose dobutamine. The presence of myocardial viability is associated with a greater incidence of events ($p < 0.05$). (From [7], with permission)

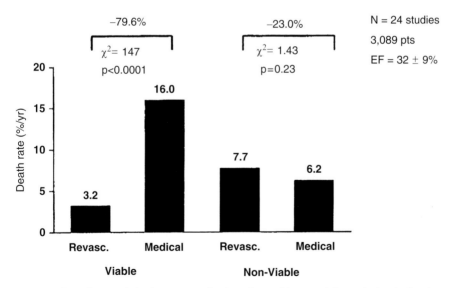

Fig. 22.3 Effect of revascularization on mortality in patients with severe left ventricular dysfunction with (*viable, left side*) and without (*nonviable, right side*) myocardial viability, assessed with one of the three main techniques: low-dose dobutamine, thallium or PET FDG scintigraphy. (From [13], with permission)

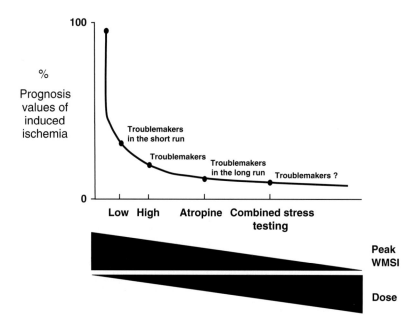

Fig. 22.4 Prognostic impact of inducible ischemia rises hyperbolically with increasing values of peak wall motion score index (*WMSI*) and decreasing doses necessary to evoke ischemia. The higher the wall motion score index, the lower the ischemic dose and the worse of prognosis

22.3
Inducible Ischemia

Tests provoking ischemia, such as exercise electrocardiography and stress scintigraphy, yield more accurate prognostic information when the result is stratified in the space and/ or time domain. The ischemic workload, i.e., the stress time necessary to induce a diagnostic modification, is the most useful prognostic information during exercise electrocardiography [4]. The severity and extension of the perfusion defect is the most important information with stress scintigraphy [5]. Stress echocardiography provides information in the time (ischemic load) and space domain (extension and severity of asynergy) [17]. The timing, extent and severity of the induced wall motion abnormality are the main determinants of the prognostic impact of stress echocardiography positivity (see also Table 22.1 of Chap. 18). As for rest function, the presence of inducible ischemia increases the risk hyperbolically with the progression of severity (Fig. 22.4). The shorter the ischemia-free stress time and the higher the wall motion score index are, the lower is the survival rate (Fig. 22.4). The prognostic effects of inducible ischemia are additive to resting left ventricular function (Fig. 22.5). However, prognosis is not destiny, and the natural history may be dramatically changed by revascularization interventions guided by the results of physiological testing. Indeed, in patients with positive stress echocardiography, ischemia-guided

Table 22.1 Single-center versus large-scale design in prognostic studies

Design	Small	Large scale
Enrollment sites	Single center	Multicenter
Patient sample size	Tens (hundreds)	Thousands
Main events considered	Revascularization	Cardiac death
Recruiting centers	Tertiary care	Primary care
Echocardiography reading	Centralized	Peripheral (quality controlled)
Domain of application	Virtual reality	True life

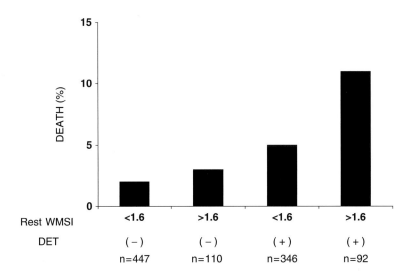

Fig. 22.5 Combined effect of resting function and inducible ischemia (with stress echocardiography) on the incidence of mortality in early postinfarction (10 days after acute myocardial infarction). Follow-up, 14.6 ± 10.2 months. *WMSI*, wall motion score index; *DET*, dipyridamole echocardiography test. EPIC update (*n* = 995). (EPIC data, adapted from [8], with permission)

revascularization reduces the risk of death by a factor of 11, while, paradoxically, the risk is three times higher in patients with negative tests and anatomy-guided revascularization [18–21] (Fig. 22.6). For pharmacological stress echocardiography, effectiveness studies (Table 22.1) have also been performed with large scale, multicenter, prospective, observational design. The Echo Persantine International Cooperative (EPIC) and Echo Dobutamine International Cooperative (EDIC) trials recruited thousands of patients, enrolled mostly by primary care cardiology centers employing stress echocardiography in their daily work for diagnostic, not academic purposes. As this large and simple clinical trial study design is produced and interpreted by cardiologists working in primary care centers, most likely dealing with real patients, real doctors, and real problems, it is more likely to provide data directly relevant to clinical practice [22].

22

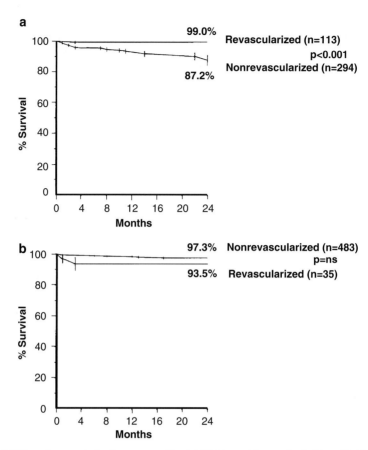

Fig. 22.6 Effect of revascularization on mortality. (**a**) Highly positive results (with an 11-fold reduction in mortality) in patients with ischemia during stress echocardiography. (**b**) Counterproductive (with threefold increase in mortality) in patients undergoing revascularization in spite of a negative stress echocardiography test. (EPIC data from [14], with permission)

22.4
Pathophysiological Heterogeneity of Different Events

In the assessment of risk stratification, disparate events such as coronary revascularization, recurrence of angina, nonfatal reinfarctions, and cardiac death are often pooled together for statistical reasons. Nevertheless, they have very heterogeneous pathophysiological mechanisms and a different clinical impact. Studies on large populations, with an adequate number of events, have pointed out that the broad definition of the term "predictor of risk" relates to widely different kinds of risk. Early after myocardial infarction, myocardial viability identifies patients at higher risk for subsequent unstable angina [7], but at lower risk of cardiac death [15, 16], since the negative impact on events related to residual ischemic instability is offset by the beneficial impact on functional recovery. Resting function is an excellent predictor of cardiac death, but it does not predict recurrence of angina, which is less frequent in conditions of more extensive dysfunction. On the other hand, inducible ischemia effectively predicts recurrence of angina (with a relative risk of 3:1) and cardiac death (with a relative risk of 4:1), but it only weakly predicts nonfatal reinfarction marginally (relative risk 2:1) [23]. These data might appear contradictory in the light of the classical theory of the progressive worsening of ischemic plaque as a cause of angina, moving from angina at rest to myocardial infarction with total occlusion. In fact, from a pathophysiological standpoint, angina and reinfarction are qualitatively different events. As for reinfarction, the occlusion of a critical, ischemia-producing plaque is asymptomatic in 50% of patients; it is often an angiographic, not a clinical event (Fig. 22.7). The occlusion of a critical coronary stenosis is the mechanism underlying 15% of infarctions; in this subgroup, the predictive power of the test might be very high, but it is diluted by the remaining 85% of reinfarctions, which occur at previously noncritical stenoses (i.e., transparent to stress echocardiography). In agreement with pathophysiological premises, the event reinfarction (which in 80% occurs independently of stenosis significance) is predicted by stress echocardiography, with a relative risk of 2.0. The ratio of fatal to nonfatal reinfarction is higher in the presence of a positive stress. Induced ischemia (imaged as the area at risk showing transient dyssynergy by stress echocardiography) inconsistently identifies the site of future infarction, although most infarctions occurring within 1 year of stress testing are in the area identified as ischemic during stress testing. When the prediction of site of infarction is the reference, stress echocardiography results are wrong in four out of ten cases (infarction occurring in a patient with a previously negative test), right in four cases (infarction occurring in the area identified as ischemic during previous stress), and right for the wrong reason in the remaining two cases (infarcted zone different from the ischemic zone identified as at risk during stress) [24]. These discrepancies cannot be considered surprising if one considers that plaque rupture, inflammation, and embolization are largely independent of plaque size, which limits coronary flow reserve and determines stress echocardiographic results. Vulnerable plaques are often angiographically invisible, and a significant number of disruption episodes that precipitate infarction occur in coronary arteries that were normal or mildly stenotic on a previous angiogram [25]. The recognition of these vulnerable, but hemodynamically subcritical plaques is out of reach even for third-generation (atropine) stress echocardiographic testing [24].

22.5
Practical Implications

Clinical evaluation will readily identify patients at high-risk: patients with complicated acute myocardial infarction (with arrhythmic, mechanical, or ischemic complications); patients with unstable angina refractory to maximal medical therapy; and patients with ischemic modification during angina suggestive of extensive multivessel coronary disease. In these patients, a good cardiologist needs little help. For most patients, on the other hand, even the best clinician will need instrumental support for an adequate risk stratification

---

22

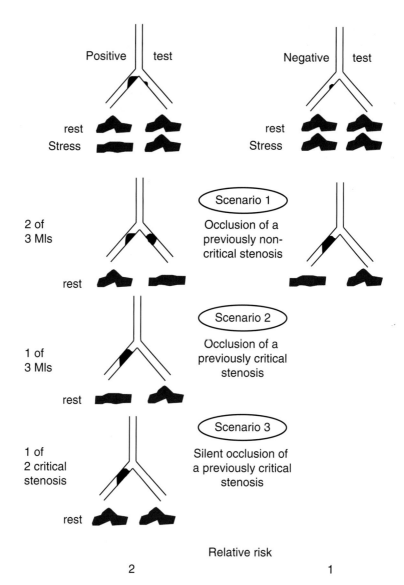

Fig. 22.7 Possible mechanisms of reinfarction. According to this theoretical model, the stress echocardiography positivity of the index test is associated with more extensive coronary artery disease, with critical stenosis in the coronary artery feeding the myocardial region with stress induced dyssynergy (*left upper panel*); coronary artery disease is more often noncritical in patients with test negativity (*right upper panel*). In keeping with angiographic data, two out of three infarctions are linked to the occlusion of a previously noncritical stenosis incapable of provoking ischemia during stress; in the patient with a positive test (scenario 1, *left panel*), a coronary stenosis different from the ischemia-producing stenosis can become occluded, with the infarction paradoxically occurring in a region different from the area at risk identified during stress. Also, in the patient with a negative stress echocardiography test, the coronary occlusion will provoke the infarction in an area with no inducible ischemia during stress (scenario 1, *right panel*). The second possibility (occurring in one-third of infarctions)

(Fig. 22.8). Resting echocardiography helps to identify patients with severe baseline dysfunction who are at high risk and in whom the search for myocardial viability becomes critical. Exercise electrocardiography is the next stress test. It is less sensitive and feasible than stress echocardiography, but the negative predictive value of a maximal test is high and the combination of a maximal exercise electrocardiographic test with a good echocardiographic function identifies a large group of patients at low risk, with an annual death rate of 1–2% [25]. It is very difficult for an imaging test to add further information to this subset [26–28]. Markedly positive exercise electrocardiography test results (see Fig. 22.3

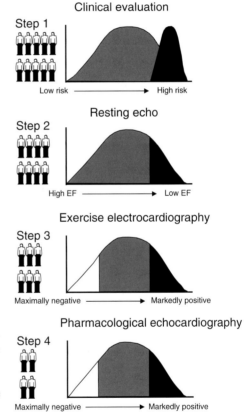

Fig. 22.8 The four-step prognostic algorithm, starting from clinical evaluation (*step 1*) and moving to resting echocardiography (*step 2*), exercise electrocardiography (*step 3*), and, when necessary, pharmacological stress echocardiography (*step 4*). *Black*, high risk; *gray shading*, intermediate risk; *white*, low risk; *EF*, ejection fraction

Fig. 22.7 (continued) is the occlusion of a coronary artery with a previously critical stenosis capable of provoking ischemia during stress; this clinical and pathological pattern occurs more frequently in patients with a previously positive stress (scenario 2, *left panel*). Another possible outcome of the critical ischemia-producing coronary stenosis is occlusion without clinical signs of myocardial infarction or regional dysfunction (scenario 3, *left panel*); the myocardium region fed by the occluded coronary keeps contracting normally

in Chap. 20) identify a group at high risk in which an imaging test might be redundant and hazardous. This subset of patients must be treated aggressively. In the rest of the patients with moderate- to high-workload positivity or equivocal or submaximal results the combined information provided by rest and pharmacological stress echocardiography results in an integrated view of the most important prognostic determinants (resting function and ischemia) that identify different subsets of patients, with an annual death risk ranging from about 1% (good resting function, no inducible ischemia) up to 20% (severe rest dysfunction, low dose, extensive inducible ischemia). A high-risk response points to the need for more invasive procedures. In the early postinfarction phase, revascularization increases the risk of death if undertaken in patients without inducible ischemia on the basis of an anatomical indication, whereas it markedly reduces this risk in patients with inducible ischemia. In patients with poor prognosis, a coronary angiography is warranted in view of a revascularization. As a rule, the steeper the decline of annual survival in the medically treated control group, the greater the benefits of revascularization [1].

22.5.1
Comparison of Invasive and Noninvasive Approaches

In the field of prognostic stratification, in the absence of carefully controlled studies, any strategy currently reflects a philosophy rather than a scientifically based method [27]. The invasive philosophy considers coronary angiography as the only essential tool; the noninvasive strategy uses a noninvasive test to indicate access to catheterization in clinically stable patients. In the invasive approach, stress echocardiography is considered as a possible candidate to break open the vicious circle of chest pain: coronary angiography revascularization; in the noninvasive approach, it is considered capable of offering insight into the main determinants of survival, i.e., function, viability, and ischemia. The noninvasive strategy can be preferred by necessity when there is restricted access to cardiac catheterization facilities, but it remains a questionable choice in the presence of unrestricted access to coronary angiography. When there is access to the invasive procedure, the question arises as to whether all patients should be catheterized and all stenoses revascularized ("angiography in all, and dilate what you can") or whether a simple stress test procedure is preferable, avoiding the further risks and discomfort of any additional procedure ("a noninvasive stress test, and back home safely") [29–31]. Risk stratification can be carried out aggressively (and expensively) or in a low-profile, less expensive manner with noninvasive testing first and medical therapy in all patients with negative stress. Only then can the noninvasive stratification strategy centered on stress echocardiography be accepted as a way of saving resources, and above all of providing patients with better treatment. Observational studies have suggested that the noninvasive method not only saves money, but may actually result in a longer survival time [18, 28]. Randomized trials show a worse outcome in patients with anatomy-guided revascularization when compared to those with ischemia guided revascularization [32–35]. For any given level of coronary anatomical angiographic disease, the impact of revascularization on survival is impressive, especially when inducible ischemia is present (see also Chap. 39). In the absence of inducible ischemia, anatomy-guided revascularization has neutral or detrimental effect on survival [36], although this may change in the era of drug-eluting stents. Nevertheless, only 9% of patients with recent myocardial infarction undergo stress testing before coronary intervention [29], but more than 40% of patients undergo angioplasty after receiving thrombolytic therapy [30]. In spite of accumulating evidence and recommendations of guidelines, the risk stratification strategy is often the result of a costly philosophical opinion rather than an evidence-based behavior.

References

1. Maseri A (1995) Determinants of prognosis: primary and secondary prevention. In: Maseri A (ed) Ischemic heart disease. Churchill Livingstone, London, pp 226–312
2. The Multicenter Postinfarction Research Group (1983) Risk stratification and survival after myocardial infarction. N Engl J Med 309:331–336
3. Di Carli MF, Davidson M, Little R, et al (1994) Value of metabolic imaging with positron emissiontomography for evaluating prognosis in patients with coronary artery disease and left ventricular dysfunction. Am J Cardiol 73:527–533
4. Gohlke H, Samek L, Betz P, et al (1983) Exercise testing provides additional prognostic information in angiographically defined subgroups of patients with coronary artery disease. Circulation 68:979–985
5. Ladenheim ML, Pollock BH, Rozanski A, et al (1986) Extent and severity of myocardial hypoperfusion as predictors of prognosis in patients with suspected coronary artery disease. J Am Coll Cardiol 7:464–471
6. Volpi A, De Vita C, Franzosi MG, et al (1993) Determinants of 6-month mortality in survivors of myocardial infarction after thrombolysis. Results of the GISSI-2 data base. The Ad hoc Working Group of the Gruppo Italiano per lo Studio della Sopravvivenza nell'Infarto Miocardico (GISSI)-2 Data Base. Circulation 88:416–429
7. Sicari R, Picano E, Landi P, et al (1997) Prognostic value of dobutamine-atropine stress echocardiography early after acute myocardial infarction. Echo Dobutamine International Cooperative (EDIC) Study. J Am Coll Cardiol 29:254–260
8. Meluzin J, Cerny J, Frelich M, et al (1998) Prognostic value of the amount of dysfunctional but viable myocardium in revascularized patients with coronary artery disease and left ventricular dysfunction. Investigators of this Multicenter Study. J Am Coll Cardiol 32:912–920
9. Senior R, Kaul S, Lahiri A (1999) Myocardial viability on echocardiography predicts long-term survival after revascularization in patients with ischemic congestive heart failure. J Am Coll Cardiol 33:1848–1854
10. Pasquet A, Robert A, D'Hondt AM, et al (1999) Prognostic value of myocardial ischemia and viability in patients with chronic left ventricular ischemic dysfunction. Circulation 100:141–148
11. Sicari R, Ripoli A, Picano E, et al, VIDA (Viability Identification with Dipyridamole Administration) Study Group (2001) The prognostic value of myocardial viability recognized by low dose dipyridamole echocardiography in patients with chronic ischaemic left ventricular dysfunction. Eur Heart J 22:837–842
12. Sicari R, Borges AC, Palagi C, et al (2002) The prognostic value of myocardial viability recognized by low dose dobutamine echocardiography in revascularized patients with chronic ischemic left ventricular dysfunction (abstract). Circulation 92:1263–1266
13. Allman KC, Shaw LJ, Hachamovitch R, et al (2002) Myocardial viability testing and impact of revascularization on prognosis in patients with coronary artery disease and left ventricular dysfunction: a meta-analysis. J Am Coll Cardiol 39:1151–1158

14. Alderman EL, Fisher LD, Litwin P, et al (1983) Results of coronary artery surgery in patients with poor left ventricular function (CASS). Circulation 68:785–795

15. Carlos ME, Smart SC, Wynsen JC, et al (1997) Dobutamine stress echocardiography for risk stratification after myocardial infarction. Circulation 95:1402–1410

16. Picano E, Sicari R, Landi P, et al (1998) Prognostic value of myocardial viability in medically treated patients with global left ventricular dysfunction early after an acute uncomplicated myocardial infarction: a dobutamine stress echocardiographic study. Circulation 98:1078–1084

17. Picano E, Severi S, Michelassi C, et al (1989) Prognostic importance of dipyridamole echocardiography test in coronary artery disease. Circulation 80:450–457

18. Picano E, Landi P, Bolognese L, et al (1993) Prognostic value of dipyridamole echocardiography early after uncomplicated myocardial infarction: a large-scale, multicenter trial. The EPIC Study Group. Am J Med 95:608–618

19. Severi S, Picano E, Michelassi C, et al (1994) Diagnostic and prognostic value of dipyridamole echocardiography in patients with suspected coronary artery disease. Comparison with exercise electrocardiography. Circulation 89:1160–1173

20. Sicari R, Pasanisi E, Venneri L, et al on behalf of the Echo-Persantine International Cooperative (EPIC) and Echo-Dobutamine International Cooperative (EDIC) Study Groups (2003) Stress echo results predict mortality: a large scale multicenter prospective international study. J Am Coll Cardiol 41:589–595

21. Cortigiani L, Dodi C, Paolini EA, et al (1998) Prognostic value of pharmacological stress echocardiography in women with chest pain and unknown coronary artery disease. J Am Coll Cardiol 32:1975–1981

22. Picano E, Ostojic M, Sicari R, et al (1997) Dipyridamole stress echocardiography: state of the art 1996. EPIC (Echo Persantine International Cooperative) Study Group. Eur Heart J 18(Suppl D):D16–D23

23. Picano E, Pingitore A, Sicari R, et al (1995) Stress echocardiographic results predict risk of reinfarction early after uncomplicated acute myocardial infarction: large-scale multicenter study. Echo Persantine International Cooperative (EPIC) Study Group. J Am Coll Cardiol 26:908–913

24. Varga A, Picano E, Cortigiani L, et al (1996) Does stress echocardiography predict the site of future myocardial infarction? A large-scale multicenter study. EPIC (Echo Persantine International Cooperative) and EDIC (Echo Dobutamine International Cooperative) Study Groups. J Am Coll Cardiol 28:45–51

25. Vilella A, Maggioni A, Vilella M et al (1995) Prognostic significance of maximal exercise testing after myocardial infarction treated with thrombolytic agents: the GISSI-2 data base. Lancet 346:523–529

26. Greco CA, Salustri A, Beccareccia F et al (1997) Prognostic value of dobutamine echocardiography early after uncomplicated acute myocardial infarction: a comparison with exercise electrocardiography. J Am Coll Cardiol 29:261–267

27. Desideri A, Bigi R, Suzzi GL et al (1999) Stress echocardiography and exercise electrocardiography for risk stratification after non-Q-wave uncomplicated myocardial infarction. Am J Cardiol 84:739–741

28. Sicari R, Landi P, Picano E, et al (2002) Exercise-electrocardiography and/or pharmacological stress echocardiography for non-invasive risk stratification early after uncomplicated myocardial infarction. A prospective international large scale multicentre study. Eur Heart J 23:1030–1037

29. Butman SM (1991) What would I want to know if my dad had a heart attack? Good sense versus dollars and cents. J Am Coll Cardiol 18:1220–1222

30. Topol EJ, Ellis SG, Cosgrove DM, et al (1993) Analysis of coronary angioplasty practice in the United States with an insurance-claims data base. Circulation 87:1489–1497

31. Rogers WS, Boulby LJ, Chandra NC, et al (1994) Treatment of myocardial infarction in the United States (1990 to 1993): observations from the National Registry of Myocardial Infarction. Circulation 90:2103–2114

32. Ellis SG, Mooney MR, George BS, et al (1992) Randomized trial of late elective angioplasty versus conservative management for patients with residual stenoses after thrombolytic treatment of myocardial infarction. Stenoses (TOPS) Study Group. Circulation 86:1400–1406

33. Madsen JK, Grande P, Saunamaki K et al (1997) Danish multicenter randomized study of invasive versus conservative treatment in patients with inducible ischemia after thrombolysis in acute myocardial infarction (DANAMI). DANish trial in Acute Myocardial Infarction. Circulation 96:748–755

34. Boden WE, O'Rourke RA, Crawford MH et al (1998) Outcomes in patients with acute non-Q wave myocardial infarction randomly assigned to an invasive as compared with a conservative management strategy. Veterans Affairs Non-Q-Wave Infarction Strategies in Hospital (VANQWISH) Trial Investigators. N Engl J Med 338:1785–1792

35. Barnett PG, Chen S, Boden WE et al (2002) Cost-effectiveness of a conservative, ischemia guided management strategy after non-Q-wave myocardial infarction: results of a randomized trial. Circulation 105:680–684

36. Smith SC Jr, Dove JT, Jacobs AK, et al, American College of Cardiology, American Heart Association Task Force on Practice Guidelines. Committee to Revise the 1993 Guidelines for Percutaneous Transluminal Coronary Angioplasty (2001) ACC/AHA guidelines of percutaneous coronary interventions (revision of the 1993 PTCA guidelines). J Am Coll Cardiol 37:2215–2239

Section 3

New Technologies and New Diagnostic Targets

New Ultrasound Technologies for Quantitative Assessment of Left Ventricular Function

23

Thomas H. Marwick, Adrian C. Borges, and Eugenio Picano

Stress echocardiography is an established and mainstream method for the diagnosis and risk stratification of patients with known or suspected coronary artery disease [1, 2]. While the overall accuracy of echocardiography-based stress echocardiography techniques is high, these methods are inherently limited by the subjective, eyeballing nature of image interpretation [3] and the learning curve [4] with relatively wide interinstitutional variability [5], unless conservative reading criteria are developed a priori through consensus [6]. In addition, the current diagnosis is based on visual assessment of systolic thickening and endocardial motion, estimating radial function, which is theoretically less sensitive to ischemia than the longitudinal and circumferential function [7]. Electrical activation disturbances (such as left bundle branch block or right ventricular pacing), hemodynamic conditions (such as right ventricular overload), or extracardiac factors (such as cardiac surgery or constrictive physiology) may affect wall motion independently of systolic thickening, making the analysis based on systolic thickening alone technically challenging [8]. Tachycardia and an increase in blood pressure may mimic ischemia, inducing a reduction of regional wall motion and thickening [9] and ventricular unloading, caused, for instance, by mitral insufficiency, which may mask ischemic wall motion abnormalities [10]. On a segmental basis, we evaluate the transmural contraction, without a selective assessment of the subendocardial function, more sensitive to ischemia than the subepicardial layer [8]. Furthermore, the current application of stress echocardiography is certainly "intelligent" (full of useful clinical information), but the results cannot be easily reduced to a "beautiful" graphical display, perceivable at a glance also by a nonspecialist of imaging. The development of an objective, quantitative method for wall motion analysis during stress testing would overcome these limitations, translating the inducible wall motion abnormality from an opinion into a number (Table 23.1). This would improve accuracy, shorten the learning curve, and improve communication of stress echocardiography results with cardiologists, ultimately strengthening the current clinical and scientific role of the technique. In addition, the quantitative assessment of left ventricular function would allow a more comprehensive

E. Picano, *Stress Echocardiography*,
© Springer-Verlag Berlin Heidelberg 2009

Table 23.1 Present reality and future promises in stress echocardiography

	What we have	What we need
Regional function	Thickening, motion	Strain
Ventricular function	Radial	Longitudinal and circumferential
Segmental function	Transmural	Subendocardial
Graphical display	"Intelligent"	"Beautiful"
Operator-dependence	High	Low
Learning curve	Long	Steep
Diagnostic gold standard	Expert opinion	Automatic number

assessment of the complex physiology of left ventricular function, which is not thoroughly described with a simple assessment of radial transmural function through endocardial motion and thickening at a single end-diastolic and end-systolic time point during the cardiac cycle. Strenuous efforts have been made in the last 30 years by bioengineers, industry, and researchers to reach the ambitious, yet elusive, target of quantitative assessment of ventricular function. Different waves of new ultrasound technologies such as M-mode for longitudinal function assessment with mitral annular plane systolic excursion (MAPSE), anatomical M-mode, tissue characterization, color kinesis (CK), tissue Doppler echocardiography (TDE), tissue Doppler strain-rate imaging (TDSRI), two-dimensional speckle tracking imaging (2D-ST), and real-time three-dimensional echocardiography (RT3D) have been proposed to overcome the limitations of conventional echocardiography [11]. Each approach can be broadly assigned to one of the four technological generations of ultrasound imaging: M-mode, 2D, tissue Doppler, and 3D (Table 23.2). Many quantitative echocardiographic techniques for regional and global contractility assessment have had promising starts, but none of them has been incorporated to date into standard praxis.

23.1
Spatial and Temporal Heterogeneity of Left Ventricular Contraction

The contraction of the heart is a complex phenomenon involving a deformation (strain) along three coordinates: radial thickening (centripetal squeeze), longitudinal (base-to-apex shortening), and circumferential shortening (torsional twist) (Fig. 23.1). Strain is a unitless quantity, and typical values of end-systolic radial, longitudinal, and circumferential deformation for normal volunteers are approximately 0.35, −0.15, and −0.20, respectively, in the midventricle, with good agreement between cardiovascular magnetic resonance (CMR) tissue tracking and quantitative echocardiographic techniques [11]. The complexity of this movement is further magnified by the physiological spatial and temporal heterogeneity observed in humans among different left ventricular segments both in resting conditions [12–14] and during stress [15, 16]. The radial strain is highest in apical and lowest in basal segments. Longitudinal strain shows the largest excursion in proximal and the mildest in apical segments. The left ventricular rotation (or circumferential strain) as viewed from the

Table 23.2 The four main approaches to quantification

	M-mode	2D	Doppler	RT3D
Biosignal	Mitral annulus	Gray-scale *B*-mode	Tissue Doppler	Segmental volume
Variable	Annulus motion	Endocardial motion	Myocardial velocity	Regional EF
Main function	Longitudinal	Radial (circumferential)	Longitudinal	Composite
Angle dependence	No	No	Yes	No
Eyeballing feedback	+++	+++	–	+++
Graphical display	Sober	Elegant	Complex	Intuitive
All segments	±	++	–	+++
First generation	MAPSE	Color kinesis	TDI	Offline 3D
Second generation	Anatomical *M*-mode	Speckle tracking	SRI	RT3D
Imaging/Analysis time	Seconds	A few minutes	Several minutes	A few minutes

RT3D real-time three-dimensional echocardiography, *MAPSE* mitral annular plane systolic excursion, *TDE* tissue Doppler echocardiography, *SRI* strain-rate imaging

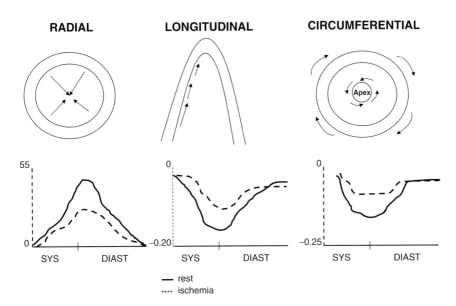

Fig. 23.1 A schematic representation of the three coordinates of left ventricular contraction: radial, longitudinal, circumferential (*upper panels*). Note the physiological heterogeneity of left ventricular contraction (expressed by the *length of arrows*). Radial thickening is higher in anterior and septal than in inferior and lateral segments. Longitudinal shortening is highest in basal and lowest in apical segments. Circumferential shortening is highest (*clockwise*) in basal, counterclockwise in apical segments (*right panel*). All three can be altered in stress-induced ischemia (*lower panels*), which provokes both a reduction and a delay (dyssynchrony) of contraction in involved segments

apex is clockwise in basal segments, and counter-clockwise in apical segments, creating the torsion or twisting motion. Toward the end of systole, a negative torsion velocity or untwisting begins, possibly as a result of the release of elastic energy accumulated in systole [11]. Systolic rotation, as a component of torsion, winds the heart muscle like a spring, setting up recoil for early diastole. Within each segment, there is also a clear vertical (transmural) gradient, with the subendocardial layers contributing to the majority of systolic thickening (radial function) [17], longitudinal shortening [18], and segmental twisting [19].

The complex 3D deformation of the heart during the cardiac cycle may not be adequately captured by investigating only radial, transmural function with regional wall thickening and motion. The presence of stress-induced ischemia reduces, up to abolishing, all three components of deformation – radial [20], longitudinal [21], and circumferential [22] – (Fig. 23.1, lower panel), but not all of them simultaneously and symmetrically. Experimentally, a reduction in overall systolic thickening (which is an index of radial function) is not the most sensitive mechanical manifestation of local ischemia: subendocardial fibers that support ventricular long-axis function are more sensitive to ischemia than the circumferential ones responsible for normal radial myocardial thickening (Fig. 23.2, right panel) [23]. This is also true in chronic heart failure, characterized by an initial phase when the longitudinal function can be reduced and the radial function supernormal, for compensatory function, yielding a normal ejection fraction, which averages longitudinal and radial function [24, 25], and is correlated only weakly with percent systolic thickening and more closely with circumferential strain [26]. This same concept may apply, in the single segment, to systolic thickening and motion, which can be normal at an initial stage when the subendocardial function is already markedly impaired (Fig. 23.3, right panel).

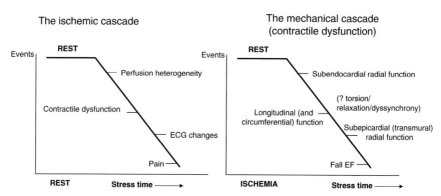

Fig. 23.2 On the *left*, the ischemic cascade, with a well-defined sequence of events, where perfusion heterogeneity is an earlier marker than regional contractile dysfunction, classically evaluated on the basis of segmental wall thickening. On the *right*, the mechanical cascade shown in its increasingly recognized complexity and heterogeneity. Segmental function indices (displayed on the *right* side of the cascade) tend to appear earlier than global function indices, with subendocardial dysfunction being earlier and more profound than subepicardial dysfunction. Among global indices, longitudinal (and probably circumferential) indices occur before radial indices. Ejection fraction reduction can appear only downstream in the cascade, since at initial stages the early depression of longitudinal function can be masked by normal, compensatory supernormal radial function

Longitudinal

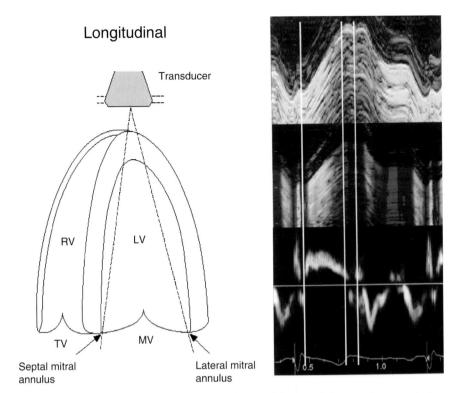

Fig. 23.3 The downward motion of the base of the ventricle toward the transducer can be imaged with mitral annular plane systolic excursion (*left*). On the *right*, the synchronous assessment of longitudinal function by *M*-mode (*upper panel*), tissue Doppler (*middle panel*), and strain-rate imaging (*lower panel*). (Adapted and modified from [7, 14])

In clinical echocardiography, we usually rely on ejection fraction (an index of global function) and percent systolic thickening (an index of regional function). Regional ejection fraction can be viewed as a composite measure of the local contribution to ejection, determined by the increased motion and deformation (circumferentially and longitudinally) of the endocardium. The regional ejection fraction increases significantly from base to apex, and remarkably, in normal hearts the regions with the highest ejection fraction show the least wall thickening [26]. On simple pathophysiological ground, we might achieve better diagnostic sensitivity for more subtle, initial myocardial disease if we also assess longitudinal function, for the global assessment, and subendocardial function, for regional segmental assessment. In the ischemic or cardiomyopathy cascade, left ventricular dysfunction might be sampled upstream of the classical, conventional markers of global and regional dysfunction used in standard conventional echocardiography [24]. The different technologies proposed for quantitative assessment of left ventricular function focus on different aspects of this functional heterogeneity (Table 23.2).

23

23.2
M-mode Echocardiography and Longitudinal Function

The assessment of longitudinal function can be obtained not only with last-generation technology, but also – and probably with even greater reproducibility – by simple *M*-mode echocardiography, measuring the mitral annulus systolic amplitude excursion (Table 23.2). Mitral ring echoes are of high amplitude and can be recorded in the large majority of patients [25]. The technical basis, *M*-mode echocardiography, is simple and widely available. The printed records can be measured directly, thus avoiding the requirement for consensus and establishing clear unities (Fig. 23.3). Values greater than 25 mm are normal, and below 20 mm are clearly abnormal. Use of different sites around the atrioventricular ring may allow the effect of induced ischemia to be localized, although not to the same extent as with the standard method. The technique detects the physiological heterogeneity of longitudinal function of the normal heart [14], the ischemia-induced alterations in longitudinal function during stress [27, 28], and the early changes in left ventricular function during cardiomyopathy [23, 24], with an accuracy similar to more trendy techniques such as TD or TDSE. No colors, no 3D reconstruction, no fancy tracings and numbers support the interpretation. As a result, the technique suffers from the widespread perception that it is in some ways out of date. Yet, according to Derek Gibson [29], older techniques should be continuously kept under review, since reintegrating them into the mainstream often brings surprising dividends.

Specifically regarding stress applications, stress ventricular long-axis demonstrates the mechanical behavior of the subendocardial layer of the myocardium. The myocardial fibers of this layer are longitudinal in orientation. They originate from the ventricular apex and insert around the circumference of the mitral and tricuspid valve rings. In systole, as they contract they bring the insertion site (mitral and tricuspid annulus) toward their origin (the apex) and in diastole they move in the opposite direction, bringing the annuli back toward the atria in early diastole and again in late diastole, during atrial contraction. Having the ability to record the long-axis function from the valve annulus movement (fibrous landmark) makes the technique highly reproducible. The same principle can be used for studying the free wall function of the right ventricle, which cannot be assessed by other stress techniques. During stress, the normal ventricle increases the amplitude and velocity and long-axis function, whereas in presence of a coronary artery stenosis the amplitude is reduced, the time to peak delayed, and some degree of incoordination appears during stress. Disturbances of the anterior and septal segments of the mitral annulus represent left anterior descending coronary artery disease. The left segments represent the circumflex artery disease, and the posterior and right ventricular free walls represent the right coronary disease. The technique has also proved useful outside coronary artery disease, for instance, in children with Mustard repair for great vessel transposition. In these patients, the right ventricular long-axis contractile reserve of the systemic right ventricle mirrors the exercise capacity [30].

There is little doubt that this simple approach has suffered from the misperception that it is in some way out of date. Unlike the competing technologies, there are no colors, no 3D reconstruction, and no fancy tracings! Nonetheless, there are some problems. First, because the test measures displacement, the percentage error may be large when the maximal displacement in a failing ventricle is ambiguous. Second, although the use of different sites around the atrioventricular ring may allow the effect of induced ischemia to be localized, annular displacement is a function of the response in the entire wall. As four of the six walls have a different coronary supply to the apical and basal segments, ischemia in one zone may be obscured by hyperkinesis in another. Third, the time course of contraction is at least as important (probably more so) as displacement in the recognition of ischemia. Finally, the reproducibility of this measure is not well defined.

23.3
Anatomical *M*-mode

The *M*-mode format is undoubtedly well suited to assess left ventricular regional function for several reasons. First, it objectively displays the motion of myocardial segments; second, it simultaneously evaluates endocardial excursion and myocardial thickening, the true marker of myocardial contraction; and third, it facilitates measurements of wall motion and thickening for quantitative analysis of function. Yet despite all these advantages, the conventional *M*-mode technique is not used in clinical stress echocardiography because its application is restricted to a limited portion of the left ventricular myocardium, namely the anterior septum and the posterior wall in the parasternal long and short axis view. Only these two walls, in fact, can be orthogonally cut by the ultrasound beam for correct *M*-mode representation of their motion. Anatomical *M*-mode is a postprocessing technique of 2D echocardiographic images designed to overcome the limitations of the conventional *M*-mode methodology (Table 23.2). A line of *M*-mode analysis can be freely oriented within the 2D sector angle regardless of the direction of the ultrasound beam. In this way, all myocardial segments can be reconstructed and displayed in *M*-mode format and their motion and thickening quantified [30]. At present, with the very high velocity of data processing and 2D frame rates provided by the current digital echocardiography scanners, the *M*-mode reconstruction can be obtained in real time, with a high degree of temporal resolution, and can be applied to multiple myocardial segments simultaneously. Specifically, the anatomical *M*-mode approach has been employed to characterize function in lateral and apical segments, which are off-axis with the standard *M*-mode approach [31]. The amount and the time to peak systolic thickening is also different in normal individuals among the six myocardial segments studied in the short-axis view, with an earlier systolic peak of the inferior and anterior septum, and the anterior wall. In the stress echocardiography setting, anatomical *M*-mode has been shown to precisely quantify the degree of myocardial ischemia [32], making it easier to measure the endocardial excursion and identify the pattern of wall motion abnormalities and incoordination [16]. However, the penetration of this technology has been limited for several reasons. Firstly, the same advantages but also the same limitations of *M*-mode apply to the technique, and one needs to visualize the wall endocardium and epicardium in systole and diastole to measure systolic thickening. Secondly, the frame rate is best in the axial rather than in the perpendicular line of view

(250 fps, as in conventional *M*-mode) and in transverse views (100 fps), leading to poorer resolution for instance in the lateral wall in the apical four-chamber approach, and particularly during stress when heart rate increases. Thirdly, the display of the technique is not so different from the old, standard, not so exciting display of the ultrasound image.

23.4
Tissue Characterization

Interest in ultrasound tissue characterization during stress echocardiography stems from experimental studies showing that transient myocardial ischemia is associated with an increased myocardial reflectivity and a blunting of the physiologic systolic–diastolic variation [33], whose amplitude mirrors the subendocardial function (Table 23.2). In accordance with the experimental background, an increased myocardial echodensity – detectable by simple videodensitometric analysis of conventionally acquired images – has been observed in several models of transient acute myocardial ischemia, induced with angioplasty, ergonovine, dipyridamole, exercise, or pacing [34, 35]. The regional gray-level amplitude increased and the blunting of cyclic gray-level (or backscatter) changes is detected well before the regional dyssynergy. The cyclic variation is of great potential interest as an ancillary marker of myocardial ischemia, since it is affected symmetrically with regional wall thickening and, compared to wall motion analysis, is less operator-dependent and therefore more quantitative. Cyclic variation is independent of motion abnormalities, which may impair the evaluation of regional wall motion in certain conditions, such as left bundle branch block or postcardiac surgery [36]. Cyclic variation can also be preserved in dyssynergic but viable myocardium, offering a clue to the identification of viable segments in ischemic cardiomyopathy [37].

In spite of the promising experimental and initial clinical results, the technique never gained clinical relevance for several reasons. First, the cyclic variation can only be observed in some myocardial regions orthogonal to ultrasound beam such as septum and inferolateral (formerly called posterior) in the parasternal short axis. Second, the technique is exquisitely sensitive to artifacts, and great care is needed in image acquisition and analysis to obtain stable data. Third, tissue characterization data change monotonously in the same way – with increased echodensity and blunting of cyclic variation – in a variety of conditions, from ischemia to fibrous conditions to hypertrophy [33], and are profoundly affected by heart rate changes, making it difficult to assess these parameters fruitfully during stresses associated with tachycardia.

23.5
Color Kinesis

Color kinesis (CK) is a method that evolved from acoustic quantification, which uses ultrasonic integrated backscatter to track endocardial motion in real time and to create an image with an improved signal-to-noise ratio [38]. CK offers an objective and automated assessment not only of global function as acoustic quantification does, but also regional function. Employing a user-defined threshold, pixel transitions between blood and tissue are detected in real time based on differences in backscatter or signal strength, allowing the automatic detection and tracking of the endocardial boundary in real time on a frame-by-frame basis and then color-encoded. Each color represents a distinct time interval within the ejection period (33 ms). The thickness of the color bands represents the degree of endocardial wall motion during that systolic interval. The end-systolic frame, therefore, provides an integrated snapshot of both the magnitude and timing of systolic wall motion [39] (Table 23.2). Qualitatively, hypokinetic segments are depicted by a thinning of the color band in the affected region (Fig. 24.9 in Chap. 24). In contrast to other more time-consuming methods, analysis of CK images takes less than 2 min per echocardiographic view.

Color kinesis has been effectively used to detect regional wall motion abnormalities at rest and during stress, both in standard images and on contrast-enhanced images, allowing a simultaneous assessment of function and perfusion [40]. While both tissue Doppler imaging and color kinesis provide quantitative information on the magnitude of regional wall motion, color kinesis can also explore apical function (where tissue Doppler velocities are too low) and adds information regarding the timing of endocardial motion in both systole and diastole and may also have a role in the assessment of regional diastolic function. Regional left ventricular delayed outward wall motion or diastolic stunning after exercise-induced ischemia can last 1 h after stress, when normal regional systolic function was completely restored [41]. However, the image quality is significantly degraded during increased heart rate, and – as always – an optimal signal is required since the image quality affects the quality of data. The method's overall accuracy and intertechnique variability are comparable to the standard conventional gray-scale image interpretation by expert readings. The method shows a modest degree of interbeat variability due to cardiac translation and respirophasic changes in image quality. Its sensitivity to careful adjustments in the lateral and time gain compensations to obtain accurate endocardial tracking makes it highly dependent on the technician's experience. There are no clear advantages over the standard black-and-white format and gray-scale reading – except for the sexier display.

23.6
Tissue Doppler Imaging

Tissue Doppler imaging color maps the tissue velocities rather than the blood velocities and is mainly used in the cardiac muscle. Myocardial velocities are considerably lower (0–30 cm s^{-1}) than blood velocities, but the amplitude of the echocardiography signal is approximately 40 dB larger than that of the blood flow. The signal processing is similar to color flow imaging, but the clutter filter is bypassed so the signal component from the relatively slow moving myocardial tissue is not removed. The imaging parameters are optimized differently and the PRF is lower in tissue Doppler imaging than in color flow imaging due to the lower velocities in the tissue compared to the blood. Color tissue Doppler imaging is therefore a new cardiac ultrasound technique, which in its current high frame rate format (>120 frames s^{-1}) can resolve all mean myocardial velocities along its scan lines [42]. The technique evaluates longitudinal function, rather than radial function as anatomical *M*-mode. The functional impairment induced by infarction and ischemia is mirrored in a reduction of peak velocity of S (systolic) wave in involved wall, although basal segments are also affected by global contractility changes. Peak systolic velocity brings back in the clinical arena the important variable of long-axis function, which is also expressed by the good old MAPSE. It is a potentially sensitive marker of ischemia, since the long axis is mostly affected by subendocardial ischemia (Table 23.2).

In addition to the physiological insight into longitudinal function of the left ventricle, the advantage of tissue Doppler would be the display, quantification, and regionality [43]. Experimental results were encouraging, proving that tissue Doppler imaging permits subtle segmental assessment of myocardial function during the cardiac cycle, is accurate compared to reference methods such as sonomicrometry [44], and is sensitive to inotropic stimulation and ischemic challenge [45]. Clinical studies show the feasibility of the TDSE, but the reproducibility of the method has been suboptimal [46], the accuracy no better than expert eye reading [47, 48], and the regional assessment is difficult in medial regions and impossible in apical regions [49].

Clinical data made clear to physiologists and bioengineers that the interrogation of regional myocardial velocities alone has major drawbacks. Firstly, as with any Doppler-derived method, the velocities measured are angle-dependent, limiting this technique to the apical views. Angle issues may be circumvented by narrowing the sector and imaging single walls. Image collection is duplicated as TDE images are collected in addition to standard *B*-mode images. These issues make TDE challenging and time-consuming, thus reducing its wider application. In addition, the longitudinal systolic wall motion at the apex is minimal, and therefore myocardial velocities are too low and variable to reliably detect apical wall motion abnormalities. Because of the physiologic base-to-apex gradient, there is a need for different regional cut-off values, which can be implemented into the software of the echocardiography machine. Tissue Doppler is further limited by cardiac translation and rotation, which may cause the myocardial segment interrogated to move away from the Doppler sample volume [50]. In order to reduce the effects of translation, strain-rate imaging, or in other words, rate or speed of deformation, has been developed by estimating spatial gradients in myocardial velocities.

23.7
Strain-Rate Imaging

Strain and strain-imaging techniques can be derived from color-coded TDI. Strain and strain-rate (rate of shortening) imaging measures the rate of myocardial deformation and has the advantage of differentiating between active and passive myocardial motion [51]. Strain and strain rate are less tethering- and translation-dependent than tissue Doppler imaging and provide better assessment of myocardial contraction with almost homogeneous values within the different segments. This is particularly important in regions with extensive infarction and scar formation, where passive motion occurs. From strain-rate curves, local strain can be extracted. Longitudinal strain can be measured in all left ventricular segments using the apical views. However, radial and circumferential strains can only be assessed in some segments, e.g., radial strain in the posterior wall and circumferential strain in the lateral wall using a parasternal short axis view (Table 23.2). Experimental studies show that parameters derived from strain-rate imaging can be helpful in identifying and quantifying ischemia-induced myocardial abnormalities and in identifying viable myocardium, whose strain rate is normalized in stunned areas following inotropic challenge with dobutamine or dipyridamole [52, 53]. These studies also suggest that indices of deformation (strain and strain rate) are better than those of displacement (myocardial velocity) in the evaluation of regional myocardial function, as they might avoid the limitations of velocity (overall heart motion, influence of adjacent segments, etc.). Unfortunately, clinical studies (Fig. 23.4) do not confirm the clear advantage suggested by experimental studies and show comparable values of strain rate and tissue velocity imaging for diagnosis of coronary artery disease and myocardial viability, and comparable accuracy compared to expert reader eyeballing interpretation [54, 55]. Only the sophisticated analysis of strain and strain-rate values, plus postsystolic shortening (which is not always pathologic under stress), plus time to onset of regional relaxation together have been shown to be accurate markers of ischemia [56]. The combination of strain and anatomic M-mode might be a promising alternative technique with prognostic value [57, 58]. The combination allows the expression of strain rate as magnitude (color-coded images instead of complex and less robust wave forms), location (apex-base direction), and timing.

The major limitation of TDSE, as for TDE, is that peak amplitudes, and to some extent phase (timing), of velocity and strain variables are influenced by the angle of the incident beam with the myocardial wall. This restricts imaging to the apical projections wherein the operator attempts to align the myocardial wall parallel to the ultrasound beam; however, this is not always possible. The technique is heavily dependent on the sonographer's expertise, has a limited reproducibility even in expert hands, loses stability with high heart rates and degraded image quality, and is unable to image apical segments (5 out of the total 17 of the left ventricle) [59]. Even in the ideal condition of patient selection, technology, and expertise, the accuracy is comparable to expert reader eyeballing interpretations [54]. In more general terms, the relatively unsatisfactory discriminating power of TDSE and TDE may stem from the very basic biophysical roots of the technique. In fact, the word "tissue Doppler" is a misnomer, since it gives the impression that only myocardial tissues are studied. The appropriate term would be "low-velocity Doppler" [50]. Any movement in the low-velocity range will be detected by tissue Doppler, and myocardial tissue movement is just one of them. In the cardiac motion there are translational, rotational, and deformational movements. Moreover, many tissues near the heart move – due to transmitted cardiac motion, vessel pulsation, respiratory motion, and involuntary muscle movements – and these interact with cardiac motion further and cause false Doppler shifts [50]. Velocity is a vector quantity and so Doppler interrogation at one point will determine the velocity of the resultant of all these movements projected in the line of the Doppler beam with angle corrections. Similarly, at a particular point there are movements in several axes and we can never predict the sum resultant vector. Even if known, the resultant is accurately recorded only if it is in line with the Doppler beam because of the inherent problems of directional bias.

23

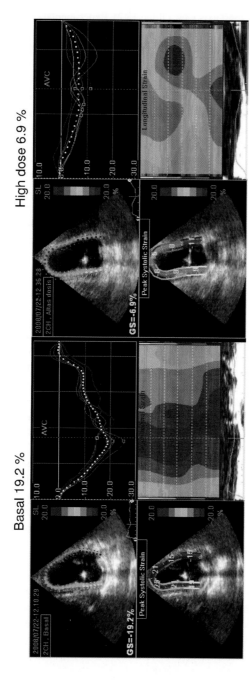

Fig. 23.4 A 2D speckle tracking image of a normal apex at rest (*left panel*) showing decreased contraction at peak dose (*right panel*). The quantitative assessment of velocity and direction of vectors by global strain helps to describe the motion information in an integrated and quantitative fashion. (Courtesy of Dr. Jorge Lowenstein)

23.8
Speckle Tracking

Two-dimensional speckle tracking (also called velocity vector imaging) is based on 2D gray-scale imaging, which is angle-independent, differently from TDI and SRI. Thus, they can be used in any projection and without paying much attention to the orientation of the heart in the imaging sector. Speckles are natural acoustic markers, seen as small and bright elements in conventional gray-scale ultrasound images. A speckle is a unique acoustic pattern resulting from the interaction of ultrasound energy with tissue. These unique patterns can be tracked automatically over periods of the cardiac cycle, thus providing information about motion and displacement of that particular region of the myocardium. The distance between selected speckles is measured simultaneously from multiple regions of interest and is a direct measure of myocardial deformation, used to derive strain and strain rate. Speckle-derived strain has obvious advantages in stress imaging. B-mode images can be collected as in usual clinical practice; therefore, there is no duplication of image acquisition. The technique eliminates the angle dependency of Doppler-based modalities. Other advantages of 2D, non-Doppler-derived strain imaging include high reproducibility and the fact that it is an automated tracking method (especially important for inexperienced observers).

It evaluates the longitudinal and circumferential, and to a lesser extent radial, dynamics of the left ventricle, differently from TDI and SRI, which mainly assesses longitudinal function [59, 60]. Speckle-derived strain has been validated experimentally with excellent results, especially for the sensitivity and reproducibility of longitudinal and circumferential strain [61]. The first clinical studies showed a high feasibility during handgrip stress [62], and with dobutamine a similar accuracy to TDI strain in the anterior, but not in the posterior circulation [63]. Some disadvantages are the lower frame rate in comparison with TDI, influenced by image quality, examination of strain rather than strain rate, and reduced combination with contrast echocardiography for enhancement of border detection [64]. As additional limitations, speckle-derived methods measure systolic strain, but not diastolic strain rates, which are evaluated by tissue Doppler techniques and may in theory be useful in detecting ischemia [64].

23.9
Three-Dimensional Echocardiography

Left ventricular volumes and LV ejection fraction can be assessed with great accuracy using real-time three-dimensional (3D) echocardiography, which has clear advantages over standard 2D echocardiography, both conceptually and practically. The technique is a major development in echocardiography over the last decade, having evolved from slow and labor-intense offline reconstruction to real-time volumetric imaging. The major advantage of this technique over more conventional 2D echocardiography is the improvement in the accuracy of the evaluation of cardiac chamber volumes, which is achieved by eliminating the need for geometric modeling and the errors caused by foreshortened views [65].

23

Another fundamental advantage of the 3D format is the advantage communicating with the patient, the other imaging specialists, and the cardiological community at large. The patient will finally leave the echocardiography laboratory with a "beautiful" picture (easy to understand for nonechocardiographers), which is also "intelligent" (full of information summarized in seductive color-coded, reasonably quantitative information), and speaking the common 3D Esperanto of all competing and complementary imaging techniques [65]. You do not need to be a radiologist to understand a 3D picture of the heart from MSCT or MRI, but you need to be a dedicated echocardiographer to try to understand a TD and TDSE. Eventually, the new technique will be faster to learn, easier to implement, and less operator-dependent in the interpretation, also based on a robust quantitative package of excursion, synchronicity, shape, and volumes.

Two types of imaging modes, full-volume and multiplane mode, can be used to acquire and analyze stress echocardiography. Both modes have their particular benefits and limitations [66]. The multiplane mode is suitable for regional wall motion analysis, since regional function can be represented as a function of time, and a series of plots is obtained representing the change in volume for each segment throughout the cycle. In the presence of ischemia, minimum volume will be reached for each segment at different times and ischemic segments will have higher end-systolic regional volumes (Fig. 23.5). A complete 3D cardiac ultrasound image acquisition can be obtained in a shorter time than with 2D echocardiography and this is a valuable advantage, especially when imaging children and adults during stress [66]. Parametric polar map displays (of the 2D data) of the timing and extent of regional contraction have been developed to simplify interpretation of results. The positive stress echocardiography response is characterized by higher dyssynchrony, greater heterogeneity, and larger end-systolic volumes than the negative stress echocardiography responses (Fig. 23.6) [67–72]. However, and in spite of this exciting potential, the overall accuracy of 3D stress echocardiography is at present no better, and the feasibility markedly lower, than 2D echocardiography [67–72]. The 3D version has a lower spatial resolution than 2D, and the resolution becomes even worse when you need it more, at faster heart rates during stress (because of 3D echocardiography's frame rate of 40 fps, compared to 100 fps for 2D). However, the 3D evaluation of volumes (plus standard assessment of heart rate and blood pressure) is ideally suited for a quantitative and accurate calculation of a set of parameters allowing a complete characterization of cardiovascular hemodynamics (including cardiac output and systemic vascular resistance), left ventricular elastance (an immaculate index of left ventricular contractility, theoretically independent of afterload and preload changes heavily affecting the ejection fraction) [73], arterial elastance [74] (essential to characterize the distal impedance of the arterial system downstream of the aortic valve), ventricular–arterial coupling (a central determinant of net cardiovascular performance in normal and pathological conditions), and diastolic function (through the diastolic mean filling rate). All these parameters were previously inaccessible or inaccurate or labor-intensive and now become, at least in principle, available in the stress echocardiography laboratory since all of them need an accurate estimation of left ventricular volumes and stroke volume, both easily derived from 3D (Table 23.3). It is expected that the technology will improve present critical areas of the technique, such as the need for transducers with higher frequencies, smaller footprints, full Doppler capabilities, and higher frame rates, especially important for stress echocardiography applications.

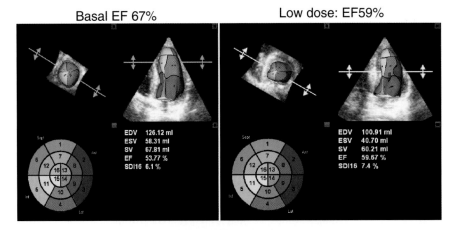

Basal EF 67%   Low dose: EF59%

High dose: EF 47%

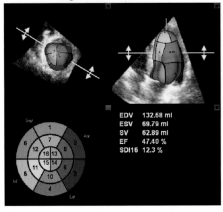

Fig. 23.5 A 3D positive stress echocardiography test. The positive test result is characterized by an area of reduced regional and global ejection fraction at peak stress (*right panel*) when compared to rest (*left panel*) and low dose (*middle panel*). A quantitative assessment of left ventricular volumes and stroke volume is possible at each stage

23.10
Protechnology Bias: A Word of Caution

At times it seems that there is a mismatch between the space devoted to new technologies in major journals and meetings and the lesser coverage of everyday practice. To a certain extent, this is inevitable if new technology is to be trialed sufficiently to understand its benefits and limitations. Nonetheless, it also risks encouraging a cult of technology – all of us, as clinical cardiologists, researchers, and scientists have a major bias in favor of

Basal: SDI 6%   Low dose: SDI 7.4%

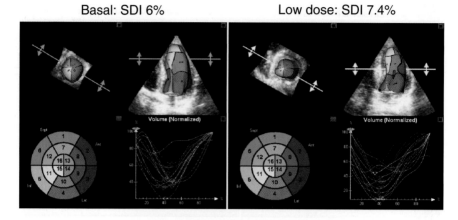

High dose: DSI 12 %

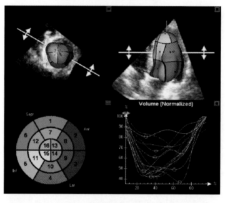

Fig. 23.6 A 3D positive stress echocardiography test with dyssynchrony assessment. The positive test result is characterized by an area of greater segmental dyssynchrony at peak stress (*right panel*) when compared to rest (*left panel*) and low dose (*middle panel*). During ischemia, the peak of contraction is reached by different segments at different time points

technology. What we need to ensure is that technology in medicine is tested scientifically, that it is applied with data relating to cost and benefit, and that it is driven by patient needs rather than market forces [75]. Efficacy studies should be considered the "seed," typically very selected patients are evaluated by a dedicated person, devoted (often full-time) to the technology, in a research-oriented setting where resources are frequently granted by the manufacturer of the technology under scrutiny. This stage – while critical to the development of new technologies – should be followed by effectiveness studies, from which the clinician should be able to discern whether the technology provides clinically relevant information that is independent of, and incremental to, simpler and less expensive tests. In the current economic and cultural milieu, the seed of effectiveness obtained under ideal conditions should not be mistaken for the "fruit" of efficacy: the value of the technique when deployed in the field [76] (Table 23.4).

Table 23.3 Cardiovascular hemodynamics derived from real-time three-dimensional echocardiography (RT3D)

Parameter	Raw RT3D data	Formula	Normal values (rest)	Normal values (stress)	Meaning
Cardiac index	SV (EDV-ESV)	SV × HR	2.5 L min⁻¹ m⁻²	× 2 (ex) × 2 (dob) × 1.5 (dip)	Cardiac pump function
Systemic vascular resistance	SV	80 × (MAP-5)/CO	900–1,300 (dyn×sec) cm⁻⁵	−30 (ex) −40 (dip)	Vascular resistance
Systemic arterial compliance	SV	SVi/PP	0.50 (mL × m⁻² mmHg)	−30% (ex) +20% (dip)	Arterial compliance
Ventricular elastance	ESV	ESP/ESV	7 mmHg mL⁻¹ m⁻²	× 2 (ex) × 1.2 (dip) × 1.5 (pac)	LV contractility
Arterial elastance	SV	ESP/SV	4 mmHg mL⁻¹ m⁻²	× 1.5 (ex) × 0.9 (dip) × 1.5 (pac)	Integration of arterial resistance, compliance and heart rate
Ventriculoarterial coupling	SV and ESV	SV/ESV Ventricular elastance/Arterial elastance	≥1.5	× 1.5 (ex) × 1.3 (dip) × 1.0 (pac)	Ventricular elastance/arterial elastance
Diastolic mean filling rate	SV	SV/diastolic time	100 ml m⁻² s⁻¹	× 3 (ex) × 1.5 (dip)	Diastolic function

ESP (end-systolic pressure) = $SPA \times 0.90$. 5 is an approximation of right atrial pressure. Diastolic time can be calculated from phonocardiogram or 2D echocardiography; with high heart rate, the diastolic time is progressively more reduced than systolic time

MAP mean arterial pressure, PP pulse pressure (systolic arterial pressure − diastolic blood pressure) CO cardiac output, DIP dipyridamole, DOB dobutamine, EX exercise, HR heart rate, PAC pacing, SPA sphygmomanometer systolic pressure, SV stroke volume

Table 23.4 New technologies between efficacy and effectiveness

	Effectiveness	Efficacy
Dictionary definition	Deployed in the field	Ideal conditions
Responsible physician	Wise, gray-haired	Research fellow in training
Scientific interest	Absent	Present
Patient	The protagonist	Part of the method
Technology	Validated	Under validation
Results	True, but unpublishable	Published, but true?
Economic induction	Absent	Present

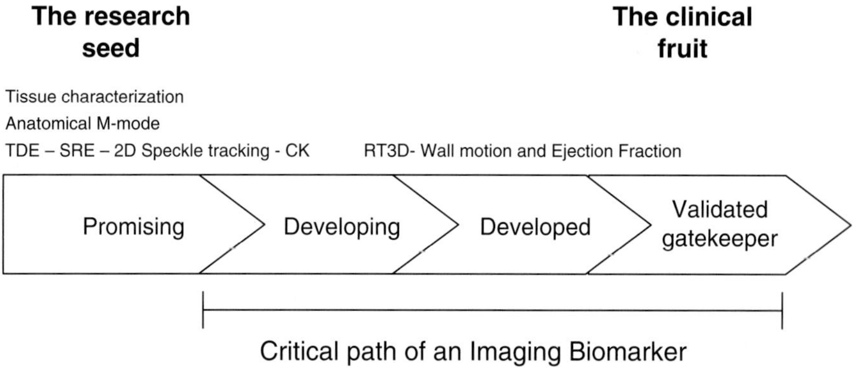

Fig. 23.7 The natural history of a new technology from initial seed of efficacy to established fruit of effectiveness

Any emerging biomarker should, like a new drug, withstand a chain of validation before arriving at clinical impact [77]. With new technologies, like new drugs, large-scale experience should be gathered before accepting the catchy definition promoted by the marketing offices as proven. The additional merits of the new technique should be weighted against the established and more easily accessible methods, and the new technologies should be assessed against other competitive imaging tools (Fig. 23.7). Only at that point will an innovation in engineering be valid in physiological terms and will it give patients the promised diagnostic help, changing an attractive technological gadget into a medical advance [78]. Some of these techniques already have a clear clinical role outside stress echocardiography applications. Tissue characterization may allow a clinically relevant characterization of "soft" (more vulnerable, lipid-rich) vs. "hard" (fibrocalcific) plaques, which can be imaged by ultrasound [79, 80]. Tissue velocity imaging is helpful for characterizing diastolic function through E/E [81, 82]. Strain-rate imaging holds promise for assessing intraventricular dyssynchrony and echocardiography-driven selection of candidate to CRT, although in this case the large-scale validation has been frankly disappointing to date [83]. RT3D is now the clinical gold standard for left ventricular mass and volume calculations and is extremely helpful in complex congenital and valvular disease [64]. However, when we come to the clinically driven practice of stress echocardiography, no technique can be considered clinically useful today, as concordantly stated by US and European guidelines [84, 85].

23.11
Conclusion – Technology and Teaching

Unfortunately, there is no easy solution to the continuing need to quantify regional function, the problem being complicated by issues of translational motion, tethering, torsional movements, image quality, and so on [86]. As stated by one of the founding fathers of modern echocardiography, Arthur Weyman, 20 years ago, "the discriminatory power of the human eye which naturally integrates space and time is very difficult to equal, and virtually impossible to surpass" [10]. This also remains true today for most modern new technologies [87]. There are important consequences for learning and research.

The first relates to the learning curve. Given the profound physiological heterogeneity of myocardial contraction, in space and time, at rest and during stress, it must be recognized that in some segments, mild-to-moderate hypokinesia is a normal variant, especially for specific segments such as inferobasal and inferior basal septum. These should not be read aggressively as a pathological finding in resting conditions and even more so during stress. Aggressive reading of mild hypokinesia, relative hypokinesia, or lack of hyperkinesia, albeit used in the past, should be abandoned since they have a slippery pathophysiological basis and, pragmatically, will lead to an exorbitant number of false-positive results [4–6].

Second, all quantitative methods have matched and rarely outperformed the accuracy and reproducibility of qualitative expert reading for stress echocardiography. They have been shown to help the less expert reader, but should be considered a means of diagnostic support rather than a replacement for expert training. However, in routine work, an eyeball reading by a trained observer remains the best, and only, way to diagnose wall motion abnormalities during stress echocardiography performed in the clinical arena. As summarized by the American Society of Echocardiography and European Association of Echocardiography recommendations [84, 85], visual assessment of left ventricular wall thickening and motion remains the standard method of interpretation of stress echocardiography, albeit with relevant interobserver and interinstitutional variability. In contrast, under resting conditions, the quantitative approach can offer obvious advantages when compared to standard eyeballing analysis for the detection of changes in longitudinal, circumferential, and radial function (e.g., in the serial assessment of changes induced by cardiotoxic interventions such as chemotherapy).

The attempt as old as echocardiography itself to translate the wall motion abnormality from an opinion into a number remains a dream for the clinical cardiologist and a nightmare for the researcher. Maintenance of a critical attitude on the part of the clinical cardiologist and sonographer faced with the forest of new technologies proposed every year by the manufacturers is essential. What has been said about Internet might be echoed by sonographers struggling with new technologies: "The adventure starts now but it is not the one that the

23

marketing experts are talking about. It is the one that you will build with your own hands. How? First, learn to use the new machines. Second, beware of those who are saying they traced the way for you. Third, avoid the traps and pitfalls, and identify the routes. No one will do it for you" [88].

References

1. Fox K, Garcia MA, Ardissino D, et al (2006) Task Force on the Management of Stable Angina Pectoris of the European Society of Cardiology, ESC Committee for Practice Guidelines (CPG). Guidelines on the management of stable angina pectoris: executive summary: the Task Force on the Management of Stable Angina Pectoris of the European Society of Cardiology. Eur Heart J 27:1341–1381
2. Gibbons RJ, Abrams J, Chatterjee K, et al, American College of Cardiology, American Heart Association Task Force on practice guidelines (Committee on the Management of Patients With Chronic Stable Angina) (2003) ACC/AHA 2002 guideline update for the management of patients with chronic stable angina – summary article: a report of the American College of Cardiology/American Heart Association Task Force on practice guidelines (Committee on the Management of Patients With Chronic Stable Angina). J Am Coll Cardiol 41:159–168
3. Picano E (1992) Stress echocardiography. From pathophysiological toy to diagnostic tool. Point of view. Circulation 85:1604–1612
4. Picano E, Lattanzi F, Orlandini A, et al (1991) Stress echocardiography and the human factor: the importance of being expert. J Am Coll Cardiol 17:666–669
5. Hoffmann R, Lethen H, Picano E, et al (1996) Analysis of interinstitutional observer agreement in interpretation of dobutamine stress echocardiograms. J Am Coll Cardiol 27:330–336
6. Varga A, Picano E, Pratali L et al (1999) Madness and method in stress echo reading. Eur Heart J 20:1271–1275
7. Henein M, Gibson D (2002) Dobutamine stress echocardiography: the long and short of it. Eur Heart J 23:520–522
8. De Castro S, Pandian NG (eds) (2000) Manual of Clinical Echocardiography. Time-Science International Medical
9. Hirshleifer J, Crawford M, O'Rourke RA, et al (1975) Influence of acute alterations in heart rate and systemic arterial pressure on echocardiographic measures of left ventricular performance in normal human subjects. Circulation 52:835–841
10. Mann DL, Gillam LD, Weyman AE (1986) Cross-sectional echocardiographic assessment of regional left ventricular performance and myocardial perfusion. Prog Cardiovasc Dis 29:1–52
11. Epstein FH (2007) MRI of left ventricular function. J Nucl Cardiol 14:729–744
12. Pandian NG, Skorton DJ, Collins SM, et al (1983) Heterogeneity of left ventricular segmental wall thickening and excursion in 2-dimensional echocardiograms of normal human subjects. Am J Cardiol 51:1667–1673
13. Falsetti HL, Marcus ML, Kerber RE, et al (1981) Quantification of myocardial ischemia and infarction by left ventricular imaging. Circulation 63:747–751
14. Mondillo S, Galderisi M, Ballo P, et al, Study Group of Echocardiography of the Italian Society of Cardiology (2006) Left ventricular systolic longitudinal function: comparison among simple M-mode, pulsed, and M-mode color tissue Doppler of mitral annulus in healthy individuals. J Am Soc Echocardiogr 9:1085–1091
15. Borges AC, Sicari R, Picano E, et al (1995) Heterogeneity of left ventricular regional wall thickening following dobutamine infusion in normal human subjects. Eur Heart J 11:1726–1730

16. Carstensen S, Ali SM, Stensgaard-Hansen FV, et al (1995) Dobutamine-atropine stress echocardiography in asymptomatic healthy individuals. The relativity of stress-induced hyperkinesia. Circulation 92:3453–3463

17. Ross J Jr (1986) Assessment of ischemic regional myocardial dysfunction and its reversibility. Circulation 74:1186–1190

18. Derumeaux G, Loufoua J, Pontier G, et al (2001) Tissue Doppler imaging differentiates transmural from nontransmural acute myocardial infarction after reperfusion therapy. Circulation 103:589–596

19. Hui L, Pemberton J, Hickey E, et al (2007) The contribution of left ventricular muscle bands to left ventricular rotation: assessment by a 2-dimensional speckle tracking method. J Am Soc Echocardiogr 20:486–491

20. Matre K, Moen CA, Fanneløp T, et al (2007) Multilayer radial systolic strain can identify subendocardial ischemia: an experimental tissue Doppler imaging study of the porcine left ventricular wall. Eur J Echocardiogr 8:420–430

21. Skulstad H, Urheim S, Edvardsen T, et al (2006) Grading of myocardial dysfunction by tissue Doppler echocardiography: a comparison between velocity, displacement, and strain imaging in acute ischemia. J Am Coll Cardiol 47:1672–1682

22. Tanaka H, Oishi Y, Mizuguchi Y, et al (2008) Contribution of the pericardium to left ventricular torsion and regional myocardial function in patients with total absence of the left pericardium. J Am Soc Echocardiogr 21:268–274

23. Henein MY, Cailes J, O'Sullivan C, et al (1995) Abnormal ventricular long-axis function in systemic sclerosis. Chest 108:1533–1540

24. Picano E (2003) Diabetic cardiomyopathy. the importance of being earliest. J Am Coll Cardiol 42:454–457

25. Henein MY, Gibson DG (1999) Long axis function in disease. Heart 81:229–231

26. Bogaert J, Rademakers FE (2001) Regional nonuniformity of normal adult human left ventricle. Am J Physiol Heart Circ Physiol 280:H610–H620

27. Duncan AM, O'Sullivan CA, Carr-White GS, et al (2001) Long axis electromechanics during dobutamine stress in patients with coronary artery disease and left ventricular dysfunction. Heart 86:397–404

28. Henein MY, Dinarevic S, O'Sullivan CA, et al (1998) Exercise echocardiography in children with Kawasaki disease: ventricular long axis is selectively abnormal. Am J Cardiol 81:1356–1359

29. Gibson D (1993) M-mode echocardiography-an obsolete technique? In: Chambers J, Monaghan MJ (eds) Echocardiography: an international review. Oxford University Press, Oxford, pp. 1–9

30. Strotmann JM, Escobar Kvitting JP, Wilkenshoff UM, et al (1999) Anatomic M-mode echocardiography: a new approach to assess regional myocardial function. A comparative in vivo and in vitro study of both fundamental and second harmonic imaging modes. J Am Soc Echocardiogr 12:300–307

31. Li W, Hornung TS, Francis DP, et al (2004) Relation of biventricular function quantified by stress echocardiography to cardiopulmonary exercise capacity in adults with Mustard (atrial switch) procedure for transposition of the great arteries. Circulation 110:1380–1386

32. Chan J, Wahi S, Cain P, et al (2000) Anatomical M-mode: a novel technique for the quantitative evaluation of regional wall motion analysis during dobutamine echocardiography. Int J Card Imaging 16:247–255

33. Mimbs JS, Bauwens D, Cohen RD, et al (1981) Effects of myocardial ischemia on quantitative ultrasonic backscatter and identification of responsible determinants. Circ Res 49:89–85

34. Picano E, Faletra F, Marini C, et al (1993) Increased echodensity of transiently asynergic myocardium in humans: a novel echocardiographic sign of myocardial ischemia. J Am Coll Cardiol 21:199–207

35. Vitale DE, Bonow RO, Gerundo G, et al (1995) Alterations in ultrasonic backscatter during exercise-induced myocardial ischemia in humans. Circulation 92:1452–1457

36. Gigli G, Maffei S, Picano E, et al (1995) Cardiac cycle-dependent gray-level variation is not distorted by abnormal septal motion after cardiac surgery: a transesophageal videodensito-metric study in humans. J Am Soc Echocardiogr 8:475–481

37. Marini C, Picano E, Varga A, et al (1996) Cyclic variation in myocardial gray level as a marker of viability in man. A videodensitometric study. Eur Heart J 17:472–479

38. Perez JE, Waggoner AD, Barzilai B, et al (1992) On-line assessment of ventricular function by automatic boundary detection and ultrasonic backscatter imaging. J Am Coll Cardiol 19:313–320

39. Lang RM, Vignon P, Weinert L, et al (1996) Echocardiographic quantification of regional left ventricular wall motion with color kinesis. Circulation 93:1877–1885

40. Mor-Avi V, Caiani EG, Collins KA, et al (2001) Combined assessment of myocardial perfusion and regional left ventricular function by analysis of contrast-enhanced power modulation images. Circulation 104:352–357

41. Ishii K, Miwa K, Sakurai T, et al (2008) Detection of postischemic regional left ventricular delayed outward wall motion or diastolic stunning after exercise-induced ischemia in patients with stable effort angina by using color kinesis. J Am Soc Echocardiogr 21:309–314

42. Sutherland GR, Stewart MJ, Grouendstroem KWE, et al (1994) Colour Doppler myocardial imaging: a new technique for assessment of myocardial function. J Am Soc Echocardiogr 7:441–458

43. Hatle L, Sutherland GR (2000) Regional myocardial function – a new approach. Eur Heart J 21:1337–1357

44. Derumeaux G, Ovize M, Loufoua J, et al (1998) Doppler tissue imaging quantitates regional wall motion during ischemia and reperfusion. Circulation 97:1970–1977

45. Gorcsan J III, Strum DP, Mandarino WA, et al (1997) Quantitative assessment of alterations in regional left ventricular contractility with color-coded tissue Doppler echocardiography: comparison with sonomicrometry and pressure-volume relations. Circulation 95:2423–2433

46. Fraser AG, Payne N, Madler CF, et al (2003) Feasibility and reproducibility of off-line tissue doppler measurement of regional myocardial function during dobutamine stress echocardiography. Eur J Echocardiogr 4:43–53

47. Madler CF, Payne N, Wilkenshoff U, et al (2003) Noninvasive diagnosis of coronary artery disease by quantitative stress echocardiography: optimal diagnostic models using off-line tissue Doppler in the MYDISE study. Eur Heart J 25:123–131

48. Pasquet A, Yamada E, Armstrong G, et al (1999) Influence of dobutamine or exercise stress on the results of pulsed-wave Doppler assessment of myocardial velocity. Am Heart J 138:753–758

49. Cain P, Short L, Baglin T, et al (2002) Development of a fully quantitative approach to the interpretation of stress echocardiography using radial and longitudinal myocardial velocities. J Am Soc Echocardiogr 15:752–767

50. Thomas G (2004) Tissue Doppler echocardiography – a case of right tool, wrong use. Cardiovasc Ultrasound 2:12

51. Fleming D, Xia X, Mc Dicken WN, et al (1994) Myocardial velocity gradients detected by Doppler imaging. Br J Radiol 799:679–688

52. Urheim S, Edvardsen T, Torp H, et al (2000) Myocardial strain by Doppler echocardiography: validation of a new method to quantify regional myocardial function. Circulation 102:1158–1164

53. Marciniak M, Claus P, Streb W, et al (2008) The quantification of dipyridamole induced changes in regional deformation in normal, stunned or infarcted myocardium as measured by strain and strain rate: an experimental study. Int J Cardiovasc Imaging 24:365–376

54. Hoffmann R, Altiok E, Nowak B, et al (2002) Strain rate measurement by Doppler echocardiography allows improved assessment of myocardial viability in patients with depressed left ventricular function. J Am Coll Cardiol 39:443–449

55. Ingul CB, Stoylen A, Slordahl SA, et al (2007) Automated analysis of myocardial deformation at dobutamine stress echocardiography: an angiographic validation. J Am Coll Cardiol 49:1651–1659

56. Voigt JU, Exner B, Schmiedehausen K, et al (2003) Strain-rate imaging during dobutamine stress echocardiography provides objective evidence of inducible ischemia. Circulation 107:2120–2126

57. Mastouri R, Mahenthiran J, Kamalesh M, Gradus-Pizlo I, Feigenbaum H, Sawada SG (2008) Prediction of ischemic events by anatomic M-mode strain rate stress echocardiography. J Am Soc Echocardiogr 21:299–306

58. Marwick TH (2008) Strain without pain: application of parametric imaging of strain rate response for the quantitation of stress echocardiography. J Am Soc Echocardiogr 21:307–308

59. Helle-Valle T, Crosby J, Edvardsen T et al (2005) New-noninvasive method for assessment of left ventricular rotation: Speckle Tracking Echocardiography. Circulation 112:3149–3156

60. Suffoletto MS, Dohi K, Cannesson M, et al (2006) Novel speckle-tracking radial strain from routine black-and-white echocardiographic images to quantify dyssynchrony and predict response to cardiac resynchronization therapy. Circulation 113:960–968

61. Amundsen BH, Helle-Valle T, Edvardsen T et al (2006) Noninvasive myocardial strain measurement by speckle tracking echocardiography: validation against sonomicrometry and tagged magnetic resonance imaging. J Am Coll Cardiol 47:789–793

62. Stefani L, Toncelli L, Di Tante V, et al (2008) Supernormal functional reserve of apical segments in elite soccer players: an ultrasound speckle tracking handgrip stress study. Cardiovasc Ultrasound 26:14

63. Hanekom L, Cho GY, Leano R, et al (2007) Comparison of two-dimensional speckle and tissue Doppler strain measurement during dobutamine stress echocardiography: an angiographic correlation. Eur Heart J 28:1765–1772

64. Abraham TP, Pinheiro AC (2008) Speckle-derived strain a better tool for quantification of stress echocardiography? J Am Coll Cardiol 51:158–160

65. Takeuchi M, Lang RM (2007) Three-dimensional stress testing: volumetric acquisitions. Cardiol Clin 25:267–272

66. Hung J, Lang R, Flachskampf F, et al, ASE (2007) 3D echocardiography: a review of the current status and future directions. J Am Soc Echocardiogr 20:213–233

67. Ahmad M, Xie T, McCulloch M, et al (2001) Real-time three-dimensional dobutamine stress echocardiography in assessment stress echocardiography in assessment of ischemia: comparison with two-dimensional dobutamine stress echocardiography. J Am Coll Cardiol 37:1303–1309

68. Matsumura Y, Hozumi T, Arai K, et al (2005) Non-invasive assessment of myocardial ischaemia using new real-time three-dimensional dobutamine stress echocardiography: comparison with conventional two-dimensional methods. Eur Heart J 26:1625–1632

69. Takeuchi M, Otani S, Weinert L, et al (2006) Comparison of contrast-enhanced real-time live 3-dimensional dobutamine stress echocardiography with contrast 2-dimensional echocardiography for detecting stress-induced wall-motion abnormalities. J Am Soc Echocardiogr 19:294–299

70. Pulerwitz T, Hirata K, Abe Y, et al (2006) Feasibility of using a real-time 3-dimensional technique for contrast dobutamine stress echocardiography. J Am Soc Echocardiogr 19:540–545

71. Eroglu E, D'hooge J, Herbots L, et al (2006) Comparison of real-time tri-plane and conventional 2D dobutamine stress echocardiography for the assessment of coronary artery disease. Eur Heart J 27:1719–1724

72. Walimbe V, Garcia M, Lalude O, et al (2007) Quantitative real-time 3-dimensional stress echocardiography: a preliminary investigation of feasibility and effectiveness. J Am Soc Echocardiogr 20:13–22

73. Bombardini T (2005) Myocardial contractility in the echo lab: molecular, cellular and patho-physiological basis. Cardiovasc Ultrasound 3:27
74. Borlaug BA, Melenovsky V, Redfield MM, et al (2007) Impact of arterial load and loading sequence on left ventricular tissue velocities in humans. J Am Coll Cardiol 50:1570–1577
75. Lown B (1997) The tyranny of technology. Hosp Pract 32:25
76. Feinstein AR (1985) Diagnostic and spectral markers. Clinical epidemiology. Saunders, Philadelphia, pp 597–631
77. US Dept of Health and human services (2004) Challenge and opportunity on the critical path of new medical products. FDA report. US Dept of Health and Human Services, Washington DC
78. Vasan RS (2006) Biomarkers of cardiovascular disease: molecular basis and practical considerations. Circulation 113:2335–2362
79. Picano E, Landini L, Distante A, et al (1985) Angle dependence of ultrasonic backscatter in arterial tissues: a study in vitro. Circulation 72:572–576
80. Kawasaki M, Bouma BE, Bressner J, et al (2006) Diagnostic accuracy of optical coherence tomography and integrated backscatter intravascular ultrasound images for tissue characterization of human coronary plaques. J Am Coll Cardiol 48:81–88
81. Nagueh SF, Middleton KJ, Kopelen HA, et al (1997) Doppler tissue imaging: a noninvasive technique for evaluation of left ventricular relaxation and estimation of filling pressures. J Am Coll Cardiol 30:1527–1533
82. Paulus WJ, Tschöpe C, Sanderson JE, et al (2007) How to diagnose diastolic heart failure: a consensus statement on the diagnosis of heart failure with normal left ventricular ejection fraction by the Heart Failure and Echocardiography Associations of the European Society of Cardiology. Eur Heart J 28:2539–2550
83. Galderisi M, Cattaneo F, Mondillo S (2007) Doppler echocardiography and myocardial dyssynchrony: a practical update of old and new ultrasound technologies. Cardiovasc Ultrasound 5:28
84. Pellikka PA, Nagueh SF, Elhendy AA, et al, American Society of Echocardiography (2007) American Society of Echocardiography recommendations for performance, interpretation, and application of stress echocardiography. J Am Soc Echocardiogr 20:1021–1041
85. Sicari R, Nihoyannopoulos P, Evangelista A, et al, European Association of Echocardiography (2008) Stress echocardiography consensus statement of the European Association of Echocardiography. Eur J Echocardiogr 9:415–437
86. Marwick TH (2003) Clinical applications of tissue Doppler imaging: a promise fulfilled. Heart 89:1377–1378
87. Picard MH, Popp RL, Weyman AE (2008) Assessment of left ventricular function by echocardiography: a technique in evolution. J Am Soc Echocardiogr 21:14–21
88. Colombo F (1996) A warning from the Internet: our freedom is at risk. La Repubblica, 8 January
89. Diamond GA (1986) Monkey business. Am J Cardiol 57:471–475
90. Berry W (1997) The unsettling of American. Sierra Club Books, San Francisco
91. Baroldi G (1995) About inflammation and atherosclerosis. G Ital Cardiol 25:241–245

Contrast Stress Echocardiography

24

Mark J. Monaghan and Eugenio Picano

24.1
Historical Background

Echocardiographic contrast agents are an important new advance in the practice of echocardiography [1, 2]. Initial attempts to better delineate endocardial borders used agitated saline, indocyanine green dye, or radiologic contrast agents. The history of myocardial contrast echocardiography (MCE) began in 1968, when an accidental injection of saline solution in the ascending aorta during an angiography examination caused the production of microbubbles that led to better echographic signals in the aorta lumen and cardiac chambers [3]. A major limitation was the large and variable size of the air bubbles, which could not transit the pulmonary circulation and opacify the left heart. The early 1990s saw the development of commercial agents with air- or gas-filled microbubbles, similar in size to red blood cells with a distribution similar to blood flow. Exciting reports described the potential of contrast echocardiography in diagnosis of coronary artery disease, the extent of risk area in acute myocardial infarction, infarct artery patency after thrombolytic therapy, microvascular integrity, myocardial viability, and coronary flow reserve. In the year 2000, three agents had been approved and at least 13 other agents were undergoing evaluation [4]. At that time, more than $ US 1 billion had been spent worldwide to develop these agents and bring them to market.

While contrast echocardiography has many important applications, the greatest utility and benefit from this technique is expected from stress echocardiography. The information provided by contrast during stress echocardiography is potentially important and tremendously versatile: from improved border recognition (Fig. 24.1a) to myocardial perfusion (Fig. 24.1b), from coronary flow velocity enhancement (Fig. 24.1c) to potentiation of regurgitant tricuspid jet velocity to analyze pulmonary artery systolic pressure (Fig. 24.1d). The addition of contrast may improve the image quality in all cases; however, it demonstrates unique advantages only in the assessment of myocardial perfusion, which

E. Picano, *Stress Echocardiography*,
© Springer-Verlag Berlin Heidelberg 2009

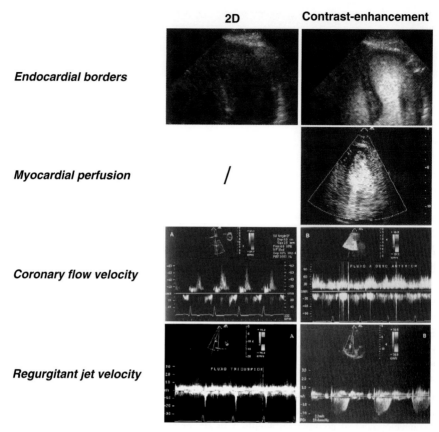

Fig. 24.1 The main potential clinical applications of contrast in the stress echocardiography laboratory: improved endocardial border definition (*first row*), myocardial perfusion (*second row*), pulsed-Doppler signal enhancement on left anterior descending coronary artery (*third row*), and enhancement of tricuspid regurgitant jet velocity for analyzing pulmonary artery systolic pressure (*last row*). On the *left*, the noncontrast 2D image; on the *right*, the contrast-enhancement image. Myocardial perfusion imaging is only possible with contrast. (Courtesy of Dr. Ana Cristina Camarozano)

has the highest potential value but unfortunately has been least convincingly validated in the clinical arena.

As a consequence, and in striking mismatch with the enormous potential, echocardiographic contrast agent perfusion analysis is today performed in only a small minority of stress studies. The main clinically driven application of contrast is the left ventricular endocardial border delineation allowing the rescue of procedures that do not provide results of diagnostic quality, especially in patients with obesity and lung disease [5]. At present three agents are licensed for left ventricular opacification and endocardial definition: Sonovue (Bracco, Italy), Definity (called Luminity in Europe, Lanthaeus medical imaging, previously Bristol-Myers Squibb, New York, NY, USA), and Optison (General Electric, Fairfield, CT, USA). In October 2007, the US FDA decided to alter the labeling of Perfluoro-containing contrast agents (perflutren lipid microspheres, Definity, and per-flutren protein-type A microspheres for injection, Optison) to include a black-box warning, contraindicating the use of echocontrast agents in patients who were acutely unwell (e.g., acute myocardial infarction or worsening congestive cardiac failure). This followed the report of 199 serious cardiopulmonary reactions, including 11 deaths, either during or shortly after the administration of contrast agents [6]. This raised strong reactions in specialist societies, strongly arguing against this FDA warning, regarded as potentially damaging to the quality of diagnosis in the echocardiography laboratory, which requires liberal use of contrast to provide the best care to each patient every day [7]. In May 2008, the FDA approved less restrictive language for the labeling of the echocardiographic perflutren-containing contrast agents. Experts vehemently disagreed with the agency's interpretation of the evidence and lamented that it would prevent use of the contrast agents in the very patients who would most benefit from them. The FDA's 2008 rewording now suggests 30 min of monitoring only in patients with pulmonary hypertension or unstable cardiopulmonary conditions, as compared with the previous label, which included monitoring for all patients. In addition, current contraindications include only "patients with known or suspected right-to-left, bidirectional or transient right-to-left cardiac shunts, or hypersensitivity to perflutren." All other contraindications ("unstable cardiopulmonary status, including unstable angina, acute myocardial infarction, respiratory failure, and recent worsening of congestive heart failure") have been removed. Stress MCE has remained on the threshold of widespread clinical acceptance for at least 20 years, and it is still there, at the crossroads between success and failure. For decades, stress MCE has been "next year's breakthrough," and we are still waiting for it to fulfill the clinical promises of bringing together wall motion and perfusion in a simple, fast, cost-effective, and user-friendly way. It should also reduce the struggle time, the time taken to obtain an adequate image in the technically challenging patient.

24.2
Pathophysiology of MCE

The pathophysiological rationale of MCE is simple and strong. The use of regional myocardial perfusion is a potentially useful diagnostic and prognostic marker of myocardial ischemia. Myocardial ischemia results in a typical cascade of events in which the various markers are hierarchically ranked on a well-defined time sequence [8]. Flow heterogeneity, especially between the subendocardial and subepicardial perfusion, is the forerunner of ischemia, followed by regional systolic dysfunction, and only at a later stage by electro-cardiographic changes and anginal pain (Fig. 24.2). The best way to unmask a perfusion defect is the use of a hyperemic stress. An epicardial coronary artery stenosis reduces the maximal flow achievable in the related territory, although the blood flow in resting conditions can be equal to that observed in regions supplied by normal coronary arteries. During hyperemia, perfusion heterogeneity will occur with lower blood flow increase in the regions supplied by the stenotic artery, even in the absence of regional ischemia (Fig. 24.3). The criterion of positivity is the presence of a reduced perfusion signal (flow tracer uptake) between different regions of the left ventricle, or in the same region between

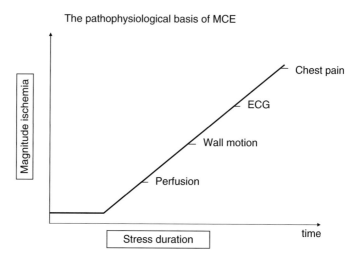

Fig. 24.2 The ischemic cascade. Perfusion abnormalities consistently precede wall motion abnormalities, theoretically supporting the use of MCE as a more sensitive diagnostic marker than systolic thickening in stress echocardiography

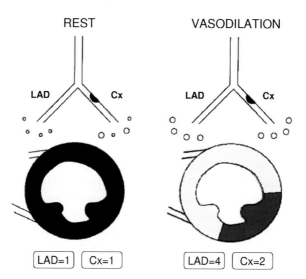

Fig. 24.3 Schematic illustration of the principle underlying myocardial perfusion imaging for the diagnosis of coronary artery disease. At rest, myocardial perfusion is homogeneous, with no differences between the territory of the normal coronary artery (*LAD* left anterior descending artery) and the diseased coronary artery territory (*Cx* left circumflex, with 80% stenosis). The resting flow image (obtained, for instance, with thallium-201 scintigraphy or contrast echocardiography) does not show any inter-region variation. However, the perfusion in the territory of the stenotic coronary artery is maintained at the price of a partial exhaustion of coronary reserve, with partial dilatation of the arteriolar bed, represented by *larger circles* located downstream from the epicardial coronary arteries.

rest and stress. The excellent spatial resolution of echocardiography makes it an ideal tool for this technique which can even detect small subendocardial perfusion defects. The use of MCE will therefore increase the sensitivity of the noninvasive diagnosis of coronary artery disease simply based on wall motion [9–13]. In addition, it will also expand the power of prognostic stratification, since the long-standing experience with other imaging methods [including cardiovascular magnetic resonance (CMR) stress and stress echocardiography with CFR assessment with pulsed-Doppler imaging of LAD)] has proved that stress-induced wall motion changes identifies those with a short-term prognosis. However, an isolated reduction in coronary flow reserve, occurring without wall motion abnormalities, may identify patients with a poorer long-term prognosis [14, 15]. In these patients, the underlying coronary anatomy may range anywhere from mild to moderate epicardial coronary artery disease (relatively frequent when patients are studied on ischemia-masking antiischemic therapy) or normal coronary anatomy but with functionally important coronary microvascular disease. These patients have prognostically important forms of microvascular disease and are often found in syndrome X, hypertension, diabetes, and also cardiomyopathy and heart transplant rejection settings [16]. It has been demonstrated in some studies that myocardial contrast positivity adds prognostic information over and above wall motion abnormalities seen during stress echocardiography [17, 18]. Obviously, the strong pathophysiological roots will generate clinically useful fruits only if the method to assess perfusion is sensitive enough, reproducible, safe, and not vulnerable to artifacts. It is also essential to use perfusion not as a "stand-alone" but rather as a "running-mate" criterion, to be added to regional wall motion assessment. In fact, perfusion (or the conceptually germane assessment of coronary flow reserve from Doppler assessment with the coronary flow velocity method) per se is unable to separate epicardial coronary artery disease from coronary microvascular disease, and if used alone will be plagued by an exorbitant number of false-positive results [16].

24.3
Physics of Microbubbles and Modalities of Administration

Today, ultrasound contrast agents may be hospital-produced or commercially produced. We now have the third-generation of commercial agents available (Table 24.1). In hospital-generated agents, contrast is used for right heart opacification and consists of an agitated

---

Fig. 24.3 (continued) The normal arteriolar tone is represented by *smaller circles* (normally vasoconstricted arterioles). During vasodilation obtained with a metabolic stimulus, such as exercise, or with a pharmacological stimulus, such as dipyridamole, the arteriolar tone is lost, causing an increase in flow that will be greater in the normal coronary artery (which, at rest, has a preserved tone in the entire arteriolar district) than in the stenotic coronary artery (with lower coronary flow reserve). Perfusion imaging will see the stenosis mirrored in the myocardium as a region with relative underconcentration of flow tracer when compared with the normal contralateral region. The septal and anterior wall appear *brighter* (due to greater echocontrast concentration) when compared with the *darker* inferoposterior wall (lower echocontrast concentration)

Table 24.1 Characteristics of echocardiography contrast agents

Production	Composition	Use	Clinical use
Agitation, zero generation	Saline solution/Emagel mixed with room air	Enhance Doppler (tricuspidal regurgitation) signal	Routine
Commercial, first generation	Polysaccharide + air	One pass only	Abandoned
Commercial, second generation	Lipid + octofluoropropane	Stable, long-lasting	Enhanced endocardial border delineation
	Plus albumin or poly-saccharide shells and sulfur–hexafluoride gas		
Commercial, third generation	Vehicle for genes and drugs	Local therapy delivery	Investigational
Commercial, fourth generation	Ligands as microbubble shells	Cells and molecular imaging	Investigational
Commercial, fifth generation	Nanotechnologies	Passive and active targeting	Investigational

saline solution containing air bubbles, which is intravenously injected. The right heart contrast is impressive, but the air quickly dissolves into the blood (Fig. 24.4, first row). The smaller bubbles that are capable of crossing the lung capillary bed do not survive long enough for imaging the left heart because the air quickly dissipates into the blood. In commercial contrast agents, persistence is achieved using an impermeable shell or a higher-density encapsulated gas that is relatively insoluble in blood (Table 24.2). In fact, gas composition is one of the most important factors in maintaining microbubble size in the circulation. First-generation commercial agents (such as Levovist) contained room air, which is 78% nitrogen; since nitrogen rapidly diffuses in blood, these microbubbles survive only a few seconds. To overcome this problem, slowly diffusing, insoluble gases (such as octofluoropropane) were incorporated into second-generation microbubbles, providing greater stability and contrast effect duration.

An exciting further development in microbubble engineering has been obtained by modifying the shell, so that it can be loaded with drugs or genes [19]. This "Trojan horse" is unloaded by destroying the microbubble in the target organ through external ultrasound. Another emerging application is the chemical remodeling of the passive external shell, which can become active, with smart ligands that can bind selectively to specific antigens or cells. This can be used with positive molecular or cellular imaging, for instance to image atherosclerotic or apoptotic cells.

Contrast agents can be administered either via a bolus injection or continuous infusion. Bolus injections have the advantages of using lower contrast volumes and are simple to administer. However, they offer result in attenuation in the image plane for a transient period and there is often only a short period, during the decay phase, when the contrast agent concentration is appropriate for analysis of myocardial blood volume. Infusions of

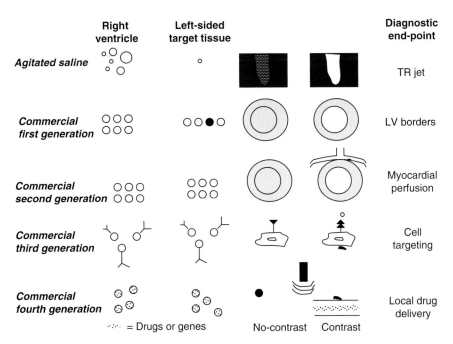

| | Right ventricle | Left-sided target tissue | | | Diagnostic end-point |

Fig. 24.4 The five different generations of contrast. The agitated preparation still has a role in right heart enhancement, for instance with tricuspid regurgitation signal for pulmonary artery systolic pressure testing in primary pulmonary hypertension during exercise. With commercial first-generation contrast, bubbles had a more uniform size and passed the pulmonary circulation, facilitating left ventricular border recognition. Stability and homogeneity were further enhanced in second-generation contrast agents, designed for myocardial contrast perfusion imaging. With third-generation agents, "smart" bubbles are aimed with regards to specific antigens, in principle allowing cellular or receptor imaging. In the fourth-generation agents, therapeutic bubbles act as Trojan horses filled with drugs and genes that can be released through external ultrasound irradiation in the target organ

contrast agents are more complex to administer and usually require a larger volume of agent. However, they need less operator involvement during the stress study and it is easier to adjust the infusion rate to optimize myocardial opacification without excessive attenuation. A constant contrast concentration is better suited to quantification of myocardial blood flow [20] and for 3D echocardiography image acquisition, which needs to be performed over several consecutive cardiac cycles.

24.4
MCE Methodology

MCE imaging technology attempts to detect contrast microbubbles in the very small quantities with which they occur in the myocardium, while suppressing the myocardial tissue signal [21]. The three main technical approaches are summarized in Table 24.3. In summary, we can use destructive high ultrasound power (high Mechanical Index, MI) power techniques, which

24

Table 24.2 The currently available second-generation microbubble contrast agents (adapted from [6])

	Sonovue	Optison	Luminity (Definity in the USA)
Gas	Sulfur hexafluoride	Perfluoropropane	Perfluoropropane
Shell composition	Predominantly phospholipid	Human albumin	Predominantly phospholipid
Mean bubble size	2–8 µm	3.0–4.5 µm	1.1–2.5 µm
Patients with side effect	11%	17%	8%
Most frequent side effects	Headache, chest pain	Headache, nausea	Headache, back pain
Manufacturer	Bracco	General Electric	Bristol-Myers Squibb

Table 24.3 Contrast imaging methods

Methods	Synonymous	Output power (MI)	Bubble destruction	Left ventricular borders	Wall motion
Harmonic power Doppler	Angiopower	High (>0.5)	+	−	−
Gray-scale harmonics	Power pulse inversion; ultra-harmonics	Low (0.2–0.5)	+	+	−
Real-time contrast imaging	Power modulation; power pulse inversion; coherent imaging	Very low (<0.1)	−	+	+

MI mechanical index

are very sensitive to contrast but provide no simultaneous wall motion information. Alternatively, we can use low-power real-time imaging, which is slightly less sensitive for myocardial contrast, but does provide wall motion information and excellent left ventricular opacification. Real-time perfusion imaging has many potential advantages. The technique is relatively easy to use, many artifacts can be avoided, and wall motion information is obtainable alongside perfusion, making this technique particularly valuable during stress echocardiography.

Myocardial perfusion can be evaluated both semiquantitatively and quantitatively. A semiquantitative contrast score is generally used: 0 = no enhancement, 1 = patchy enhancement, 2 = homogeneous enhancement (Fig. 24.5). A contrast score index may be calculated by dividing the sum of the contrast scores for each segment by the number of segments analyzed. Quantitative software programs can be used to obtain off-line analysis of the refilling curves [22]. Once injection of a myocardial contrast agent has occurred, within a few seconds, the agent will be present within the myocardial capillaries, and once a steady state is achieved the signal intensity represents the myocardial blood volume (A). The rate of increase in intensity following bubble destruction with several high-energy pulses represents red blood cell velocity (β) and the product of $A\times\beta$ is proportional

Analysis of MCE

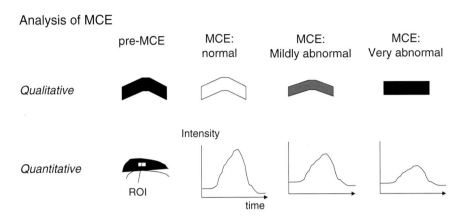

Fig. 24.5 The two possible types of analysis of MCE signal: qualitative (*upper row*) or quantitative (*lower row*). The qualitative analysis focuses on the presence and homogeneity of opacification. The quantitative analysis creates a time–intensity curve based on a region of interest in the myocardium, and estimates flow from the steepness of the filling phase and amplitude of the signal (higher flows identified by steeper rise and brighter intensity)

to myocardial blood flow (Fig. 24.6). Dedicated software can automatically construct background-subtracted plots of peak myocardial contrast intensity, A, and the slope of the replenishment curve depicting mean microbubble velocity, β reserve, and myocardial blood flow, can be derived. Coronary flow reserve (i.e., stress myocardial blood flow/rest myocardial blood flow) can then be calculated from regions of interest in segments perfused by each of the three coronary arteries.

Stress testing with MCE requires consideration of the choice of the stress. Ideally, the technique needs a maximal vasodilatory stimulus to expand the dynamic range of differentiation between normally perfused and hypoperfused regions. This clearly favors vasodilators when compared to dobutamine or exercise, since the former creates a three- to fourfold increase in coronary flow reserve, as opposed to only a two- to threefold with dobutamine or even maximal exercise [23]: Fig. 24.7. The adopted stressor should also optimize the ischemic potential of the simultaneous wall motion assessment, and therefore high doses are required [24, 25]. Vasodilatory stresses also have the clear advantage of minimally degrading the image quality, which is significantly reduced by dobutamine [26] and, to a greater extent, by exercise [27]. This is always important in stress echocardiography, since image quality is the major determinant of test accuracy and reproducibility [28, 29]. It is even more important with stress contrast, since the technique is exquisitely sensitive to artifacts, due to attenuation, variable ultrasound scan planes, and heart rate increase. During stress, a regional wall motion abnormality accompanied by a transient perfusion defect unequivocally localizes myocardial ischemia (Fig. 24.8). The superior image quality of contrast pharmaceutical stress echocardiography is also ideally suited for the combination of wall motion, perfusion, and quantitation with new technologies such as color kinesis (Fig. 24.9), 3D, or speckle tracking, all techniques in which the signal-to-noise ratio must be excellent for robust endocardial border recognition during stress [30, 31].

24

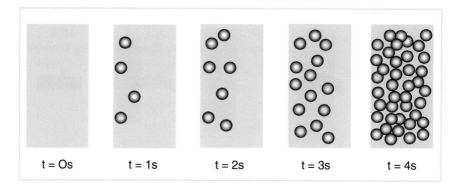

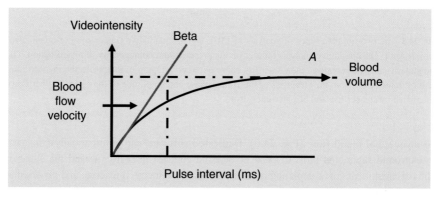

Fig. 24.6 a Time to filling of myocardium by bubbles, in resting conditions and without significant obstruction. **b** Relationship between blood volume and flow velocity with quantitative estimation of myocardial blood flow through a combination of beta (flow velocity) and A (blood volume)

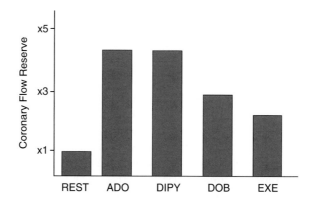

Fig. 24.7 The vasodilatory effect (ordinates, times resting flow = 1) over time (*x-axis*) for four different stressors. Vasodilators (adenosine or dipyridamole, which accumulates endogenous adenosine) are stronger hyperemic stressors than exercise or dobutamine

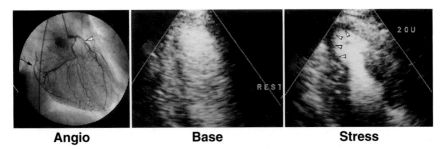

| Angio | Base | Stress |

Fig. 24.8 An example of an inducible inferior and apical myocardial perfusion defect (*arrowheads*) during dobutamine stress echocardiography following a 0.3-ml bolus intravenous injection of Optison. These images were obtained in real time at frame rates of more than 25 Hz and pulse inversion Doppler. The subsequent coronary angiogram (left main injection) demonstrates that the right coronary artery fills from the left main injection because of a 100% right coronary stenosis. In addition, there is a long left anterior descending stenosis (*arrows*). (Courtesy of Dr. Thomas Porter)

24.5
Limitation of Stress MCE

Minor limitations include the need for an intravenous line, usually not required for baseline studies or exercise stress echocardiography but already present in pharmacological stress echocardiography. To analyze contrast, considerable expertise is needed as well as additional software, and it takes time and diligence to learn how to use them. It is said that 30% of stress echocardiographic studies are nondiagnostic, and this may be true with posttreadmill exercise, but certainly it is not the common experience with semisupine exercise or pharmacological stress echocardiography, when native second harmonic or contrast imaging is used [32]. The major limitations can be grouped into economic, methodological, clinical, and safety reasons.

Patent issues, cost, reimbursement, difficult regulatory issues, and a smaller market than originally envisaged has led a number of contrast agent manufacturers to review their position. Some agents have been withdrawn from development and some put on hold. Instrument manufacturers have been reflecting on their substantial investment in contrast imaging technology.

The cost of contrast varies, but in Europe is around €50 and in the USA around $100 per exam. It is reimbursed in some states in the USA, but not in others; however, the possibility of reimbursement is not per se a reason to do it. Finally, it is true that contrast improves endocardial border detection, but it may create disturbing noise and blooming if you want to add to wall motion the evaluation of coronary flow reserve in the left anterior descending coronary artery [24]. It is not separately reimbursed in most countries and this makes the stress echocardiography (receiving a flat reimbursement of €150–400) less economical if contrast is added. In addition, new ultrasound technology such as native tissue harmonic imaging has reduced the need for contrast for border enhancement in technically difficult patients, and the use of coronary flow reserve evaluation with pulsed Doppler techniques

24

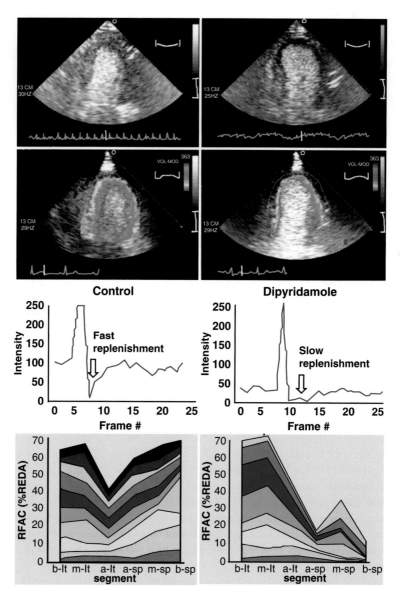

Fig. 24.9 Simultaneous quantitative assessment of myocardial perfusion and function during an adenosine stress test. *Top left*: The presence of uniform intramyocardial contrast enhancement and color kinesis (CK) bands of uniform thickness qualitatively indicate normal myocardial perfusion and function at rest, respectively. *Right*: Diminished intramyocardial contrast in the apex together with thinning of the CK color bands in the same segments qualitatively indicate a dipyridamole-induced apical perfusion defect and wall motion abnormality. *Bottom*: Videointensity curves and CK histograms obtained from the above images. *Left*: Quantitative assessment of normal myocardial perfusion and function at rest. The videointensity curve demonstrates rapid intramyocardial contrast replenishment after a high energy ultrasound impulse, while the CK histogram demonstrates normal RFAC in

has allowed a convenient dual CFR and wall motion imaging without contrast. Furthermore, in some centers – including Pisa and London – the easy access to CMR makes stress-CMR a very convenient and reliable option in patients who would otherwise have been candidates for MCE stress [33].

The routine utilization of MCE contrast has been hampered by a number of factors. These include what can appear to be a bewildering array if contrast administration techniques, imaging techniques, and analysis techniques, combined with a paucity of adequate training available to help ensure operators maximize the potential use of the methodology. Furthermore, there has been a lack of large multicenter studies providing the clinical evidence to support the routine use of myocardial contrast. Two perfusion agents are currently undergoing evaluation by the FDA and both have been subjected to multicenter studies involving approximately 800 patients each. The data on one of these agents (Imagify-Acusphere) have been presented in abstract format and will soon be published. The study demonstrates that the agent has almost identical accuracy to SPECT for the detection of obstructive coronary artery disease when angiography is used as the comparator. Once agents like this have a product license for perfusion imaging, it will make vasodilative stress MCE an easy and rapid functional test that will change the face of stress echocardiography.

Finally, it has become increasingly clear that ultrasound contrast, like all contrast agents, is not completely safe [34, 35]. Clinical studies also show that contrast injection can be accompanied in 10–20% of cases by increased subclinical release of cardiac biomarkers, especially when high mechanical index contrast echocardiography is used, while low-mechanical index real-time imaging appears to be safer [36–38]. Recent studies (Mann 2008, JACC) in over 8,000 patients have clearly demonstrated that the risk–benefit ratio of contrast use strongly favors its utilization in appropriate patients. The risks were clearly overstated in the FDA original 2007 warning [6, 7, 39]; however, it is appropriate that the risk and medical and legal aspects be considered in the final balance of using MCE in stress echocardiography [40].

24.6
Contrast Stress Echocardiography: The Current Indications

The current consensus on the appropriate and inappropriate indications for contrast in the stress echocardiography laboratory is summarized in Table 24.4. An additional useful application of contrast is the potentiation of tricuspid regurgitation signal in patients in whom the pulmonary artery systolic pressure has to be evaluated during stress, for instance, in patients with valvular disease during exercise. For this application, it is sufficient to

Fig. 24.9 (continued) all myocardial segments. *Right:* Dipyridamole-induced an apical myocardial perfusion defect with corresponding apical and septal hypokinesis. The segmental videointensity curve demonstrates a slow rate of intramyocardial contrast replenishment following high-energy ultrasound destruction, reflecting a perfusion abnormality. The CK histogram below quantifies the percentage reduction in RFAC in the apex and septum. (Courtesy of Dr. Roberto Lang) RFAC, Regional Fractional Area Change; REDA, Regional End-Diastolic Area

Table 24.4 Appropriate and inappropriate use of contrast in stress echocardiography

	Appropriate	Uncertain	Inappropriate
≥2 Contiguous segments unreadable	√		
Pulsed-Doppler CFR velocity, perfusion imaging		√	
<2 Contiguous segments unreadable			√

use agitated saline contrast, since no transpulmonary crossing of the agent is required. The recommended application of commercial contrast to stress echocardiography is for endocardial border enhancement, which should be used whenever there are suboptimal resting or peak stress images [41, 42]. According to the recent 2008 recommendations on stress echocardiography appropriateness criteria released by the American College of Cardiology Foundation, the use of contrast is appropriate when two or more contiguous segments are unreadable on a stress echocardiogram [43]. Intravenous contrast for left ventricular opacification improves endocardial border definition and may salvage an otherwise suboptimal study. Left-sided contrast agents are also helpful to improve measurement reproducibility for suboptimal studies and correlation with other imaging techniques.

A few caveats regarding the clinically oriented use of contrast agents deserve mention, as suggested by the American Society of Echocardiography [44]. The mechanical index should be lowered to decrease the acoustic power of the ultrasound beam, which reduces bubble destruction. The image should be focused on the structure of interest. Excessive shadowing may be present during the initial phase of bubble transit and often the contrast imaging occurs some time after the first appearance of contrast in the left ventricle during bolus administration. Some centers have reported the routine use of contrast in almost 90% of stress studies [45], mainly because of the consistent improvement in endocardial definition and interpreter confidence when contrast is used. The most appealing application of stress echocardiography is myocardial contrast perfusion imaging – where we await the licensing of agents specifically manufactured for this purpose. Theoretically, it might have greater sensitivity, but certainly lower specificity, than wall motion analyses unless both techniques are used together [46]. Its use instead of SPECT scintigraphy would reduce the radiation burden to the individual patient, consisting in 500–1,250 chest X-rays per scintigraphy, with a cancer risk of 1 in 1,000: 1 in 500 exposed subjects [47, 48]. This would also have a very favorable impact on the population risk [49], since 10 million stress scintigraphy procedures per year only in the US implies 20,000 new cancers per year due to stress SPECT perfusion imaging [48, 49]. The sonic, medical and economic advantage of ultrasound perfusion imaging would be immense. However, it is not recommended for clinical use by either the 2007 American Society of Echocardiography [41] or the 2008 European Association of Echocardiography [42]. Other exciting applications of contrast for cell or molecular imaging [50] or for drug or gene delivery [51] remain investigational at present.

References

1. Kaul S (1997) Myocardial contrast echocardiography: 15 years of research and development. Circulation 96:3745–3760
2. Rakhit DJ, Becher H, Monaghan M, et al (2007) The clinical applications of myocardial contrast echocardiography. Eur J Echocardiogr 8:S24–S29
3. Gramiak R, Shah PM (1968) Echocardiography of the aortic root. Invest Radiol 3:356–66
4. Rakowski H (2000) Reimbursement for contrast echocardiography: don't burst the bubble. J Am Soc Echocardiogr 13:19A–20A
5. Bhatia VK, Senior R (2008) Contrast echocardiography: evidence for clinical use. J Am Soc Echocardiogr 21:409–416
6. Information for Healthcare Professionals Micro-bubble contrast agents (Marketed as Definity [Perflutren Lipid Microsphere]) Injectable Suspension and Opison (perflutren protein-type a microspheres for injection): FDA ALERT [10/2007]. http://www.fda.gov/cder/drug/Infosheets/HCP/microbubbleHCP.htm
7. Lester SJ, Miller FA Jr, Khandheria BK (2008) Contrast echocardiography: beyond a black box warning? J Am Soc Echocardiogr 21:417–418
8. Nesto RW, Kowalchuk GJ (1987) The ischemic cascade: temporal sequence of hemodynamic, electrocardiographic and symptomatic expressions of ischemia. Am J Cardiol 59:23C–30C
9. Porter TR, Xie F, Silver M, et al (2001) Real-time perfusion imaging with low mechanical index pulse inversion Doppler imaging. J Am Coll Cardiol 37:748–753
10. Shimoni S, Zoghbi WA, Xie F, et al (2001) Real-time assessment of myocardial perfusion and wall motion during bicycle and treadmill exercise echocardiography: comparison with single photon emission computed tomography. J Am Coll Cardiol 37:741–747
11. Elhendy A, O'Leary EL, Xie F, et al (2004) Comparative accuracy of real-time myocardial contrast perfusion imaging and wall motion analysis during dobutamine stress echocardiography for the diagnosis of coronary artery disease. J Am Coll Cardiol 44:2185–2191
12. Peltier M, Vancracynest D, Pasquet A, et al (2004) Assessment of the physiologic significance of coronary disease with dipyridamole real-time myocardial contrast echocardiography. Comparison with technetium-99m sestamibi single-photon emission computed tomography and quantitative coronary angiography. J Am Coll Cardiol 43:257–264
13. Moir S, Haluska BA, Jenkins C, et al (2004) Incremental benefit of myocardial contrast to combined dipyridamole-exercise stress echocardiography for the assessment of coronary artery disease. Circulation 110:1108–1113
14. Rigo F, Sicari R, Picano E, et al (2008) The additive prognostic value of wall motion abnormalities and coronary flow reserve during dipyridamole stress echo. Eur Heart J 29:79–88
15. Cortigiani L, Sicari R, Picano E, et al (2007) Additional prognostic value of coronary flow reserve in diabetic and nondiabetic patients with negative dipyridamole stress echocardiography by wall motion criteria. J Am Coll Cardiol 50:1354–1361
16. Picano E, Palinkas A, Amyot R (2001) Diagnosis of myocardial ischemia in hypertensive patients. J Hypertens 19:1177–1183
17. Tsutsui JM, Elhendy A, Anderson JR, et al (2005) Prognostic value of dobutamine stress myocardial contrast perfusion echocardiography. Circulation 112:1444–1450
18. Tsutsui JM, Xie F, Cloutier D, et al (2008) Real-time dobutamine stress myocardial perfusion echocardiography predicts outcome in the elderly. Eur Heart J 29:377–385
19. Moos S, Odabashian J, Jasper S, et al (2000) Incorporating ultrasound contrast in the laboratory: a series on contrast echocardiography, article 1. J Am Soc Echocardiogr 13:240–247

24

20. Burgess P, Moore V, Bednarz J, et al (2000) Performing an echocardiographic examination with a contrast agent: a series on contrast echocardiography, article 2. J Am Soc Echocardiogr 13:629–634

21. McCulloch M, Gresser C, Moos S, et al (2000) Ultrasound contrast physics: a series on contrast echocardiography, article 3. J Am Soc Echocardiogr 13:959–967

22. Wei K, Jayaweera AR, Firoozan S, et al (1998) Quantification of myocardial blood flow with ultrasound-induced destruction of microbubbles administered as a constant venous infusion. Circulation 97:473–483

23. Iskandrian AE (2007) A new generation of coronary vasodilators in stress perfusion imaging. Am J Cardiol 99:1619–1620

24. Rigo F (2005) Coronary flow reserve in stress-echo lab. From pathophysiologic toy to diagnostic tool. Cardiovasc Ultrasound 3:8

25. Picano E, Molinaro S, Pasanisi E (2008) The diagnostic accuracy of pharmacological stress echocardiography for the assessment of coronary artery disease: a meta-analysis. Cardiovasc Ultrasound 6:30

26. Sochowski RA, Yvorchuk KJ, Yang Y, et al (1995) Dobutamine and dipyridamole stress echocardiography in patients with a low incidence of severe coronary artery disease. J Am Soc Echocardiogr 8:482–487

27. Beleslin BD, Ostojic M, Stepanovic J, et al (1994) Stress echocardiography in the detection of myocardial ischemia. Head-to-head comparison of exercise, dobutamine, and dipyridamole tests. Circulation 90:1168–1176

28. Picano E, Lattanzi F, Orlandini A, et al (1991) Stress echocardiography and the human factor: the importance of being expert. J Am Coll Cardiol 17:666–669

29. Hoffmann R, Lethen H, Marwick T, et al (1996) Hoffmann Analysis of interinstitutional observer agreement in interpretation of dobutamine stress echocardiograms. J Am Coll Cardiol 27:330–6

30. Mor-Avi V, Caiani EG, Collins KA, et al (2001) Combined assessment of myocardial perfusion and regional left ventricular function by analysis of contrast-enhanced power modulation images. Circulation 104:352–7

31. Nemes A, Geleijnse ML, Krenning BJ, et al (2007) Usefulness of ultrasound contrast agent to improve image quality during real-time three-dimensional stress echocardiography. Am J Cardiol 99:275–278

32. Caidahl K, Kazzam E, Lidberg J, et al (1998) New concept in echocardiography: harmonic imaging of tissue without use of contrast agent. Lancet 352:1264–1270

33. Pingitore A, Lombardi M, Picano E, et al (2008) Head to head comparison between perfusion and function during accelerated high-dose dipyridamole magnetic resonance stress for the detection of coronary artery disease. Am J Cardiol 101:8–14

34. Ay T, Havaux X, Van Camp G, et al (2001) Destruction of contrast microbubbles by ultrasound: effects on myocardial function, coronary perfusion pressure, and microvascular integrity. Circulation 104:461–466

35. Miller DL, Li P, Dou C, et al (2005) Influence of contrast agent dose and ultrasound exposure on cardiomyocyte injury induced by myocardial contrast echocardiography in rats. Radiology 237:137–143

36. Borges AC, Walde T, Reibis RK, et al (2002) Does contrast echocardiography with Optison induce myocardial necrosis in humans? J Am Soc Echocardiogr 15:1080–1086

37. Knebel F, Schimke I, Eddicks S, et al (2005) Does contrast echocardiography induce increases in markers of myocardial necrosis, inflammation and oxidative stress suggesting myocardial injury? Cardiovasc Ultrasound 3:21

38. Vancraeynest D, Kefer J, Hanet C, et al (2007) Release of cardiac bio-markers during high mechanical index contrast-enhanced echocardiography in humans. Eur Heart J 28:1236–1241

39. Stiles S (2008) FDA backpedals on warnings in Echo-contrast labelling. Heartwire. Nedscape Today, May 13

40. Ryan T (2008) A message to ASE members. Echocardiographer as patient advocate: lessons from the contrast debate. J Am Soc Echocardiogr 21:A29

41. Pellikka PA, Nagueh SF, Elhendy AA, et al, American Society of Echocardiography (2007) American Society of Echocardiography recommendations for performance, interpretation, and application of stress echocardiography. J Am Soc Echocardiogr 20:1021–1041

42. Sicari R, Nihoyannopoulos P, Evangelista A, et al, European Association of Echocardiography (2008) Stress echocardiography expert consensus statement: European Association of Echocardiography (EAE) (a registered branch of the ESC). Eur J Echocardiogr 415–437

43. Douglas PS, Khandheria B, Stainback RF, et al, American College of Cardiology Foundation Appropriateness Criteria Task Force, American Society of Echocardiography, American College of Emergency Physicians, American Heart Association, American Society of Nuclear Cardiology, Society for Cardiovascular Angiography and Interventions; Society of Cardiovascular Computed Tomography, Society for Cardiovascular Magnetic Resonance (2008) ACCF/ASE/ACEP/AHA/ASNC/SCAI/SCCT/SCMR 2008 appropriateness criteria for stress echocardiography: a report of the American College of Cardiology Foundation Appropriateness Criteria Task Force, American Society of Echocardiography, American College of Emergency Physicians, American Heart Association, American Society of Nuclear Cardiology, Society for Cardiovascular Angiography and Interventions, Society of Cardiovascular Computed Tomography, and Society for Cardiovascular Magnetic Resonance: endorsed by the Heart Rhythm Society and the Society of Critical Care Medicine. Circulation 117:1478–1497

44. Lang RM, Bierig M, Devereux RB, et al, Chamber Quantification Writing Group, American Society of Echocardiography's Guidelines and Standards Committee, European Association of Echocardiography (2005) Recommendations for chamber quantification: a report from the American Society of Echocardiography's Guidelines and Standards Committee and the Chamber Quantification Writing Group, developed in conjunction with the European Association of Echocardiography, a branch of the European Society of Cardiology. J Am Soc Echocardiogr 18:1440–1463

45. Picano E (1992) Stress echocardiography. From pathophysiological toy to diagnostic tool. Circulation 85:1604–1612

46. Picano E (2003) Stress echocardiography: a historical perspective. Am J Med 114:126–30

47. Douglas PS (2002) What are the top 10 reasons not to use a contrast? J Am Soc Echocardiogr 15:19A

48. Picano E (2004) Informed consent and communication of risk from radiological and nuclear medicine examinations: how to escape from a communication inferno. BMJ 329:849–851

49. Picano E (2004) Sustainability of medical imaging. BMJ 328:578–580

50. Villanueva FS, Wagner WR, Vannan MA, Narula J (2004) Targeted ultrasound imaging using microbubbles. Cardiol Clin 22:283–298

51. Tsutsui JM, Xie F, Porter RT (2004) The use of microbubbles to target drug delivery. Cardiovasc Ultrasound 2:23

52. Monaghan MJ (2003) Contrast echocardiography: from left ventricular opacification to myocardial perfusion. Are the promises to be realised? Heart 89:1389–1390

Diastolic Stress Echocardiography

25

Maurizio Galderisi and Eugenio Picano

Stress echocardiography is an established and mainstream method for the diagnosis and risk stratification of patients with known or suspected coronary artery disease [1, 2]. While the accuracy and clinical usefulness of echocardiography in assessment of regional and global systolic function is undisputed, the assessment of diastolic function is important, but it remains difficult by echocardiography at rest [3, 4], and even more during stress [5, 6]. In spite of the many unsolved conceptual and methodological issues, there are three reasons for the still high interest of the cardiological and echocardiography community in diastolic stress echocardiography: (1) experimental [7–9] and clinical [10–12] studies clearly show that acute diastolic dysfunction is an early event in the ischemic cascade, even earlier than regional systolic dysfunction, which remains the cornerstone of clinical diagnosis with stress echocardiography [13]; (2) diastolic dysfunction can accompany systolic dysfunction, but its presence and severity adds risk to the negative prognostic value of resting [14] or stress-induced systolic dysfunction [15]; and (3) in a high proportion of patients, "diastolic" heart failure is the dominant form of dysfunction, without any detectable systolic dysfunction at rest and during stress [16].

According to European Society of Cardiology 2007 guidelines, in presence of clinical symptoms, mainly dyspnea, and normal left ventricular (LV) systolic function with normal LV volumes, the diagnosis can be achieved by combining standard transmitral Doppler (transmitral E velocity), pulsed tissue Doppler of the mitral annulus (early diastolic velocity = e′) and clinical biochemistry criteria. Diastolic heart failure will be diagnosed in the presence of the E/e′ ratio >15 + BNP >300 and excluded with E/E′ ratio <8 and BNP <200 [17]. However, it is not infrequent for the patient to fall within a gray zone of indeterminate values (Fig. 25.1). In these patients, resting echocardiography may help with indirect, supportive signs showing structural changes frequently associated with LV diastolic dysfunction, such as left atrial dilation (left atrial volume index>28 mL m^{-2}) [18] and LV hypertrophy, but obviously a more direct documentation of diastolic dysfunction would be most helpful. These patients are the main clinical target of diastolic stress echocardiography.

E. Picano, *Stress Echocardiography*,
© Springer-Verlag Berlin Heidelberg 2009

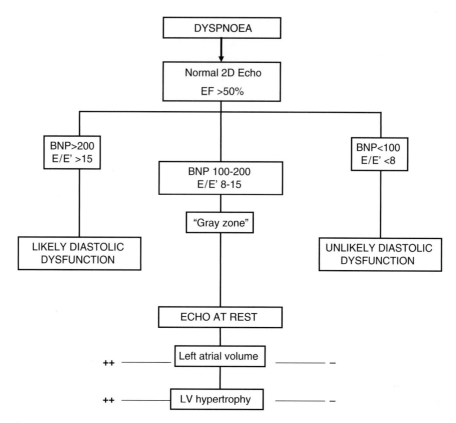

Fig. 25.1 The diagnostic algorithm for diastolic heart failure proposed by the European Society of Cardiology in 2007. Transthoracic echocardiography has a central role and is the imaging test of choice in excluding systolic dysfunction (normal ejection fraction and left ventricular volumes) and in including diastolic dysfunction, through direct, specific signs (E/e′ increase) and indirect, supportive signs (left atrial dilation and left ventricular hypertrophy). (Modified from [17])

25.1
Pathophysiological Basis of Diastolic Dysfunction

From a pathophysiological standpoint, LV diastolic function should always be viewed as a two-dimensional (2D) problem, including not only LV filling pressures but also LV volumes. ESC criteria establish a cut-off value of wedge pressure greater than 15 mmHg and LV end-diastolic pressure (LVEDP) greater than 15 mmHg to clearly document LV diastolic heart failure [17]. However, for any given pressure, LV end-diastolic volume is also important. In fact, at normal LV filling pressure, the normal heart shows end-diastolic volumes necessary to grant the adequate stroke volume. The stiff heart of diastolic dysfunction has similar volumes at higher pressures or, alternatively, normal pressures and smaller volumes. Any stress on the heart, including a simple tachycardia, is also a

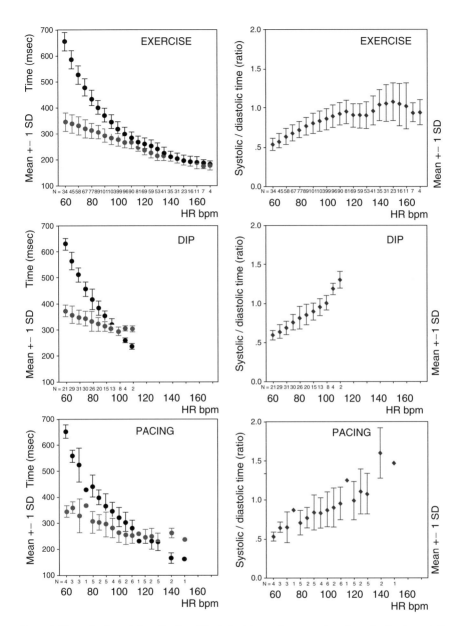

Fig. 25.2 The reduction of diastolic time (*black dots*) is much steeper than the reduction in systolic time (*red dots*) during tachycardia associated with exercise (*upper left panel*), dipyridamole (*middle left panel*), or pacing (*lower left panel*). The ratio between systolic and diastolic tissue increases during exercise (*right upper panel*), dipyridamole (*middle right panel*) and pacing (*lower right panel*)

powerful diastolic stress, since the same filling must be achieved in a much shorter time (Fig. 25.2). The positive lusitropic (improved myocardial relaxation) effects of adrenergic stress (or exercise) determine better filling in a shorter time, and in fact the normal diastolic

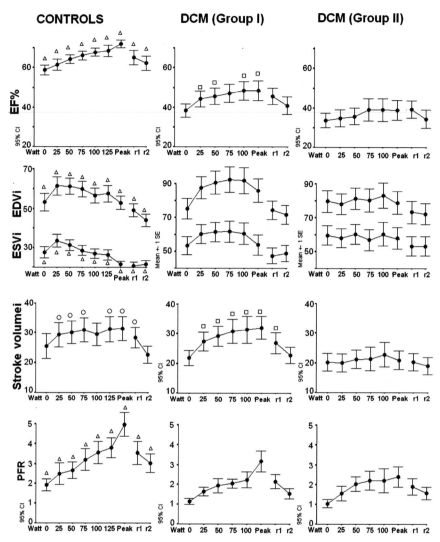

Fig. 25.3 Changes in left ventricular volume during exercise in controls, dilated cardiomyopathy patients with relatively good (Group I) and relatively poor (Group II) prognosis with exercise. The end diastolic volume is increased only in normal and Group I dilated cardiomyopathy patients. (Modified from [19]) DCM, dilated cardiomyopathy; EF, Ejection Fraction; ESVi, end-systolic volume index; EDVi, end-diastolic volume index; Stroke Volume i, stroke volume index; PFR, peak filling rate

response to stress is a reduction of LV end-systolic volume (due to an increase in contractility) and an increase in end-diastolic volume, normally occurring in the early phases of exercise, and then a plateau at intermediate to high levels of stress, up to a point when the diastolic reserve is exhausted and LV filling declines [19] (Fig. 25.3). This decline in LV filling can occur at lower heart rates in ventricles with diastolic dysfunction. The lower the diastolic filling, the lower the stroke volume, and, for any given level of systolic dysfunction, the worse the prognosis.

25.2
The Echocardiography Assessment of Diastolic Function

The four grades of LV diastolic function can be summarized as in Fig. 25.4 [20]. The assessment of diastolic function has been made easier, simpler, and more accurate by combining the transmitral E velocity with the E′ derived from pulsed tissue Doppler, i.e., the E/e′ ratio [21], which is obtained more often, more rapidly, and more easily than pulmonary blood flow and transmitral flow during Valsalva [22], which are alternative ways to separate a normal from a pseudonormal pattern. Left atrial volume is also useful as a marker of the severity and duration of diastolic dysfunction [18, 23], perhaps obviating the need for more complex characterization of diastolic function and filling pressures with Doppler echocardiography. Doppler indexes reflect LV filling pressures at one point in time, whereas increased left atrial size may better reflect the memory of the same filling pressures, i.e., the cumulative effect of filling pressures over time, in a way conceptually similar to glycated hemoglobin in diabetes. As a single assessment of glycemia is affected by dietary factors such as the sugar intake immediately prior to testing, Doppler index changes are affected by loading conditions unrelated to true LV diastolic dysfunction, and an increase in heart rate or a preload increase induced for instance by nitrates may induce a pseudorestrictive pattern. The integration of structural, 2D-based parameters on left atrial

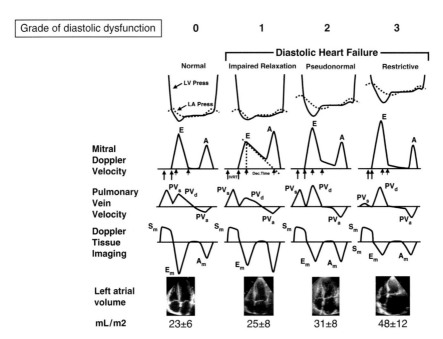

Fig. 25.4 The severity of diastolic dysfunction (from 0 = absent to 3 = severe) titrated by a combination of transthoracic echocardiography assessed with Doppler, tissue Doppler, and 2D indices. (Modified from [20])

remodeling and functional, Doppler-based markers of altered filling offers a comprehensive picture of diastolic dysfunction.

The assessment of LV diastolic function at rest has independent and additive prognostic value [24] over resting and stress-induced systolic dysfunction. The worse combination is represented by a LV diastolic restrictive pattern [25] with lack of contractile reserve in dilated cardiomyopathy patients [26] or a dilated left atrium with inducible ischemia in coronary artery disease patients [27].

The abnormal diastolic stress echocardiographic response is characterized by lower LV cavity dilation, higher E/e′ values, and possibly increases in pulmonary arterial systolic pressure (PASP) and ultrasound lung comet (ULC), surrogate signs of diastolic dysfunction mirrored in backward failure with pulmonary congestion up to interstitial lung edema [28, 29]. However, the clinical data supporting this framework are scanty to date. In a more advanced phase of LV diastolic restrictive dysfunction, the stress should be aimed at unloading the ventricle and improving the lusitropic properties: a viability test of diastole. For this purpose, the nitroprusside test can be useful [30].

25.3
Clinical Results

The ratio of transmitral E (peak early diastolic velocity) to pulsed tissue Doppler-derived e′ of the mitral annulus can be used to estimate LV filling pressures at rest and during exercise. Healthy individuals will show a similar increase in mitral E and annular e′, such that the ratio has no or minimal change with exercise. Patients with impaired LV relaxation develop an increase in LV filling pressures with exercise as a result of tachycardia and the abbreviated diastolic filling period. Accordingly, transmitral peak E velocity increases. However, given the minimal effect of preload on annular e in the presence of impaired relaxation, annular e′ remains reduced. Therefore, the E/e′ ratio increases with exercise in patients with diastolic dysfunction [31, 32]. Diastolic stress echocardiography has been demonstrated to be feasible using supine bicycle exercise [31] and is based on the assumption that the ratio of early diastolic transmitral velocity to early diastolic tissue velocity correlates with invasively measured LVDP during exercise [31, 32]. The algorithms to interpret the exercise-induced changes of the E/e′ ratio are summarized in Fig. 25.5 [31]: the three different responses to exercise have a different meaning and the passage from normal to abnormal LV filing pressure is crucial to unmask patients who cannot be appropriately defined by simple Doppler assessment at rest. Diastolic stress echocardiography has been applied in several clinical settings, including patients with normal systolic function [33] and with myocardial diastolic relaxation at rest [34], patients with ischemic heart disease [35], diabetic patients [36], and those with hypertrophic cardiomyopathy [37].

The methodological approach during stress is less clearly standardized and issues remain on feasibility, accuracy, and prognostic value. The parameters should be the same as at rest, but the two-key signal of transmitral flow and annular velocities are extremely sensitive to tachycardia, which leads to diastolic wave fusion making the tracings impossible to read and to loading condition changes that can make them difficult to interpret (Figs. 25.6 and 25.7). The E/e′ ratio is somewhat correlated to increase in LV end-diastolic pressure, but it

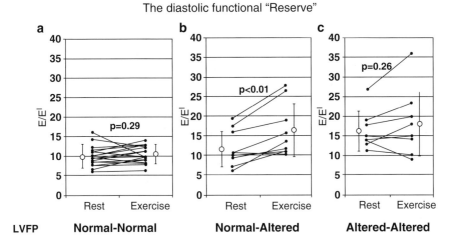

Fig. 25.5 The three possible changes of the E/e′ ratio during exercise. (Modified from [31])

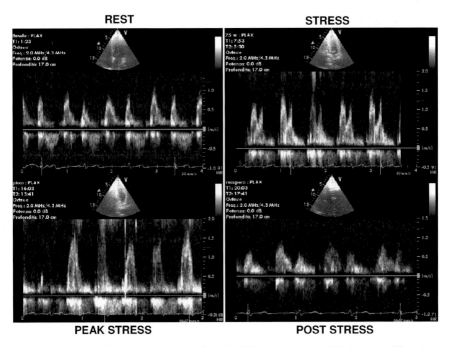

Fig. 25.6 Transmitral flow velocity tracing at baseline (*left upper panel*) and during stress. There is an obvious fusion of waves of mitral flow profile at high heart rate (*lower left panel*). The flow becomes readable again in the recovery phase (*lower right panel*)

Septal Mitral Annulus

REST   **STRESS**

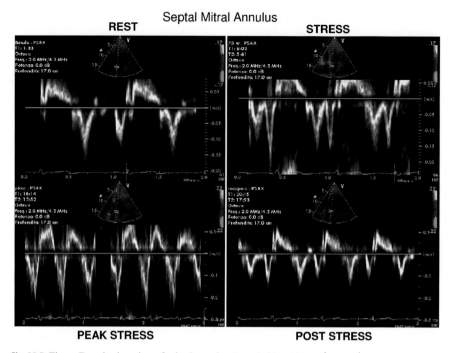

PEAK STRESS   **POST STRESS**

Fig. 25.7 Tissue Doppler imaging of mitral annulus (septal side). The 2 E′ and A′ waves are clearly distinguishable at rest and in the recovery phase, but are fused (and uninterpretable) at peak stress

can usually be measured only at submaximal levels of stress or in the recovery phase. The ventricular volumes are easy to obtain from 2D apical 4- and 3-chamber views with the Simpson biplane method, and may benefit substantially from real-time three-dimensional (RT3D) technology, which provides more information (avoiding geometric assumptions and foreshortened views inherent to the 2D approach) in less imaging time. However, they have been virtually ignored to date in the assessment of diastolic function during stress echocardiography, whereas they are a known key player in diagnosis with radionuclide angiography [38].

According to ASE guidelines on stress echocardiography released in 2008, diastolic stress echocardiography might be useful "for the evaluation of patients with dyspnea of possible cardiac origin" [39]. This evaluation is especially important in patients without inducible wall motion abnormalities, in whom dyspnea can be an angina equivalent, and in patients in whom the diagnosis of diastolic heart failure can be ascertained by the findings of resting transthoracic echocardiography, as described above. When stress testing is needed, the recommended stress is exercise, which is necessary to evoke dyspnea independent of inducible ischemia, and the semisupine approach allows the acquisition of Doppler recordings during exercise. Doppler assessment of the mitral inflow velocities should be assessed at rest, during exercise, and in the recovery when the E and A velocities are no longer fused. Doppler recordings should be acquired at a sweep speed of 100 mm s^{-1}.

There are conceptual and practical limitations to the above methodology. They include atrial fibrillation, technically challenging imaging windows, and limited validation. It remains to be seen how abnormalities in regional function influence the accuracy of a single site measurement (septal or lateral) of e′. Using pulsed tissue Doppler, early diastolic velocities are usually lower at the septal portion of the mitral annulus, where the alignment of the Doppler scan is optimal, and higher at the lateral corner where the Doppler alignment is suboptimal, but the signal is free of the influence of right ventricular longitudinal motion [40, 41]. More importantly, the value of reduced LV end-diastolic volume reserve, coupled with E/e′, remains to be evaluated as a marker of diastolic dysfunction. This approach requires two coordinates (volume and pressures) instead of one to be correctly described. Also PASP might offer ancillary, supportive information, since diastolic failure during stress induces a backward failure with pulmonary congestion. PASP is also important per se in the work-up of patients with dyspnea of unknown origin, since for instance a rise in PASP in the absence of diastolic dysfunction and valvular or other pulmonary disease can be found in patients with primary or secondary pulmonary hypertension as an initial stage of the disease, when resting values are still normal [29].

At present, we still need more data collected in a more comprehensive fashion in patients where they are more meaningful. To document diastolic dysfunction in patients with established resting systolic or diastolic dysfunction is probably of limited value. It would be more important to establish the diagnostic and prognostic correlates, and the true feasibility, of integrated (ventricular pressures and volumes, PASP and ultrasound lung comets) diastolic stress echocardiography in the subset of challenging patients such as those in the present diagnostic gray zone of diastolic heart failure. These studies are conspicuously missing to date but will determine the ultimate clinical role of the promising, challenging, yet innovative diastolic stress echocardiography.

25.4
A Roadmap to the Future

It is now possible, at least in theory, to test an array of candidate markers prospectively for the characterization of LV diastolic function during stress (Table 25.1). It is also possible to outline for diastolic dysfunction different stages of natural history, corresponding to different stages of severity, as clearly coded with stress echocardiography for systolic dysfunction: normal (at rest and during stress), initial damage (normal at rest, abnormal during stress), advanced damage (abnormal at rest; fixed abnormality during a diastolic unloading stress), and irreversible damage (abnormality at rest, fixed with an unloading stress) (Table 25.2). At most advanced stages of overt diastolic dysfunction, stress echocardiography may help in unmasking fixed vs. reversible patterns, the latter being less prognostically malignant. A restrictive fixed pattern is more dangerous than a restrictive reversible pattern, which can be at least partially normalized by nitroprusside infusion [42].

Compared to the conceptually germane systolic dysfunction, the pathophysiological basis of diastolic dysfunction is more complex, the technical approach more difficult, stresses less well standardized, and clinical experience largely immature. Still, there is

25

Table 25.1 Diastolic function during stress: the challenge continues

	Normal	Diastolic dysfunction
2D (RT3D)		
LV ED volume	↑	↔
Left atrium	↔	↑
Pulsed-wave Doppler (TDI)		
E/e'	↔	↑
CW Doppler (TR)		
PASP	↔	↑

Potential use in patients with dyspnea of *possible* cardiac origin
Still limited validation. Exercise is still the recommended stress (*ASE guidelines 2007*)
CW continuous wave, *RT3D* real-time three-dimensional, *LV* left ventricular, *ED*, *TDI* , *TR* , *PASP* pulmonary arterial systolic pressure 2D (RT3D), Pulsed-wave Doppler (TDI), CW Doppler (TR) in bold.
Legend: *ED* end-diastole, *TDI* Tissue Doppler imaging. *TR* Tricuspid regurgitation

Table 25.2 Stages of diastolic dysfunction

	Rest	Stress	Which stress	Key parameter
Stage I (normal)	Normal	Normal	Exercise	E/E'
Stage II (initial)	Normal	Abnormal	Exercise	E/E'
Stage III (advanced)	Abnormal	Normal	Nitroprusside	E wave DT
Stage IV (irreversible)	Abnormal	Abnormal	Nitroprusside	E wave DT

DT deceleration time

little doubt that diastolic dysfunction exists: it is clinically and prognostically important in CAD and in many other patients such as cardiomyopathy, valvular, and congenital heart disease patients, and echocardiography must find a better way to study it.

References

1. Gibbons RJ, Abrams J, Chatterjee K, et al; American College of Cardiology; American Heart Association Task Force on practice guidelines (Committee on the Management of Patients With Chronic Stable Angina) (2003) ACC/AHA 2002 guideline update for the management of patients with chronic stable angina-summary article: a report of the American College of Cardiology/American Heart Association Task Force on practice guidelines. [Committee on the Management of Patients With Chronic Stable Angina]. J Am Coll Cardiol 41:159K–168K
2. Fox K, Garcia MA, Ardissino D, et al (2006) Task Force on the Management of Stable Angina Pectoris of the European Society of Cardiology; ESC Committee for Practice Guidelines (CPG). Guidelines on the management of stable angina pectoris: executive summary: the Task Force on the Management of Stable Angina Pectoris of the European Society of Cardiology. Eur Heart J 27:1341–1381

3. Appleton CP, Hatle LK, Popp RL (1988) Relation of transmitral flow velocity patterns to left ventricular diastolic function: new insights from a combined hemodynamic and Doppler echocardiographic study. J Am Coll Cardiol 12:426–440

4. Lang RM, Bierig M, Devereux RB, et al; Chamber Quantification Writing Group; American Society of Echocardiography's Guidelines and Standards Committee; European Association of Echocardiography (2005) Recommendations for chamber quantification: a report from the American Society of Echocardiography's Guidelines and Standards Committee and the Chamber Quantification Writing Group, developed in conjunction with the European Association of Echocardiography, a branch of the European Society of Cardiology. J Am Soc Echocardiogr 18:1440–1463

5. Pellikka PA, Nagueh SF, Elhendy AA, et al; American Society of Echocardiography (2007) American Society of Echocardiography recommendations for performance, interpretation, and application of stress echocardiography. J Am Soc Echocardiogr 20:1021–1041

6. Sicari R, Nihoyannopoulos P, Evangelista A, et al (2008) Stress echocardiography consensus statement of the European Association of Echocardiography. Eur J Echocardiogr 9:415–437

7. Gaasch WH, Levine HJ, Quinones MA, et al (1976) Left ventricular compliance: mechanisms and clinical implications. Am J Cardiol 38:645–653

8. Glantz SA, Parmley WW (1978) Factors which affect the diastolic pressure-volume curve. Circ Res 42:171–180

9. Mor-Avi V, Vignon P, Koch R, et al (1997) Segmental analysis of color kinesis images: new method for quantification of the magnitude and timing of endocardial motion during left ventricular systole and diastole. Circulation 95:2082–2097

10. Labovitz AJ, Pearson AC (1987) Evaluation of left ventricular diastolic function: clinical relevance and recent Doppler echocardiographic insights. Am Heart J 114:836–851

11. Chierchia S, Patrono C, Distante A, et al (1982) Effects of intravenous prostacyclin in variant angina. Circulation 65:470–477

12. Picano E, Simonetti I, Carpeggiani C, et al (1989) Regional and global biventricular function during dipyridamole stress testing. Am J Cardiol 63:429–432

13. Picano E (1992) Stress echocardiography. From pathophysiological toy to diagnostic tool. Circulation 85:1604–1612

14. Pinamonti B, Lenarda AD, Nucifora G, et al (2007) Incremental prognostic value of restrictive filling pattern in hypertrophic cardiomyopathy: a Doppler echocardiographic study. Eur J Echocardiogr 9:466–471

15. Pratali L, Otasevic P, Picano E (2005) The additive prognostic value of restrictive pattern and dipyridamole-induced contractile reserve in idiopathic dilated cardiomyopathy. Eur J Heart Fail 7:844–851

16. Galderisi M (2005) Diastolic dysfunction and diastolic heart failure: diagnostic, prognostic and therapeutic aspects. Cardiovasc Ultrasound 3:9

17. Paulus WJ, Tschöpe C, Sanderson JE, et al (2007) How to diagnose diastolic heart failure: a consensus statement on the diagnosis of heart failure with normal left ventricular ejection fraction by the Heart Failure and Echocardiography Associations of the European Society of Cardiology. Eur Heart J 28:2539–2550

18. Lang RM, Bierig M, Devereux RB, et al (2005) Chamber Quantification Writing Group; American Society of Echocardiography's Guidelines and Standards Committee; European Association of Echocardiography. Recommendations for chamber quantification: a report from the American Society of Echocardiography's Guidelines and Standards Committee and the Chamber Quantification Writing Group, developed in conjunction with the European Association of Echocardiography, a branch of the European Society of Cardiology. J Am Soc Echocardiogr 8:1440–1463

19. Bombardini T, Picano E, Neglia D et al (2008) Prognostic value of left-ventricular and peripheral vascular performance in patients with dilated cardiomyopathy. J Nucl Cardiol 15:353–362

20. Pritchett AM, Mahoney DW, Jacobsen SJ, et al (2005) Diastolic dysfunction and left atrial volume: a population-based study. J Am Coll Cardiol 45:87–92

21. Ommen SR, Nishimura RA, Appleton CP, et al (2008) Clinical utility of Doppler echocardiography and tissue Doppler imaging in the estimation of left ventricular filling pressures: a comparative simultaneous Doppler-catheterization study. Circulation 102:1788–1794

22. Bess RL, Khan S, Rosman HS, et al (2006) Technical aspects of diastology: why mitral inflow and tissue Doppler imaging are the preferred parameters? Echocardiography 23:332–339

23. Tsang TS, Abhayaratna WP, Barnes ME, Miyasaka Yet al (2006) Prediction of cardiovascular outcomes with left atrial size: is volume superior to area or diameter? J Am Coll Cardiol 47:1018–1023

24. Bella JN, Palmieri V, Roman MJ, et al (2002) Mitral ratio of peak early to late diastolic filling velocity as a predictor of mortality in middle-aged and elderly adults: the Strong Heart Study. Circulation 105:1928–1933

25. Pinamonti B, Di Lenarda A, Sinagra G, et al (1993) Restrictive left ventricular filling pattern in dilated cardiomyopathy assessed by Doppler echocardiography: clinical, echocardiographic and hemodynamic correlations and prognostic implications. Heart Muscle Disease Study Group. J Am Coll Cardiol 22:808–815

26. Pratali L, Rigo F, Picano E et al (2005) The additive prognostic value of restrictive pattern and dipyridamole-induced contractile reserve in idiopathic dilated cardiomyopathy. Eur J Heart Fail 7:844–851

27. Bangalore S, Yao SS, Chaudhry FA (2007) Role of left atrial size in risk stratification and prognosis of patients undergoing stress echocardiography. J Am Coll Cardiol 50:1254–1262

28. Agricola E, Picano E, Oppizzi M, et al (2006) Assessment of stress-induced pulmonary interstitial edema by chest ultrasound during exercise echocardiography and its correlation with left ventricular function. J Am Soc Echocardiogr 19:457–463

29. Agricola E, Oppizzi M, Pisani M, et al (2004) Stress echocardiography in heart failure. Cardiovasc Ultrasound 2:11

30. Capomolla S, Pozzoli M, Opasich C, Febo O, et al (1997) Dobutamine and nitroprusside infusion in patients with severe congestive heart failure: hemodynamic improvement by discordant effects on mitral regurgitation, left atrial function, and ventricular function. Am Heart J 134:1089–1098

31. Ha JW, Oh JK, Pellikka PA, et al (2005) Diastolic stress echocardiography: a novel noninvasive diagnostic test for diastolic dysfunction using supine bicycle exercise Doppler echocardiography. J Am Soc Echocardiogr 8:63–68

32. Burgess MI, Jenkins C, Sharman JE, et al (2006) Diastolic stress echocardiography: hemodynamic validation and clinical significance of estimation of ventricular filling pressure with exercise. J Am Coll Cardiol 47:1891–1900

33. Talreja DR, Nishimura RA, Oh JK (2007) Estimation of left ventricular filling pressure with exercise by Doppler echocardiography in patients with normal systolic function: a simultaneous echocardiographic-cardiac catheterization study. J Am Soc Echocardiogr 20:477–479

34. Ha JW, Choi D, Park S, et al (2008) Left ventricular diastolic functional reserve during exercise in patients with impaired myocardial relaxation at rest. Heart [Epub ahead of print]

35. Podolec P, Rubís P, Tomkiewicz-Pajak L, et al (2008) Usefulness of the evaluation of left ventricular diastolic function changes during stress echocardiography in predicting exercise capacity in patients with ischemic heart failure. J Am Soc Echocardiogr 21:834–840

36. Ha JW, Lee HC, Kang ES, et al (2007) Abnormal left ventricular longitudinal functional reserve in patients with diabetes mellitus: implication for detecting subclinical myocardial dysfunction using exercise tissue Doppler echocardiography. Heart 93:1571–1576

37. Ha JW, Ahn JA, Kim JM, Choi EYet al (2006) Abnormal longitudinal myocardial functional reserve assessed by exercise tissue Doppler echocardiography in patients with hypertrophic cardiomyopathy. J Am Soc Echocardiogr 19:1314–1319

38. Meine TJ, Hanson MW, Borges-Neto S (2004) The additive value of combined assessment of myocardial perfusion and ventricular function studies. J Nucl Med 45:1721–1724

39. Douglas PS, Khandheria B, Stainback RF, et al; American College of Cardiology Foundation Appropriateness Criteria Task Force; American Society of Echocardiography; American College of Emergency Physicians; American Heart Association; American Society of Nuclear Cardiology; Society for Cardiovascular Angiography and Interventions; Society of Cardiovascular Computed Tomography; Society for Cardiovascular Magnetic Resonance. ACCF/ASE/ACEP/AHA/ASNC/SCAI/SCCT/SCMR (2008) Appropriateness criteria for stress echocardiography: a report of the American College of Cardiology Foundation Appropriateness Criteria Task Force, American Society of Echocardiography, American College of Emergency Physicians, American Heart Association, American Society of Nuclear Cardiology, Society for Cardiovascular Angiography and Interventions, Society of Cardiovascular Computed Tomography, and Society for Cardiovascular Magnetic Resonance: endorsed by the Heart Rhythm Society and the Society of Critical Care Medicine. Circulation 117:1478–1497

40. Sohn DW, Chai IH, Lee DJ, et al (1997) Assessment of mitral annulus velocity by Doppler tissue imaging in the evaluation of left ventricular diastolic function. J Am Coll Cardiol 30:474–480

41. Innelli P, Sanchez R, Marra F, et al (2008) The impact of aging on left ventricular longitudinal function in healthy subjects: a pulsed tissue Doppler study. Eur J Echocardiogr 9:241–249

42. Pozzoli M, Traversi E, Cioffi G, et al (1997) Loading manipulations improve the prognostic value of Doppler evaluation of mitral flow in patients with chronic heart failure. Circulation 95:1222–1230

Endothelial Function in the Stress Echocardiography Laboratory

26

Eugenio Picano

26.1
Introduction

Endothelial dysfunction is an early stage of atherosclerotic disease [1], which may progress to impairment in coronary flow reserve in the intermediate stage and then to stress-induced dysfunction in the advanced stages (Fig. 26.1). The challenge of endothelial function can be obtained through a physical (postischemic dilation) and a pharmacological (nitrate-induced vasodilation) challenge. Technologically, the assessment of endothelial function employs the same basic echocardiography hardware of stress echocardiography testing, with a higher frequency transducer [1]. Similar know-how and training are also required for accurate measurements of two-dimensional (2D) echocardiography images and Doppler signals from the brachial artery. The additional technological and cultural burden required to implement the technique is high for a hypertension specialist or a cardiologist without echocardiography training and only modest for a cardiologist already skilled in echocardiography. The endothelial function is attractive for a cardiologist because of the potential it has to supply important pathophysiological, diagnostic, and prognostic information currently missed by our noninvasive testing modalities. Endothelial dysfunction is a key factor in the onset and development of atherosclerosis, hypertension, and heart failure, as it is also a serious candidate to bridge the gap between hemodynamic atherosclerotic burden and occurrence of clinical events [2]. It is placed exactly in the physiological scotoma of stress echocardiography, which somewhat measures the functional or hemodynamic impact of a coronary stenosis [3] but is unable to assess the status of endothelial function, allegedly responsible for many catastrophic cardiovascular events.

Endothelial dysfunction is also and mainly a biomarker of atherosclerosis. In 2001, a working group of the National Institutes of Health standardized the definition of a biomarker as a "characteristic that is objectively measured and established as an indicator of normal biological pathologic processes, pathogenic processes, or pharmacologic responses to a therapeutic intervention" [4]. A biomarker may be measured on a biosample (such as

E. Picano, *Stress Echocardiography*,
© Springer-Verlag Berlin Heidelberg 2009

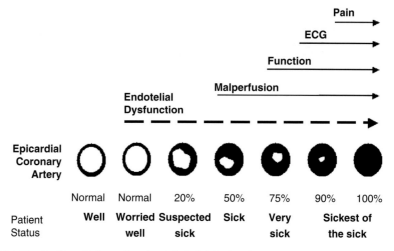

Fig. 26.1 The timeline of atherosclerosis. Endothelial dysfunction occurs early in the natural history of atherosclerosis

a blood test, for instance, the D-dimer as a biomarker of vulnerable blood) or it may be an imaging test (for instance, echocardiogram for vulnerable myocardium). A simplistic way to think of biomarkers (including endothelial dysfunction) is as indicators of a disease trait (risk factor or risk marker), a disease state (preclinical or clinical), or a disease rate (progression). Biomarkers may also serve as surrogate end points. Although there is limited consensus on this issue, a surrogate end point is one that can be used as an outcome in clinical trials to evaluate the safety and effectiveness of therapies in lieu of measurements of true outcome of interest. Surrogate end points (for instance, endothelial dysfunction in hypertensives in lieu of major cardiovascular events) have the advantage that they may be gathered in a shorter time frame and with less expense than end points such as morbidity and mortality, which require large clinical trials for evaluation. A biomarker will be of clinical value only if it is accurate, it is reproducibly obtained in a standardized fashion, it is acceptable to the patient, it is easy to interpret by the clinician, it has high sensitivity and specificity for the outcome it is expected to identify, and it explains a reasonable proportion of the outcome independent of established predictors (in case of atherosclerosis, Framingham Heart Study risk score) [4]. As a biomarker of atherosclerosis, endothelial dysfunction assessed by brachial ultrasound meets only some of these criteria (Table 26.1), and the deceptively simple methodology and pathophysiologically sweet appearance of the technique may harbor, at the present stage of technology and knowledge, substantial inaccuracies.

26.2
Historical Background

Endothelial surface totals about $27,000 \, m^2$, an extension similar to a football field, and represents the largest epithelial surface of the body. It was long considered "little more than a sheet of nucleated cellophane," according to the definition of Florey, the Nobel

Table 26.1 Ultrasound biomarkers for identifying the vulnerable patient (adapted and modified from [4])

	Methodology standardized	Methodology available/ convenient	Linked to disease progression	Addictive to FHS risk score	Tracks with disease treatments
Arterial vulnerability					
• Structural markers (carotid IMT)	++	+	++	+	+
• Functional markers (endothelial dysfunction)	+	+	?	?	+
Myocardial vulnerability					
• Structural markers (LVH, LV dysfunction)	++	++	++	?	++
• Functional markers (stress echo)	++	++	++	++	++

++ Good evidence, + some evidence, ? unknown or ambiguous data
LVH left ventricular hypertrophy, *LV* left ventricle, *FHS* Framingham heart study

Prize winner for medicine for his work on penicillin. Actually, the endothelium not only serves as a nonthrombogenic diffusion barrier to the migration of substances in and out of the bloodstream, but also as the largest and most active paracrine organ of the body, producing potent vasoactive, anticoagulant, procoagulant, and fibrinolytic substances [4]. In 1992, the journal *Science* dedicated the cover page to nitric oxide (NO), referring to it as the molecule of the year. In that very same year, Celermejer proposed a novel method to assess endothelial function in a totally noninvasive way through ultrasound assessment of postischemic hyperemia in the forearm [5]. This postischemic flow-mediated vasodilation is largely mediated by NO. Clinical assessment of endothelial function shifted from the venous occlusion plethysmographic method, exclusively used by a few research-oriented centers mostly interested in hypertension and clinical pharmacology, to the widespread availability of the echocardiography laboratory, crowded by cardiologists, who expect clinically relevant information from the technique [6]. The plethysmographic technique is complex, time-consuming, technically demanding, and invasive, requiring highly skilled expertise and intra-arterial scalar administration of acetylcholine (to assess endothelial function) and nitroprusside (to assess endothelium-independent vasodilation) [6]. The ultrasonic technique immediately showed potential for much broader applications, repeated assessment and large-scale diagnostic and prognostic validations. Both plethysmographic and ultrasonic techniques assess endothelial function in the brachial artery. With invasive cardiac catheterization, endothelial function can be assessed in the coronary artery segments by measuring the vasoconstrictor response to intracoronary acetylcholine administration [4] (Table 26.2).

26

Table 26.2 Methods to assess endothelial function in humans

	Intracoronary angiography	Brachial artery ultrasound	Venous occlusion plethysmography
Target endothelium	Coronary	Systemic	Systemic
Arterial catheterization	Yes (coronary)	No	Yes (brachial)
Radiation exposure	Yes	No	No
Intra-arterial acetylcholine	Yes (intracoronary)	No	Yes (intrabrachial)
Endothelium-dependent stimulus	Pharmacological (acetylcholine)	Physical (postischemic hyperemia)	Pharmacological (acetylcholine)
Intra-arterial nitrates	Yes (intracoronary)	No	Yes (intrabrachial)
Endothelium-independent stimulus	Coronary nitrates	Sublingual nitrates	Intra-arterial nitroprusside
Risk	Yes	No	Yes
Dedicated hardware	No	No	Yes
Cost	Very high	Low	High
Time required	Hours	Minutes	Hours
Key parameter	Coronary diameter	Brachial diameter	Brachial resistance
Setting	Catheterization lab	Echocardiography lab	Clinical pharmacology
Interest	Pathophysiology	Clinical and Pathophysiology	Pathophysiology

26.3
Physiology of Normal Endothelium

The endothelium lies between the lumen and the vascular smooth muscle (Fig. 26.2). Although it is only one cell layer thick, it senses changes in hemodynamic forces, or blood-borne signals by membrane receptor mechanisms, and is able to respond to physical and chemical stimuli by synthesis or release of a variety of vasoactive and thromboregulatory molecules or growth factors [7]. These are secreted into the lumen or abluminally toward the smooth muscle, affecting vessel tone and growth (Fig. 26.2). In addition to its universal functions, the endothelium may have organ-specific roles (such as control of myocardial contractility by coronary artery and endocardial endothelium) that are differentiated for various parts of the body [7]. As a result of their unique location, endothelial cells experience three primary mechanical forces: pressure, created by the hydrostatic forces of blood within the blood vessel; circumferential stretch or tension, created as a result of defined intercellular connections between the endothelial cells that exert longitudinal forces on the cell during vasomotion; and shear stress, the dragging friction force created by blood flow [8]. Of these forces, shear stress appears to be a particularly important hemodynamic force because it stimulates the release of vasoactive substances (including NO) and changes gene expression, cell metabolism, and cell morphology (Fig. 26.3). Many blood

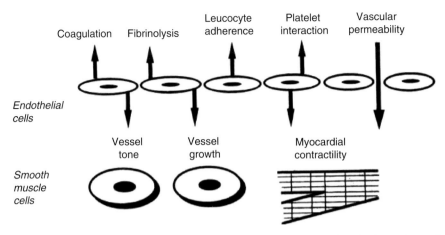

Fig. 26.2 The functional versatility of the endothelial cell. Factors secreted into the lumen (*upward arrows*) include prostacyclin and t-PA, which influence coagulation. Cell surface adhesion molecules (such as intercellular adhesion molecules-1, ICAM-1) and vascular cell adhesion molecule-1 (VCAM-1) regulate leukocyte adhesion. Factors secreted abluminally (toward the smooth muscle, *downward arrows*) may influence vessel tone and growth. Coronary artery and endocardial endothelium may also influence myocardial contractility. (From [7], with permission)

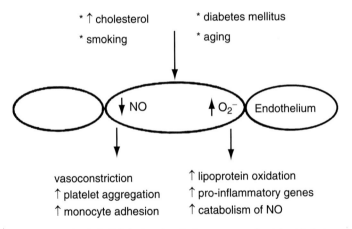

Fig. 26.3 A radical view of endothelial dysfunction. In the presence of certain risk factors, endothelial cells may produce less nitric oxide (NO) or more oxygen-derived free radicals (such as O_2^-) or both. This may lead to a variety of proischemic or proatherogenic effects. (From [7], with permission)

vessels respond to an increase in flow, or more precisely shear stress, by dilating (Fig. 26.3). This phenomenon is designated flow-mediated dilation. The principal mediator of flow-mediated vasodilation is endothelium-derived NO produced by endothelial nitric oxide synthase (eNOS), although other mediators such as endothelium-derived prostanoids or the putative endothelium-derived hyperpolarizing factor can cause vasodilation if NO

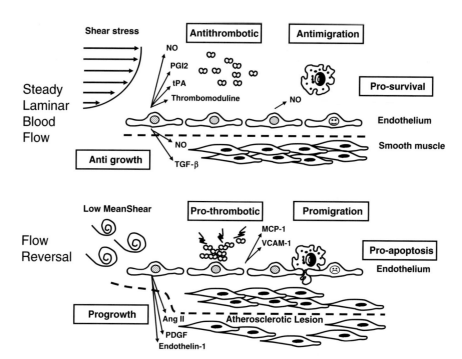

Fig. 26.4 Endothelial cell biology and shear stress. Steady laminar shear stress promotes release of factors from endothelial cells that inhibit coagulation, migration of leukocytes, and smooth muscle proliferation, while simultaneously promoting endothelial cell survival. Conversely, low shear stress and flow reversal favor the opposite effects, thereby contributing to the development of atherosclerosis. (From [8], with permission)

is deficient. The biological link between endothelial damage and atherosclerosis may be related to the decreased arterial bioavailability of NO. In the presence of certain risk factors, endothelial cells may produce less NO or more oxygen-derived free radicals (such as O_2), or both. These changes may in turn result in certain proischemic or proatherogenic effects (Fig. 26.4). The reduced bioavailability of NO translates into impaired flow-mediated vasodilation, which becomes a biomarker of depressed endothelial function.

26.4
Methodology of Endothelium-Dependent Flow-Mediated Vasodilation

The ultrasound technique for assessing endothelial function is attractive because it is non-invasive and allows repeated measurements. However, it also has technical and interpretative limitations [9, 10]. Until recently, the clinical instability of the technique had been magnified by absolute methodological deregulation on how to collect and interpret data. When evaluating endothelial function, these important factors should be taken into consideration:

1. Location of the occlusion device (upper vs. lower arm)
2. Duration of the brachial artery occlusion (5 min vs. 10 min)
3. Timing for detection of peak hyperemia
4. Portion of cardiac cycle during which brachial diameter should be measured
5. Time of day
6. Dominant or nondominant arm testing
7. Ongoing vasoactive medications
8. How best to evaluate vessel diameter
9. What form of nitrates should be used
10. Which are the normal reference values

In 2002, this methodological tower of Babel was replaced by the guidelines issued by the International Brachial Artery Reactivity Task Force [9], which aimed to minimize the sources of variability associated with patient, acquisition, analysis, and interpretation (Fig. 26.5). Because the magnitude of brachial artery diameter change is a fraction of a millimeter, the technique requires extreme accuracy in the methodology. According to these guidelines,

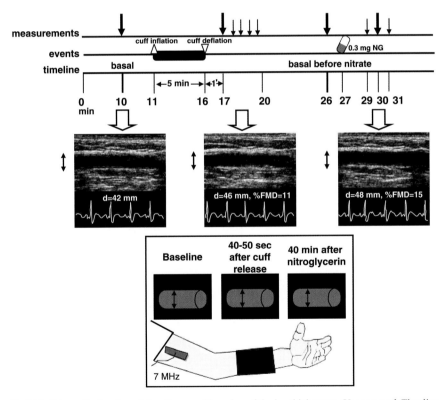

Fig. 26.5 Schematic drawing of the ultrasound imaging of the brachial artery. *Upper panel*: Timeline of events. *Middle panel*: Ultrasound imaging of the brachial artery. *Lower panel*: Cuff and transducer position. (Modified from [10], with permission)

26

the patient should fast for at least 8 h before the study. All vasoactive medications should be withheld for at least four half-lives, if possible. A linear array transducer with a minimum frequency of 7 MHz is used to acquire images with sufficient resolution for subsequent analysis. The brachial artery is imaged above the antecubital fossa in the longitudinal plane. A segment with clear anterior and posterior intimal interfaces between the lumen and vessel wall is selected for continuous 2D gray-scale imaging. After baseline rest image acquisition, arterial occlusion is created by cuff inflation to suprasystolic pressure, typically 50 mmHg above systolic pressure for 5 min. Lower-arm occlusion is preferred, since upper-arm occlusion is technically more challenging for accurate data acquisition, because the image is distorted by collapse of the brachial artery and shift in soft tissue. At least 10 min of rest is needed after reactive hyperemia before another image is acquired to reflect the reestablished baseline conditions. An exogenous NO donor, such as a single high dose (0.4 mg) of nitroglycerin spray or sublingual tablet is administered. Peak vasodilation occurs 3–4 min after nitroglycerin administration. Nitroglycerin should not be given to individuals with clinically significant bradycardia or hypotension. Variability during analysis is lowest when there is an average of three diameter measurements along a segment of the vessel. Such measurements should be obtained at baseline, during hyperemia (at least at 60 s, better every 30 s from 30 to 120 s after release, to circumvent the problem of temporal variability of response), again at baseline and 4 min after exogenous nitrates. The available technology now also makes it possible to acquire multiple images of the brachial artery automatically, using the ECG signal as a trigger. Arterial diameter is measured automatically using computer edge-detection techniques, making it possible to examine the entire time course of brachial dilation in response to reactive hyperemia (Fig. 26.6). In addition to errors related to improper techniques, it is important to be aware of a host of factors that cause intrinsic

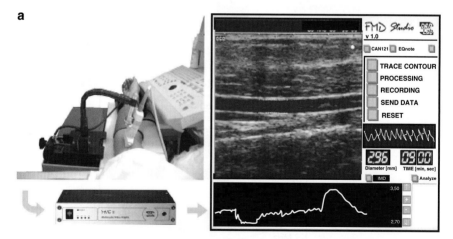

Fig. 26.6 Showing the automated edge-detection system (a), with on-line visual feedback on the quality of the detected signal. Brachial artery flow-mediated vasodilation is obtained with a brachial artery diameter measured using an operator-independent, automated software (Prototype by Marcello Demi, Institute of Clinical Physiology, Pisa, Italy). In panel b, two examples are shown, of a normal (*upper panel*) and an abnormal (*lower panel*) endothelial function

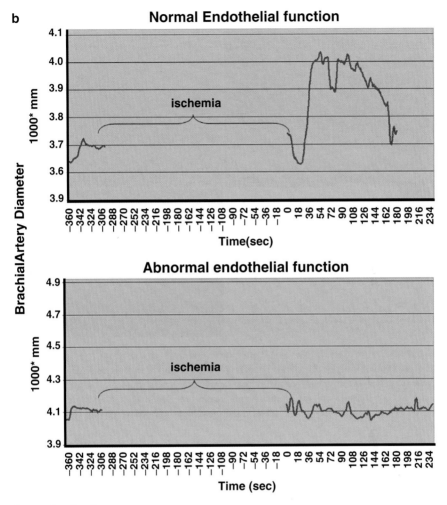

Fig. 26.6 (continued)

variability in flow-mediated vasodilation, including mental or physical stress, recent intake of a meal, medications including vitamins, exogenous hormones, cyclic changes related to the menstrual cycle in females, age, and body weight [10].

26.5
Diagnostic Value of Endothelial Dysfunction for Detection of Coronary Artery Disease

The integration of endothelial function in the stress testing laboratory has already provided some clinically relevant information. The electrocardiographic ischemic response during stress testing is in fact highly predictive of an altered systemic endothelial

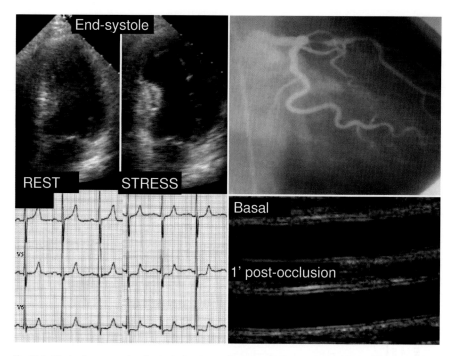

Fig. 26.7 Illustrative example of a typical pattern of test results in a patient with significant proximal stenosis of the left anterior descending artery (*right upper panel*). Exercise stress echocardiography testing (with representative end-systolic frames) reveals a dyskinetic septoapical segment (*left upper panel*) and significant ST-segment depression at peak stress (*lower left panel*); depressed brachial artery flow-mediated vasodilation (FMD) is also displayed on the *lower right panel*. (From [13], with permission)

dysfunction. This endothelial dysfunction can occur with normal (Fig. 26.7) or stenotic (Fig. 26.8) coronary arteries. The electrocardiographic information is therefore considered a misleading false-positive response compared to an angiographic standard, but a true-positive result when a physiologically relevant gold standard such as endothelial dysfunction is considered [11–16]. However, the diagnostic accuracy of endothelial dysfunction for noninvasively predicting coronary artery disease is poor, and there is no correlation between presence and extent of angiographically assessed coronary artery disease and percent flow-mediated vasodilation (Fig. 26.9). This cannot be surprising since flow-mediated vasodilation is impaired, independently of underlying coronary artery disease, in patients with coronary risk factors such as hypercholesterolemia [17], hypertension [18], smoking [19], diabetes mellitus [20], hyperhomocysteinemia [21], and aging [22]. In addition, lipid-lowering therapy [23], antioxidants [24], estrogen replacement [25], and treatment with angiotensin-enzyme inhibitors or receptor blockers [26] have each been shown to improve the flow-mediated vasodilation response, but cannot affect anatomically significant coronary artery disease.

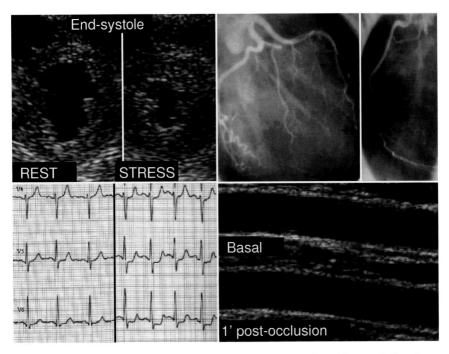

Fig. 26.8 Illustrative example of a typical pattern of test results in a patient with an anginal syndrome and normal coronary angiogram (*right upper panel*). Dipyridamole stress echocardiography testing (with representative end-systolic frames) reveals hyperkinetic wall motion response at peak stress (*left upper panel*), but significant ST-segment depression at peak stress (*left lower panel*); brachial artery FMD confirmed systemic endothelial dysfunction (*right lower panel*). (From [13], with permission)

26.6
Prognostic Value of Endothelial Dysfunction

The prognostic value of endothelial dysfunction is founded on a strong pathophysiological basis but supported, at present, by only weak clinical evidence, at least in patients with known or suspected coronary artery disease. From the pathophysiological viewpoint, the mechanism by which endothelial dysfunction may lead to cardiac events is multifactorial. One possible mechanism is myocardial ischemia secondary to endothelial dysfunction, even in the absence of obstructive coronary artery disease. Patients with abnormal coronary endothelial function often show a positive stress perfusion scintigraphy [14, 27, 28]. Another possible mechanism by which coronary endothelial dysfunction may contribute to cardiac events is through acceleration of coronary atherosclerosis, as evidenced by the development of obstructive coronary artery disease. This is also supported by the observation that in cardiac transplant patients, coronary endothelial dysfunction precedes the development of coronary atherosclerosis [29]. A number of studies have examined the prognostic value of endothelial assessment in predicting subsequent cardiovascular event risks, and ten of them were pooled in a 2005 meta-analysis [30] (Fig. 26.10). Studies have

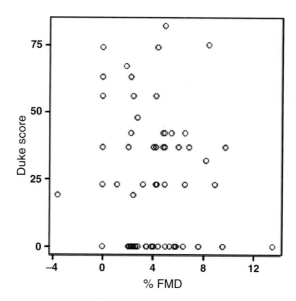

Fig. 26.9 Scatter plot diagram for angiographically assessed Duke score (*y-axis*) and percent flow mediated vasodilation (% FMD, *x-axis*) fails to show any significant relationship. (From [13], with permission)

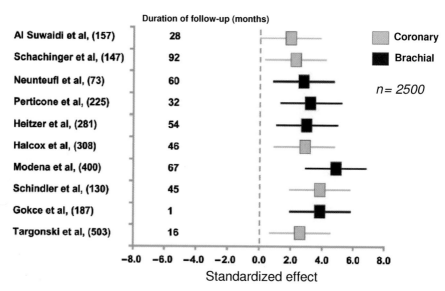

Fig. 26.10 A 2005 meta-analysis showing the capability of endothelial dysfunction to predict future cardiovascular events. In parenthesis, number of patients in each study (From [30])

differences in the method (brachial artery ultrasound, venous plethysmography with intra-brachial injection, or intracoronary Doppler flow wire), cohort of patients studied (those with established atherosclerosis vs. those with risk factors for cardiovascular disease), and design (with or without comparison with established clinical or echographic risk predictors, such as stress-induced wall motion abnormalities or carotid intima-media thickness). Taken together, these studies suggest the presence of a pathogenetic and prognostic link between (coronary or systemic) endothelial dysfunction and cardiovascular disease. In particular, the patients with relatively preserved endothelial function have a very low risk, a finding consistent with the growing evidence that endothelial dysfunction contributes to the pathogenesis of cardiovascular disease. However, these studies have also revealed that, in general, measures of endothelial function do not have additional prognostic yield in patients at high risk [31–45] (Fig. 26.11).

The ability of flow-mediated vasodilation to provide prognostic information in individuals of intermediate to low risk, independent of more standard risk-specific approaches, remains to be established. As a matter of fact, there are conceptual and pragmatic limitations in the use of endothelial dysfunction as a marker of risk. First, there is only a weak ($r = 0.36$), albeit significant, relationship between endothelial function (assessed by ultrasound in the brachial artery) and coronary endothelial function (assessed invasively by intracoronary acetylcholine and quantitative coronary angiography) [46]. Second, endothelial responses are heterogeneous within the same coronary artery or within the

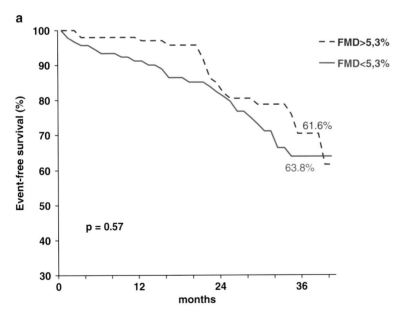

Fig. 26.11 Kaplan–Meier survival curves in patients with known or suspected coronary artery disease, whose prognosis cannot be separated on the basis of FMD values (**a**), but is clearly distinguished on the basis of echocardiographically assessed left ventricular hypertrophy (LVH, **b**) and ejection fraction (FE, **c**). (Adapted from [45])

26

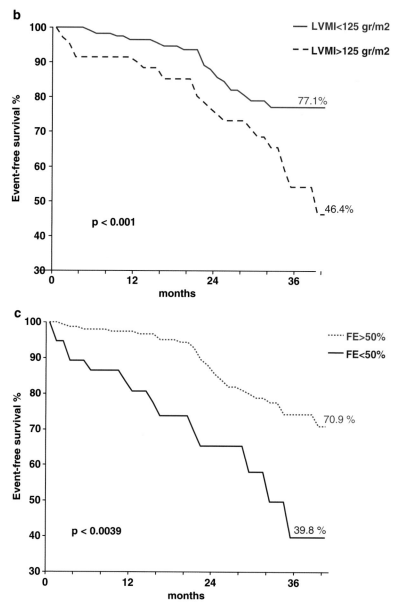

Fig. 26.11 (continued)

same patient [47], and a brachial artery endothelial function cannot be realistically considered a good predictor of endothelial function of the entire coronary tree, and much less of the endothelial function in the vulnerable coronary plaque. In the football field of endothelial layer, we are not measuring the endothelial function in the box, which is the critical region for events, but rather near the sidelines, far away from the core of the clinical action. Third, some of these studies were retrospective in nature [33]; others included highly selected patient populations with a high number of adverse events when compared to the population usually enrolled in trials [34]; in still others the same prognostic value of coronary endothelial dysfunction was shown by much simpler – and theoretically much less robust – assessment of endothelium-independent vasodilation by nitrates [31]. In one study, the prognostic value of systemic endothelial dysfunction was lost after adjusting for presence and extent of angiographically assessed coronary artery disease [35]. In another study [39], there was no prognostic difference between patients with severely (<4%) to only mildly (4–8%) depressed flow-mediated vasodilation, although both these groups had worse prognosis than patients with preserved (>8%) endothelium-dependent vasodilation. Fourth, at present, there is no clear prospective evidence for prognostic benefit after improving endothelial function, although a recent study in postmenopausal hypertensive women shows that a significant improvement in endothelial function may be obtained after 6 months of antihypertensive therapy and clearly identifies patients who possibly have a more favorable prognosis [37].

26.7
Clinical Implications and Future Perspectives

Much more data are needed at this point to establish the clinical place, if any, of endothelial function in our diagnostic and prognostic flow charts. Despite its simple appearance, ultrasound assessment of brachial artery reactivity is technically challenging and has a significant learning curve [10]. The technique has the potential to offer an individual biological dosimeter of risk exposure through endothelial function [48], to identify early stages of atherosclerotic process [49], and to monitor interventions or therapy-induced changes in endothelial function in patients with heart disease [50], but it also skill- and labor-intensive and not easily used in routine clinical practice. Furthermore, interreader variability has led to difficulties replicating data and quantifying the real magnitude of the response [10]. For the clinical purpose of identifying asymptomatic patients at high risk who might be candidates for more intensive, evidence-based medical interventions that reduce cardiovascular disease risk, the evaluation of carotid intima-media thickness [51] might be a more robust option in the setting of carotid ultrasonography, which is already established in the cardiovascular ultrasound laboratory, traditionally used to evaluate the presence of obstructive atherosclerosis in the setting of symptomatic cerebrovascular disease or asymptomatic carotid bruit [10]. The carotid scan is presently recommended for risk assessment on patients at intermediate cardiovascular risk, i.e., patients with a 6–20% 10-year risk of myocardial infarction or coronary heart disease who do not have established coronary heart disease. In the near future, an effort should be made in order to study endothelial function in clinically critical districts, such as coronary, cerebral, and pulmonary circulation. This will make the base of the current diagnostic pyramid of atherosclerosis even more solid and attractive (Fig. 26.12), which makes it possible to track the natural history of atherosclerosis at an early stage [52, 53], certainly more susceptible to a reversal than a flow-limiting, ischemia-producing plaque determining stress echocardiographic positivity.

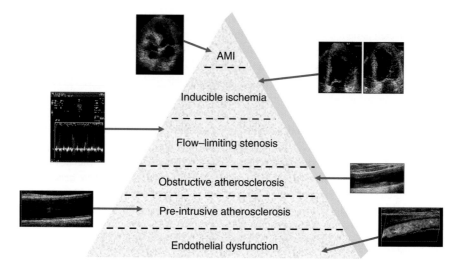

Fig. 26.12 The pyramid of atherosclerosis and the ultrasound imaging tools devoted to each of the segments of the disease: from the asymptomatic, clinically silent large base of the pyramid (endothelial dysfunction by brachial artery ultrasound) to the clinically obvious tip of the pyramid, represented by the baseline regional left ventricular dysfunction. *AMI* acute myocardial infarction

References

1. Greenland P, Abrams J, Aurigemma GP, et al (2000) Prevention conference V: beyond secondary prevention: identifying the high-risk patient for primary prevention: non-invasive tests of atherosclerotic burden. Writing Group III. Circulation 101:E16–E22
2. Ross R (1999) Atherosclerosis – an inflammatory disease. N Engl J Med 340:115–126
3. Anderson TJ (1999) Assessment and treatment of endothelial dysfunction in humans. J Am Coll Cardiol 34:631–638
4. Vasan RS (2006) Biomarkers of cardiovascular disease. Molecular basis and practical considerations. Circulation 113:2335–2362
5. Celermajer DS, Sorensen KE, Gooch VM, et al (1992) Non-invasive detection of endothelial dysfunction in children and adults at risk of atherosclerosis. Lancet 340:1111–1115
6. Wilkinson IB, Webb DJ (2001) Venous occlusion plethysmography in cardiovascular research: methodology and clinical applications. Br J Clin Pharmacol 52:631–646
7. Celermajer DS (1997) Endothelial dysfunction: does it matter? Is it reversible? J Am Coll Cardiol 30:325–333
8. Traub O, Berk BC (1998) Laminar shear stress: mechanisms by which endothelial cells transducer an atheroprotective force. Arterioscler Thromb Vasc Biol 18:677–685
9. Corretti MC, Anderson TJ, Benjamin EJ, et al (2002) Guidelines for the ultrasound assessment of endothelial-dependent flow mediated vasodilation of the brachial artery: a report of the International Brachial Artery Reactivity Task Force. J Am Coll Cardiol 39:257–265
10. Roman MJ, Naqvi TZ, Gardin JM, et al, American Society of Echocardiography, Society for Vascular Medicine and Biology (2006) Clinical application of noninvasive vascular ultrasound in cardiovascular risk stratification: a report from the American society of echocardiography and the society of vascular medicine and biology. Vasc Med 11:201–11

11. Virdis A, Ghiadoni L, Lucarini A, et al (1996) Presence of cardiovascular structural changes in essential hypertensive patients with coronary microvascular disease and effects of long term treatment. Am J Hypertens 9:361–369
12. Lekakis JP, Papamichael CM, Vemmos CN, et al (1998) Peripheral vascular endothelial dysfunction in patients with angina pectoris and normal coronary arteriograms. J Am Coll Cardiol 31:541–546
13. Palinkas A, Toth E, Amyot R, et al (2002) The value of ECG and echocardiography during stress testing for identifying systemic endothelial dysfunction and epicardial artery stenosis. Eur Heart J 23:1587–1595
14. Kuvin JT, Patel AR, Sliney KA, et al (2001) Peripheral vascular endothelial function testing as a noninvasive indicator of coronary artery disease. J Am Coll Cardiol 38:1843–1849
15. Rigo F, Pratali L, Palinkas A, et al (2002) Coronary flow reserve and brachial artery reactivity in patients with chest pain and "false positive" exercise-induced ST segment depression. Am J Cardiol 89:1141–1144
16. Cannon RO 3rd (1996) The heart in hypertension. Thinking small. Am J Hypertens 9:406–408
17. Vogel RA, Corretti MC, Plotnick GD (1996) Changes in flow-mediated brachial artery vasoactivity with lowering of desirable cholesterol levels in healthy middle-aged men. Am J Cardiol 77:37–40
18. Li J, Zhao SP, Li XP, et al (1997) Non-invasive detection of endothelial dysfunction in patients with essential hypertension. Int J Cardiol 61:165–169
19. Celermajer DS, Sorensen KE, Georgakopoulos D, et al (1993) Cigarette smoking is associated with dose-related and potentially reversible impairment of endothelium-dependent dilation in healthy young adults. Circulation 8:2149–2155
20. McNally PG, Watt PAC, Rimmer T, et al (1994) Impaired contraction and endothelium-dependent relaxation in isolated resistance vessels from patients with insulin-dependent diabetes mellitus. Clin Sci (Colch) 87:31–36
21. Tawakol A, Rorbjorn O, Gerhard M, et al (1997) Hyperhomocyst(e)inemia is associated with impaired endothelium- dependent vasodilation in humans. Circulation 95:1119–1121
22. Taddei S, Virdis A, Mattei P, et al (1995) Aging and endothelial function in normotensive subjects and patients with essential hypertension. Circulation 91:1981–1987
23. de Jongh S, Lilien MR, op't Roodt J, et al (2002) Early statin therapy restores endothelial function in children with familial hypercholesterolemia. J Am Coll Cardiol 40:2117–2121
24. Plotnick GD, Corretti MC, Vogel RA (1997) Effect of antioxidant vitamins on the transient impairment of endothelium-dependent brachial artery vasoactivity following a single high-fat meal. JAMA 278:1682–1686
25. Koh KK, Cardillo C, Bui MN, et al (1999) Vascular effects of estrogen and cholesterol-lowering therapies in hypercholesterolemic postmenopausal women. Circulation 99:354–360
26. Wilmink HW, Banga JD, Hijmering M, Erkelens WD, Stroes ES, Rabelink TJ (1999) Effect of angiotensin-converting enzyme inhibition and angiotensin II type 1 receptor antagonism on postprandial endothelial function. J Am Coll Cardiol 34:140–145
27. Zeiher AM, Krause T, Schachinger V, et al (1995) Impaired endothelium-dependent vasodilation of coronary resistance vessels is associated with exercise-induced myocardial ischemia. Circulation 91:2345–2352
28. Hasdai D, Gibbons RJ, Holmes DR Jr, et al (1997) Coronary endothelial dysfunction in humans is associated with myocardial perfusion defects. Circulation 96:357–362
29. Fish ED, Nable EG, Selwin AP, et al (1988) Responses of coronary arteries of cardiac transplant patients to acetylcholine. J Clin Invest 81:21–31
30. Lerman A, Zeiher (2005) Endothelial function: cardiac events. Circulation 111(3):363–8
31. Suwaidi JA, Hamasaki S, Higano ST, et al (2000) Long-term follow-up of patients with mild coronary artery disease and endothelial dysfunction. Circulation 101:948–954
32. Schächinger V, Britten MB, Zeiher AM (2000) Prognostic impact of coronary vasodilator dysfunction on adverse long-term outcome of coronary heart disease. Circulation 101:1899–1906

33. Neunteufl T, Heher S, Katzenschlager R, et al (2000) Late prognostic value of flow-mediated dilation in the brachial artery of patients with chest pain. Am J Cardiol 86:207–210

34. Perticone F, Ceravolo R, Pujia A, et al (2001) Prognostic significance of endothelial dysfunction in hypertensive patients. Circulation 104:191–196

35. Heitzer T, Schlinzig T, Krohn K, et al (2001) Endothelial dysfunction, oxidative stress, and risk of cardiovascular events in patients with coronary artery disease. Circulation; 104:2673–2678

36. Halcox JP, Schenke WH, Zalos G, et al (2002) Prognostic value of coronary vascular endothelial dysfunction. Circulation 106:653–658

37. Modena MG, Bonetti L, Coppi F, et al (2002) Prognostic role of reversible endothelial dysfunction in hypertensive postmenopausal women. J Am Coll Cardiol 40:505–510

38. Schindler TH, Hornig B, Buser PT, et al (2003) Prognostic value of abnormal vasoreactivity of epicardial coronary arteries to sympathetic stimulation in patients with normal coronary angiograms. Arterioscler Thromb Vasc Biol 23:495–501

39. Gokce N, Keaney JF Jr, Hunter LM, et al (2002) Risk stratification for postoperative cardiovascular events via noninvasive assessment of endothelial function: a prospective study. Circulation 105:1567–1572

40. Targonski PV, Bonetti PO, Pumper GM, et al (2003) Coronary endothelial dysfunction is associated with an increased risk of cerebrovascular events. Circulation 107:2805–2809

41. Fathi R, Haluska B, Isbel N, et al (2004) The relative importance of vascular structure and function in predicting cardiovascular events. J Am Coll Cardiol 43:616–623

42. Frick M, Suessenbacher A, Alber HF, et al (2005) Prognostic value of brachial artery endothelial function and wall thickness. J Am Coll Cardiol 46:1006–1010

43. Yeboah J, Crouse JR, Hsu FC, et al (2007) Brachial flow-mediated dilation predicts incident cardiovascular events in older adults: the Cardiovascular Health Study. Circulation 115:2390–2397

44. Shimbo D, Grahame-Clarke C, Miyake Y, et al (2007) The association between endothelial dysfunction and cardiovascular outcomes in a population-based multi-ethnic cohort. Atherosclerosis 192:197–203

45. Venneri L, Varga A, Picano E, et al (2007) The elusive prognostic value of systemic endothelial function in patients with chest pain syndrome. Int J Cardiol 119:109–111

46. Anderson TJ, Uehata A, Gerhard MD, et al (1995) Close relation of endothelial function in the human coronary and peripheral circulations. J Am Coll Cardiol 26:1235–1241

47. El-Tamimi H, Mansour M, Wargovich TJ, et al (1994) Constrictor and dilator responses to intracoronary acetylcholine in adjacent segments of the same coronary artery in patients with coronary artery disease. Circulation 89:45–51

48. Poggianti E, Venneri L, Picano E, et al (2003) Aortic valve sclerosis is associated with systemic endothelial dysfunction. J Am Coll Cardiol 41:136–141

49. Morelos M, Amyot R, Picano E et al (2001) Effect of coronary bypass and cardiac valve surgery on systemic endothelial function. Am J Cardiol 87:364–366

50. Fábián E, Varga A, Picano E, et al (2004) Effect of simvastatin on endothelial function in cardiac syndrome X patients. Am J Cardiol 94:652–655

51. Pignoli P, Tremoli E, Poli A, et al (1986) Intimal plus medial thickness of the arterial wall: a direct measurement with ultrasound imaging. Circulation 74:1399–1406

52. Gaeta G, De Michele M, Cuomo S, et al (2000) Arterial abnormalities in the offspring of patients with premature myocardial infarction. N Engl J Med 343:840–846

53. Cuomo S, Guarini P, Gaeta G, et al (2002) Increased carotid intima-media thickness in children-adolescents, and young adults with a parental history of premature myocardial infarction. Eur Heart J 23:1345–1350

In Front of The Patient:
Clinical Applications in Different
Patient Subsets

Special Subsets of Angiographically Defined Patients: Normal Coronary Arteries, Single-Vessel Disease, Left Main Coronary Artery Disease, Patients Undergoing Coronary Revascularization

Eugenio Picano and Rosa Sicari

27.1
Normal Coronary Arteries

In patients undergoing coronary angiography for investigation of chest pain, the incidence of normal or near-normal coronary arteriographic findings varies between 10 and 20% [1]. In general, patients without significant epicardial coronary artery disease have an excellent prognosis, but not all nonsignificant stenoses are created prognostically equal, since coronary events are rare in patients with smooth, normal arteriograms, sixfold more frequent in patients with mild (0–20% stenosis) and 15-fold more frequent in patients with moderate (20–40%, and still nonsignificant) lesions [2]. Even with most conservative reading criteria, stress echocardiography positivity occurs in 10–20% of patients with angiographically nonsignificant coronary artery disease [3]. The presence of minor, nonsignificant coronary angiographic abnormalities is four times more frequent in patients with an abnormal stress echocardiogram than in patients with a normal one (Fig. 27.1). At long-term (9 years) follow-up, hard events are ten times more frequent in patients with positive stress echocardiographic results than in those with negative stress echocardiographic results [3]. The "anatomical lies" of stress echocardiography, i.e., false-positive responses occurring in patients with nonsignificant epicardial coronary artery disease, can be turned into "prognostic truths" when long-term outcome is considered. Milder forms of reduction in regional coronary flow reserve and/or abnormal coronary microcirculatory function may occur in patients with angiographically normal coronary arteries and may give rise to a positive perfusion scan [4], as described in the alternative ischemic cascade [5]. More advanced degrees of reduction in coronary flow reserve may lead to subendocardial underperfusion above the threshold necessary to trigger a critical ischemic mass evoking the transient dyssynergy. The prerequisite of stress echocardiography positivity is true myocardial ischemia.

E. Picano, *Stress Echocardiography*,
© Springer-Verlag Berlin Heidelberg 2009

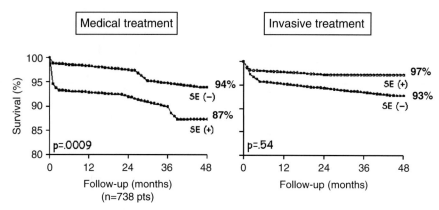

Fig. 27.1 Cumulative rates of survival free of hard cardiac events (death and nonfatal infarction) in patients with single-vessel disease treated medically ($n = 494$) or invasively ($n = 260$). Patients had pharmacological stress echocardiography with dipyridamole ($n = 576$) or dobutamine ($n = 178$). Among medically treated patients, event-free survival was worse in those with positive results on pharmacological stress echocardiography than in those with negative results; this indicates the usefulness of pharmacological stress echocardiography in risk stratification of patients in an angiographically benign subgroup. No difference in survival was seen between invasively treated patients with positive results and invasively treated patients with negative results, which suggests that ischemia-guided revascularization can exert a maximal prognostic beneficial effect in these patients. (Modified from [7])

27.2
Single-Vessel Disease

The natural history of patients with single-vessel disease is generally benign, but heterogeneous [6]. The 4-year infarction-free survival rate is higher for a negative stress echocardiography than for a positive stress echocardiography result in medically, but not invasively treated patients (Fig. 27.2). Moreover, a significant higher 4-year infarction-free survival rate is found in invasively vs. medically treated patients with a positive, but not in those with a negative stress echocardiography test result [7]. The prognostic value of stress echocardiography test results outperforms the impact of the degree of stenosis (50, 75, 90 or 100%) and location of disease (left anterior descending, left circumflex, or right coronary artery), which are recognized as powerful prognostic predictors. These data conflict with the practice of performing coronary revascularization on the basis of coronary anatomical findings only, without preprocedural evaluation of the patient by noninvasive stress testing. This practice is a very frequent and particularly disturbing therapeutic option, overloading the health care system [8] and conflicting with the recommendation of the American College of Cardiology/American Heart Association Guidelines. According to these guidelines a preprocedural demonstration of myocardial ischemia is necessary, since to date there is no evidence that coronary revascularization is effective in reducing either mortality or subsequent myocardial infarction in patients with single-vessel disease [9].

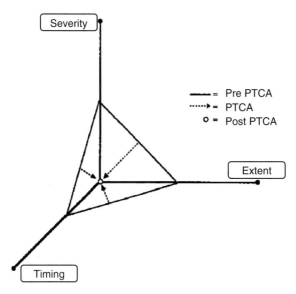

Fig. 27.2 A completely successful percutaneous transluminal coronary angioplasty (*PTCA*). Following the intervention, the stress echocardiography test result becomes completely negative, ideally placed at the origin of the system of coordinates localizing the stress-induced ischemia. (Modified from [50])

27.3
Left Main Coronary Artery Disease

Significant left main artery stenosis is the single most prognostically important lesion involving the coronary arteries. In patients with left main coronary artery stenosis, regardless of the presence of symptoms, surgery can significantly improve survival as compared to medical therapy. Left main coronary artery disease is a formal contraindication to any further form of stress testing (see Table 27.1 of Chap. 18). Nevertheless, since testing is often done before coronary angiography, several series have reported on stress echocardiography results in this subset of patients. The overall picture is that pharmacological stress testing is reasonably safe with dipyridamole [10], dobutamine, or exercise [11], and although no pathognomonic response for left main coronary artery disease can be recognized, the stress echocardiography pattern in the time and space domain is characterized by a shorter stress time, greater extent and severity of the induced dyssynergy, more frequent antidote resistance, and longer recovery time. All these conditions should raise the suspicion of left main equivalent coronary artery disease and warrant urgent coronary angiography.

Table 27.1 Indications to stress echocardiography after coronary revascularization (PCI or CABG)

	Appropriate	Uncertain	Inappropriate
Symptomatic:			
• Evaluation of chest pain syndrome	√		
• Not in the early postprocedure period	√		
Asymptomatic:			
• ≥5 years after CABG		√	
• ≥2 years after PCI		√	
• <2 years after PCI			√
• <5 years after CABG			√

PCI percutaneous coronary intervention, *CABG* coronary artery bypass graft

27.4
Patients Undergoing Coronary Revascularization

Coronary artery revascularization with either coronary artery bypass surgery or percutaneous transluminal coronary angioplasty is an effective therapeutic procedure in the management of properly selected patients with coronary artery disease. For patient selection and assessment of procedure efficacy, a functional evaluation of stenosis is mandatory. As stated by Gruntzig at the dawn of the angioplasty era, "imaging postcatheterization permits evaluation of the physiologic significance of an observed lesion and to determine the potential effect of dilatation on perfusion distal to the lesion" [31]. In addition, a preangioplasty imaging evaluation "provides a baseline for noninvasive postangioplasty monitoring of the procedure's success. As with the patient who has undergone bypass surgery, subjective symptoms are usually a good guide, but are not sufficient for the longitudinal evaluation of the procedure" [31]. The practical impact of stress echocardiography in assessing revascularization procedures has been shown both in coronary artery bypass surgery [32–36] and in coronary angioplasty [37–49]. The main tasks of physiological testing in revascularized patients can be summarized as follows:

1. Anatomical identification of disease and geographical localization, with physiological assessment of stenosis of intermediate anatomical severity and identification of target lesion in multivessel disease
2. Risk stratification to identify asymptomatic patients more likely to benefit, in terms of survival, from a revascularization procedure
3. Identification of myocardial viability in region with dyssynergy at rest
4. Identification of restenosis or graft occlusion or disease progression

According to the conceptual framework outlined in Fig. 17.1 in Chap. 17, it is also easy to assess the results of the revascularization procedure, which may be completely successful (with disappearance of inducible ischemia; Fig. 27.3) or partially successful (with persisting inducible ischemia; Fig. 27.4). The timing of postangioplasty stress echocardiography

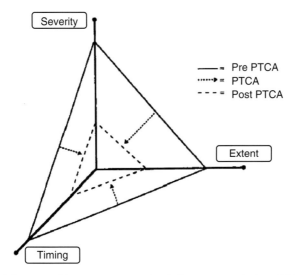

Fig. 27.3 A partially successful percutaneous transluminal coronary angioplasty (*PTCA*). The severity of the ischemic response is proportional to the *area of the triangle*, whose vertices are placed on the coordinates of ischemia. The area obviously shrinks following intervention, but the test remains positive, suggesting a primary failure, an incomplete revascularization, or an early restenosis. (Modified from [50])

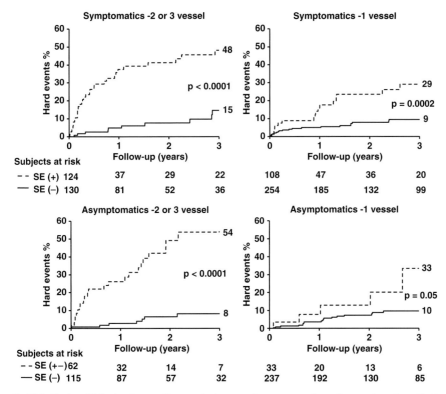

Fig. 27.4 Kaplan–Meier hard event-free survival curves for symptomatic and asymptomatic patients with multivessel and single-vessel disease, separated on the basis of the presence (*SE+*) and absence (*SE−*) of inducible ischemia. Number of patients per year is shown

varies widely, ranging from 24 h to 1 week in the various studies [36–49]. All of these studies demonstrated a comparable reduction in stress echocardiography positivity rates, ranging from 70 to 100% before and from 10 to 30% after angioplasty [50]. Stress echocardiography testing performed early after percutaneous transluminal coronary angioplasty does not seem to suffer from the reduced specificity that limits the usefulness of perfusion stress testing in this setting [51] and can be linked to the transient reduction in coronary flow reserve for reversible microvascular damage [5].

The possible physiological benefit on the regional coronary reserve determined by revascularization appears to be the most likely explanation for the improvement in stress test results. A consistently positive stress echocardiography test after angioplasty has an unfavorable prognostic implication, placing the patient in a subset at high risk for recurrence of symptoms [43, 47]. After a successful percutaneous coronary intervention, stress echocardiography positivity (with exercise, dobutamine, or dipyridamole) adds prognostic information to clinical and resting echocardiography parameters both in symptomatic and asymptomatic patients, independently of underlying coronary anatomy (Fig. 27.4). The limited, or even total, lack of improvement in the test response after angiographically successful angioplasty may have several explanations [50]. The residual stenosis may be anatomically insignificant and yet hemodynamically important because there is a poor correlation between the percentage of lumen reduction and regional flow reserve, particularly very early after angioplasty. Restenosis may be difficult to recognize on postangioplasty angiograms because of the apparent improvement in luminal dimensions secondary to extravasation of contrast into the media to the plaque, with fissuring and dissection.

References

1. Schwartz L, Bourassa MG (2001) Evaluation of patients with chest pain and normal coronary angiograms. Arch Intern Med 161:1825–1833
2. Proudfit WL, Albert VG, Bruschke MD, et al (1980) Clinical course of patients with normal or slightly or moderately abnormal coronary angiograms: 10-year follow-up of 521 patients Circulation 62:712–717
3. Bigi R, Cortigiani L, Bax JJ, et al (2002) Stress echocardiography for risk stratification of patients with chest pain and normal or slightly narrowed coronary arteries. J Am Soc Echocardiogr 15:1285–1289
4. Zeiher AM, Krause T, Schachinger V, et al (1995) Impaired endothelium-dependent vasodilation of coronary resistance vessels is associated with exercise-induced myocardial ischemia. Circulation 91:2345–2352
5. Picano E, Palinkas A, Amyot R (2001) Diagnosis of myocardial ischemia in hypertensive patients. J Hypert 19:1177–1183
6. Parisi AF, Folland ED, Hartigan P (1992) A comparison of angioplasty with medical therapy in the treatment of single-vessel coronary artery disease. N Engl J Med 326:10–16
7. Cortigiani L, Picano E, Landi P, et al on behalf of the Echo Persantine (EPIC) and Echo Dobutamine (EDIC) International Cooperative Study Groups (1998) Value of pharmacological stress echocardiography in risk stratification of patients with single-vessel disease: a report from the Echo-Persantine and Echo-Dobutamine International Cooperative studies. J Am Coll Cardiol 32:69–74

8. Topol EJ, Ellis SG, Cosgrowe D, et al (1993) Analysis of coronary angioplasty practice in the United States with an insurance-claims data base. Circulation 87:1489–1497

9. Smith SC Jr, Dove JT, Jacobs AK, et al, American Heart Association Task Force on Practice Guidelines. Committee to Revise the 1993 Guidelines for Percutaneous Transluminal Coronary Angioplasty (2001) ACC/AHA guidelines of percutaneous coronary interventions (revision of the 1993 PTCA guidelines) – executive summary. J Am Coll Cardiol 37:2215–2239

10. Andrade MJ, Picano E, Pingitore A, et al on behalf of the EPIC Study Group –Subproject "Left Main Detection" (1994) Dipyridamole stress echocardiography in patients with severe left main coronary artery narrowing. Am J Cardiol 73:450–455

11. Attenhofer CH, Pellikka PA, Oh JK, et al (1996) Comparison of ischemic response during exercise and dobutamine echocardiography in patients with left main coronary artery disease. J Am Coll Cardiol 27:1171–1177

12. Boersma E, Poldermans D, Bax JJ, et al, DECREASE Study Group (Dutch Echocardiographic Cardiac Risk Evaluation Applying Stress Echocardiography) (2001) Predictors of cardiac events after major vascular surgery: role of clinical characteristics, dobutamine echocardiography, and beta-blocker therapy. JAMA 285:1865–1873

13. Shaw LJ, Eagle KA, Gersh BJ, et al (1996) Meta-analysis of intravenous dipyridamole-thallium- 201 imaging (1985 to 1994) and dobutamine echocardiography (1991 to 1994) for risk stratification before vascular imaging. J Am Coll Cardiol 27:787–798

14. Tischler MD, Lee TH, Hirsch AT, et al (1991) Prediction of major cardiac events after peripheral vascular surgery using dipyridamole echocardiography. Am J Cardiol 68:593–597

15. Sicari R, Picano E, Lusa AM, et al on behalf of the EPIC Study Group – Subproject "Risk Stratification Before Major Vascular Surgery"(1995) The value of dipyridamole echocardiography in risk stratification before vascular surgery. A multicenter study. Eur Heart J 16:842–847

16. Rossi E, Citterio F, Vescio MF, et al (1998) Risk stratification of patients undergoing peripheral vascular revascularization by combined resting and dipyridamole echocardiography. Am J Cardiol 82:306–310

17. Pasquet A, D'Hondt AM, Verhelst R, et al (1998) Comparison of dipyridamole stress echocardiography and perfusion scintigraphy for cardiac risk stratification in vascular surgery patients. Am J Cardiol 82:1468–1474

18. Sicari R, Ripoli A, Picano E, et al (1999) On behalf of the EPIC study group. Perioperative prognostic value of dipyridamole echocardiography in vascular surgery: a large-scale multicenter study on 509 patients. Circulation 100(Suppl 2):269–274

19. Zamorano J, Duque A, Baquero M, et al (2002) Stress echocardiography in the pre-operative evaluation of patients undergoing major vascular surgery. Are results comparable with dipyridamole versus dobutamine stress echo? Rev Esp Cardiol 55:121–126

20. Lane RT, Sawada SG, Segar DS, et al (1991) Dobutamine stress echocardiography for assessment of cardiac risk before noncardiac surgery. Am J Cardiol 68:976–977

21. Lalka SG, Sawada SG, Dalsing MC, et al (1992) Dobutamine stress echocardiography as a predictor of cardiac events associated with aortic surgery. J Vasc Surg 15:831–842

22. Davila-Roman VG, Waggoner AD, Sicard GA, et al (1993) Dobutamine stress echocardiography predicts surgical outcome in patients with an aortic aneurysm and peripheral vascular disease. J Am Coll Cardiol 21:957–963

23. Eichelberger JP, Schwarz KQ, Black ER, et al (1993) Predictive value of dobutamine echocardiography just before noncardiac vascular surgery. Am J Cardiol 72:602–607

24. Poldermans D, Fioretti PM, Forster T, et al (1993) Dobutamine stress echocardiography for assessment of perioperative cardiac risk in patients undergoing major vascular surgery. Circulation 87:1506–1512

25. Kertai MD, Boersma E, Sicari R et al (2002) Which stress test is superior for perioperative cardiac risk stratification in patients undergoing major vascular surgery? Eur J Vasc Endovasc Surg 24:222–229

26. Poldermans D, Arnese M, Fioretti PM, et al (1997) Sustained prognostic value of dobutamine stress echocardiography for late cardiac events after major noncardiac vascular surgery. Circulation 195:53–58

27. Sicari R, Ripoli A, Picano E et al on behalf of the EPIC (Echo Persantine International Cooperative) Study Group (2002) Long-term prognostic value of dipyridamole echocardiography in vascular surgery: a large-scale multicenter study. Coron Artery Dis 13:49–55

28. Institute for Clinical Systems Improvement (2001) Cardiac stress test supplement. http://www.ICI.org

29. Schechter D, Bocher M, Berlatzky Y, et al (1994) Transient neurological events during dipyridamole stress test: an arterial steal phenomenon? J Nucl Med 35:1802–1804

30. Molnar T, Zambo K, Schmidt E, et al (2000) Dipyridamole test in the early detection of cerebrovascular disorders? Orv Hetil 141:2717–2722

31. Gruntzig AR, Senning A, Siegenthaler WE (1979) Nonoperative dilatation of coronary-artery stenosis: percutaneous transluminal coronary angioplasty. N Engl J Med 301:61–68

32. Sawada SG, Judson WE, Ryan T, et al (1989) Upright bicycle exercise echocardiography after coronary artery bypass grafting. Am J Cardiol 64:1123–1129

33. Biagini IA, Maffei S, Baroni M, et al (1990) Early assessment of coronary reserve after bypass surgery by dipyridamole transesophageal echocardiographic stress test. Am Heart J 120:1097–1101

34. Bongo AS, Bolognese L, Sarasso G, et al (1991) Early assessment of coronary artery bypass graft patency by high-dose dipyridamole echocardiography. Am J Cardiol 67:133–136

35. Crouse LJ, Vacek JL, Beauchamp GD, et al (1992) Exercise echocardiography after coronary artery bypass grafting. Am J Cardiol 70:572–576

36. Bjoernstad K, Aakhus S, Lundbom J, et al (1993) Digital dipyridamole stress echocardiography in silent ischemia after coronary artery bypass grafting and/or after healing of acute myocardial infarction. Am J Cardiol 72:640–646

37. Labovitz AJ, Lewen M, Kern MJ, et al (1989) The effects of successful PTCA on left ventricular function: assessment by exercise echocardiography. Am Heart J 117:1003–1008

38. Massa D, Pirelli S, Gara E, et al (1989) Exercise testing and dipyridamole echocardiography test before and 48h after successful coronary angioplasty: prognostic implications. Eur Heart J 10(Suppl G):13–17

39. Picano E, Pirelli S, Marzilli M, et al (1989) Usefulness of high-dose dipyridamole echocardiography test in coronary angioplasty. Circulation 80:807–815

40. Broderick T, Sawada S, Armstrong WF, et al (1990) Improvement in rest and exercise-induced wall motion abnormalities after coronary angioplasty: an exercise echocardiographic study. J Am Coll Cardiol 15:591–599

41. Aboul-Enein H, Bengston JR, Adams DB, et al (1991) Effect of the degree of effort on exercise echocardiography for the detection of restenosis after coronary artery angioplasty. Am Heart J 122:430–437

42. Pirelli S, Danzi GB, Alberti A, et al (1991) Comparison of usefulness of high-dose dipyridamole echocardiography and exercise electrocardiography for detection of asymptomatic restenosis after coronary angioplasty. Am J Cardiol 67:1335–1338

43. Pirelli S, Massa D, Faletra F, et al (1991) Exercise electrocardiography versus dipyridamole echocardiography testing in coronary angioplasty. Early functional evaluation and prediction of angina recurrence. Circulation 83(Suppl 3):38–42

44. McNeil AT, Fioretti PM, Al-Said SM, et al (1992) Dobutamine stress echocardiography before and after coronary angioplasty. Am J Cardiol 69:740–745

45. Akosah KO, Porter TR, Simon R, et al (1993) Ischemia-induced regional wall motion abnormality is improved after coronary angioplasty: demonstration by dobutamine stress echocardiography. J Am Coll Cardiol 21:584–589

46. Mertes H, Erbel R, Nixdorff U, et al (1993) Exercise echocardiography for the evaluation of patients after nonsurgical coronary artery revascularization. J Am Coll Cardiol 21:1087–1093

47. Dagianti A, Rosanio S, Penco M et al (1997) Clinical and prognostic usefulness of supine bicycle exercise echocardiography in the functional evaluation of patients undergoing elective percutaneous transluminal coronary angioplasty. Circulation 95:1176–84

48. Pirelli S, Danzi GB, Massa D, et al (1993) Exercise thallium scintigraphy versus high-dose dipyridamole echocardiography testing for detection of asymptomatic restenosis in patients with positive exercise tests after coronary angioplasty. Am J Cardiol 71:1052–1056

49. Hecht HS, DeBord L, Shaw R, et al (1993) Usefulness of supine bicycle stress echocardiography for detection of restenosis after percutaneous transluminal coronary angioplasty. Am J Cardiol 71:293–296

50. Varga A, Picano E (1996) Evaluation of immediate and long-term results of intervention by echocardiography: can restenosis be predicted? Kluwer, Dordrecht, The Netherlands, pp 387–399

51. Miller DD, Verani MS (1994) Current status of myocardial perfusion imaging after percutaneous transluminal coronary angioplasty. J Am Coll Cardiol 24:260–266

52. Cortigiani L, Sicari R, Bigi R et al (2008) Usefulness of stress echocardiography for risk stratification of patients after percutaneous coronary intervention. Am J Cardiol 102:1170–1174

Special Subsets of Electrocardiographically Defined Patients: Left Bundle Branch Block, Right Bundle Branch Block, Atrial Fibrillation

28

Eugenio Picano and Lauro Cortigiani

28.1
Left Bundle Branch Block

Left bundle branch block is a frequent, etiologically heterogeneous, clinically challenging, and diagnostically hostile entity. Approximately 2% of patients referred for cardiac stress testing show stable or intermittent left bundle branch block [1]. Although left bundle branch block is a recognized predictor of unfavorable cardiac outcome [2–4], the prognosis is primarily determined by the underlying cardiac pathology, including coronary artery disease, hypertension, idiopathic dilated cardiomyopathy, and aortic valve stenosis [5, 6]. The presence of left bundle branch block makes the ECG uninterpretable for ischemia and, therefore, a stress imaging technique is necessary. The presence of an abnormal sequence of left ventricular activation determines increased diastolic extravascular resistances in left bundle branch block [7] (Fig. 28.1), with lower and slower diastolic coronary flow, accounting clinically for the observed reduction in coronary flow reserve in patients with left bundle branch block [8] (Fig. 28.2), or reasonable pathophysiological substrate of the stress-induced defect often observed by perfusion imaging in patients with normal coronary arteries [9]. The altered electrical activation also affects septal wall motion, which may range anywhere between a normal and a paradoxical movement (Fig. 28.3). Normal thickening is observed in the presence of a less abnormal activation sequence (QRS duration<150 ms) and preserved contraction capability. The paradoxical wall motion is more frequent, with a markedly abnormal activation sequence (QRS>150 ms) and/or septal fibrosis (Fig. 28.3). In spite of the difficulty posed by the abnormal wall motion, stress echocardiography is the best option for the diagnosis of coronary artery disease [10–12] (Fig. 28.4): it is more specific than perfusion imaging [10, 12] and its sensitivity is good, albeit reduced in the left anterior descending territory only in presence of a dyskinetic septum in the baseline echocardiogram [11]. The prognostic value of stress echocardiography is excellent, additive when

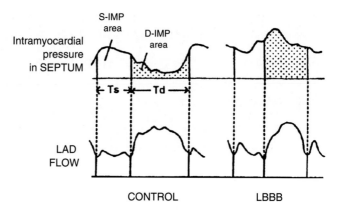

Fig. 28.1 The experimental data obtained with intramyocardial pressure (*IMP*) monitoring and left anterior descending (*LAD*) flowmetry in the dog. With normal conduction (*left panel*), the coronary flow is mostly diastolic, during the phase of cardiac cycle when extravascular resistances (expressed by intramyocardial pressure) are lowest. The induction of left bundle branch block (*LBBB*) increases diastolic resistances and reduces coronary flow. S, systolic; D, diastolic (Modified from [7])

compared to clinical and resting echocardiography variables, and especially pronounced in patients without previous myocardial infarction [13] (Fig. 28.5).

28.2
Right Bundle Branch Block

Right bundle branch block is present in 2% of patients with chronic coronary artery disease and in 3% of subjects referred for noninvasive assessment of coronary artery disease [1]. Although patients with right bundle branch block and no clinical evidence of cardiovascular disease generally have a favorable outcome [3, 6, 9], right bundle branch block in subjects with chronic coronary artery disease is predictive of a more severe left ventricular dysfunction, extensive coronary artery disease, and a mortality rate that is approximately twice as high [4]. Stress echocardiography is an excellent diagnostic choice since right bundle branch block does not affect regional wall motion. In addition, it provides an efficient prognostic stratification, additive to simple resting electrocardiogram parameters such as left anterior fascicular block [14]. In populations referred to pharmacological stress echocardiography testing, three levels of risk are identified on the basis of stress echocardiography results and presence or absence of left anterior fascicular block: a low risk, in the case of no ischemia and no left anterior fascicular block (almost 50% of the entire population); an intermediate risk in the case of ischemia or left anterior fascicular block only; and a high risk in the case of both ischemia and left anterior fascicular block (Fig. 28.6) [14].

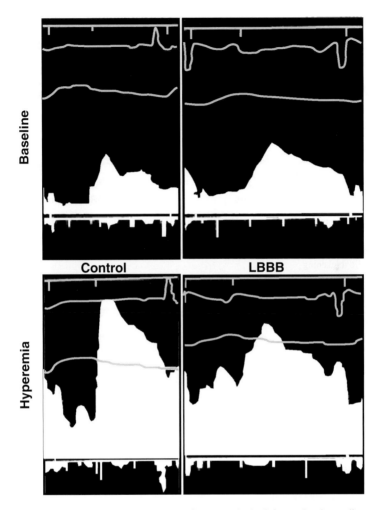

Fig. 28.2 The clinical data obtained with Doppler flowmetry in the left anterior descending coronary artery at baseline (*upper panels*) and following hyperemia (*lower panels*) with adenosine. Compared to normal conduction (*left panel*), the presence of left bundle branch block (*LBBB*) is associated with a lower and slower diastolic coronary flow velocity, especially during hyperemia. (Modified from [8])

28.3
Atrial Fibrillation

The prevalence of atrial fibrillation increases with the age of the population, being less than 1% in subjects under the age of 60 and greater than 5% in those over the age of 70 [15, 16]. Approximately 70% of individuals with atrial fibrillation are between 65 and 85 years old [17]. Coronary artery disease is one of the most common cardiovascular conditions associated with atrial fibrillation, present in 18% of chronic cases [18]. Although exercise electrocardiography is the cornerstone of noninvasive diagnostic techniques, in

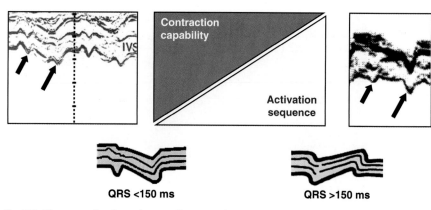

Fig. 28.3 The two major determinants of interventricular septal motion in left bundle branch block: contraction capability and activation sequence. Paradoxical wall motion is more frequent with wide QRS and/or septal fibrosis. *Small arrow* indicates early systolic septal beaking; *large arrow* indicates peak systolic thickening

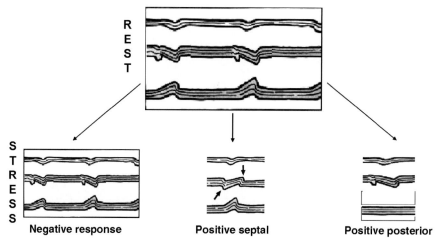

Fig. 28.4 Different types of wall motion response during stress (*lower panels*) in a patient with left bundle branch block, showing early systolic downward septal motion or beaking with normal wall motion at rest (*upper panel*). During stress, the response can be negative (*lower left panel*), with normal to increased septal motion and thickening. The stress can induce an ischemic response on the septum (*middle panel*): in this case, both motion and thickening are reduced. The stress can also induce ischemia in a region different from the septum (*lower right panel*). This location of ischemia does not raise special interpretation problems in patients with left bundle branch block. Induced ischemia depending on the pacing mode (arterial vs. ventricular pacing), in ventricular pacing mode depending on the site of stimulation

the presence of atrial fibrillation it shows several limitations. In particular, advanced age and other clinical conditions that limit the patient's functional capacity (including heart failure and bronchopulmonary disease) can reduce the feasibility of the test in patients

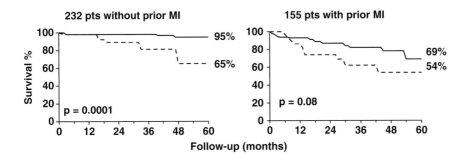

Fig. 28.5 Kaplan–Meier survival curves according to the absence (−) or presence (+) of ischemia at stress echocardiography (*SE*) and the absence (*left panel*) or presence (*right panel*) of previous myocardial infarction. (Modified from [13], with permission)

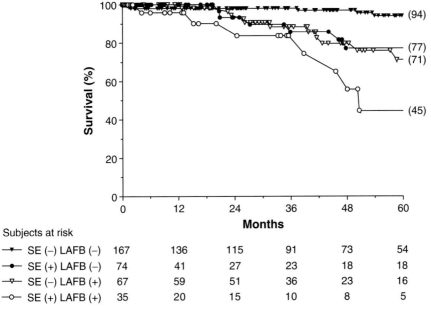

Fig. 28.6 Kaplan–Meier survival curves according to the absence (−) or presence (+) of ischemia at stress echocardiography (*SE*) and the absence (−) or presence (+) of left anterior fascicular block (*LAFB*) on the resting electrocardiogram. All patients had right bundle branch block. (Modified from [14])

with atrial fibrillation. In addition, atrial fibrillation is often associated with factors lowering the specificity of exercise-induced ECG changes, such as hypertension [18], left ventricular hypertrophy [19], and digitalis therapy [20, 21].

28

Very short diastolic intervals can contribute to false-positive responses during exercise testing in atrial fibrillation, since the diastolic perfusion of the subendocardium is impaired [22]. Stress echocardiography is an effective modality for investigating atrial fibrillation patients. In spite of the pronounced chronotropic response and, therefore, the lower doses administered [23, 24], dobutamine stress echocardiography provides useful diagnostic [23] and prognostic [23, 24] information in these patients. Moreover, the prognostic value of the test is comparable in patients with atrial fibrillation and sinus rhythm [24]. As for the safety of dobutamine stress in atrial fibrillation, conflicting results have been reported. While no dobutamine-induced adverse effects were observed in a series of 92 patients [23], a significant greater occurrence of cardiac arrhythmias was described in 69 patients with atrial fibrillation compared to controls with sinus rhythm [24]. No data are available at this time on stress echocardiography using vasodilator agents in atrial fibrillation.

References

1. Hesse B, Diaz LA, Snader CE, et al (2001) Complete bundle branch block as an independent predictor of all-cause mortality: report of 7,073 patients referred for nuclear exercise testing. Am J Med 110:253–259
2. Rotman M, Triebwasser JH (1975) A clinical and follow-up study of right and left bundle branch block. Circulation 51:477–485
3. Fahy GJ, Pinski SL, Miller DP, et al (1996) Natural history of isolated bundle branch block. Am J Cardiol 77:1185–1190
4. Freedman RA, Alderman EL, Sheffield LT, et al (1987) Bundle branch block in patients with chronic coronary artery disease: angiographic correlates and prognostic significance. J Am Coll Cardiol 10:73–80
5. Haft JI, Herman MV, Gorlin R (1971) Left bundle branch block. Etiologic, hemodynamic and ventriculographic considerations. Circulation 43:279–283
6. Schneider JF, Thomas HE Jr, Sorlie P, et al (1981) Comparative features of newly acquired left and right bundle branch block in the general population: the Framingham study. Am J Cardiol 47:931–940
7. Ono S, Nohara R, Kambara H, et al (1992) Regional myocardial perfusion and glucose metabolism in experimental left bundle branch block. Circulation 85:1125–1131
8. Skalidis EI, Kochiadakis GE, Koukouraki SI, et al (1999) Phasic coronary flow pattern and flow reserve in patients with left bundle branch block and normal coronary arteries. J Am Coll Cardiol 33:1338–1346
9. Hayat SA, Dwivedi G, Jacobsen A, et al (2008) Effects of left bundle-branch block on cardiac structure, function, perfusion, and perfusion reserve: implications for myocardial contrast echocardiography versus radionuclide perfusion imaging for the detection of coronary artery disease. Circulation 117:1832–41
10. Mairesse GH, Marwick TH, Arnese M, et al (1995) Improved identification of coronary artery disease in patients with left bundle branch block by use of dobutamine stress echocardiography and comparison with myocardial perfusion tomography. Am J Cardiol 76:321–325
11. Geleijnse ML, Vigna C, Kasprzak JD, et al (2000) Usefulness and limitations of dobutamine atropine stress echocardiography for the diagnosis of coronary artery disease in patients with left bundle branch block. A multicentre study. Eur Heart J 21:1666–1673

12. Vigna C, Stanislao M, De Rito V, et al (2001) Dipyridamole stress echocardiography vs dipyridamole sestamibi scintigraphy for diagnosing coronary artery disease in left bundle-branch block. Chest 120:1534–1539

13. Cortigiani L, Picano E, Vigna C, et al on behalf of the EPIC and EDIC study groups (2001) Prognostic value of pharmacologic stress echocardiography in patients with left bundle branch block. Am J Med 110:361–369

14. Cortigiani L, Bigi R, Gigli G et al (2003) Prognostic significance of intraventricular conduction defects in patients undergoing stress echocardiography for suspected coronary artery disease. Am J Med 15:126–132

15. Wolf PA, Abbott RD, Kannel WB (1991) Atrial fibrillation as an independent risk factor for stroke: the Framingham Study. Stroke 22:983–988

16. Furberg CD, Psaty BM, Manolio TA, et al (1994) prevalence of atrial fibrillation in elderly subjects (the Cardiovascular Health Study). Am J Cardiol 74:236–241

17. Feinberg WM, Blackshear JL, Laupacis A, et al (1995) Prevalence, age distribution, and gender of patients with atrial fibrillation: analysis and implications. Arch Intern Med 155:469–473

18. Scheler S, Motz W, Strauer BE (1994) Mechanism of angina pectoris in patients with systemic hypertension and normal epicardial coronary arteries by arteriogram. Am J Cardiol 73:478–482

19. Wroblewski EM, Pearl FJ, Hammer WJ, et al (1982) False positive stress tests due to undetected left ventricular hypertrophy. Am J Epidemiol 115:412–417

20. Kawai C, Hultgren HN (1964) The effect of digitalis upon exercise electrocardiogram. Am Heart J 80:409–413

21. Levy S, Maarek M, Coumel P, et al (1999) Characterization of the different subsets of atrial fibrillation in general practice in France: the ALFA study. Circulation 99:3028–3035

22. Ellestad MH (1986) Stress testing. Principles and practice, 3rd edn. Davis, Philadelphia, p 279

23. Hobday TJ, Pellikka PA, Attenhofer Jost CH, et al (1998) Chronotropic response, safety, and accuracy of dobutamine stress echocardiography in patients with atrial fibrillation and known or suspected coronary artery disease. Am J Cardiol 82:1425–1427

24. Poldermans D, Bax JJ, Elhendy A, et al (2001) Long-term prognostic value of dobutamine stress echocardiography in patients with atrial fibrillation. Chest119:144–149

Special Subsets of Clinically Defined Patients: Elderly, Women, Outpatients, Chest Pain Unit, Noncardiac Vascular Surgery

29

Rosa Sicari, Gigliola Bedetti, and Eugenio Picano

29.1
Elderly Patients

Individuals over 65 years of age account for 12% of the total population in the USA, twice the proportion 20 years ago. This group is expected to increase by 20% in the next decade and is predicted to constitute more than 20% of the population in the year 2030. Coronary artery disease accounts for two-thirds of all deaths in subjects over 65 years of age. More than 50% of all patients admitted to the hospital with acute myocardial infarction are older than 65. Therefore, identifying patients at high risk for future cardiac events is a particularly important and recurrent clinical problem [1]. Pharmacological stress echocardiography, with dipyridamole [2–4], dobutamine [4–7], or adenosine [6], has proved to work efficiently in elderly patients both for diagnosis and prognosis. Nevertheless, elderly patients with positive stress echocardiography test results tended to receive less coronary angiography and fewer revascularization procedures when compared to the overall population [2]. The prevalence of revascularization procedures in the group with a positive dipyridamole echocardiography was 28% in the overall study group, but only 15% in the elderly group. A relatively advanced age seems to exert a protective effect in the physician's decision concerning intervention, but this policy in time may adversely affect outcome, since a dramatic change in the natural history can be achieved by properly targeted interventions strategically oriented by the results of physiological testing. With current advances in surgical techniques and intraoperative myocardial protection, elderly patients with multivessel disease and even significant baseline dysfunction can undergo coronary artery bypass surgery with a low in-hospital mortality rate and an excellent short-term survival rate. Therefore, one may never be too old for risk stratification [1]: such risk stratification can safely and effectively be achieved by pharmacological stress echocardiography [4].

E. Picano, *Stress Echocardiography*,
© Springer-Verlag Berlin Heidelberg 2009

29.2
Women

The diagnostic accuracy of the exercise electrocardiographic stress test is definitely lower in women than in men, mostly for the low specificity (Fig. 29.1). In other words, a negative maximal test result in a woman with an interpretable ECG is reasonably accurate in excluding the possibility of coronary artery disease, but a positive test result is not sufficient to include the diagnosis. To make the diagnosis of coronary artery disease in women even more challenging, perfusion imaging also suffers from frequent false-positive results, due to physiological facts (reduction of flow reserve in syndrome X, mostly affecting female patients) and artifacts (breast attenuation) [8]. In contrast, stress echocardiography has proven equally diagnostically efficient in male and female subjects when combined with dipyridamole [9], exercise [10, 11], or dobutamine [12–14]. The prognostic value of stress echocardiography is high in women [15–19] and higher than exercise ECG, especially in the subset with positive or ambiguous response [20]. In contrast to ECG stress test and perfusion imaging, stress echocardiography is an "equal opportunity" test, with no difference in diagnostic and prognostic accuracy between males and females. When exercise electrocardiography gives positive or ambiguous results, stress echocardiography is warranted [19]. For the diagnosis of coronary artery disease, stress echocardiography is more specific than perfusion imaging and provides an accurate prognostic stratification, additive and incremental over clinical and exercise electrocardiography variables [20]. Prognosis is at least comparable in men and women with ischemia compared to those without ischemia at stress echocardiography (Fig. 29.2) [21]. The proposed policy to screen asymptomatic women at risk (for instance, diabetics) with perfusion scintigraphy and/or with 64-slice multislice computed tomography (MSCT) [22, 23] is questionable, since it ignores the radiation burden (500–1,500 chest X-rays) and the cancer risk (1 in 400 to 1 in 1,000) of

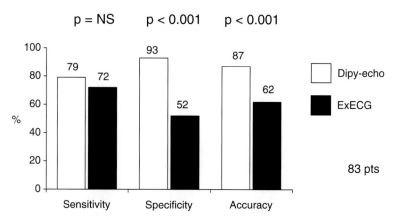

Fig. 29.1 Graphic display of the analyzed variables for the exercise electrocardiography test (*black bars*) and the dipyridamole echocardiography test (*white bars*) in a group of 68 women without previous myocardial infarction. (From [9])

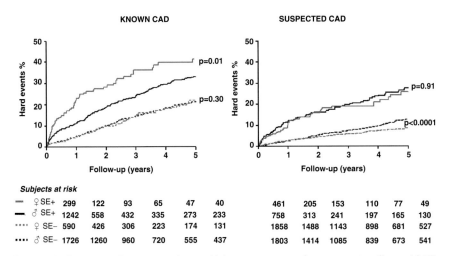

Fig. 29.2 Hard-event rate for women and men with known or suspected coronary artery disease (*CAD*), separated on the basis of presence (+) or absence (−) of ischemia at stress echocardiography. Number of patients per year is shown. (Adapted from [21])

radiation. This risk is 37% higher in women than in men, mainly because of the high radio-sensitivity of breast [24]. Guidelines and good clinical practice should incorporate the long-term cancer risk in the risk–benefit assessment of various diagnostic options in all patients at all ages of life, but especially in women of younger age [24–26].

29.3
Outpatients

In industrial countries, outpatient investigations account for more than 85% of the increasing costs of the total workload. Also in these patients, exercise electrocardiography testing remains the most effective and safest diagnostic exam. For both clinical and economic reasons, stress echocardiography should not in general replace stress ECG as a screening method [27]. In patients with nondiagnostic or ambiguous test results, stress echocardiography testing in properly selected patients can be effectively performed in outpatients, with excellent safety and risk stratification capability [28–30] (Fig. 29.3).

29.4
Chest Pain Unit Patients

A patient arrives at the emergency room complaining of chest pain. After careful physical examination, serial ECG, and blood chemistry testing, the patient is discharged home. In one out of ten cases, the patient suffers from cardiac death and/or myocardial infarction

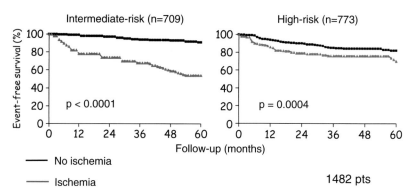

Fig. 29.3 Kaplan–Meier survival curves (considering hard events as an end point) in patients stratified according to presence (*ischemia*) or absence (*no ischemia*) of wall motion abnormalities during pharmacological stress echocardiography (with either dipyridamole or dobutamine). The separation is more obvious in patients with intermediate risk on the basis of clinical presentation (*left panel*), when compared to patients with high risk (*right panel*). (Modified from [30])

within the next month. Another patient arrives at the same emergency room complaining of chest pain. Physical examination, serial ECG, and blood chemistry testing are not sufficient to exclude myocardial ischemia. He is admitted to the hospital and discharged after 1 week with the diagnosis of anxiety. Every day, these two characters play their part on the stage of the emergency department. In the United States, approximately six million people annually undergo evaluation at the emergency department for acute chest pain: more than 50% of them are admitted to the hospital [31]. Roughly 2–10% of patients with acute myocardial infarction (AMI) are inadvertently discharged from the emergency department. The missed diagnosis accounts for 20% of indemnities for malpractice in the United States. On the other hand, inappropriate admission of noncardiac chest pain is an enormous, avoidable cost for society and loss of time for the patient. Unnecessary admission to coronary care units costs over 2,000 per day, and imposes both undue stress and potential morbidity on patients [31]. To help the cardiologist (and the patient) find the narrow pathway between risks of inappropriate discharges and the cost of aggressive admission policy, stress testing before discharge can be helpful. Patients who are more likely to benefit from testing are those with low to intermediate probability of angina on clinical grounds (Fig. 29.4), since those with typical chest pain should be admitted anyway and referred to coronary angiography. In those patients with low-to-intermediate probability, stress testing is an effective choice (Fig. 29.5). Stress testing can be performed with exercise electrocardiography, which is, as always, an excellent option with a very good negative predictive value for events in patients who can exercise maximally and who have an interpretable ECG [32], not a frequent finding in the chest pain unit. Nuclear perfusion imaging can be an alternative, but it is always complex and it can be logistically demanding in the emergency department [32]. The nuclear isotopes are strictly regulated by the Nuclear Regulatory Commission. The emergency physician may only inject the isotopes provided that he or she has undergone the necessary radiation training. Additionally, the patient has to be moved from the emergency department to a radioisotope-approved

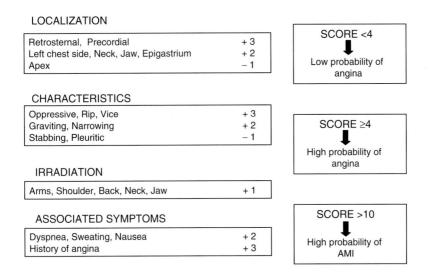

LOCALIZATION

Retrosternal, Precordial	+ 3
Left chest side, Neck, Jaw, Epigastrium	+ 2
Apex	– 1

CHARACTERISTICS

Oppressive, Rip, Vice	+ 3
Graviting, Narrowing	+ 2
Stabbing, Pleuritic	– 1

IRRADIATION

| Arms, Shoulder, Back, Neck, Jaw | + 1 |

ASSOCIATED SYMPTOMS

| Dyspnea, Sweating, Nausea | + 2 |
| History of angina | + 3 |

SCORE <4
↓
Low probability of angina

SCORE ≥4
↓
High probability of angina

SCORE >10
↓
High probability of AMI

Fig. 29.4 Chest pain score in chest pain unit. Patients with low to intermediate score are suitable candidates for stress echocardiography. Patients with typical chest pain (score>10) should be directly admitted to the coronary care unit. AMI, acute myocardial infarction (From [55])

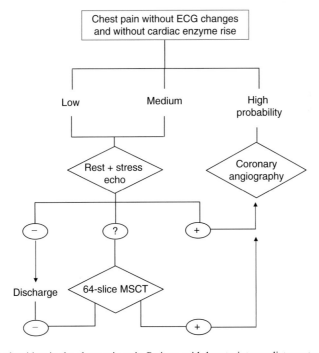

Chest pain without ECG changes and without cardiac enzyme rise

Low   Medium   High probability

Rest + stress echo

Coronary angiography

–   ?   +

Discharge   64-slice MSCT

–   +

Fig. 29.5 The algorithm in the chest pain unit. Patients with low-to-intermediate pretest probability, negative serial cardiac markers, negative electrocardiogram, negative resting and stress echocardiography can be discharged. Patients with positivity of at least one of these markers should be admitted with high probability of acute coronary syndrome

area for the duration of the scan. The simple resting echocardiography can be performed at bedside and can by itself clarify the diagnostic problem by showing a newly onset regional wall motion dysfunction (often detectable in the absence of diagnostic electrocardiographic changes) or other noncoronary causes of chest pain, such as aortic dissection, hypertrophic cardiomyopathy, mitral valve prolapse, pulmonary embolism, or pericardial effusion [33]. After the resting echocardiography has ruled out a possible cause of chest pain, stress echocardiography can be performed on-line, since the technology and know-how of echocardiography are already available at the bedside [34]. Patients with positive stress echocardiography results are admitted to the coronary care unit and almost invariably they are found to have coronary artery disease at angiography. An ischemia-guided revascularization with angioplasty is the most frequent therapeutic choice. The majority of patients had a negative stress echocardiography test result (i.e., with no inducible ischemia and no wall motion abnormalities) and were discharged home, usually without experiencing cardiac events in the subsequent 1 year of follow-up (Table 29.1). In other words, out of ten patients – who were otherwise ready for discharge – at least one has true myocardial ischemia detected by stress echocardiography. This patient can be identified and referred to coronary angiography to be revascularized. The remaining nine patients have a negative test result and can be discharged, with a probability lower than 1% of having a heart attack in the following 12 months [34–42].

In the chest pain unit, the cardiologist can find the narrow pathway between inappropriate discharge and inappropriate admissions by adding resting and stress echocardiography to the conventional clinical electrocardiography and blood chemistry testing. This would be an economically convenient, biohazard-free, and ecologically compatible imaging technique making it possible to abate costs and improve quality of health care in the critical setting of the emergency department [42].

Patients with chest pain and equivocal or normal ECGs and negative cardiac enzyme studies may be considered for stress perfusion scintigraphy [43], Coronary Artery Calcium Score assessment [44, 45], or noninvasive coronary angiography by MSCT [46–48]. The high sensitivity and negative predictive value may allow early discharge of those patients with nondiagnostic ECG and negative scans. However, the radiation burden would be

Table 29.1 Stress echo in chest pain unit

Author, year	Stress of choice	Patients (n)	Mean follow-up (months)	NPV (%)	Rate of positivity
Trippi et al. (1996)	Dobutamine	139	3	98.5	8/139 (5%)
Colon et al. (1998)	Exercise	108	12.8	99	8/108 (7%)
Gelejinse et al. (2000)	Dobutamine	80	6	95	36/80 (45%)
Orlandini et al. (2000)	Dipyridamole	177	6	99	5/177 (%)
Buchsbaum et al. (2001)	Exercise	145	6	99.3	5/145 (3%)
Bholasingh et al. (2003)	Dobutamine	377	6	96	26/377 (7%)
Bedetti et al. (2004)	Dipyridamole	552	13	98.8	50/552 (10%)
Conti et al. (2005)	Exercise	503	6	97	99/503 (20%)

NPV negative predictive value

considerably different for individual patients [24, 25] and the population [28] for each of the four different imaging strategies. Each year, roughly 6 million patients arrive at the emergency room for chest pain in the United States only [31]. Therefore, the (not insignificant) radiation dose and cancer risk for the individual patient become a significant population burden. A stress scintigraphy with thallium gives a dose of 1,250 chest X-rays, and with sestamibi a does of 600 X-rays. A coronary artery calcium scan and a 64-slice MSCT expose the patient to a dose of 100 and 750 chest X-rays, respectively. The corresponding cancer risk per exam for a 50-year-old patient is 1 in 500 for thallium, 1 in 1,000 for a sestamibi, 1 in 5,000 for a coronary artery calcium scan, and 1 in 750 for MSCT. The individual risk multiplied for 6 million admissions each year translates into a population risk of around 1,000 (Coronary Artery Calcium Score), 6,000 (sestamibi), 10,000 (MSCT) to 15,000 (thallium) new cancers each year [23–26, 51, 52]. The recent White Paper of the American College of Radiology identified the ER as a key setting for inappropriate and exorbitant radiation exposure [53, 54]. The efficiency of our diagnostic strategies should be weighted against the long-term risks, which is part of the very same definition of appropriateness [55]. If this is done, there is little doubt that stress echocardiography has decisive advantages for playing a central role in the noninvasive strategy in the ER. Also for stress echocardiography, however, the ER is a frequent source of inappropriate indications [56, 57] (Table 29.2). The most appropriate indication remains the patient with low-to-intermediate pretest probability [31, 47, 52]: MSCT might be chosen as a second-line noninvasive test, as proposed in Fig. 29.5, for intermediate-risk patients in whom stress echocardiography is unfeasible or gives ambiguous results. In high-risk patients, direct referral to coronary angiography is warranted. Cardiac magnetic resonance is promising in patients with acute coronary syndrome in the emergency department [58], but its application is currently limited by restricted access. In perspective, it would become an ideal choice in patients with nondiagnostic or ambiguous stress echocardiography results.

Table 29.2 Stress echocardiography in acute coronary syndrome

	Appropriate	Uncertain	Inappropriate
Intermediate pretest probability (no dynamic ST changes *and* serial cardiac enzymes negative)	√		
Risk assessment without recurrent symptoms or signs of heart failure	√		
Pt with prior positive perfusion scintigraphy or positive MSCT		√	
Low pretest probability, ECG interpretable and able to exercise			√
Routine evaluation prior to hospital discharge (in asymptomatic post-PCI patient)			√
High pretest probability of CAD			√
ECG ST elevation			√

MSCT multislice computed tomography, *ECG* electrocardiogram, *PCI* percutaneous coronary intervention, *CAD* coronary artery disease

29.5
Noncardiac Vascular Surgery

Perioperative ischemia is a frequent event in patients undergoing major noncardiac vascular or general surgery. From a clinical standpoint, it is well known that multidistrict disease, especially at the coronary level, is a severe aggravation of the operative risk. From a pathophysiological point of view, surgery creates conditions able to unmask coronary artery disease. Prolonged hypotension, hemorrhages, and hemodynamic stresses caused by aortic clamping and unclamping during major vascular surgery are the most relevant factors endangering the coronary circulation with critical stenoses. From the epidemiological standpoint, coronary disease is known to be the leading cause of perioperative mortality and morbidity following vascular and general surgery [59]. The diagnostic/therapeutic corollary of these considerations is that coronary artery disease – and therefore the perioperative risk – in these patients has to be identified in an effective way preoperatively. This is not feasible in an accurate way with either clinical scores (such as Detsky's or Goldman's score) or rest echocardiography. It is necessary to perform ischemic-provocative tests and, of these, pharmacological stress echocardiography appears to be the ideal first choice (more feasible than exercise electrocardiography, less expensive but more accurate than nuclear scintigraphy) [60]. The experience with either dipyridamole [61–66] or dobutamine [67–73] univocally indicates that these tests have a very high and comparable negative predictive value (between 90 and 100%); a negative test result is associated with a very low incidence of cardiac events and allows a safe surgical procedure [74–76]. The positive predictive value is at least comparable with stress echocardiography when compared to perfusion imaging (Fig. 29.6). The risk stratification capability is high for perioperative events and

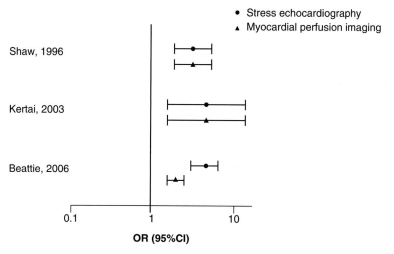

Fig. 29.6 Forest plot depicting the odds ratio (*OR*) for hard cardiac events (death and myocardial infarction) of three meta-analyses comparing (dobutamine or dipyridamole) stress echocardiography and myocardial perfusion imaging. (Modified from [60])

also remains excellent for long-term follow-up [77, 78]. To date, it appears reasonable to perform coronary revascularization before peripheral vascular surgery in the presence of a markedly positive result of stress echocardiography. A more conservative approach – with watchful cardiological surveillance coupled with pharmacological cardioprotection with β-blockers – can be adopted in patients with less severe ischemic responses during stress [79]. Risk stratification with pharmacological stress echocardiography should be probably targeted to patients over 70 years of age, with current or prior angina pectoris, and previous myocardial infarction and heart failure (Table 29.3). In other patients, the event rate under β-blocker therapy is so low that an indiscriminate risk stratification policy with stress echocardiography is probably untenable (Table 29.4). Interestingly, clearly inappropriate indications for preoperative risk stratification before noncardiac surgery (intermediate risk

Table 29.3 Noncardiac surgery: procedural and patient's risk

	Surgery risk		
	High risk	**Intermediate risk**	**Low risk**
Predictors	Unstable coronary syndromes Decompensated heart failure	Mild angina Prior myocardial infarction Compensated heart failure	Advanced age Rhythm other than sinus Low functional capacity
Procedures	Aortic and peripheral artery surgery Prolonged surgical procedures	Carotid endarterectomy Orthopedic surgery Prostate surgery Chest or abdomen	Breast Cataract Endoscopic
Risk level (cardiac death or myocardial infarction)	>5%	1–5%	<1%

Table 29.4 Stress echocardiography in noncardiac surgery

	Appropriate	Uncertain	Inappropriate
High-risk surgery + intermediate-risk patient (poor exercise tolerance ≤4 METS and/or >3 risk factors)	√		
Intermediate-risk surgery + intermediate-risk patient (poor exercise tolerance ≤4 METS and/ or ≥3 risk factors)		√	
Intermediate-risk surgery + low-risk patient (good exercise tolerance)			√
Low-risk surgery + intermediate-risk patient			√
High-risk surgery + asymptomatic up to 1 year after normal catheterization, noninvasive test, or previous revascularization			√

METS maximal exercise tolerance

surgery in patients with good exercise capacity, and low risk surgery) account for 25% of all inappropriate testing in large-volume stress echocardiography laboratories [53, 54], and therefore this field provides a key opportunity for quality improvement and targeted educational programs to achieve measurable improvements in results.

References

1. Beller GA (1992) Are you ever too old to be risk stratified? J Am Coll Cardiol 19:1399–401
2. Camerieri A, Picano E, Landi P, et al on behalf of the EPIC study group (1993) The prognostic value of dipyridamole echocardiography test early after myocardial infarction in elderly patients. J Am Coll Cardiol 22:1809–1815
3. Ferrara N, Leosco D, Abete P, et al (1991) Dipyridamole echocardiography as a useful and safe test in the assessment of coronary artery disease in the eldeyrl. J Am Geriatr Soc 39:993–999
4. Cortigiani L, Bigi R, Sicari R, et al (2007)Prognostic implications of dipyridamole or dobutamine stress echocardiography for evaluation of patients > or = 65 years of age with known or suspected coronary heart disease. Am J Cardiol 99:1491–1495
5. Poldermans D, Fioretti PM, Boersma E, et al (1994) Dobutamine-atropine stress echocardiography in elderly patients unable to perform an exercise test. Hemodynamic characteristics, safety, and prognostic value. Arch Intern Med 154:2681–2686
6. Anthoupolus LP, Bonou MS, Kardaras FG, et al (1996) Stress echocardiography in elderly patients with coronary artery disease. Applicability, safety and prognostic value of dobutamine and adenosine echocardiography in elderly patients J Am Coll Cardiol 28:52–59
7. Bonou M, Benroubis A, Kranidis A, et al (2001) Functional and prognostic significance of silent ischemia during dobutamine stress echocardiography in the elderly. Coron Artery Dis 12:499–506
8. Douglas PS, Ginsburg GS (1996) The evaluation of chest pain in women. N Engl J Med 334:1311–1315
9. Masini M, Picano E, Lattanzi F, et al (1988) High-dose dipyridamole-echocardiography test in women: correlation with exercise-electrocardiography test and coronary arteriography. J Am Coll Cardiol 12:682–685
10. Sawada SG, Ryan T, Fineberg NS, et al (1989) Exercise echocardiographic detection of coronary artery disease in women. J Am Coll Cardiol 14:1440–1447
11. Marwick TH, Anderson T, Williams MJ, et al (1995) Exercise echocardiography is an accurate and cost-efficient technique for detection of coronary artery disease in women. J Am Coll Cardiol 26:335–341
12. Ho YL, Wu CC, Huang PJ, et al (1998) Assessment of coronary artery disease in women by dobutamine stress echocardiography: comparison with stress thallium-201 single-photon emission computed tomography and exercise electrocardiography. Am Heart J 135:655–662
13. Elhendy A, van Domburg RT, Bax JJ, et al (1998) Noninvasive diagnosis of coronary artery stenosis in women with limited exercise capacity: comparison of dobutamine stress echocardiography and 99mTc sestamibi single-photon emission CT. Chest 114:1097–1104
14. Dionisopoulos PN, Collins JD, Smart SC, et al (1997) The value of dobutamine stress echocardiography for the detection of coronary artery disease in women. J Am Soc Echocardiogr 10:811–817
15. Cortigiani L, Dodi C, Paolini EA, et al (1998) Prognostic value of pharmacological stress echocardiography in women with chest pain and unknown coronary artery disease. J Am Coll Cardiol 32:1975–1981

16. Heupler S, Mehta R, Lobo A, et al (1997) Prognostic implications of exercise echocardiography in women with known or suspected coronary artery disease. J Am Coll Cardiol 30:414–420

17. Davar JI, Brull DJ, Bulugahipitiya S, et al (1999) Prognostic value of negative dobutamine stress echo in women with intermediate probability of coronary artery disease. Am J Cardiol 83:100–102

18. Arruda-Olson AM, Juracan EM, Mahoney DW, et al (2002) Prognostic value of exercise echocardiography in 5,798 patients: is there a gender difference? J Am Coll Cardiol 39:625–631

19. Cortigiani L, Gigli G, Vallebona A, et al (2001) The stress echo prognostic gender gap. Eur J Echocardiogr 2:132–138

20. Dodi C, Cortigiani L, Masini M, et al (2001) The incremental prognostic value of pharmacological stress echo over exercise electrocardiography in women with chest pain of unknown origin. Eur Heart J 22:145–152

21. Cortigiani L, Sicari R, Bigi R, et al (2009) Prognostic value of stress echocardiography in men and women with known or suspected coronary artery disease. Am J Cardiol in press

22. Mieres JH, Shaw LJ, Arai A, et al; Cardiac Imaging Committee, Council on Clinical Cardiology, and the Cardiovascular Imaging and Intervention Committee, Council on Cardiovascular Radiology and Intervention, American Heart Association (2005) Role of noninvasive testing in the clinical evaluation of women with suspected coronary artery disease: consensus statement from the Cardiac Imaging Committee, Council on Clinical Cardiology, and the Cardiovascular Imaging and Intervention Committee, Council on Cardiovascular Radiology and Intervention, American Heart Association. Circulation 111:682–696

23. Bax JJ, Bonow RO, Tschöpe D, et al; Global Dialogue Group for the Evaluation of Cardiovascular Risk in Patients With Diabetes (2006) The potential of myocardial perfusion scintigraphy for risk stratification of asymptomatic patients with type 2 diabetes. J Am Coll Cardiol 48:754–760

24. Health Risks from Exposure to Low Levels of Ionizing Radiation: BEIR VII Phase 2 (2006) www.nap.edu/books/030909156X/html

25. Picano E (2003) Stress echocardiography: a historical perspective. Special Article. Am J Med 114:126–130

26. Picano E (2004) Informed consent and communication of risk from radiological and nuclear medicine examinations: how to escape from a communication inferno. Education and Debate. BMJ 329:849–851

27. Grunig E, Mereles D, Benz A, et al (2002) Contribution of stress echocardiography to clinical decision making in unselected ambulatory patients with known or suspected coronary artery disease. Int J Cardiol 84:179–185

28. Gordon BM, Mohan V, Chapekis AT, et al (1995) An analysis of the safety of performing dobutamine stress echocardiography in an ambulatory setting. J Am Soc Echocardiogr 8:15–20

29. Cortigiani L, Lombardi M, Landi P, et al (1998) Risk stratification by pharmacological stress echocardiography in a primary care cardiology centre. Experience in 1082 patients. Eur Heart J 19:1673–1680

30. Cortigiani L, Picano E, Coletta C, et al, on behalf of Echo Persantine International Cooperative (EPIC) Study Group; Echo Dobutamine International Cooperative (EDIC) Study Group (2001) Safety, feasibility, and prognostic implications of pharmacologic stress echocardiography in 1482 patients evaluated in an ambulatory setting. Am Heart J 141:621–629

31. Stein RA, Chaitman BR, Balady GJ, et al (2000) Safety and utility of exercise testing in emergency room chest pain centers: an advisory from the Committee on Exercise, Rehabilitation, and Prevention, Council on Clinical Cardiology, American Heart Association. Circulation 102:1463–1467

32. Mather PJ, Shah R (2001) Echocardiography, nuclear scintigraphy, and stress testing in the emergency department evaluation of acute coronary syndrome. Emerg Med Clin North Am 19:339–349

33. Zabalgoitia M, Ismaeil M (2000) Diagnostic and prognostic use of stress echo in acute coronary syndromes including emergency department imaging. Echocardiography 17:479–493

34. Trippi JA, Lee KS, Kopp G, et al (1997) Dobutamine stress tele-echocardiography for evaluation of emergency department patients with chest pain. J Am Coll Cardiol 30:627–632

35. Colon PJ 3rd, Cheirif J (1999) Long-term value of stress echocardiography in the triage of patients with atypical chest pain presenting to the emergency department. Echocardiography 16:171–177

36. Geleijnse ML, Elhendy A, Kasprzak JD, et al (2000) Safety and prognostic value of early dobutamine-atropine stress echocardiography in patients with spontaneous chest pain and a non-diagnostic electrocardiogram. Eur Heart J 21:397–406

37. Orlandini A, Tuero E, Paolasso E, et al (2000) Usefulness of pharmacologic stress echocardiography in a chest pain center. Am J Cardiol 86:1247–1250

38. Buchsbaum M, Marshall E, Levine B, et al (2001) Emergency department evaluation of chest pain using exercise stress echocardiography. Acad Emerg Med 8:196–199

39. Bholasing h R, Cornel JH, Kamp O, et al (2003) Prognostic value of predischarge dobutamine stress echocardiography in chest pain patients with a negative cardiac troponin T. J Am Coll Cardiol 41:596–602

40. Bedetti G, Pasanisi E, Tintori G, et al (2005) Stress echo in chest pain unit: the SPEED trial. Int J Cardiol 102:461–467

41. Conti A, Paladini B, Toccafondi S, et al (2005) Effectiveness of a multidisciplinary chest pain unit for the assessment of coronary syndromes and risk stratification in the Florence area. Am Heart J 144:630–635

42. Sicari R, Nihoyannopoulos P, Evangelista A, et al (2008); European Association of Echocardiography (2008) Stress echocardiography expert consensus statement: European Association of Echocardiography (EAE) (a registered branch of the ESC). Eur J Echocardiogr 9:415–437

43. Marcassa C, Bax JJ, Bengel F, et al; European Council of Nuclear Cardiology (ECNC); European Society of Cardiology Working Group 5 (Nuclear Cardiology and Cardiac CT); European Association of Nuclear Medicine Cardiovascular Committee (2008) Clinical value, cost-effectiveness, and safety of myocardial perfusion scintigraphy: a position statement. Eur Heart J 29:557–563

44. Budoff MJ, Achenbach S, Blumenthal RS, et al; American Heart Association Committee on Cardiovascular Imaging and Intervention; American Heart Association Council on Cardiovascular Radiology and Intervention; American Heart Association Committee on Cardiac Imaging, Council on Clinical Cardiology (2006) Assessment of coronary artery disease by cardiac computed tomography: a scientific statement from the American Heart Association Committee on Cardiovascular Imaging and Intervention, Council on Cardiovascular Radiology and Intervention, and Committee on Cardiac Imaging, Council on Clinical Cardiology. Circulation 114:1761–1791

45. Greenland P, Bonow RO, Brundage BH, et al; American College of Cardiology Foundation Clinical Expert Consensus Task Force (ACCF/AHA Writing Committee to Update the 2000 Expert Consensus Document on Electron Beam Computed Tomography); Society of Atherosclerosis Imaging and Prevention; Society of Cardiovascular Computed Tomography (2007) ACCF/AHA 2007 clinical expert consensus document on coronary artery calcium scoring by computed tomography in global cardiovascular risk assessment and in evaluation of patients with chest pain: a report of the American College of Cardiology Foundation Clinical Expert Consensus Task Force (ACCF/AHA Writing Committee to Update the 2000 Expert

Consensus Document on Electron Beam Computed Tomography) developed in collaboration with the Society of Atherosclerosis Imaging and Prevention and the Society of Cardiovascular Computed Tomography. J Am Coll Cardiol 49:378–402

46. Haberl R, Tittus J, Böhme E, et al (2005) Multislice spiral computed tomographic angiography of coronary arteries in patients with suspected coronary artery disease: an effective filter before catheter angiography? Am Heart J 149:1112–1119

47. Goldstein JA, Gallagher MJ, O'Neill WW, et al (2007) A randomized controlled trial of multislice coronary computed tomography for evaluation of acute chest pain. J Am Coll Cardiol 49:863–871

48. Bonello L, Armero S, Jacquier A, et al (2008) Non-invasive coronary angiography for patients with acute atypical chest pain discharged after negative screening including maximal negative treadmill stress test. A prospective study. Int J Cardiol Mar 24

49. Schroeder S, Achenbach S, Bengel F, et al; Working Group Nuclear Cardiology and Cardiac CT; European Society of Cardiology; European Council of Nuclear Cardiology (2008) Cardiac computed tomography: indications, applications, limitations, and training requirements: report of a Writing Group deployed by the Working Group Nuclear Cardiology and Cardiac CT of the European Society of Cardiology and the European Council of Nuclear Cardiology. Eur Heart J 29:531–556

50. Bluemke DA, Achenbach S, Budoff M, et al (2008) Noninvasive coronary artery imaging: magnetic resonance angiography and multidetector computed tomography angiography: a scientific statement from the American heart association committee on cardiovascular imaging and intervention of the council on cardiovascular radiology and intervention, and the councils on clinical cardiology and cardiovascular disease in the young. Circulation 118:586–606

51. Einstein AJ, Henzlova MJ, Rajagopalan S (2007) Estimating risk of Cancer associated with radiation exposure from 64-slice computed tomography coronary angiography. JAMA 298:317–323

52. Picano E (2005) Economic and biological costs of cardiac imaging. Cardiovasc Ultrasound 3:13

53. Amis ES Jr, Butler PF, Applegate KE, et al (2007) American College of Radiology. American College of Radiology white paper on radiation dose in medicine. J Am Coll Radiol 4:272–284

54. Brenner DJ, Hall EJ (2007) Computed tomography – an increasing source of radiation exposure. N Engl J Med 357:2277–2284

55. Douglas PS, Khandheria B, Stainback RF, et al; American College of Cardiology Foundation Appropriateness Criteria Task Force; American Society of Echocardiography; American College of Emergency Physicians; American Heart Association; American Society of Nuclear Cardiology; Society for Cardiovascular Angiography and Interventions; Society of Cardiovascular Computed Tomography; Society for Cardiovascular Magnetic Resonance. ACCF/ASE/ACEP/AHA/ASNC/SCAI/SCCT/SCMR (2008) 2008 appropriateness criteria for stress echocardiography: a report of the American College of Cardiology Foundation Appropriateness Criteria Task Force, American Society of Echocardiography, American College of Emergency Physicians, American Heart Association, American Society of Nuclear Cardiology, Society for Cardiovascular Angiography and Interventions, Society of Cardiovascular Computed Tomography, and Society for Cardiovascular Magnetic Resonance: endorsed by the Heart Rhythm Society and the Society of Critical Care Medicine. Circulation 117:1478–1497

56. Picano E, Pasanisi E, Brown J, et al (2007) A gatekeeper for the gatekeeper: inappropriate referrals to stress echocardiography. Am Heart J 154:285–290

57. Gibbons RJ, Miller TD, Hodge D, et al (2008) Application of appropriateness criteria to stress single-photon emission computed tomography sestamibi studies and stress echocardiograms in an academic medical center. J Am Coll Cardiol 51:1283–1289

58. Cury RC, Shash K, Nagurney JT, et al (2008) Cardiac magnetic resonance with T2-weighted imaging improves detection of patients with acute coronary syndrome in the emergency department. Circulation 118(8):837–844

59. Fleisher LA, Beckman JA, Brown KA, et al (2007) ACC/AHA 2007 Guidelines on perioperative cardiovascular evaluation and care for noncardiac surgery: Executive summary: a report of the American College of Cardiology/American Heart Association Task Force on Practice Guidelines (Writing committee to revise the 2002 guidelines on perioperative cardiovascular evaluation for noncardiac surgery) developed in collaboration with the American Society of Echocardiography, American Society of Nuclear Cardiology, Heart Rhythm Society, Society of Cardiovascular Anesthesiologists, Society for Cardiovascular Angiography and Interventions, Society for Vascular Medicine and Biology, and Society for Vascular Surgery. J Am Coll Cardiol 50:1707–1732

60. Poldermans D et al (2009) Preoperative cardiac risk assessment and perioperative cardiac management in non cardiac surgery: the task force on for preoperative cardiac risk assessment and perioperative cardiac management in non-cardiac surgery of the European Society of Cardiology. Eur Heart J

61. Tischler MD, Lee TH, Hirsch AT, et al (1991) Prediction of major cardiac events after peripheral vascular surgery using dipyridamole echocardiography. Am J Cardiol 68:593–597

62. Sicari R, Picano E, Lusa AM, et al (1995) The value of dipyridamole echocardiography in risk stratification before vascular surgery. A multicenter study. The EPIC (Echo Persantine International Study) Group-Subproject: risk stratification before major vascular surgery. Eur Heart J 16:842–847

63. Rossi E, Citterio F, Vescio MF, et al (1998) Risk stratification of patients undergoing peripheral vascular revascularization by combined resting and dipyridamole echocardiography. Am J Cardiol 82:306–310

64. Pasquet A, D'Hondt AM, Verhelst R, et al (1998) Comparison of dipyridamole stress echocardiography and perfusion scintigraphy for cardiac risk stratification in vascular surgery patients. Am J Cardiol 82:1468–1474

65. Sicari R, Ripoli A, Picano E, et al on behalf of the EPIC study group (1999) Perioperative prognostic value of dipyridamole echocardiography in vascular surgery: a large-scale multicenter study on 509 patients. Circulation 100(Suppl 19):II269–II274

66. Zamorano J, Duque A, Baquero M, et al (2002) Stress echocardiography in the pre-operative evaluation of patients undergoing major vascular surgery. Are results comparable with dipyridamole versus dobutamine stress echo? Rev Esp Cardiol 55:121–126

67. Lane RT, Sawada SG, Segar DS, et al (1991) Dobutamine stress echocardiography for assessment of cardiac risk before noncardiac surgery. Am J Cardiol 68:976–977

68. Lalka SG, Sawada SG, Dalsing MC, et al (1992) Dobutamine stress echocardiography as a predictor of cardiac events associated with aortic surgery. J Vasc Surg 15:831–842

69. Davila-Roman VG, Waggoner AD, Sicard GA, et al (1993) Dobutamine stress echocardiography predicts surgical outcome in patients with an aortic aneurysm and peripheral vascular disease. J Am Coll Cardiol 21:957–963

70. Eichelberger JP, Schwarz KQ, Black ER, et al (1993) Predictive value of dobutamine echocardiography just before noncardiac vascular surgery. Am J Cardiol 72:602–607

71. Poldermans D, Fioretti PM, Forster T, et al (1993) Dobutamine stress echocardiography for assessment of perioperative cardiac risk in patients undergoing major vascular surgery. Circulation 87:1506–1512

72. Karagiannis SE, Feringa HH, Vidakovic R, et al (2007) Value of myocardial viability estimation using dobutamine stress echocardiography in assessing risk preoperatively before noncardiac vascular surgery in patients with left ventricular ejection fraction < 35%. Am J Cardiol 99:1555–1559

73. Boersma E, Poldermans D, Bax JJ, et al; DECREASE Study Group (Dutch Echocardiographic Cardiac Risk Evaluation Applying Stress Echocardiography) (2001) Predictors of cardiac events after major vascular surgery: role of clinical characteristics, dobutamine echocardiography, and beta-blocker therapy. JAMA 285:1865–1873

74. Shaw LJ, Eagle KA, Gersh BJ, et al (1996) Meta-analysis of intravenous dipyridamole-thallium-201 imaging (1985 to 1994) and dobutamine echocardiography (1991 to 1994) for risk stratification before vascular imaging. J Am Coll Cardiol 27:787–798

75. Kertai MD, Boersma E, Bax JJ, et al (2003) A meta-analysis comparing the prognostic accuracy of six diagnostic tests for predicting perioperative cardiac risk in patients undergoing major vascular surgery. Heart 89:1327–1334

76. Beattie WS, Abdelnaem E, Wijeysundera DN (2006) A meta-analytic comparison of preoperative stress echocardiography and nuclear scintigraphy imaging. Anesth Analg 102:8–16

77. Poldermans D, Arnese M, Fioretti PM, et al (1997) Sustained prognostic value of dobutamine stress echocardiography for late cardiac events after major noncardiac vascular surgery. Circulation 195:53–58

78. Sicari R, Ripoli A, Picano E, et al on behalf of the EPIC (Echo Persantine International Cooperative) Study Group (2002) Long-term prognostic value of dipyridamole echocardiography in vascular surgery: a large-scale multicenter study. Coron Artery Dis 13:49–55

79. Bonow RO (2008) Is appropriateness appropriate? J Am Coll Cardiol 51:1290–1291

Microvascular Disease

30

Paolo G. Camici and Eugenio Picano

30.1
Background

The link between myocardial ischemia and obstructive atherosclerosis of the epicardial coronary arteries is well established, and coronary angiography has proven the relationship between the severity and extent of coronary artery disease and patient survival. More recently, however, coronary microvascular abnormalities have been described in patients with normal coronary angiograms and different clinical conditions (Table 30.1). In some of these conditions, the abnormalities of the microvasculature represent important markers of risk and may even contribute to the pathogenesis of myocardial ischemia, thus becoming therapeutic targets [1]. Currently, no technique allows the direct visualization of the coronary microcirculation in vivo in humans. Several measurements that rely on the quantification of blood flow through the coronary circulation are commonly used to describe the function of the microvasculature in patients with normal coronary angiograms. These methods include positron emission tomography (PET), cardiovascular magnetic resonance (CMR), and echocardiography methods. The latter measure blood flow ultrasonographically, according to the Doppler principle, in an invasive, semi-invasive, or totally noninvasive way with intracoronary, transesophageal, or transthoracic Doppler echocardiography, respectively. In patients with coronary artery disease, the extent of the reduction in coronary/myocardial blood flow and flow reserve is directly, albeit only grossly, related to the severity of stenosis, whereas in subjects with angiographically normal arteries it is a marker of microvascular dysfunction. With last-generation ultrasound technology and advanced expertise, dual imaging (function and flow) stress echocardiography provides simultaneous insight into regional and global left ventricular function and coronary flow reserve, both necessary for the diagnostic and prognostic characterization of the heterogeneous population of patients with chest pain and angiographically normal coronary arteries [2].

Clinically, the term "chest pain with normal coronary angiogram" has been used to encompass a broad range of conditions. Patients often had coronary artery disease ranging from minimal disease to coronary stenosis up to 50% of luminal diameter and different comorbidities including diabetes and arterial hypertension [3]. A more homogeneous

E. Picano, *Stress Echocardiography*,
© Springer-Verlag Berlin Heidelberg 2009

30

Table 30.1 The pathophysiological and clinical spectrum of microvascular disease (adapted from [1])

	Alterations	Causes
Structural	Luminal obstruction	Microembolization in ACS or after revascularization
		Infiltrative heart disease (e.g., Anderson-Fabry cardiomyopathy)
	Vascular wall infiltration	
	Vascular remodeling	HCM, arterial hypertension
		Aortic stenosis, arterial hypertension
	Vascular rarefaction	
		Aortic stenosis, arterial hypertension
	Perivascular fibrosis	
		Systemic sclerosis
Functional	Endothelial dysfunction	Smoking, hyperlipidemia, diabetes
	Dysfunction of smooth muscle cell	HCM, arterial hypertension
	Autonomic dysfunction	Coronary recanalization
Extravascular	Extravascular compression	Aortic stenosis, HCM, arterial hypertension, acute transplant rejection
	Reduction in diastolic perfusion time	Aortic stenosis

ACS acute coronary syndrome, *HCM* hypertrophic cardiomyopathy

set of patients would be defined if the following exclusion criteria are employed (Table 30.2): absence of even minimal irregularities on the arteriogram (since these patients have minor forms of coronary artery disease, and the prognosis of even a 20% stenosis is clearly worse than a normal coronary angiogram) [4]; absence of regional or global wall motion abnormalities on resting echocardiogram or of left bundle branch block either on the resting or exercise electrocardiogram (which identify patients who may develop dilated cardiomyopathy during follow-up) [5]; no evidence of diabetes mellitus, arterial hypertension, hyperlipidemia, valve disease (including mitral valve prolapse), and epicardial artery spasm. Clinical history electrocardiogram and resting transthoracic echocardiogram are therefore essential for identifying patients with true cardiac syndrome X that probably represent no more than 10% of all patients with chest pain and supposedly normal coronary arteries. The term "syndrome X" (originally the Group X in the 1973 paper by Arbogast and Bourassa) was coined to stress the uncertainty over the pathophysiology of chest pain [6]. This name is still appropriate, since from the pathophysiological point of view things are far from clear, and it remains unclear whether the chest pain in these patients is ischemic or nonischemic in nature.

Table 30.2 Chest pain with "normal" coronary arteries: more than syndrome X

Appropriate nosography	Nonsmooth coronary arteries)	Resting regional or global LV dysfunction, LBBB	Coronary vasospasm	LV hypertrophy, MVP, diabetes, hypertension	LVOT obstruction	Normal CFR	CFR ↓ (<2.0)	Metabolic or mechanical ischemia
Minor, initial CAD (30%)	√							
Early possible cardiomyopathy		√						
Variant angina			√					
Secondary microvascular disease				√				
LVOTO (dynamic LV obstruction)					√			
Normal CFR (microvascular disease disproven)						√		
Microvascular disease (cardiac syndrome X)							√	
True ischemia with microvascular disease								√

LV left ventricle, *LBBB* left bundle branch block, *MVP* mitral valve prolapse, *LVOT* left ventricular outflow tract, *CFR* coronary flow reserve, *CAD* coronary artery disease, *LVOTO* left ventricular ourflow tract obstruction

30

30.2
Pathophysiology of Microvascular Angina

Several conditions can be clustered together in the syndrome of microvascular disease, characterized by normal epicardial coronary arteries and reduction in coronary flow reserve, in the absence of epicardial coronary artery vasospasm [1]. Microvascular disease may also coexist with epicardial coronary artery stenosis, since a reduced vasodilator response in nonstenosed coronary arteries has been observed in patients with single-vessel disease [7] and in normal, non-infarct-related coronary arteries early after an acute myocardial infarction [8]. Therefore, abnormalities of small distal coronary vessels may contribute to determining an altered coronary flow reserve in patients with ischemic heart disease, independent of atherosclerotic coronary stenoses, and may at least partially account for the elusive link between the anatomical severity of coronary stenoses and clinical symptoms [1]. Reversible alterations in the coronary microcirculation have also been described soon after coronary angioplasty, where they may account for the relatively high rate of false-positive results on electrocardiography and perfusion imaging testing [9]. Microvascular disease can also be a codeterminant of the reduced coronary flow reserve found outside coronary artery disease, in dilated cardiomyopathy [10], hypertrophic cardiomyopathy [11], or in patients with secondary left ventricular hypertrophy, e.g., hypertension and aortic stenosis [12]. In all these conditions, coronary flow reserve impairment is often independent of the degree of left ventricular hypertrophy and the typical behavior of microvascular disease during stress testing is the frequent induction of chest pain, ST-segment depression, and perfusion abnormalities without regional or global wall motion changes (Fig. 30.1). The sequence of events is therefore strikingly different from the

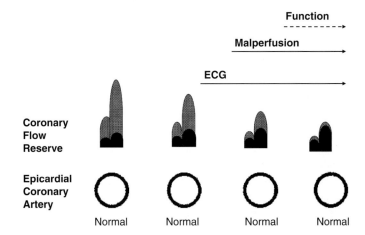

Fig. 30.1 The features of microvascular disease consist of normal epicardial coronary arteries (even when observed by intravascular ultrasound: *lower row*) and reduced coronary flow reserve (by Doppler tracing showing a spectrum of coronary hyperemic responses, from normal – *left* – to abolished – *far right*). Chest pain and ECG changes are frequent during stress, especially when flow reserve is reduced, whereas echocardiography changes (*dashed lines*) are only very rarely observed. (Modified from [2])

Table 30.3 Classic and alternative cascade during stress testing

	Classic	Alternative
Clinical models	Coronary stenosis	Microvascular disease
Epicardial coronary anatomy	Stenotic	Normal
Coronary flow reserve	Depressed	Depressed
Stress: chest pain	Present	Present
Stress: ST depression	Present	Present
Stress: dyssynergy	Present	Usually absent
Experimental model	Yes	No

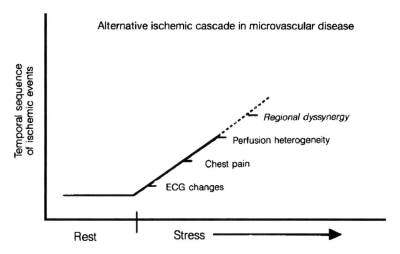

Fig. 30.2 In the model of microvascular disease (reduction in coronary flow reserve with normal epicardial arteries), such as that found in syndrome X or left ventricular hypertrophy, anginal pain and ST-segment changes usually appear in the absence of any detectable wall dysfunction. (Modified from [2])

classic ischemic cascade found during stress testing in the presence of a coronary stenosis (Table 30.3). The alternative ischemic cascade is illustrated in Fig. 30.2 and is derived from pragmatic clinical experience [2]. It integrates, in diagnostic practice, the classical monolithic concept of ischemic cascade. While the classic ischemic cascade was a clear laboratory phenomenon that waited 30 years for a clinical application, which became obvious in the era of cardiac imaging, the alternative ischemic cascade is a clear clinical finding disclosed by cardiac imaging techniques and still in search of a good laboratory model [2].

As Kemp wrote 30 years ago, many findings in syndrome X "like the clues in the first half of an Agatha Christie novel, may not be readily understandable, but we can be certain they are important" [13]. The very same ischemic nature of chest pain and ST-segment depression in cardiac syndrome X patients remains uncertain [14–17]. In theory, true ischemia might develop in spite of normal coronary arteries. Maseri et al. have proposed that in these patients focal ischemia in small myocardial regions scattered throughout the myocardium and caused by prearteriolar dysfunction might explain the paradox of angina and ST-segment depression provoked by physical or pharmacological stress [18]. In keeping with this interpretation, Cannon and Epstein first hypothesized that the site of abnormally elevated resistances (in patients with reduced coronary flow reserve) is intramural, upstream from the endocardium–epicardium branching point, which is not visualized by coronary angiography [19] (Fig. 30.3). According to their hypothesis, the abnormal resistance to flow would result in maximal dilation of subendocardial arterioles in the rest conditions because of the concomitant higher metabolic demand of the subendocardium. The putative mechanism of the steal as a response to pharmacological or metabolic stimuli, such as dipyridamole or pacing or exercise, would be related to the inability of subendocardial arterioles to dilate further compared with a "normal" dilation of the subepicardial arterioles and the consequent decrease in pressure downstream from the site of increased resistance, with reduction of flow to the subendocardium. The concept of intramural steal cannot be considered proved to date, since we lack consistent and convincing evidence – on the basis of perfusion, metabolic, or mechanical markers – of the truly ischemic nature of ischemic-like stress-induced

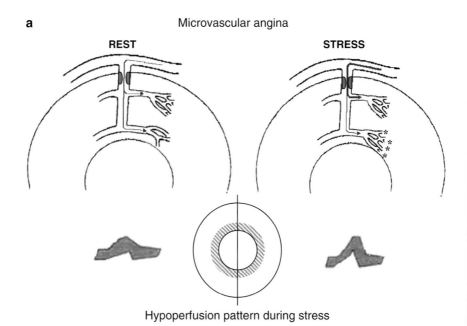

Fig. 30.3 Schematic representation of transmural coronary hemodynamics (*upper panels*), regional wall motion thickening (*lower panels*), and myocardial ischemia transmural distribution (*middle panels*) in syndrome X (**a**) and in epicardial stenosis (**b**). Induced myocardial hypoperfusion is more horizontally diffuse in syndrome X, and more transmurally extended in CAD: only in the latter case of critical mass of ischemic myocardium is reached. (Redrawn and modified from the original hypothesis of Epstein and Cannon [19])

b   Coronary Artery Disease

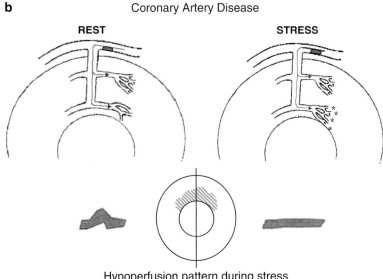

Hypoperfusion pattern during stress

Fig. 30.3 (continued)

chest pain and ST-segment changes [3]. We must keep an open mind on this issue, waiting for more conclusive evidence. However, it is important to emphasize that normal left ventricular function consistently recorded during stress echocardiography is not incompatible with true myocardial ischemia, since the presence or absence of abnormal wall motion appears to be related to the amount of subendocardial tissue rendered ischemic, with minor degrees of transmural involvement (onion skin-like ischemia) or patchy myocardial ischemia (leopard skin-like ischemia), less likely to produce regional dysfunction [2]. In fact, for minimal flow reductions, abnormalities of regional systolic function are subtle and certainly below the threshold of detection by echocardiography. The appreciation of a regional dysfunction by two-dimensional (2D) echocardiography requires a critical ischemic mass of at least 20% of transmural wall thickness and about 5% of the total myocardial mass [20–22]. These experimental data have a clinical correlate. It is well known that even under ideal imaging conditions a subendocardial infarction – not ischemia, infarction – can be accompanied in 20% of cases by a perfectly normal/hyperkinetic regional and global wall thickening [23, 24]. In addition, we now know that regional thickening and motion – which are the cornerstone of clinical echocardiography – express radial function, which can be still normal when longitudinal and/or circumferential function are clearly impaired during less severe ischemia, as shown recently applying new echocardiography technologies (such as myocardial velocity imaging and speckle tracking) to experimental models of stress-induced ischemia [25–26]. In summary, sticking to the very definition of myocardial ischemia proposed by John Ross Jr. ("ischemia is a reduction in myocardial blood flow sufficient to cause a decrease in myocardial contraction" [27]), we can conclude that stress echocardiographic findings in syndrome X are yet another clue in the first half of this novel: we can be certain they are important, but at present they are not sufficient to find the culprit, which was smart enough not to leave ischemia fingerprints on the stress echocardiography based on regional wall motion and thickening.

30.3
Stress Echocardiographic Findings in Cardiac Syndrome X

There are three main findings during stress echocardiography in syndrome X: (1) regional and global left ventricular hyperkinesia (but regional wall motion abnormalities are described in roughly 10% of patients); (2) reduced coronary flow reserve on mid-distal left anterior descending coronary arteries in about 20% of patients (but reserve is normal in the majority of patients) (3) stress-induced intraventricular pressure gradient (in appro-ximately 5–10% of patients). In cardiac syndrome X, the peculiar pattern during stress echocardiography is the regional and global left ventricular hyperkinesia with ST-segment depression and chest pain, consistently observed during dipyridamole [28], exercise [29], and dobutamine [30, 31]. The stress-induced hyperkinesis is coherent with the original report by Arbogast and Bourassa in 1973 with pacing left ventriculography [6, 13]. Coronary flow reserve can be measured during Doppler-transthoracic vasodilator stress echocardio-graphy on mid-distal left anterior descending coronary artery, semi-simultaneously with wall motion imaging, and shows a reduced (<2.0) coronary flow reserve in one out of five syndrome X patients, in the absence of wall motion abnormalities. The left ventricle is hyperdynamic during stress (too good to be ischemic) (Fig. 30.4), but perfusion changes are often found with perfusion scans [32, 33] and coronary flow reserve by transthoracic echocardiography can be normal (Fig. 30.5) or impaired (Fig. 30.6). CMR may show strictly subendocardial underperfusion during stress and metabolic abnormalities consistent with ischemia in at least 30% of cases but with some inconsistency of results across different laboratories [14–17].

Another stress echocardiographic finding has been observed with increasing frequency – when it is looked for – especially, but not only, in patients with left ventricular hypertrophy or young athletes [34–36]. In these subjects, symptoms such as chest pain or syncope typically occur during exercise. Resting echocardiography is within normal limits, as always in microvascular angina, coronary reserve can be normal, but exercise induces ST-segment depression and a significant (>50 mmHg) intraventricular gradient (Fig. 30.7). In these subjects, the abnormality detected during effort is not among the diagnoses that contraindicate participation in competitive sports according to the recommendations of the 36th Bethesda Conference [37] and the European Society of Cardiology [38]. It has been suggested that, in presence of a history of chest pain or syncope during exercise, the athletes should be advised to suspend sports activity [36]. In theory, this subgroup of patients might especially benefit from β-blocker therapy, which determines an inconstant benefit in the general population of patients with micro-vascular angina [14]. A similar left ventricular outflow tract obstruction has been described during dobutamine infusion in patients with chest pain that develop significantly higher intraventricular gradients [39–41]. Not surprisingly, treatment with the β-blockers bisoprolol resulted in a reduction of angina score, as well as normalization of intraventricular flow velocities [41].

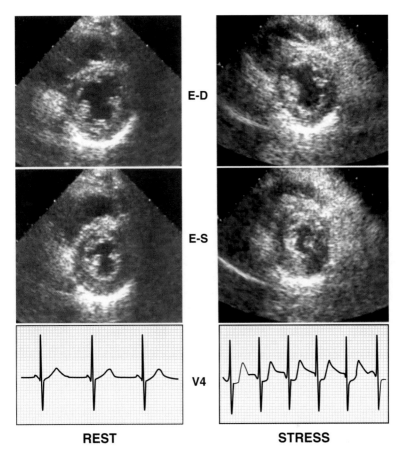

Fig. 30.4 Parasternal short-axis section of the left ventricle at the papillary muscle level under basal conditions (*left*) and after dipyridamole infusion (*right*). Despite ST-segment depression induced by dipyridamole, regional asynergy is not detectable. *E-D* end-diastole, *E-S* end-systole. This patient had a positive exercise electrocardiography test for both chest pain and ST-segment depression. Coronary angiography showed a normal coronary artery tree. (Modified from [28])

30.4
The Prognostic Heterogeneity of Chest Pain with Angiographically Normal Coronary Arteries

On a more pragmatic ground, it is generally considered that chest pain with the angiographic label of normal coronary arteries readily identifies a prognostically benign subset [42, 43], but with substantial heterogeneity. First, not all the patients with a history of chest pain, normal resting function, and normal coronary arteries have microvascular disease [1]. In fact, at least two other broad categories can contribute to the finding of normal coronary arteries: variant angina, which can certainly be overlooked if not considered,

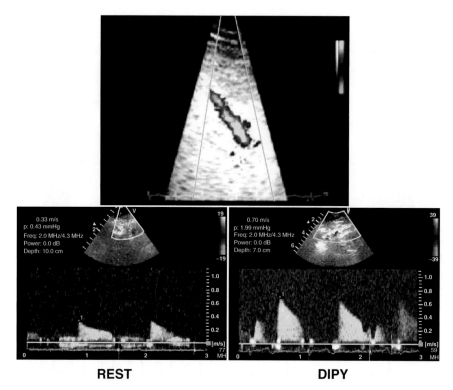

Fig. 30.5 Sample of coronary arteries assessment in patients with normal coronary arteries. Visualization of coronary flow in the mid-distal portion of left anterior descending artery using color Doppler flow mapping in the *upper panel*. Peak flow diastolic velocity was 33 cm s^{-1} under basal conditions (*lower left panel*) and 70 cm s^{-1} after dipyridamole infusion (*lower right panel*), with a normal coronary arteries value (2.1). (Courtesy of Dr. Fausto Rigo)

and a noncardiac origin of chest pain, as can be found in anxiety, psychotic disorders, and esophageal disease. Table 30.4 reports several clues that can aid in the often difficult recognition of these three noncardiac conditions. Second, even considering only patients with microvascular disease, as a group, it is true that these patients indeed have a good prognosis, but with some heterogeneity. Out of nine patients, six had no evidence of wall motion abnormalities and had a preserved coronary flow reserve (>2.0). The prognosis of these patients was found to be excellent (<0.5% hard event-rate per year). At the other end of the spectrum, 10% of patients showed stress-induced regional wall motion abnormalities. In these patients, the event-rate was threefold higher [44]. These patients are "wolves in sheep's clothing" (Fig. 30.8). Between the two extremes, we found about 20% of patients without wall motion abnormalities but with reduced coronary flow reserve (<2.0), with an intermediate hard-event rate (Fig. 30.9) [45]. The situation can be schematically represented as in Fig. 30.10: out of nine patients with identical clinical and angiographic presentation, and, as a group, supposedly good prognosis, six have excellent, two have good, and one has a poor prognosis. As always, stress echocardiography helps identify the pathophysiological heterogeneity hidden behind apparently similar clinical, stress electro-cardiographic, and angiographic presentations.

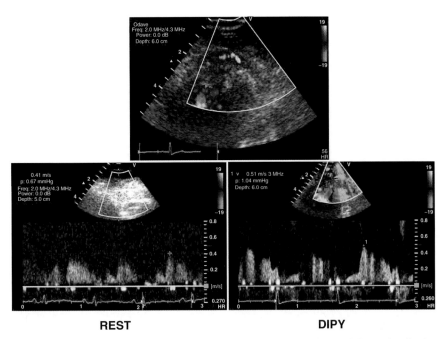

Fig. 30.6 Sample of coronary flow reserve assessment in patients with abnormal CFR. Visualization of coronary flow in the mid-distal portion of left anterior descending artery using color Doppler flow mapping in the *upper panel*. Peak flow diastolic velocity was 41 cm s^{-1} under basal conditions (*lower left panel*) and 51 cm s^{-1} after dipyridamole infusion (*lower right panel*), with an abnormal coronary flow reserve value (1.2). (Courtesy of Dr. Fausto Rigo)

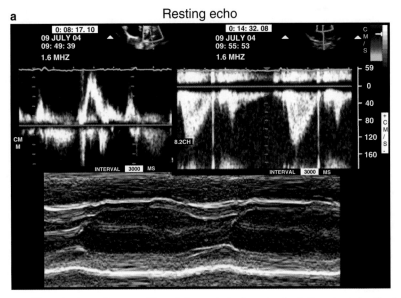

Fig. 30.7 a Normal echocardiogram without left ventricular hypertrophy. **b** Exercise test with alteration in ST segment in DII, DIII, and AF. **c** At peak exercise, systolic anterior movement of mitral valve and significant intraventricular gradient was detected. (Courtesy of Cotrim et al [36])

b   Exercise-ECG

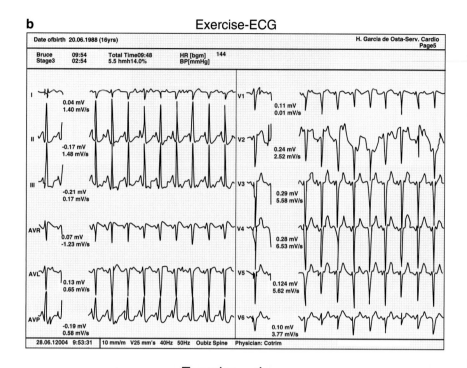

c   Exercise-echo

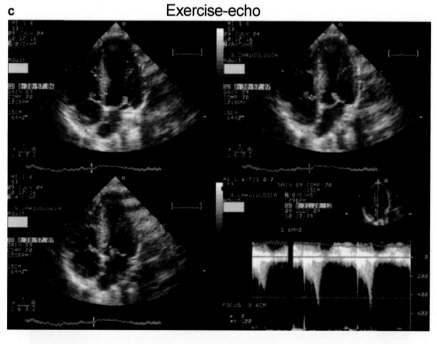

Fig. 30.7 (continued)

Table 30.4 Clues for the recognition of noncardiac conditions

	Microvascular disease	Variant angina	Noncardiac chest pain
Pathogenesis	Small-vessel alteration	Epicardial artery spasm	Anxiety, esophageal spasm, etc.
Chest pain pattern	On effort, emotion, at rest	At night, with palpitations and/or lipothymia	Nitrate sensitive or resistant, lasting second to hours
	Nitrate-resistant	Lasting up to 10 min, nitrate-sensitive	Localized or retrosternal
Resting LV function	Normal	Usually normal	Normal
Ergonovine test	Negative	Positive	Negative
Exercise stress test	Positive	Negative or positive	Negative
Stress test			
Chest pain	Yes	No	No or yes
ST segment	Yes	No	No
Perfusion changes	Frequent	No	Usually no
Echocardiographic changes	No	No	No
Coronary angiography	Normal	Normal (irregularities frequent)	Normal
ICUS	Frequently normal	Alterations on spasm site	Normal
Therapy	Trial and error	Nitrates and Ca^{2+} blockers	None

ICUS intracoronary ultrasound, *LV* left ventricle

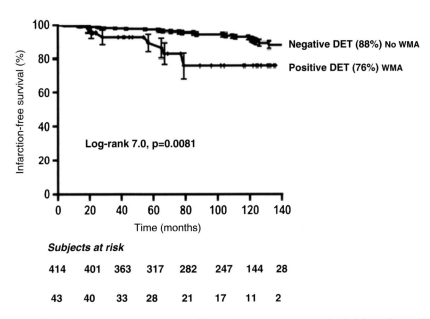

Fig. 30.8 Kaplan–Meier survival curves (considering hard events as an end point) in patients with presence *(DET+)* and absence *(DET−)* of wall motion abnormalities during dipyridamole stress and angiographically normal or near-normal coronary arteries. Survival is worse in patients with inducible ischemia. (Modified from [44])

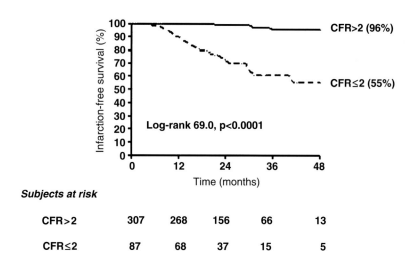

Fig. 30.9 Kaplan–Meier survival curves (considering hard cardiac events as an end point) in patients stratified according to normal (CFR>2) or abnormal (CFR<2) coronary flow reserve at Doppler echocardiography during DET. Survival rate in CFR>2 is significantly different from CFR<2 ($p<0.0001$). The best survival is observed in patients with normal coronary flow reserve; the worst survival is observed in patients with impaired coronary flow reserve. (Modified from [45])

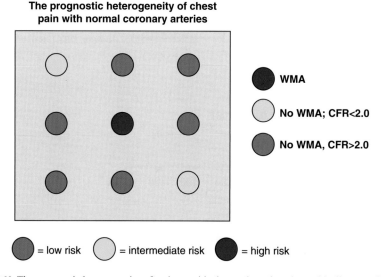

Fig. 30.10 The prognostic heterogeneity of patients with chest pain and angiographically normal coronary arteries. Although the prognosis as a group is good, there is considerable heterogeneity. Prognosis is less good in patients (one out of nine) with inducible wall motion abnormalities, and poor in patients with inducible regional wall motion abnormalities

These results are coherent with a recent meta-analysis [46] showing that patients with chest pain and angiographically nonsignificant coronary artery stenoses may have a prognosis that is not as benign as commonly thought. In fact, even in the absence of true ischemia associated with stress-induced wall motion abnormalities, coronary endothelial dysfunction, presence of left ventricular hypertrophy, and evidence of coronary microvascular dysfunction have been linked to adverse outcome [47].

30.5
The Diagnostic Flow Chart in Microvascular Angina

Stress echocardiography can play a key role in the diagnostic identification of the pathophysiological and prognostic heterogeneity underlying angina with normal coronary arteries. A stress for induction of coronary vasospasm (with ergometrine or hyperventilation) is required to exclude this condition as the cause of the symptoms [48], especially in patients with a clinical presentation suggestive of coronary vasospasm: angina also at rest and with highly variable exercise tolerance; marked seasonal and circadian variation, with worsening in springtime and early morning, worsening with β-blockers; association with palpitations and syncope; and ongoing therapy with methergin, 5-fluoromacil, or sumatriptan (Fig. 30.11). After ruling out coronary vasospasm in selected patients, stress echocardiography is again useful to stratify three risk groups: low risk (no wall motion abnormalities; normal

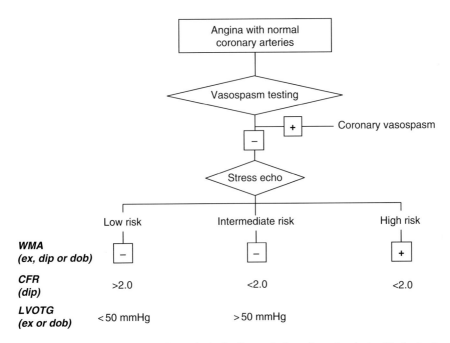

Fig. 30.11 The role of stress echocardiography in the diagnostic flow-chart of patients with chest pain and normal coronary arteries

coronary artery flow reserve); intermediate risk (no wall motion abnormalities, reduced coronary flow reserve); and high risk (inducible wall motion abnormalities). Wall motion can be easily assessed with all stresses (exercise, dobutamine, dipyridamole), whereas the evaluation of coronary flow is best performed with vasodilators (dipyridamole or adenosine). In patients at low risk, a special subset – to be systematically looked for in symptomatic athletes – at probably higher risk are those developing a significant intraventricular gradient during exercise or dobutamine. In them, sports activity can be theoretically at greater risk and β-blockers might be warranted, possibly with a more consistent therapeutic benefit that in the overall population, although certainly more data are needed at this point.

In conclusion, the patient with known or suspected cardiac syndrome X will benefit from the versatility of resting and stress echocardiography. In the screening phase, resting transthoracic echocardiography is helpful to rule out possible causes of angina with normal coronary arteries: left ventricular hypertrophy with or without valvular heart disease, mitral valve prolapse, regional or global left ventricular dysfunction, and left ventricular outflow tract obstruction. Following the initial screening, stress echocardiography can kill three birds with one stone: identification of wall motion, coronary flow reserve, and dynamic intraventricular obstruction with a single technique. A refined diagnostic and prognostic characterization of the different subsets will eventually allow targeting specific therapies on strictly selected patients, more likely to benefit from a tailored approach than with blind carpet bombing on the basis of nonspecific clinical and angiographic criteria.

References

1. Camici PG, Crea F (2007) Coronary microvascular dysfunction. N Engl J Med 356:830–840
2. Picano E, Palinkas A, Amyot R (2001) Diagnosis of myocardial ischemia in hypertensive patients. J Hypertens 19:1177–1183
3. Camici PG (2007) Is the chest pain in cardiac syndrome X due to subendocardial ischaemia? Eur Heart J 28:1539–1540
4. Kemp HG, Kronmal RA, Vlietstra RE, et al (1986) Seven year survival of patients with normal or near normal coronary arteriograms: a CASS registry study. J Am Coll Cardiol 7:479–483
5. Opherk D, Schuler G, Wetterauer K, et al (1989) Four-year follow-up study in patients with angina pectoris and normal coronary arteriograms ("syndrome X"). Circulation 80:1610–1666
6. Arbogast R, Bourassa MG (1973) Myocardial function during atrial pacing in patients with angina pectoris and normal coronary arteriograms. Comparison with patients having significant coronary artery disease. Am J Cardiol 32:257–263
7. Uren NG, Marraccini P, Gistri R, et al (1993) Altered coronary vasodilator reserve and metabolism in myocardium subtended by normal arteries in patients with coronary artery disease. J Am Coll Cardiol 22:650–658
8. Uren NG, Crake T, Lefroy DC, et al (1994) Reduced coronary vasodilator function in infarcted and normal myocardium after myocardial infarction. N Engl J Med 33:222–227
9. Miller DD, Verani MS (1994) Current status of myocardial perfusion imaging after percutaneous transluminal coronary angioplasty. J Am Coll Cardiol 24:260–266
10. Neglia D, Parodi O, Gallopin M, et al (1995) Myocardial blood flow response to pacing tachycardia and to dipyridamole infusion in patients with dilated cardiomyopathy without overt heart failure. A quantitative assessment by positron emission tomography. Circulation 92:796–804

11. Camici P, Chiriatti G, Lorenzoni R, et al (1991) Coronary vasodilation is impaired in both hypertrophied and nonhypertrophied myocardium of patients with hypertrophic cardiomyopathy: a study with nitrogen-13 ammonia and positron emission tomography. J Am Coll Cardiol 17:879–886

12. Scheler S, Motz W, Strauer BE (1994) Mechanism of angina pectoris in patients with systemic hypertension and normal epicardial coronary arteries by arteriogram. Am J Cardiol 73:478–482

13. Kemp HG (1973) Left ventricular function in patients with the anginal syndrome and normal coronary arteriograms. Am J Cardiol 32:375

14. Panting JR, Gatehouse PD, Yang GZ, et al (2002) Abnormal subendocardial perfusion in cardiac syndrome X detected by cardiovascular magnetic resonance imaging. N Engl J Med 346:1948–1953

15. Lanza GA, Buffon A, Sestito A, et al (2008) Relation between stress-induced myocardial perfusion defects on cardiovascular magnetic resonance and coronary microvascular dysfunction in patients with cardiac syndrome X. J Am Coll Cardiol 51:466–472

16. Buchthal SD, den Hollander JA, Merz CN, et al (2000) Abnormal myocardial phosphorus-31 nuclear magnetic resonance spectroscopy in women with chest pain but normal coronary angiograms. N Engl J Med 342:829–835

17. Vermeltfoort IA, Bondarenko O, Raijmakers PG, et al (2007) Is subendocardial ischaemia present in patients with chest pain and normal coronary angiograms? A cardiovascular MR study. Eur Heart J 28:1554–1558

18. Maseri A, Crea F, Kaski JC, et al (1991) Mechanisms of angina pectoris in syndrome X. J Am Coll Cardiol 17:499–506

19. Epstein SE, Cannon RO (1986) Site of increased resistance to coronary flow in patients with angina pectoris and normal coronary arteries. J Am Coll Cardiol 8:459–461

20. Lieberman AN, Weiss JL, Jugdutt BI, et al (1981) Two-dimensional echocardiography and infarct size: relationship of regional wall motion and thickening to the extent of myocardial infarction in the dog. Circulation 63:739–746

21. Falsetti HL, Marcus ML, Kerber RE, et al (1981) Quantification of myocardial ischemia and infarction by left ventricular imaging. Circulation 63:747–751

22. Armstrong WF (1988) Echocardiography in coronary artery disease. Prog Cardiovasc Dis 30:267–288

23. Carpeggiani C, L'Abbate A, Marzullo P (1989) Multiparametric approach to diagnosis of non-Q-wave acute myocardial infarction. Am J Cardiol 63:404–408

24. Thygesen K, Alpert JS, White HD; Joint ESC/ACCF/AHA/WHF Task Force for the Redefinition of Myocardial Infarction (2007) Universal definition of myocardial infarction. Circulation 116:2634–2653

25. Abraham TP, Pinheiro AC (2008) Speckle-derived strain a better tool for quantification of stress echocardiography? J Am Coll Cardiol 51:158–160

26. Reant P, Labrousse L, Lafitte S, et al (2008) Experimental validation of circumferential, longitudinal, and radial 2-dimensional strain during dobutamine stress echocardiography in ischemic conditions. J Am Coll Cardiol 51:149–157

27. Ross J Jr, Hearse DJ (1994) Myocardial ischemia can we agree on a definition for the 21st century? Cardiovasc Res 28:1737–1744

28. Picano E, Lattanzi F, Masini M, et al (1987) Usefulness of dipyridamole-echocardiography test for the diagnosis of syndrome X. J Am Cardiol 60:508

29. Nihoyannopoulos P, Kaski JC, Crake T, et al (1991) Absence of myocardial dysfunction during stress in patients with syndrome X. J Am Coll Cardiol 19:1463–1470

30. Lanzarini L, Previtali M, Fetiveau R, et al (1994) Results of dobutamine stress echocardiography in patients with syndrome X. Int J Card Imaging 10:145–148

31. Panza JA, Laurienzo JM, Curiel RV, et al (1997) Investigation of the mechanism of chest pain in patients with angiographically normal coronary arteries using transesophageal dobutamine stress echocardiography. J Am Coll Cardiol 29:293–301

32. Berger BC, Abramowitz R, Park CH,et al (1983) Abnormal thallium-201 scans in patients with chest pain and angiographically normal coronary arteries. Am J Cardiol 52:365–370

33. Tweddel AC, Martin W, Hutton I (1992) Thallium scans in syndrome X. Br Heart J 68:48–50

34. Peteiro J, Monserrat L, Castro Beiras A (1999) Labile subaortic obstruction during exercise stress echocardiography. Am J Cardiol 84:1119–23

35. Lau K, Navarijo J, Stainback F (2001) Pseudo-false-positive exercise treadmill testing. Tex Heart Inst J 28:308–311

36. Cotrim C, Almeida AG, Carrageta M (2007) Clinical significance of intraventricular gradient during effort in an adolescent karate player. Cardiovasc Ultrasound 5:39

37. Maron B, Zipes D (2005) 36th Bethesda Conference. Introduction: eligibility recommendations for competitive athletes with cardiovascular abnormalities – general considerations. J Am Coll Cardiol 45:1318–21

38. Corrado D, Pelliccia A, Bjørnstad H, et al (2005) Study Group of Sport Cardiology of the Working Group of Cardiac Rehabilitation and Exercise Physiology and the Working Group of Myocardial and Pericardial Diseases of the European Society of Cardiology. Cardiovascular pre-participation screening of young competitive athletes for prevention of sudden death: proposal for a common European protocol. Consensus statement of Study Group of Sport Cardiology of the Working Group of Cardiac Rehabilitation and Exercise Physiology and Working Group of Myocardial and Pericardial Diseases of European Society of Cardiology. Eur Heart J 26:516–524

39. Tousoulis D, Crake T, Lefroy DC, et al (1993) Left ventricular hypercontractility and ST segment depression in patients with syndrome X. J Am Coll Cardiol 22:1607–1613

40. Christiaens L, Duplantier C, Alla J, et al (2001) Normal coronary angiogram and dobutamine-induced left ventricular obstruction during stress echocardiography: a higher hemodynamic responsiveness to dobutamine. Echocardiography 18:285–290

41. Madaric J, Bartunek J, Verhamme K, et al (2005) Hyperdynamic myocardial response to beta-adrenergic stimulation in patients with chest pain and normal coronary arteries. J Am Coll Cardiol 46:1270–1275

42. Papanicolaou MN, Califf RM, Hlatky MA et al (1986) Prognostic implications of angiographically normal and insignificantly narrowed coronary arteries. Am J Cardiol 58:1181–1187

43. Lichtlen PR, Bargheer K, Wenzlaff P (1995) Long-term prognosis of patients with anginalike chest pain and normal coronary angiographic findings. J Am Coll Cardiol 25:1013–1018

44. Sicari R, Palinkas A, Pasanisi E, et al (2005) Long-term survival of patients with chest pain syndrome and angiographically normal or near-normal coronary arteries: the additional prognostic value of dipyridamole-echocardiography test. Eur Heart J 26:2136–2141

45. Rigo F, Gherardi S, Cortigiani L, et al (2007) Long-term survival of patients with chest pain syndrome and angiographically normal or near-normal coronary arteries. Eur Heart J (abstract Suppl)

46. Bugiardini R, Merz NB (2005) Angina with "normal" coronary arteries – a changing philosophy. JAMA 293:477–484

47. von Mering GO, Arant CB, Wessel TR, et al; National Heart, Lung, and Blood Institute (2004) Abnormal coronary vasomotion as a prognostic indicator of cardiovascular events in women: results from the National Heart, Lung, and Blood Institute-Sponsored Women's Ischemia Syndrome Evaluation (WISE). Circulation 109:722–725

48. Maseri A (1986) Role of coronary spasm in symptomatic and silent myocardial ischemia. J Am Coll Cardiol 9:249–262

Hypertension

31

Eugenio Picano

31.1
Background

Uncontrolled and prolonged elevation of blood pressure can lead to a variety of changes in the myocardial structure, coronary vasculature, and conduction system of the heart. These changes can lead to the development of left ventricular hypertrophy, coronary artery disease, various conduction system diseases, and systolic or diastolic dysfunction of the myocardium, which manifest clinically as angina or myocardial infarction, cardiac arrhythmias (especially atrial fibrillation), and congestive heart failure. Patients with angina have a high tolerance for hypertension. Hypertension is an established risk factor for the development of coronary artery disease, almost doubling the risk [1]. Transthoracic echocardiography is especially helpful for an initial risk stratification, and identifies four key variables of recognized prognostic value [2]: (1) left ventricular hypertrophy, especially of the concentric type; (2) left atrial dilatation, often occurring in the absence of valvular heart disease or systolic dysfunction and may correlate with the severity of diastolic dysfunction; (3) diastolic dysfunction, common in hypertension, and usually, but not invariably, accompanied by left ventricular hypertrophy [3]; and (4) systolic dysfunction (Table 31.1).

To the information provided by resting transthoracic echocardiography and stress echocardiography adds critically important pathophysiologic, diagnostic, and prognostic information.

31.2
Pathophysiology

Arterial hypertension can provoke a reduction in coronary flow reserve through several mechanisms, which may overlap in the individual patient: coronary artery disease, left ventricular hypertrophy, and microvascular disease [4] (Fig. 31.1). Abnormal coronary flow reserve has been demonstrated in patients with essential hypertension, despite the presence of angiographically normal arteries and the absence of left ventricular hypertrophy [5].

E. Picano, *Stress Echocardiography*,
© Springer-Verlag Berlin Heidelberg 2009

Table 31.1 Rest and stress echocardiography for risk stratification in hypertensive subjects with normal resting left ventricular function

	Higher risk	Lower risk
Resting echocardiography		
LVH (g m ^{2})	>125	<125
LA (mm^2)	>4.5	<4.5
DD (grade)	2–3	0–1
RWT	>0.45	<0.45
Stress echocardiography		
WMA	Yes	No
CFR	<2.0	>2.0

CFR coronary flow reserve, *DD* diastolic dysfunction (from 0 = absent to 3 = severe), *LA* left atrial volume (in apical biplane view), *LVH* left ventricular hypertrophy (by ASE-cube method), *RWT* relative wall thickness, *WMA* wall motion abnormalities

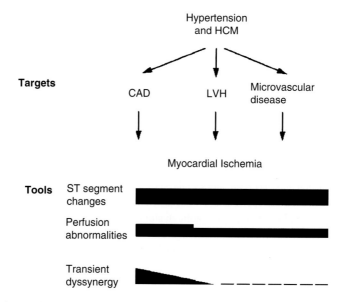

Fig. 31.1 Three main targets of hypertension: coronary artery disease (*CAD*), left ventricular hypertrophy (*LVH*), and microvascular disease. All three of these conditions can provoke stress-induced ST-segment depression and perfusion abnormalities, but only CAD evokes transient dyssynergy. (Modified from [9])

This observation has been attributed to both the remodeling of vascular and extravascular structures and to coronary hemodynamic alterations. The former includes remodeling of intramural arterioles and interstitial fibrosis, and leads to a decreased density of vessels in the coronary microvasculature, whereas the latter is characterized by increased extravascular compressive forces and elevated systolic and diastolic wall stress and impaired relaxation. Coronary microvascular dysfunction in patients with hypertension is not necessarily related to the presence or degree of left ventricular hypertrophy [6, 7].

31.3
Diagnosis of Coronary Artery Disease

The noninvasive diagnosis of coronary artery disease in hypertensive individuals is particularly challenging for the cardiologist, because the coexistence of hypertension dramatically lowers the specificity of exercise electrocardiography and perfusion scintigraphy [8, 9]. Experience with diagnostic tests in these patients led to the frustrating conclusion in the prestress echocardiographic era that "no non-invasive screening test has been found to adequately discriminate between hypertensive patients with and without associated atherosclerosis" [10]. Furthermore, all exercise-dependent tests also show a markedly lowered feasibility in hypertensive patients; severe hypertension during the resting condition is a contraindication to exercise testing, and even in mild to moderate hypertension, the first step of exercise can induce an exaggerated hypertensive response that limits effort tolerance [10]. Stress echocardiography tests have proven to have a higher specificity than ECG [11, 12] or perfusion stress testing [13, 14], with a similar sensitivity (Fig. 31.2). In addi-

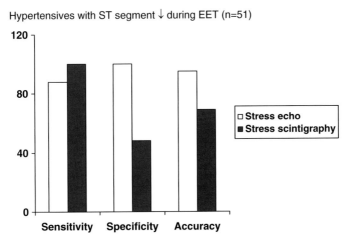

Fig. 31.2 Histogram showing sensitivity, specificity, accuracy, negative predictive value (NPV) and positive predictive value (PPV) of dipyridamole stress test with atropine (*black bars*) and exercise thallium perfusion scintigraphy (*white bars*) for coronary artery disease detection in hypertensive patients with chest pain and positive exercise test. *EET* exercise thallium perfusion scintigraphy. (Modified from [14])

31

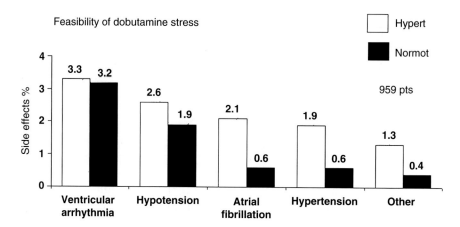

Fig. 31.3 Safety and tolerability profile of dobutamine stress testing in a large cohort of normotensive (*black bars*) and hypertensive patients (*white bars*): all side effects are more frequent in hypertensive subjects. (Modified from [15])

tion, pharmacological stresses have a significantly higher feasibility than exercise stress testing [11], especially with vasodilator testing, which does not evoke the often limiting hypertensive response that can be associated with dobutamine stress [15] (Fig. 31.3). The exaggerated systolic blood pressure rise is also a frequent determinant of wall motion abnormalities during exercise, lowering the specificity of the test [16]. Dipyridamole is less vulnerable to false-positive wall motion abnormalities since there is little or no systolic blood pressure rise during stress [17].

31.4
Prognostic Stratification

During stress, we have three signals of potential value in hypertensive patients: ST-segment depression, wall motion abnormalities, and coronary flow reserve. The pathophysiological significance of stress-induced, ischemic-like electrocardiographic changes remains uncertain [18]. This stress pattern is often found in these patients with normal coronary arteries and hyperkinetic wall motion. The electrocardiographic changes may merely represent nonspecific, innocent alterations or may reflect true subendocardial hypoperfusion. Such ischemic-like electrocardiographic changes occurring with angiographically normal coronary arteries have been associated with a reduced coronary flow reserve [19], a higher incidence of spontaneously occurring or stress-induced ventricular arrhythmias [20], higher values of left ventricular mass index, and, when left ventricular mass is normal, more pronounced structural and functional changes in systemic arterioles [21]. Regression of structural changes of systemic arterioles achieved with any form of antihypertensive therapy is paralleled by the electrocardiographic negativity of a previously positive ECG stress test result [22, 23].

As with microvascular angina, resting and stress echocardiography can be very helpful for risk stratification in patients with chest pain and angiographically normal coronary arteries. The prognostic value of stress-induced wall motion abnormalities is strong and extensively documented. Hypertensive patients with inducible wall motion abnormalities (with or without underlying coronary artery disease) are at higher risk than those without [24–26] (Fig. 31.4). Within the subset with no wall motion abnormalities, patients with reduced coronary flow reserve assessed with transthoracic echocardiography are at intermediate risk (Fig. 31.5) and patients with neither wall motion abnormalities nor coronary flow reserve are at lowest risk [27] (Fig. 31.6).

When compared to other stress imaging techniques with comparable prognostic value, such as myocardial perfusion scintigraphy, stress echocardiography has three clear advantages: lower cost (approximately 1:3 compared with perfusion scintigraphy) [28, 29]; higher specificity (which is important to avoid a number of useless coronary angiographies) [13, 14], also maintained in challenging subsets such as patients with right bundle branch block [30]; and, most importantly, lack of radiation exposure, ranging from a dose equivalence of 500–1,500 chest X-rays for a stress scintigraphy with sestamibi or thallium, respectively, or 700–1,500 chest X-rays for cardiac computed tomography [31–33]. These

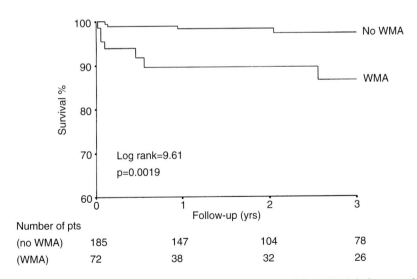

Fig. 31.4 The prognostic value of inducible wall motion abnormalities (*WMA*) in hypertensive patients. (Modified from [24])

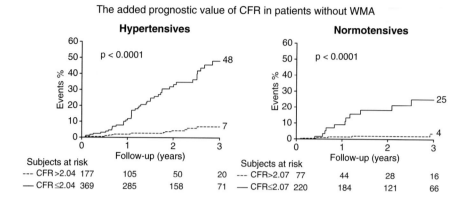

Fig. 31.5 The prognostic value of reduced coronary flow reserve (*CFR*) in hypertensives (*left panel*), and normotensives (*right panel*) with reduced coronary flow reserve. (Modified from [28])

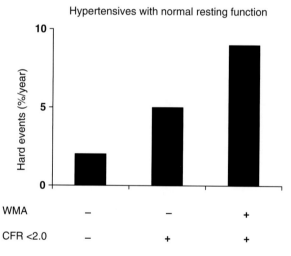

Fig. 31.6 Risk stratification in hypertensive patients based on the simple parameters: wall motion abnormalities (*WMA*) and reduction in coronary flow reserve (*CFR* <2.0). Both parameters can be identified during a single stress echocardiography test ("two birds with one stone"), more easily with a vasodilator stress

aspects are especially important in our cost-conscious and risk-conscious era, in particular if we consider that serial examinations are required in these patients since the results of a negative test are no longer valid after 12–24 months, and every test adds cost to cost, dose to dose, and risk to risk [34]. Stress echocardiography today appears to offer an advantageous trade-off between the top priority of granting the optimal care for our patients with the emerging need to optimize the economic and biological sustainability of our diagnostic strategies [35] (Figs. 31.6 and 31.7).

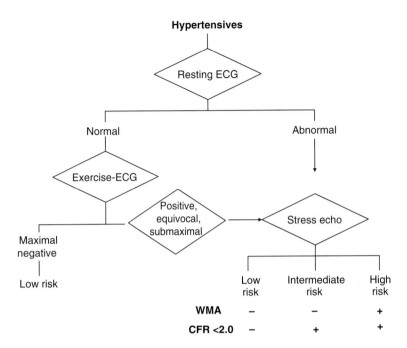

Fig. 31.7 The proposed diagnostic algorithm in hypertensive patients. Exercise electrocardiography remains the most informative first-line test, because of the wealth of information (blood pressure response, arrhythmias, exercise tolerance) provided beyond ST-segment changes. The negative predictive value is high in patients with interpretable and normal ECG at rest. In patients with abnormal or equivocal stress ECG findings, and in patients with resting ECG abnormalities, a stress imaging test is indicated as a gatekeeper to coronary angiography

References

1. Mancia G, De Backer G, Dominiczak A, et al; The task force for the management of arterial hypertension of the European Society of Hypertension, The task force for the management of arterial hypertension of the European Society of Cardiology (2007). 2007 Guidelines for the management of arterial hypertension: The Task Force for the Management of Arterial Hypertension of the European Society of Hypertension (ESH) and of the European Society of Cardiology (ESC). Eur Heart J 28:1462–1536
2. de Simone G, Schillaci G, Palmieri V, et al (2000) Should all patients with hypertension have echocardiography? J Hum Hypertens 14:417–421
3. Galderisi M (2005) Diastolic dysfunction and diastolic heart failure: diagnostic, prognostic and therapeutic aspects. Cardiovasc Ultrasound 3:9
4. Marcus ML (1989) Importance of abnormalities in coronary flow reserve to the pathophysiology of left ventricular hypertrophy secondary to hypertension. Clin Cardiol 12:IV34–IV35
5. Strauer BE (1979). Ventricular function and coronary hemodynamics in hypertensive heart disease. Am J Cardiol 44:999–1006

6. Opherk D, Mall G, Zebe H, et al (1984) Reduction of coronary reserve: a mechanism for angina pectoris in patients with arterial hypertension and normal coronary arteries. Circulation 69:1–7

7. Brush JE Jr, Cannon RO III, Schenke WH, et al (1988). Angina due to coronary microvascular disease in hypertensive patients without left ventricular hypertrophy. N Engl J Med 319: 1302–1307

8. Vogt M, Motz W, Strauer BE (1992). Coronary haemodynamics in hypertensive heart disease. Eur Heart J 13(Suppl D):44–49

9. Lucarini AR, Picano E, Lattanzi F, et al (1991) Dipyridamole-echocardiography stress testing in hypertensive patients. Target and tools. Circulation 83(Suppl III):68

10. Prisant LM, Frank MJ, Carr AA, et al (1987) How can we diagnose coronary heart disease in hypertensive patients? Hypertension 10:467–472

11. Picano E, Lucarini AR, Lattanzi F, et al (1988) Dipyridamole echocardiography in essential hypertensive patients with chest pain. Hypertension 12:238–243

12. Lucarini AR, Lattanzi F, Picano E, et al (1989) Dipyridamole-echocardiography test in essential hypertensives with chest pain and angiographically normal coronary arteries. Am J Hypertens 2:120–123

13. Fragasso G, Lu C, Dabrowski P, et al (1999). Comparison of stress/rest myocardial perfusion tomography, dipyridamole and dobutamine stress echocardiography for the detection of coronary disease in hypertensive patients with chest pain and positive exercise test. J Am Coll Cardiol 34:441–447

14. Astarita C, Palinkas A, Nicolai E, et al (2001) Dipyridamole-atropine stress echocardiography versus exercise SPECT scintigraphy for detection of coronary artery disease in hypertensives with positive exercise test. J Hypertens 19:495–502

15. Cortigiani L, Zanetti L, Bigi R, et al (2002) Safety and feasibility of dobutamine and dipyridamole stress echocardiography in hypertensive patients. J Hypertens 20:1423–1429

16. Ha JW, Juracan EM, Mahoney DW, et al (2002). Hypertensive response to exercise: a potential cause for new wall motion abnormality in the absence of coronary artery disease. J Am Coll Cardiol 39:323–327

17. Picano E, Palinkas A, Amyot R (2001) Diagnosis of myocardial ischemia in hypertensive patients. J Hypertens 19:1177–1183

18. Picano E, Lucarini AR, Lattanzi F, et al (1990) ST segment depression elicited by dipyridamole infusion in asymptomatic hypertensive patients. Hypertension 16:19–25

19. Strauer BE, Schwartzkopff B, Kelm M (1998) Assessing the coronary circulation in hypertension. J Hypertens 16:1221–1233

20. Lucarini AR, Picano E, Bongiorni MG, et al (1991) Increased prevalence of ventricular arrhythmias in essential hypertensives with dipyridamole-induced ischemic-like S-T segment changes. J Hypertens 9:839–844

21. Virdis A, Ghiadoni L, Lucarini A, et al (1996) Presence of cardiovascular structural changes in essential hypertensive patients with coronary microvascular disease and effects of long-term treatment. Am J Hypertens 9:361–369

22. Lucarini AR, Picano E, Salvetti A (1992) Coronary microvascular disease in hypertensives. Clin Exp Hypertens A 14:55–66

23. Cannon RO 3rd (1996) The heart in hypertension. Thinking small. Am J Hypertens 9:406–408

24. Cortigiani L, Paolini EA, Nannini E (1998) Dipyridamole stress echocardiography for risk stratification in hypertensive patients with chest pain. Circulation 98:2855–2859

25. Marwick TH, Case C, Sawada S, et al (2002) Prediction of outcomes in hypertensive patients with suspected coronary disease. Hypertension 39:1113–1118

26. Bigi R, Bax JJ, van Domburg RT, et al (2005) Simultaneous echocardiography and myocardial perfusion single photon emission computed tomography associated with dobutamine stress to

   predict long-term cardiac mortality in normotensive and hypertensive patients. J Hypertens
   23:1409–1415
27. Rigo F, Cortigiani L, Gherardi S, et al (2008) Coronary flow reserve in hypertensives: the best
   diagnostic and prognostic cut-off values. Eur Heart J (abstract Suppl)
28. Gibbons RJ, Balady GJ, Bricker JT, et al; American College of Cardiology/American Heart
   Association Task Force on Practice Guidelines (Committee to Update the 1997 Exercise Testing
   Guidelines) (2002) ACC/AHA 2002 guideline update for exercise testing: summary article:
   a report of the American College of Cardiology/American Heart Association Task Force on
   Practice Guidelines (Committee to Update the 1997 Exercise Testing Guidelines). Circulation.
   106:1883–1892
29. Picano E (2005). Economic and biological costs of cardiac imaging. Cardiovasc Ultrasound
   3:13
30. Cortigiani L, Bigi R, Rigo F, et al; Echo Persantine International Cooperative Study Group
   (2003) Diagnostic value of exercise electrocardiography and dipyridamole stress echocardiography in hypertensive and normotensive chest pain patients with right bundle branch block.
   J Hypertens 21:2189–2194
31. Picano E (2003) Stress echocardiography: a historical perspective. Special Article. Am J Med
   114:126–130
32. Picano E (2004) Sustainability of medical imaging. Education and Debate. BMJ 328:578–580
33. Picano E (2004) Informed consent and communication of risk from radiological and nuclear
   medicine examinations: how to escape from a communication inferno. Education and debate.
   BMJ 329:849–851
34. Picano E, Vano E, Semelka R, et al (2007). The American College of Radiology white paper
   on radiation dose in medicine: deep impact on the practice of cardiovascular imaging. Cardiovasc Ultrasound 5:37
35. Brenner DJ, Hall EJ (2007). Computed tomography – an increasing source of radiation exposure.
   N Engl J Med 357:2277–2284

Diabetes

32

Eugenio Picano and Lauro Cortigiani

Coronary artery disease is the leading cause of mortality and morbidity in patients with diabetes. Approximately one-half of deaths are attributed to coronary artery disease in diabetic patients, whose risk of myocardial infarction or cardiac death is two- to fourfold greater than in nondiabetic patients [1]. Moreover, cardiac events are as frequent in diabetic patients without evidence of coronary artery disease as in nondiabetic patients with known coronary artery disease [2]. Recent studies with electron beam computed tomography have shown that subclinical atherosclerosis is common in patients with diabetes, and studies with myocardial perfusion scintigraphy (with single-photon emission tomography) or stress echocardiography have demonstrated that between 25 and 50% of asymptomatic diabetic patients have ischemia during exercise or pharmacological stress and that a substantial proportion of these patients go on to develop major cardiovascular events within several years [2, 3]. The increased risk associated with diabetes calls for effective prevention and risk stratification strategies to optimize therapeutic interventions [3]. Clearly, asymptomatic diabetic patients include a subset of individuals at high risk of cardiovascular disease who would benefit from improved risk stratification beyond that possible with risk factor scoring systems alone [4]. Exercise testing is of limited value in the diabetic population because exercise capacity is often impaired by peripheral vascular [5] or neuropathic disease [6]. Furthermore, test specificity on electrocardiographic criteria is less than ideal because of the high prevalence of hypertension and microvascular disease [7]. Stress imaging, and in particular stress echocardiography, can play a key role in the optimal identification of the high-risk diabetic subset, also minimizing the economic and biologic costs of diagnostic screening, since stress echocardiography costs three times less than a perfusion scintigraphy and is a radiation-free technique without long-term oncogenic risks [8].

32.1
Pathophysiology

Diabetes mellitus can provoke cardiac damage at four levels: coronary macrovascular disease, autonomic cardiomyopathy, diabetic cardiomyopathy, and coronary microvascular disease (Fig. 32.1). These syndromes are rarely found in isolated form in individual patients, but

E. Picano, *Stress Echocardiography*,
© Springer-Verlag Berlin Heidelberg 2009

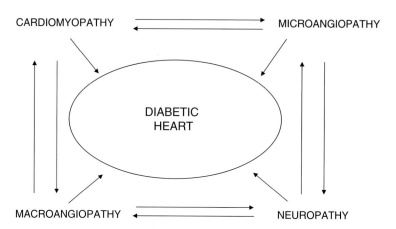

Fig. 32.1 The four aspects of damage in the diabetic heart: autonomic neuropathy, diabetic cardiomyopathy, coronary microangiopathy, coronary macroangiopathy. The four pathways – albeit pathogenetically distinct – cross-talk. For instance, microangiopathy may codetermine neuropathy – through vas nervorum involvement – and at the coronary level, may impair coronary flow reserve, amplifying the impact of an epicardial coronary artery stenosis

more often overlap and potentiate each other. In particular, diabetes mellitus induces coronary structural [9] and functional [10, 11] microvascular abnormalities, which are associated with coronary endothelial dysfunction and impairment in coronary flow reserve, even in the absence of epicardial coronary artery disease [12]. In young subjects with uncomplicated diabetes, there is a marked coronary microvascular dysfunction in response to adenosine infusion (primarily reflecting aberrant endothelium-independent vasodilation) and to the cold pressor test (primarily reflecting endothelium-dependent vasodilation) [13].

32.2
Diagnosis of Coronary Artery Disease

The coronary microangiopathy component can amplify the effects of coronary macroangiopathy, which is a major complication of diabetes. Coronary, cerebral, and peripheral vascular diseases are the causes of death in 75% of adult diabetic subjects. The coexistence of epicardial coronary artery stenosis with microangiopathy can explain the low specificity of perfusion imaging compared to stress echocardiography in the detection of coronary artery disease in asymptomatic (and symptomatic diabetic patients [14–21]). In fact, the typical behavior of microvascular disease during stress testing is the frequent induction of ST-segment depression and perfusion abnormalities, with true reduction in coronary flow reserve without regional or global wall motion changes [8]. In practical terms, this means that in patients with normal baseline ECG results, the negative predictive value of a maximal exercise ECG is satisfactory, but in all patients with positive or ambiguous ECG and/or chest pain findings, a stress echocardiography test is warranted. In diabetic patients, stress echocardiography has shown a higher specificity than perfusion imaging but suffers from a higher rate of false-positive results, possibly due to the coexistence of cardiomyopathy in many patients [21].

32.3
Prognostic Stratification

Risk stratification of diabetic patients is a major objective for the clinical cardiologist, given their increased risk for coronary artery disease [1]. Resting echocardiography is already important for this purpose, since there is a distinct "cardiomyopathy cascade" (Fig. 32.2) with higher risk levels – and higher degrees of cardiomyopathic involvement – identified by left atrial dilatation [22], diastolic dysfunction [23], and impaired longitudinal function [24], which all may coexist with normal ejection fraction [25].

Stress echocardiography has shown powerful risk stratification capabilities in diabetics. In patients with overt resting ischemic cardiomyopathy, the presence of myocardial viability recognized by dobutamine echocardiography independently predicts improved outcome following revascularization in nondiabetics as well as in diabetic patients following revascularization [26]. Also in patients with normal resting left ventricular function, a clear refinement of prognosis can be obtained with stress echocardiography, first and foremost on the basis of classical wall motion abnormalities [27–32], which place the patients in a high-risk subset for cardiovascular events (Fig. 32.3). The incremental prognostic information pro-

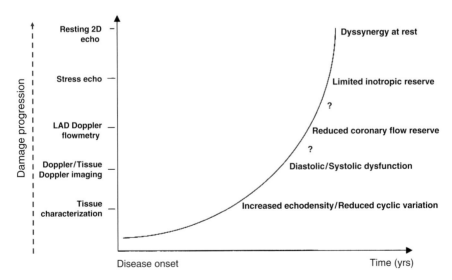

Fig. 32.2 Cardiomyopathy cascade. In the sequence of events, changes in diastolic function and alternations in longitudinal function of the left ventricle (such as reduction in mitral annulus plane systolic excursion by *M*-mode or reduction in systolic velocity by myocardial tissue Doppler or strain rate imaging) precede by years or decades the reduction of ejection fraction. (From [25])

32

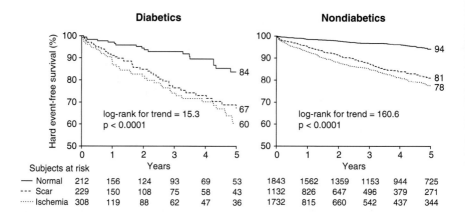

Fig. 32.3 Kaplan–Meier event-free survival curves in diabetics (*left*) and nondiabetics (*right*). In patients without scar and inducible wall motion abnormalities, the prognosis is excellent in nondiabetics, but still poor in diabetics in whom a better stratification is needed. (From [33])

vided by stress echocardiography is highest in patients with intermediate-to-high threshold positive exercise electrocardiography test results [33]. However, in diabetic patients – differently from nondiabetic subjects – a negative test result based solely on wall motion criteria is associated with less benign outcome in the presence of diabetes [32] (Fig. 32.3). In these patients, coronary flow reserve evaluated simultaneously with wall motion during vasodilation stress testing by transthoracic Doppler echocardiography adds independent prognostic information [34] (Fig. 32.4). In particular, a normal coronary flow reserve off therapy is associated with better and similar survival both in the diabetic and nondiabetic population. Explanations for reduced coronary flow reserve in the absence of stress-induced wall motion abnormalities include mild-to-moderate epicardial coronary artery stenosis, severe epicardial artery stenosis in presence of antiischemic therapy, and severe microvascular coronary disease in presence of patent epicardial coronary arteries [34].

32.4
The Diagnostic Flow Chart in Diabetics

The general diagnostic flow chart in diabetics (both symptomatic and intermediate-to-high risk asymptomatic) can be summarized as in Fig. 32.5. After the exercise stress test, a stress imaging test is often warranted. In the literature, strategies based on perfusion imaging (with thallium or sestamibi) have been proposed, even in guidelines and in young or middle-aged women. For instance, the Swiss Society of Endocrinology-Diabetology recommends screening for coronary artery disease for diabetic patients with two or more additional cardiovascular risk factors, and the recommended test for screening is either stress echocardiography or myocardial perfusion imaging [35]. Nearly 10 years ago, the American Diabetes Association recommended exercise tolerance testing alone in asymptomatic patients with two or more coronary artery disease risk factors or an abnormal resting electrocardiogram. However, the recommendation is not based on hard evidence but rather is the consensus of an

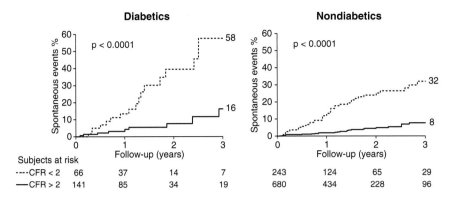

Fig. 32.4 Kaplan–Meier survival curve event rate for diabetic and nondiabetic patients with coronary flow reserve (*CFR*)>2 or ≤2, normal resting echocardiography, and negative stress echocardiography by wall motion criteria. (From [34])

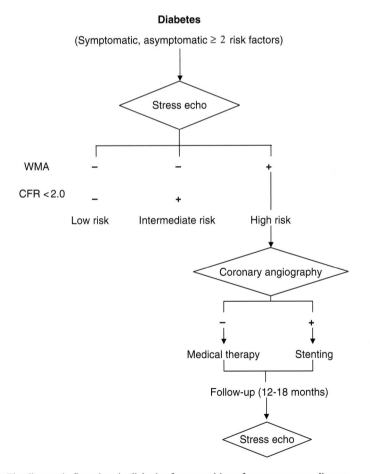

Fig. 32.5 The diagnostic flow chart in diabetics for recognition of coronary artery disease

32

expert panel. The recognized finding that 10–15% of asymptomatic diabetics indeed have coronary artery disease have led to proposing stress imaging for a more effective risk stratification [36]. However, the economic and long-term risk burden is especially important due to recent accumulation of suggestive evidence that percutaneous coronary revascularization may not provide additive benefit to intensive medical management in patients with stable coronary artery disease [4]. Therefore, we currently recommend that testing for atherosclerosis or ischemia be reserved for those in whom medical treatment goals cannot be met and for selected individuals in whom there is strong clinical suspicion of very-high-risk coronary artery disease [4]. Even in these individuals, techniques with substantial radiation exposure – albeit recommended by authorities – such as myocardial scintigraphy or cardiac computed tomography should be used with great wisdom and prudence, and stress echocardiography is by far a more sustainable option [8]. The information obtained with the two different approaches is more or less the same for the physician, but certainly not for the patient and society, since small individual risks multiplied by a million examinations translate into significant population risks [37]. The radiation dose is 500–1,500 chest X-rays for every scintigraphy or 50–1,500 chest X-rays for each cardiac computed tomography scan. The long-term risk of cancer for these procedures is not insignificant (1 in 500 for a single thallium scan), higher in women (1 in 350 for a 35-year-old woman) and cumulative: every test adds dose to dose, risk to risk, and cost to cost. In addition, patient acceptance of testing is higher when no radiation exposure is involved [38]. The issue of economic and biological sustainability is especially important in diabetic patients, since the results of testing are thought to no longer be valid after 12–18 months and serial examinations are regularly needed in these patients [39]. The same diagnostic efficacy can be achieved with stress echocardiography, if possible with combined wall motion and coronary flow reversible assessment simultaneously evaluated with a single stress (a "two birds with a stone" approach). Patients with wall motion abnormalities are at high risk and should be referred to coronary angiography for ischemia-driven revascularization. Patients without wall motion abnormalities and after reduction in coronary flow reserve are at intermediate risk and should be treated aggressively with tight metabolic control, maximal antiischemic therapy, and a more frequent follow-up by noninvasive stress testing [32]. Patients with neither wall motion abnormalities nor reduction in coronary flow reserve are at low risk and can be managed conservatively. These approaches will optimize the quality of screening for coronary artery disease but at the same time minimize the costs and the radiation burden of a diagnostic "carpet bombing" still of questionable benefit in asymptomatic diabetes.

References

1. Ryden L, Standl E, Bartnik M, et al; Task Force on Diabetes and Cardiovascular Diseases of the European Society of Cardiology (ESC); European Association for the Study of Diabetes (EASD) (2007) Guidelines on diabetes, pre-diabetes, and cardiovascular diseases: executive summary. Eur Heart J 28:88–136
2. Berry C, Tardif J-C, Bourassa MG (2007) Coronary heart disease in patients with diabetes. Part I: recent advances in prevention and non-invasive management. J Am Coll Cardiol 49:631–642
3. Bax JJ, Bonow RO, Tschöpe D, et al; Global Dialogue Group for the Evaluation of Cardiovascular Risk in Patients With Diabetes (2006) The potential of myocardial perfusion scintigra-

phy for risk stratification of asymptomatic patients with type 2 diabetes. J Am Coll Cardiol 48:754–760

4. Bax JJ, Young LH, Frye RL, et al; ADA (2007) Screening for coronary artery disease in patients with diabetes. Diabetes Care 30:2729–2736

5. Akbari CM, LoGerfo FW (1999) Diabetes and peripheral vascular disease. J Vasc Surg 30:373–384

6. May O, Arildsen H, Damsgaard EM, et al (2000) Cardiovascular autonomic neuropathy in insulin-dependent diabetes mellitus: prevalence and estimated risk o coronary heart disease in the general population. J Intern Med 248:483–491

7. Picano E, Pálinkás A, Amyot R (2001) Diagnosis of myocardial ischemia in hypertensive patients. J Hypertens 19:1177–1183

8. Picano E (2003) Stress echocardiography: a historical perspective. Am J Med 114:126–130

9. Factor SM, Okun EM, Minase T (1980) Capillary microaneurysms in the human diabetic heart. N Engl J Med 302:384–388

10. Strauer BE, Motz W, Vogt M, et al (1997) Evidence for reduced coronary flow reserve in patients with insulin-dependent diabetes. A possible cause for diabetic heart disease in man. Exp Clin Endocrinol Diabet 105:15–20

11. Nahser PJ Jr, Brown RE, Oskarsson H, et al (1995) Maximal coronary flow reserve and metabolic coronary vasodilation in patients with diabetes mellitus. Circulation 91:635–640

12. Nitenberg A, Valensi P, Sachs R, et al (1993) Impairment of coronary vascular reserve and ACh-induced coronary vasodilation in diabetic patients with angiographically normal coronary arteries and normal left ventricular systolic function. Diabetes 42:1017–1025

13. Di Carli MF, Janisse J, Grunberger G, et al (2003) Role of chronic hyperglycemia in the pathogenesis of coronary microvascular dysfunction in diabetes. J Am Coll Cardiol. 41:1387–1393

14. Bates JR, Sawada SG, Segar DS, et al (1996) Evaluation using dobutamine stress echocardiography in patients with insulin-dependent diabetes mellitus before kidney and/or pancreas transplantation. Am J Cardiol 77:175–179

15. Hennessy TG, Codd MB, Kane G et al (1997) Evaluation of patients with diabetes mellitus for coronary artery disease using dobutamine stress echocardiography. Coron Artery Dis 8:171–174

16. Elhendy A, Domburg RT van, Poldermans D, et al (1998) Safety and feasibility of dobutamine-atropine stress echocardiography for the diagnosis of coronary artery disease in diabetic patients unable to perform an exercise stress test. Diabetes Care 21:1797–1802

17. Gaddi O, Tortorella G, Picano E, et al (1999) Diagnostic and prognostic value of vasodilator stress echocardiography in asymptomatic type 2 diabetic patients with positive exercise thallium scintigraphy: a pilot study. Diabet Med 16:762–766

18. Lin K, Stewart D, Cooper S, et al (2001) Pre-transplant cardiac testing for kidney–pancreas transplant candidates and association with cardiac outcomes. Clin Transplant 15:269–275

19. Penfornis A, Zimmermann C, Boumal D, et al (2001) Use of dobutamine stress echocardiography in detecting silent myocardial ischaemia in asymptomatic diabetic patients: a comparison with thallium scintigraphy and exercise testing. Diabet Med 18:900–905

20. Coisne D, Donal E, Torremocha F, et al (2001) Dobutamine stress echocardiography response of asymptomatic patients with diabetes. Echocardiography 18:373–379

21. Griffin ME, Nikookam K, Teh MM, et al (1998) Dobutamine stress echocardiography: false positive scans in proteinuric patients with type 1 diabetes mellitus at high risk of ischaemic heart disease. Diabet Med 15:427–430

22. Bangalore S, Yao SS, Chaudhry FA (2007) Role of left atrial size in risk stratification and prognosis of patients undergoing stress echocardiography. J Am Coll Cardiol 50:1254–1262

23. Galderisi M (2006) Diastolic dysfunction and diabetic cardiomyopathy: evaluation by Doppler echocardiography. J Am Coll Cardiol 48:1548–1551

24. Fang ZY, Najos-Valencia O, Leano R, et al (2003) Patients with early diabetic heart disease demonstrate a normal myocardial response to dobutamine. J Am Coll Cardiol 41:1457–1465

25. Picano E (2003) Diabetic cardiomyopathy: the importance of being earliest. Editorial comment. J Am Coll Cardiol 41:1465–1471
26. Cortigiani L, Sicari R, Desideri A, et al; VIDA (Viability Identification with Dobutamine Administration) Study Group (2007) Dobutamine stress echocardiography and the effect of revascularization on outcome in diabetic and non-diabetic patients with chronic ischaemic left ventricular dysfunction. Eur J Heart Fail 9:1038–1043
27. Elhendy A, Arruda AM, Mahoney DW, et al (2001) Prognostic stratification of diabetic patients by exercise echocardiography. J Am Coll Cardiol 37:1551–1557
28. Bigi R, Desideri A, Cortigiani L, et al (2001) Stress echocardiography for risk stratification of diabetic patients with known or suspected coronary artery disease. Diabetes Care 24:1596–1601
29. Kamalesh M, Matorin R, Sawada S (2002) Prognostic value of a negative stress echocardiographic study in diabetic patients. Am Heart J 2002 143:163–168
30. Marwick TH, Case C, Sawada S, et al (2002) Use of stress echocardiography to predict mortality in patients with diabetes and known or suspected coronary artery disease. Diabetes Care 25:1042–1048
31. Sozzi F, Elhendy A, Rizzello V, et al (2007) Prognostic significance of myocardial ischemia during dobutamine stress echocardiography in asymptomatic patients with diabetes mellitus and no prior history of coronary events. Am J Cardiol 99(9):1193–1195
32. Cortigiani L, Bigi R, Sicari R, et al (2006) Prognostic value of pharmacological stress echocardiography in diabetic and nondiabetic patients with known or suspected coronary artery disease. J Am Coll Cardiol 47:605–610
33. Cortigiani L, Bigi R, Sicari R, et al (2007) Comparison of prognostic value of pharmacologic stress echocardiography in chest pain patients with versus without diabetes mellitus and positive exercise electrocardiography. Am J Cardiol 100:1744–1749
34. Cortigiani L, Rigo F, Gherardi S, et al (2007) Additional prognostic value of coronary flow reserve in diabetic and nondiabetic patients with negative dipyridamole stress echocardiography by wall motion criteria. J Am Coll Cardiol. 50:1354–1361
35. Hurni CA, Perret S, Monbaron D, et al (2007) Coronary artery disease screening in diabetic patients: how good is guideline adherence? Swiss Med Wkly 137:199–204
36. Heller GV (2005) Evaluation of the patient with diabetes mellitus and suspected coronary artery disease. Am J Med 118:9S–14S
37. Picano E (2004) Sustainability of medical imaging. Education and debate. BMJ 328:578–580
38. Picano E (2004) Informed consent and communication of risk from radiological and nuclear medicine examinations: how to escape from a communication inferno. BMJ 329:849–851
39. Picano E (2005) Economic and biological costs of cardiac imaging. Cardiovasc Ultrasound 3:13

Stress Echocardiography in Dilated Cardiomyopathy

33

Eugenio Picano

Heart failure is a progressive, lethal syndrome characterized by accelerating deterioration [1]. Its estimated prevalence in the USA is around 2.0%, with an increased prevalence of 6–10% in patients over 65 years of age [2]. The prognosis of heart failure is uniformly poor if the underlying problem cannot be rectified; half of all patients carrying a diagnosis of heart failure will die within 4 years, and in patients with severe heart failure, more than 50% will die within 1 year [2]. The actual rate of deterioration is highly variable and depends on the nature and causes of the overload, the age of the patient, and many other factors (Fig. 33.1). Following a period of asymptomatic left ventricular dysfunction that can last more than a decade, survival after the onset of significant symptoms averages about 5 years [3]. Stress echocardiography has a role in initial and advanced stages (Fig. 33.2). In formulating the 2001 document, also endorsed in the 2005 document, the ACC/AHA guidelines developed a new approach to the classification of heart failure, identifying four stages: stage A (at high risk, but without structural heart disease, e.g., hypertension), stage B (structural heart disease but without signs and symptoms of heart failure, e.g., previous myocardial infarction or asymptomatic valvular heart disease), stage C (structural heart disease with current or prior symptoms of heart failure), and stage D (refractory heart failure requiring specialized interventions). According to this staging approach, which is conceptually similar to that achieved by staging in other diseases such as cancer, patients would be expected either not to advance at all or to advance from one stage to the next, unless progression of the disease was slowed or stopped by treatment. The recent realization that therapies aimed at symptomatic heart failure may improve outcomes in patients with asymptomatic left ventricular dysfunction has increased the importance of recognizing and treating patients with the asymptomatic stage A and B condition, possibly even more frequent than overt heart failure. In the early stage, in patients with normal left ventricular function, a reduced inotropic reserve can unmask initial damage. In advanced stages, stress echocardiography complements resting echocardiography, identifying a heterogenous prognostic profile that underlies a similar resting echocardiographic pattern (Table 33.1).

E. Picano, *Stress Echocardiography*,
© Springer-Verlag Berlin Heidelberg 2009

33

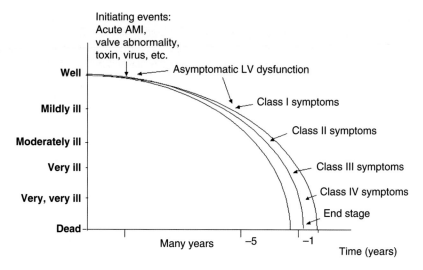

Fig. 33.1 The natural history of cardiomyopathy. (Modified from [3])

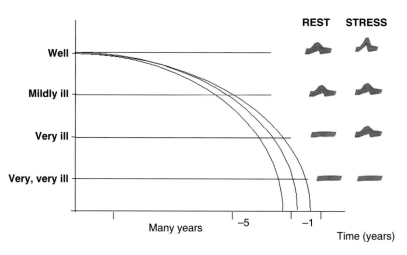

Fig. 33.2 The role of stress echocardiography in prognostic titration of cardiomyopathy. At an early stage, baseline function is normal but inotropic reserve is depressed. At an advanced stage, the baseline function is depressed but there is inotropic reserve. At a very advanced stage, the resting function is depressed and the inotropic response is abolished

33.1
Incipient or Latent Cardiomyopathy

Some patients are exposed to potentially cardiotoxic conditions, such as chemotherapy in cancer or iron overload in thalassemia. The clinical natural history of these conditions is characterized by a very short interval between the onset of cardiac symptoms and end-stage cardiac failure. The detection of preclinical cardiac involvement can be important in order to start more aggressive therapy. There are two possible, and not mutually exclusive, approaches for the early detection of incipient myocardial damage when ejection fraction is still normal. The first possibility is to assess longitudinal function, impaired at an earlier stage of disease than ejection fraction, which may remain normal due to supernormal compensatory radial function. The selective early impairment of longitudinal global function can be easily measured with *M*-mode mitral annulus plane systolic excursion or with myocardial velocity imaging, as decreased systolic S wave velocity of basal (septal and/or lateral) segments with tissue Doppler and/or strain-rate imaging. The early reduction in longitudinal function, with normal ejection fraction, has been described in several conditions, from systemic sclerosis [4] to diabetic [5] or hypertensive [6] cardiomyopathy.

The second approach is to assess the segmental and global contractile reserve during inotropic challenge. The rationale of applying stress echocardiography in these conditions is that structural impairments of the myocardial wall can be subtle enough so as not to impair resting systolic function, but severe enough to blunt or even exhaust the contractile response to the inotropic stimulation. At low doses ($\leq 10\,\mu g\ kg^{-1}$ per min), dobutamine selectively stimulates β-1 myocardial receptors, determining a mild, sustained inotropic stimulation with little if any effect on either systemic hemodynamic parameters or loading conditions. With these low dobutamine doses, the lower basal wall shows a blunted increase in percent systolic thickening, or in peak systolic velocity on myocardial velocity imaging, which helps detect early damage. The blunted regional cardiac contractile reserve (Fig. 33.2) has also proved useful in detecting subtle forms of cardiac involvement in several diseases, such as doxorubicin chemotherapy [7], thalassemia [8], diabetic [9], or hypertrophic cardiomyopathy [10]. In all these conditions, the reduction in myocardial contractile reserve – best observed with dobutamine stress – is also accompanied by impaired coronary flow reserve, best detected today by vasodilator stress combined with pulsed Doppler of the mid-distal left anterior descending coronary artery [11]. The reduction of coronary flow reserve at a very early clinical stage, when symptoms are absent or minimal and left ventricular ejection fraction is normal at baseline [12], has been described in several clinical conditions such as systemic sclerosis [13], and diabetic [14] or hypertensive [15] heart disease. Contractile reserve focuses on the myocytes, whereas coronary

Table 33.1 Stress echocardiography response and the four stages of dilated cardiomyopathy

Disease class (ACC/AHA)	Stage of disease	Resting global function (EF)	Longitudinal function	Stress function	Coronary flow reserve
A	Absent	Normal	Normal	Normal	Normal
B	Initial	Normal	Abnormal	Blunted hyperkinesia	↓ →
C	Overt	Abnormal	Very abnormal	Functional recovery	↓
D	Advanced	Abnormal	Very abnormal	No functional recovery	↓↓

EF ejection fraction

flow reserve assessed the coronary microcirculation. Both impaired contractile reserve and decreased coronary flow reserve are therefore very early, and possibly diagnostically relevant, markers of initial cardiomyopathy, at a stage when any form of intervention (lifestyle or drugs) is more likely to be efficacious (Table 33.1).

33.2
Dilated Cardiomyopathy

Dilated cardiomyopathy is a condition that predominantly affects ventricular systolic function. Nevertheless, indices of global systolic dysfunction as measured at rest are inadequate for depicting the severity of the disease and are poorly correlated with symptoms, exercise capacity, and prognosis [16]. In contrast, the assessment of contractile reserve by pharmacological challenge, rather than baseline indices, is an important means of quantifying the degree of cardiac impairment and refining prognostic prediction [17]. In general, all of the twelve available studies on several hundred patients have shown a beneficial effect of a preserved inotropic response on prognosis, although disparate methodology, selection criteria (including both idiopathic and ischemic dilated cardiomyopathy) and prognostic end point were utilized [18–30]. The contractile reserve can be identified through wall motion index improvement (greater than 0.20) or with a reduction of end-systolic volume during stress. A specific application has been proposed in patients with long-lasting atrial fibrillation and dilated cardiomyopathy. Atrial fibrillation can cause a reversible form of dilated cardiomyopathy, with restoration of normal left ventricular function after cardioversion to sinus rhythm. The distinction between idiopathic dilated cardiomyopathy and tachycardiomyopathy is important because restoration of sinus rhythm leads to a significant improvement in left ventricular function only in the latter case [19].

The dobutamine infusion protocol is similar to the one followed in patients with ischemic heart disease, but without atropine administration. In patients with dilated cardiomyopathy and heart failure, a lack of increase in left ventricular function is associated with higher mortality (Fig. 33.3). However, limiting minor side effects occur in about 10–20% of these patients, who have a depressed ejection fraction and are more vulnerable to an arrhythmic side effect of the drug. In patients with contraindications to or submaximal, nondiagnostic dobutamine stress echocardiography, alternative tests may offer comparable information. Dipyridamole may elicit a prognostically meaningful increase in function, comparable to that provided with the more arrhythmogenic dobutamine [31]. With dipyridamole, the prognostic information is further expanded by the assessment of coronary flow reserve on the left anterior descending artery (Fig. 33.4) and, when possible, the posterior descending right coronary artery. The prognosis is worse in patients with coronary flow reserve on LAD less than 2 [32] and worst when the coronary flow reserve is depressed in both coronaries [33]. The prognostic information derived from stress echocardiography can be added on the top of the versatility of data provided by resting transthoracic echocardiography. A reduced tricuspid annulus plane systolic excursion and increased pulmonary artery systolic pressure may further worsen the prognostic outlook (Table 33.2), dominated by the "deadly quartet": (1) dilated (end-systolic volume >90 ml m^{-2})

Survival (%)

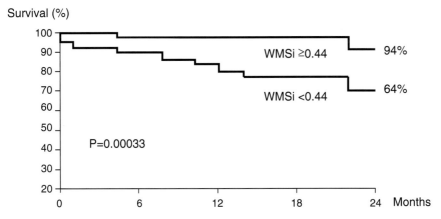

Fig. 33.3 Kaplan–Meier survival curves in patients with dilated cardiomyopathy separated on the basis of preserved (Δ WMSI>0.44) or impaired (Δ WMSI<0.44) left ventricular contractile reserve during dobutamine stress. (Modified from [24])

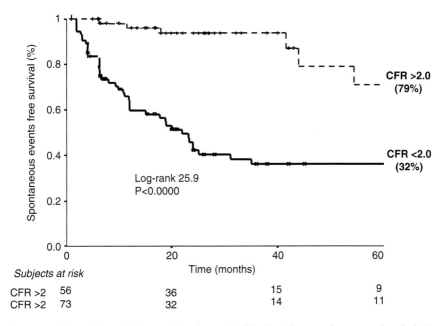

Fig. 33.4 Kaplan–Meier survival curves in patients with dilated cardiomyopathy separated on the basis of normal (CFR>2.0) or depressed (CFR<2.0) coronary flow reserve. (Modified from [32])

left ventricle, (2) severe mitral insufficiency, (3) diastolic restrictive pattern (or E/e value>15), and (4) increased extravascular lung water detectable as ultrasound lung comets on chest sonography [34, 35].

Table 33.2 Prognosis in dilated cardiomyopathy: from bad to worse

	M-mode	2D	Color	CW	Pulsed TDI	Chest
TAPSE	√					
LV end-systolic volume		√				
Mitral insufficiency			√			
PASP increase				√		
E/e (restrictive)					√	
ULC						√

PASP pulmonary artery systolic pressure, *TDI* tissue Doppler imaging, *TAPSE* tricuspid annular plane systolic excursion, *ULC* ultrasound lung comets

33.3
Differentiation Between Ischemic and Nonischemic Dilated Cardiomyopathy

The detection of coronary artery disease in a patient with global left ventricular dysfunction and dilatation has important therapeutic and prognostic implications. The diagnosis of ischemic cardiomyopathy may either be straightforward or impossible on a noninvasive basis. At one end of the clinical spectrum, the ischemic etiology is obvious when an unequivocal history of ischemic heart disease and infarction can be collected. As a rule, several episodes of myocardial necrosis have progressively reduced pump function. After repeated infarctions, marked global dysfunction ensues, anginal symptoms are reduced and progressively replaced by dyspnea. At the other end of the clinical spectrum, ischemic cardiomyopathy can be completely superimposable on an idiopathic form with signs and symptoms of congestive heart failure. Dyspnea can be an angina equivalent, and on the other hand angina may be present in idiopathic and absent in ischemic cardiomyopathy. Several noninvasive clues to this differentiation have been proposed (Table 33.3). Ischemic patients more frequently show akinetic segments and a more elliptical shape at resting echocardiography, a smaller and less compromised right ventricle, and larger stress-induced defects during perfusion imaging, with scintigraphy or echocardiography. Encouraging results have also been reported with dobutamine stress echocardiography. Of particular value is the biphasic response in at least two segments and/or the extensive ischemic response [36–38]. However, all stress-imaging clues concerning the distinction between ischemic and idiopathic cardiomyopathy cannot always be considered clinically significant, although they have been reported to be statistically significant in some studies. Cardiomyopathy is one of the most frequent sources of false-positive ischemic response and no wall motion abnormalities can be evoked in an ischemic cardiomyopathy when fibrosis is extensive. Cardiovascular magnetic resonance can be more helpful, identifying a subendocardial–transmural regional pattern in ischemia as opposed to a patchy, diffuse scar pattern in nonischemic dilated cardiomyopathy. Coronary angiography (or its noninvasive counterpart of multislice computed tomography) is quite often the only way to firmly establish the differential diagnosis between ischemic and idiopathic cardiomyopathy.

Table 33.3 Differential diagnosis of dilated cardiomyopathy

	Ischemic	Nonischemic
History of infarction	Yes/no	No
Resting echocardiography: regional abnormality	Yes/no	No/yes
Stress echocardiography: inducible abnormalities	Yes/no	No/yes
CMR	Subendocardial transmural scar	Patchy, subepicardial fibrosis
MSCT	Severe CAD	Normal

CAD coronary artery disease, *CMR* cardiac magnetic resonance, *MSCT* multislice computed tomography

In these patients, the role of stress echocardiography is mainly focused on the prognostic stratification dictating the therapy. In ischemic cardiomyopathy, only the presence of significant (four or more left ventricular segments) contractile reserve warrants a prognostically beneficial revascularization [39].

33.4
Stress Echocardiography and Cardiac Resynchronization Therapy

Cardiac resynchronization therapy (CRT) is a promising technique in patients with end-stage heart failure. Current selection criteria include New York Heart Association class III or IV heart failure, left ventricular ejection fraction 35% or less, and wide QRS complex (>120 ms). The majority of patients selected according to these criteria respond well to CRT, but 30% (by echocardiographic criteria) do not respond. The most frequently used clinical marker is the improvement of one grade or more in NYHA class; the most frequently used echocardiographic marker is an antiremodeling effect defined as a reduction of 15% or more in left ventricular end-systolic volume [40]. In the majority of patients, there is full agreement between clinical and echocardiographic response, but 25% of patients show discordant results, more often with clinical but not echocardiographic response. The large number of nonresponders for a costly, risky, and demanding therapy such as CRT led researchers to look for better selection criteria (Figs. 33.5 and 33.6). In the failing heart, cardiac dyssynchrony is present on three levels: (1) atrioventricular, (2) interventricular (right vs. left ventricle), and (3) intraventricular (within the left ventricle). Echocardiography can assess intra- and interventricular dyssynchrony. The assessment of interventricular dyssynchrony is simple, standardized, and reproducible but basically useless [40]; the assessment of intraventricular dyssynchrony is complex, deregulated with dozens of different methods proposed in the last 10 years, suffers from higher variability [41], and is equally worthless [42]. *M*-mode echocardiography is the simplest technique, and a short axis view is used to measure the so-called septal-to-posterior wall motion delay, the interval between the systolic excursion of the anteroseptum and of the inferolateral wall [41]. Unfortunately, with this method only two segments (out of 17!) are sampled and the

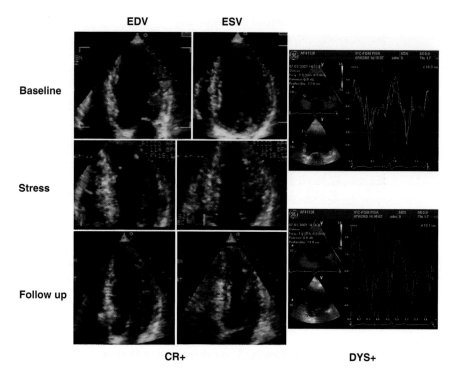

Fig. 33.5 An example of a CRT responder. Echocardiographic four-chamber view at rest, at peak stress and at follow-up of a patient with contractile reserve (*CR+*) (*left*) and tissue Doppler criteria of intra-ventricular dyssynchrony (*Rest DYS+*) (*right*). EDV, end-diastolic volume; ESV, end-systolic volume. (Modified from [44])

parameter cannot be assessed in 50% of patients, when the septum is akinetic, especially in ischemic cardiomyopathy. Tissue Doppler imaging (TDI) is probably the most popular technique for assessing LV dyssynchrony. It measures peak systolic velocities in different regions of the myocardium and the time intervals between electrical activity (the QRS complex) and mechanical activity (segmental peak systolic velocity). The 2-, 4- or 11-segment approach has been used (the apical segments are unreadable with this technique). Tissue synchronization imaging is more visually oriented. It automatically calculates the peak systolic velocities from TDI and displays them as a color map, for direct visualization of the early activated segments (displayed in green) and late activated segments (displayed in red). With strain imaging – and more specifically with strain-rate imaging measures of the rate of myocardial deformation – the extent of left ventricular dyssynchrony is assessed by measuring time to peak systolic strain. With real-time three-dimensional (RT3D) echocardiography, a series of plots is obtained representing the change in volume for each segment throughout the cycle. However, in the presence of left ventricular dyssynchrony, minimum volume will be reached for each segment at different times, and the extent of this dispersion reflects the left ventricular dyssynchrony [40, 41]. Responders have a higher systolic dyssynchrony than nonresponders.

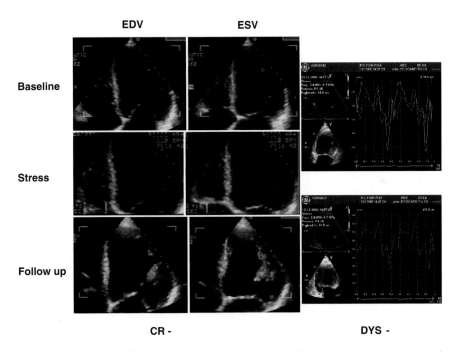

Fig. 33.6 An example of a CRT nonresponder. Echocardiographic four-chamber view at rest, at peak stress, and at follow-up of a patient without contractile reserve (*CR−*) (*left*) without tissue Doppler criteria of intraventricular dyssynchrony (*Rest DYS−*) (*right*). (Modified from [44])

At present, TDI is probably the most popular technique for assessing LV dyssynchrony [40, 41], but not the most useful, since all proposed parameters tested in the multicenter PROSPECT trial failed, adding nothing to clinical and ECG stratification [42].

Recently, disappointment with the mechanical dyssynchrony approach led several investigators to integrate the electrical approach with a more functional approach. In fact, it is probably unrealistic to expect a response to CRT if there is not enough muscle to be resynchronized. In other words, it is unlikely that home comfort will benefit from a brand-new electric system if there are no walls and no ceiling left. Indeed, this so-called functional approach appears to be much more gratifying in selecting candidates for CRT. In patients with depressed ejection fraction, lack of a substantial (five segments or more) viability response to dobutamine stress echocardiography is invariably associated with a lack of response to CRT [43, 44]. This is the same pattern that has been described in ischemia cardiomyopathy patients undergoing revascularization [39] or cardiomyopathy patients on β-blockers or other medical therapy [45] or low-flow, low-gradient aortic stenosis patients undergoing aortic valve replacement [46]. The beneficial effect of medical, mechanical, or electrical therapy in heart failure patients requires the presence of a critical mass of target tissue: "No muscle, no party!" [47]. Also, this shift in diagnostic forms from electrical synchronicity to functional reserve dramatically simplifies the screening of the CRT candidate; stress echocardiography is simpler, much faster, and more reproducible

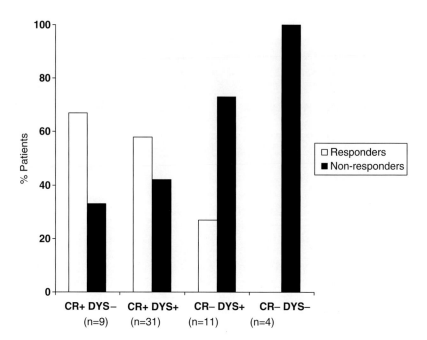

Fig. 33.7 Responders to cardiac Resynchronization Therapy are selected on the basis of contractile reserve more efficiently than with dyssynchrony (Modified from [44])

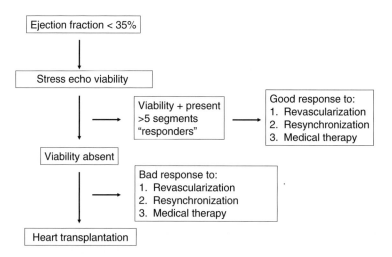

Fig. 33.8 The importance of being viable in patients with depressed ejection fraction. Whatever the underlying disease, response to therapy is dependent upon underlying presence of myocardial viability. The type of therapy obviously depends on the underlying etiology: coronary revascularization in coronary artery disease, aortic valve replacement in low-flow, low-gradient aortic stenosis, cardiac resynchronization therapy in nonischemic cardiomyopathy. (Modified from [48])

than CRT criteria. Echocardiographic evaluation of dyssynchrony may add something to the risk stratification, but only in patients with viability. This approach can be made even simpler and more quantitative in CRT, when the single most important stress echocardiographic parameter is variation in end-systolic volume, which today can be estimated even more accurately with RT3D. This stress echocardiography-driven approach to selection of CRT responders is now mature and ready for large-scale validation (Figs. 33.7 and 33.8).

References

1. Swedberg K, Cleland J, Dargie H, et al; Task Force for the Diagnosis and Treatment of Chronic Heart Failure of the European Society of Cardiology (2005) Guidelines for the diagnosis and treatment of chronic heart failure: executive summary (update 2005): The Task Force for the Diagnosis and Treatment of Chronic Heart Failure of the European Society of Cardiology. Eur Heart J 26:1115–1140

2. Hunt SA, Abraham WT, Chin MH, et al; American College of Cardiology; American Heart Association Task Force on Practice Guidelines; American College of Chest Physicians; International Society for Heart and Lung Transplantation; Heart Rhythm Society (2005) ACC/AHA 2005 Guideline Update for the Diagnosis and Management of Chronic Heart Failure in the Adult: a report of the American College of Cardiology/American Heart Association Task Force on Practice Guidelines (Writing Committee to Update the 2001 Guidelines for the Evaluation and Management of Heart Failure): developed in collaboration with the American College of Chest Physicians and the International Society for Heart and Lung Transplantation: endorsed by the Heart Rhythm Society. Circulation 112:e154–e235

3. Katz AM (2001) Heart failure. Pathophysiology, molecular biology and clinical management. Lippincott Williams and Wilkins, Philadelphia

4. Henein MY, Cailes J, O'Sullivan C, et al (1995) Abnormal ventricular long-axis function in systemic sclerosis. Chest 108:1533–1540

5. Fang ZY, Najos-Valencia O, Leano R, et al (2003) Patients with early diabetic heart disease demonstrate a normal myocardial response to dobutamine. J Am Coll Cardiol 42:446–53

6. Kobayashi T, Tamano K, Takahashi M, et al (2003) Myocardial systolic function of the left ventricle along the long axis in patients with essential hypertension: a study by pulsed tissue Doppler imaging. J Cardiol 41:175–182

7. Klewer SE, Goldberg SJ, Donnerstein RL, et al (1992) Dobutamine stress echocardiography: a sensitive indicator of diminished myocardial function in asymptomatic doxorubicin-treated long-term survivors of childhood cancer. J Am Coll Cardiol 19:394–401

8. Mariotti E, Agostini A, Angelucci E, et al (1996) Reduced left ventricular contractile reserve identified by low dose dobutamine echocardiography as an early marker of cardiac involvement in asymptomatic patients with thalassemia major. Echocardiography 13:463–472

9. Ha JW, Lee HC, Kang ES, et al (2007) Abnormal left ventricular longitudinal functional reserve in patients with diabetes mellitus: implication for detecting subclinical myocardial dysfunction using exercise tissue Doppler echocardiography. Heart 93:1571–1576

10. Kawano S, Ilda K, Fujeda K, et al (1995) Response to isoproterenol as a prognostic indicator of evolution from hypertrophic cardiomyopathy to a phase resembling dilated cardiomyopathy. J Am Coll Cardiol 25:687–692

11. Picano E (2003) Diabetic cardiomyopathy. The importance of being earliest. J Am Coll Cardiol 42:454–457

12. Neglia D, Parodi O, Gallopin M, et al (1995) Myocardial blood flow response to pacing tachycardia and to dipyridamole infusion in patients with dilated cardiomyopathy without overt heart failure. A quantitative assessment by positron emission tomography. Circulation 92:796–804

13. Montisci R, Vacca A, Garau P, et al (2003) Detection of early impairment of coronary flow reserve in patients with systemic sclerosis. Ann Rheum Dis 62:890–893

14. Galderisi M, Capaldo B, Sidiropulos M, et al (2007) Determinants of reduction of coronary flow reserve in patients with type 2 diabetes mellitus or arterial hypertension without angiographically determined epicardial coronary stenosis. Am J Hypertens 20:1283–1290

15. Bartel T, Yang Y, Müller S, et al (2002) Noninvasive assessment of microvascular function in arterial hypertension by transthoracic Doppler harmonic echocardiography. J Am Coll Cardiol 39:2012–2018

16. Agricola E, Oppizzi M, Pisani M, et al (2004) Stress echocardiography in heart failure. Cardiovasc Ultrasound 2:11

17. Neskovic AN, Otasevic P (2005) Stress-echocardiography in idiopathic dilated cardiomyopathy: instructions for use. Cardiovasc Ultrasound 3:3

18. Nagaoka H, Isobe N, Kubota S, et al (1997) Myocardial contractile reserve as prognostic determinant in patients with idiopathic dilated cardiomyopathy without overt heart failure. Chest 111:344–350

19. Paelinck B, Vermeersch P, Stockman D, et al (1999) Usefulness of low-dose dobutamine stress echocardiography in predicting recovery of poor left ventricular function in atrial fibrillation dilated cardiomyopathy. Am J Cardiol 83:1668–1671

20. Naqvi TZ, Goel RK, Forrester JS, et al (1999) Myocardial contractile reserve on dobutamine echocardiography predicts late spontaneous improvement in cardiac function in patients with recent onset idiopathic dilated cardiomyopathy. J Am Coll Cardiol 34:1537–1544

21. Kitaoka H, Takata J, Yabe T, et al (1999) Dobutamine stress echocardiography can predict the improvement of left ventricular systolic function in dilated cardiomyopathy. Heart 81:523–527

22. Scrutinio D, Napoli V, Passantino A, et al (2000) Low-dose dobutamine responsiveness in idiopathic dilated cardiomyopathy: relation to exercise capacity and clinical outcome. Eur Heart J 21:927–934

23. Paraskevaidis IA, Adamopoulos S, Kremastinos DT (2001) Dobutamine echocardiographic study in patients with nonischemic dilated cardiomyopathy and prognostically borderline values of peak exercise oxygen consumption: 18-month follow-up study. J Am Coll Cardiol 37:1685–1691

24. Pratali L, Picano E, Otasevic P, et al (2001) Prognostic significance of dobutamine echocardiography test in idiopathic dilated cardiomyopathy. Am J Cardiol 88:1374–1378

25. Pinamonti B, Perkan A, Di Lenarda A, et al (2002) Dobutamine echocardiography in idiopathic dilated cardiomyopathy: clinical and prognostic implications. Eur J Heart Fail 4:49–61

26. Drozdz J, Krzeminska-Pakula M, Plewka M, et al (2002) Prognostic value of low-dose dobutamine echocardiography in patients with idiopathic dilated cardiomyopathy. Chest 121:1216–1222

27. Otasevic P, Popovic ZB, Vasiljevic JD, et al (2006) Head-to-head comparison of indices of left ventricular contractile reserve assessed by high-dose dobutamine stress echocardiography in idiopathic dilated cardiomyopathy: five-year follow up. Heart 92:1253–1258

28. Williams MJ, Odabashian J, Lauer MS, et al (1996) Prognostic value of dobutamine echocardiography in patients with left ventricular dysfunction. J Am Coll Cardiol 27:132–139

29. Marron A, Schneeweiss A (1997) Prognostic value of noninvasively obtained left ventricular contractile reserve in patients with severe heart failure. J Am Coll Cardiol 29:422–428

30. Pratali L, Otasevic P, Rigo F, et al (2005) The additive prognostic value of restrictive pattern and dipyridamole-induced contractile reserve in idiopathic dilated cardiomyopathy. Eur J Heart Fail 7:844–851

31. Pratali L, Otasevic P, Neskovic A, et al (2007) DIP Prognostic value of pharmacologic stress echocardiography in patients with idiopathic dilated cardiomyopathy: a prospective, head-to-head comparison between dipyridamole and dobutamine test. J Card Fail 13:836–842

32. Rigo F, Gherardi S, Galderisi M, et al (2006) The prognostic impact of coronary flow-reserve assessed by Doppler echocardiography in non-ischaemic dilated cardiomyopathy. Eur Heart J 27:1319–1323

33. Rigo F, Richieri M, Pasanisi E, et al (2003) Usefulness of coronary flow reserve over regional wall motion when added to dual-imaging dipyridamole echocardiography. Am J Cardiol 91:269–273

34. Pinamonti B, Zecchin M, Di Lenarda A, et al (1997) Persistence of restrictive left ventricular filling pattern in dilated cardiomyopathy: an ominous prognostic sign. J Am Coll Cardiol 29:604–612

35. Frassi F, Gargani L, Tesorio P, et al (2007) Prognostic value of extravascular lung water assessed with ultrasound lung comets by chest sonography in patients with dyspnea and/or chest pain. J Card Fail 13:830–835

36. Sharp SM, Sawada SG, Segar DS, et al (1994) Dobutamine stress echocardiography: detection of coronary artery disease in patients with dilated cardiomyopathy. J Am Coll Cardiol 24:934–939

37. Vigna C, Russo A, De Rito V, et al (1996) Regional wall motion analysis by dobutamine stress echocardiography to distinguish between ischemic and non-ischemic dilated cardiomyopathy. Am Heart J 131:537–543

38. Cohen A, Chauvel C, Benhalima B, et al (1997) Is dobutamine stress echocardiography useful for noninvasive differentiation of ischemic from idiopathic dilated cardiomyopathy? Angiology 48:783–793

39. Allman KC, Shaw LJ, Hachamovitch R, et al (2002) Myocardial viability testing and impact of revascularization on prognosis in patients with coronary artery disease and left ventricular dysfunction: a meta-analysis. J Am Coll Cardiol 39:1151–1158

40. Galderisi M, Cattaneo F, Mondillo S (2007) Doppler echocardiography and myocardial dyssynchrony: a practical update of old and new ultrasound technologies. Cardiovasc Ultrasound 5:28

41. Gorcsan J 3rd, Abraham T, Agler DA, et al; American Society of Echocardiography Dyssynchrony Writing Group (2008) Echocardiography for cardiac resynchronization therapy: recommendations for performance and reporting–a report from the American Society of Echocardiography Dyssynchrony Writing Group endorsed by the Heart Rhythm Society. J Am Soc Echocardiogr 21:191–213

42. Chung ES, Leon AR, Tavazzi L, et al (2008) Results of the Predictors of Response to CRT (PROSPECT) Trial. Circulation 2008 117:2608–2616

43. Da Costa A, Thévenin J, Roche F, et al (2006) Prospective validation of stress echocardiography as an identifier of cardiac resynchronization therapy responders. Heart Rhythm 3:406–413

44. Ciampi Q, Pratali L, Citro R, et al (2009) Identification of responders to CRT by stress echo: no contractile reserve, no party. Eur J Heart, in press

45. Jourdain P, Funck F, Fulla Y, et al (2002) Myocardial contractile reserve under low doses of dobutamine and improvement of left ventricular ejection fraction with treatment by carvedilol. Eur J Heart Fail 4:269–276

46. Schwammenthal E, Vered Z, Moshkowitz Y, et al (2001) Dobutamine echocardiography in patients with aortic stenosis and left ventricular dysfunction: predicting outcome as a function of management strategy. Chest 119:1766–1777

47. Ciampi Q, Villari B (2007) Role of echocardiography in diagnosis and risk stratification in heart failure with left ventricular systolic dysfunction. Cardiovasc Ultrasound 5:34

Stress Echocardiography in Hypertrophic Cardiomyopathy

34

Eugenio Picano

34.1
Background

Hypertrophic cardiomyopathy (HCM) is a clinically heterogeneous but relatively common autosomal dominant genetic heart disease (1 in 500 of the general population for the disease phenotype recognized by echocardiography) that probably is the most frequently occurring cardiomyopathy [1]. HCM is characterized morphologically and defined by a nonhypertrophied, nondilated left ventricle in the absence of another systemic or cardiac disease that is capable of producing the magnitude of wall thickening evident (e.g., systemic hypertension, aortic valve stenosis). Clinical diagnosis is customarily made with two-dimensional echocardiography by detection of otherwise unexplained LV wall thickening, usually in the presence of a small LV cavity, after suspicion is raised by the clinical profile or as a part of family screening. Most HCM patients have the propensity to developing dynamic obstruction to LV outflow under resting or physiologically provocable conditions, produced by systolic anterior motion of the mitral valve with ventricular septal contrast [1]. HCM is caused by a variety of mutations encoding contractile proteins of the cardiac sarcomeres, and – in a minority of cases – nonsarcomeric proteins. This genetic diversity is compromised by considerable intragenic heterogeneity, with more than 400 individual mutations now identified. The genetic heterogeneity only partially accounts for the clinical heterogeneity of the presentation, which may range anywhere from sudden death to progressive heart failure to a completely asymptomatic condition. The strongest risk factors are a family history of sudden death, a personal history of cardiac arrest or recurrent syncope, multiple-repetitive nonsustained ventricular tachycardia, and adverse genotype. Resting adds to clinical stratification by assessing massive left ventricular hypertrophy (>30 mm), intraventricular obstruction (>50 mmHg), and wall thinning in serial evaluations over time (Fig. 34.1). On the top of this established information, stress echocardiography is now increasingly used to offer a substantial contribution to risk stratification of these patients, which remains a formidable challenge for the clinician [2].

E. Picano, *Stress Echocardiography*,
© Springer-Verlag Berlin Heidelberg 2009

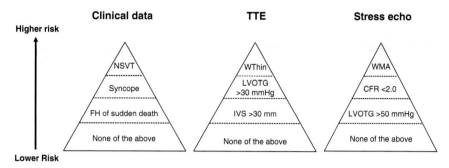

Fig. 34.1 The pyramid of risk in hypertrophic cardiomyopathy (HCM) according to simple clinical assessment (*left panel*), resting transthoracic echocardiography (*middle panel*), and stress echocardiography (*right panel*) parameters. For each pyramid, three main factors are identified. *CFR* coronary flow reserve, *IVS* interventricular septal thickness, *LVOTG* left ventricular outflow tract gradient, *WMA* wall motion abnormalities, *FH* Family history, *NSVT* non-sustained ventricular tchycardia, *Wthin* Wall thinning at serial resting echo evaluation

34.2
Pathophysiology

Symptoms and signs of myocardial ischemia are often found in patients with HCM, despite the presence of angiographically normal coronary arteries (Fig. 34.2). Myocardial ischemia can contribute to some of the severe complications of HCM including ventricular arrhythmias, sudden death, progressive left ventricular remodeling, and systolic dysfunction. Coronary flow reserve is severely blunted not only in the hypertrophied septum, but also in the less hypertrophied left ventricular free wall [3]. The severity of microvascular dysfunction is an independent prediction of long-term deterioration and death from cardiovascular causes [4]. As in other models of microvascular disease, such as cardiac syndrome X or arterial hypertension [5], ST-segment changes and perfusion abnormalities are frequently elicited during stress in the absence of inducible wall motion abnormalities (Fig. 34.3), which remain a specific hallmark of epicardial coronary artery disease [6].

However, stress-induced ST-segment depression and perfusion abnormalities are probably not innocent even with normal coronary arteries: they are associated with reduced flow reserve [7], subendocardial underperfusion, and, most importantly, an adverse prognosis. Myocardial malperfusion detected by stress scintigraphy is frequently related to cardiac arrest and syncope in young patients with HCM [8]. Stress-induced ischemic-like electrocardiographic changes, in the absence of wall motion abnormalities, are also frequently related to syncope and/or left ventricular dilatation in adult patients with HCM and normal coronary arteries [9] (Fig. 34.4).

Fig. 34.3 Two-dimensional end-diastolic (*E-D, upper row*) and end-systolic (*E-S, second row*) frames of a parasternal long-axis view following dipyridamole infusion, showing a normal/hyperkinetic motion of intraventricular septum and inferolateral wall. In the *lower row*, pulsed Doppler of mid-distal left anterior descending coronary artery shows a blunted increase in coronary artery flow velocity during stress (rest = 38, peak = 67, cm/s, CFR = 1.25)

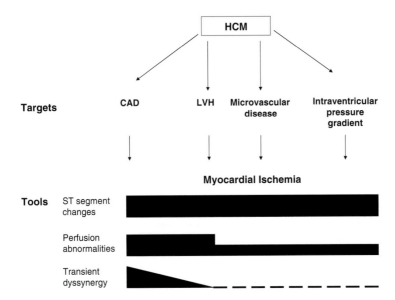

Fig. 34.2 The four main pathways to myocardial ischemia in hypertrophic cardiomyopathy (*HCM*): epicardial coronary artery disease (*CAD*); left ventricular hypertrophy; microvascular disease; intraventricular dynamic obstruction. Only CAD induces stress-induced wall motion abnormalities, but all four mechanisms may induce a reduction in coronary flow reserve

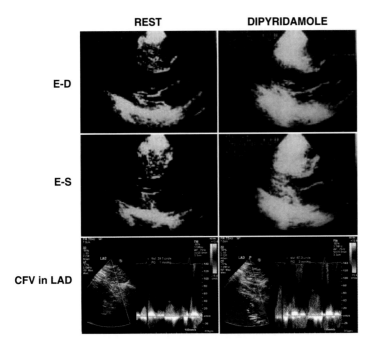

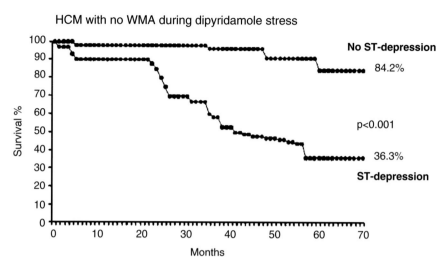

Fig. 34.4 Kaplan–Meier curve indicating the cumulative event-free survival rates in patients with a positive dipyridamole ECG test (*DET*+) and in patients with a negative dipyridamole ECG test (*DET*−). All these patients had angiographically normal coronary arteries and no wall motion abnormality during the dipyridamole test. FH, Family history; NSVT, non-sustained ventricular tchycardia; Within, wall thinning at serial resting echo evaluation (Modified from [9])

34.3
Stress Echocardiographic Findings in HCM

According to the pathophysiological background, stress echocardiography can recognize three important, distinct risk markers in HCM patients: the transient regional wall motion abnormality; the reduction in coronary flow reserve in absence of wall motion changes; and the dynamic intraventricular pressure gradient.

Angina and myocardial ischemia can occur in patients with HCM independently of angiographically assessed atherosclerotic coronary artery disease, which nevertheless can be present in 20–30% of HCM patients with a history of chest pain [10]. For the purposes of noninvasive identification of underlying coronary artery disease, wall motion abnormalities are equally sensitive and substantially more specific than perfusion abnormalities and ST-segment depression, as has been consistently observed in all models of primary or secondary coronary microvascular angina [10]. Stress echocardiography based on wall motion abnormalities is therefore the test of choice [11] and patients with inducible wall motion abnormalities will have the greatest benefit from an ischemia-driven revascularization. After ruling out wall motion abnormalities (and therefore functionally significant underlying coronary artery disease), stress echocardiography may offer invaluable information on coronary flow reserve and underlying microvascular disease. With a last-generation "two birds with one stone" protocol, both function and coronary flow reserve can be caught with a single stress (accelerated, fast high-dose dipyridamole). Even in absence of inducible

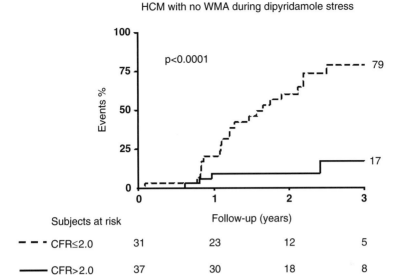

Fig. 34.5 Kaplan–Meier curve indicating the cumulative event-free survival rates in patients with reduced (*CFR>2.0*) and preserved (*CFR>2.0*) coronary flow reserve. All these patients had angiographically normal coronary arteries and no wall motion abnormality during dipyridamole test. (Modified from [12])

wall motion abnormalities, a reduced coronary flow reserve identifies a relatively higher risk subgroup (Fig. 34.5) [12]. In these patients, the absence of wall motion abnormalities does not necessarily contradict the ischemic nature of chest pain and ST-segment depression. In fact, the presence or absence of abnormal wall motion appears to relate to the account of ischemic subendocardial tissue, minor degrees of transmural involvement are less likely to reach the critical mass of ischemic tissue needed to determine wall motion and thickening abnormalities [6]. The third possible finding during stress is the development of a critical intraventricular pressure gradient (>50 mmHg) (Fig. 34.6), which identifies yet another mechanism – beyond coronary artery disease and microvascular dysfunction – possibly responsible for symptoms (chest pain and dyspnea) in HCM patients [13, 14]. An exercise-induced gradient greater than 50 mmHg may be responsible for ischemia (through increased extravascular compression forces) and dyspnea (with increased endoventricular diastolic pressure). These findings may have a potential, although not proven, therapeutic interest, possibly with "obstructions" more likely to benefit from β-blockade.

The stress for coronary artery disease detection can be exercise, dobutamine, or dipyridamole; the best stress for coronary flow reserve assessment is dipyridamole (or adenosine) [15], and the most suitable one to unmask a latent, albeit physiologically important, intraventricular gradient is exercise – even better if the echocardiography scan is performed in the more physiologic orthostatic position – rather than in left lateral decubitus [14]. Another approach of potential value in risk stratification in patients with HCM is the evaluation of the inotropic reserve after low-dose challenge with catecholamines, i.e., isoproterenol.

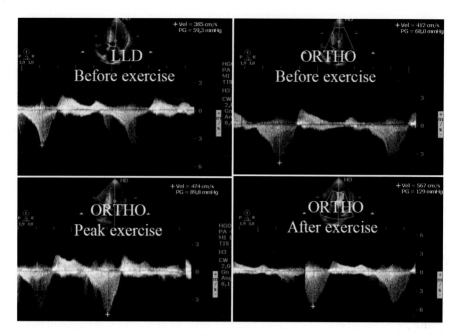

Fig. 34.6 Left ventricular outflow tract gradient during exercise in a patients with hypertrophic cardiomyopathy. (From [14])

A blunted increase in regional systolic thickening to low-dose adrenergic stimulation can predict a long-term adverse progression toward left ventricular dilatation [16].

34.4
Conclusion

Stress echocardiography can play a key role in the diagnostic and prognostic stratification of the HCM patient, identifying three distinct patterns: high-risk wall motion abnormalities, which dictate ischemia-driven revascularization; intermediate-risk reduction in coronary flow reserve warranting aggressive medical therapy; intermediate-risk patients with intraventricular gradients most likely to benefit from β-blockade; and low-risk patients with none of these features, in whom no specific intervention other than watchful waiting is warranted if the patient is asymptomatic (Fig. 34.7).

An additional advantage of stress echocardiography over alternative techniques is its low cost, wide availability, versatility, and radiation-free nature, most important in young patients often in need of several examinations over time. For instance, a thallium scan is associated with a radiological dose exposure of about 1,500 chest X-rays, with a risk of cancer of 1 in 400 in a 50-year-old man, and 1 in 200 in a 20-year-old woman [17–19]. Although more data are warranted at this point, stress echocardiography promises to offer an increasingly important contribution to the management of HCM patients.

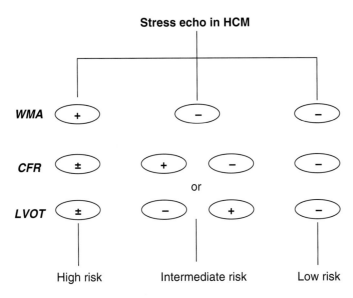

Fig. 34.7 The possible role of stress echocardiography in risk stratification of HCM patients with indeterminate risk. CFR, coronary flow reserve; HCM, hypertrophic cardiomyopathy; LVOT, left functional outflow tract obstruction

References

1. Maron BJ, Towbin JA, Thiene G, et al; American Heart Association; Council on Clinical Cardiology, Heart Failure and Transplantation Committee; Quality of Care and Outcomes Research and Functional Genomics and Translational Biology Interdisciplinary Working Groups; Council on Epidemiology and Prevention (2006) Contemporary definitions and classification of the cardiomyopathies: an American Heart Association Scientific Statement from the Council on Clinical Cardiology, Heart Failure and Transplantation Committee; Quality of Care and Outcomes Research and Functional Genomics and Translational Biology Interdisciplinary Working Groups; and Council on Epidemiology and Prevention. Circulation 113:1807–1816
2. Spirito P, Maron BJ (2001) Sudden death and hypertrophic cardiomyopathy. Lancet 357: 1975–1976
3. Camici P, Chiriatti G, Lorenzoni R, et al (1991) Coronary vasodilation is impaired in both hypertrophied and nonhypertrophied myocardium of patients with hypertrophic cardiomyopathy: a study with nitrogen-13 ammonia and positron emission tomography. J Am Coll Cardiol 17:879–886
4. Cecchi F, Olivotto I, Gistri R, et al (2003) Coronary microvascular dysfunction and prognosis in hypertrophic cardiomyopathy. N Engl J Med 349:1027–1035
5. Camici PG, Crea F (2007) Coronary microvascular dysfunction. N Engl J Med 356:830–840
6. Picano E, Pálinkás A, Amyot R (2001) Diagnosis of myocardial ischemia in hypertensive patients. J Hypertens 19:1177–1183
7. Camici PG, Chiriatti G, Picano E, et al (1992) Noninvasive identification of limited coronary flow reserve in hypertrophic cardiomyopathy. Coronary Artery Dis 3:513–521

8. Dilsizian V, Bonow RO, Epstein SE, et al (1993) Myocardial ischemia detected by thallium scintigraphy is frequently related to cardiac arrest and syncope in young patients with hypertrophic cardiomyopathy. J Am Coll Cardiol 22:796–804

9. Lazzeroni E, Picano E, Morozzi L, et al for the Echo Persantine Italian Cooperative (EPIC) Study group, Subproject Hypertrophic Cardiomyopathy (1997) Dipyridamole-induced ischemia as a prognostic marker of future adverse cardiac events in adult hypertrophic cardiomyopathy. Circulation 96:4268–4272

10. Cokkinos DV, Krajcer Z, Leachman RD (1985) Coronary artery disease in hypertrophic cardiomyopathy. Am J Cardiol 55:1437–1438

11. Lazzeroni E, Picano E, Dodi C, et al (1995) Dipyridamole echocardiography for diagnosis of coexistent coronary artery disease in hypertrophic cardiomyopathy. Echo-Persantine International Cooperative (EPIC) Study Group – Subproject Hypertrophic Cardiomyopathy. Am J Cardiol 75:810–813

12. Cortigiani L, Rigo F, Gherardi S, Galderisi M, Sicari R, Picano E (2008) Prognostic implications of coronary flow reserve in left anterior descending coronary artery in hypertrophic cardiomyopathy. Am J Cardiol 102:926–932

13. Maron MS, Olivotto I, Zenovich AG, et al (2006) Hypertrophic cardiomyopathy is predominantly a disease of left ventricular outflow tract obstruction. Circulation 114:2232–2239

14. Cotrim C, Loureiro MJ, Simões O, et al (2005) Evaluation of hypertrophic obstructive cardiomyopathy by exercise stress echocardiography. New methodology. Rev Port Cardiol 24:1319–1327

15. Sicari R, Niohyannopoulos P, Evangelista A, et al (2008) Stress echocardiography consensus statement of the European Association of Echocardiography. Eur J Echocardiogr 9:415–437

16. Kawano S, Ilda K, Fujeda K, et al (1995) Response to isoproterenol as a prognostic indicator of evolution from hypertrophic cardiomyopathy to a phase resembling dilated cardiomyopathy. J Am Coll Cardiol 25:687–692

17. Picano E (2003) Stress echocardiography: a historical perspective. Am J Med 114:126–130

18. Picano E (2004) Informed consent and communication of risk from radiological and nuclear medicine examinations: how to escape from a communication inferno. Education and debate. BMJ 329:849–851

19. Picano E (2004) Sustainability of medical imaging. Education and debate. BMJ 328:578–580

Stress Echocardiography After Cardiac Transplantation

35

Eugenio Picano, Tonino Bombardini, and Giorgio Arpesella

35.1
Background

Cardiac transplantation is an increasingly important treatment for end-stage cardiac disease, but rejection continues to be a major complication [1]. Rejection can be either acute or chronic (Table 35.1). Acute rejection is a major problem in the first year following cardiac transplantation. It is characterized by normal epicardial coronary arteries, with a concomitant restriction in coronary flow reserve [2], a pathophysiological hallmark of microvascular disease, as has been described in other situations such as syndrome X or hypertension with normal coronary arteries [3, 4]. In particular, during acute cardiac rejection, the reversible reduction of coronary reserve could be the result of the limitation of vasodilation due to functional abnormalities such as metabolically or immunologically related decreased responsiveness of vascular wall to vasodilator stimuli or to structural abnormalities, for example, interstitial edema or cellular infiltration [2]. Immunosuppressive treatment can resolve structural and functional abnormalities and restore the normal coronary flow reserve [2].

Cardiac allograft vasculopathy (CAV) is a major factor limiting long-term prognosis after heart transplantation [1]. In several respects, the disease differs from atherosclerotic coronary artery disease. The mechanism is thought to be immune-mediated. An early manifestation of CAV is thickening of the vessel wall, with progression to diffuse involvement of the vessel in the longitudinal direction or development of more focal, localized stenosis [5–7]. Small-vessel disease is also common, and contributes to the reduction in coronary flow reserve [8, 9, 10] and unfavorable outcome [11, 12]. The disease may develop rapidly within months and the clinical diagnosis of CAV is difficult. As the transplanted heart is surgically denervated and remains without functionally relevant reinnervation in most patients, angina pectoris does not usually occur. Several noninvasive tests have proven to be of limited value for the detection of CAV [13–16]. This may be explained by some of the specific features of CAV and by the specific alterations of cardiac physiology in heart transplant recipients. For example, exercise electrocardiography is a priori restricted to a minority of transplant recipients due to the high prevalence of (most commonly right) bundle branch block and

Table 35.1 Heart transplant rejection

	Acute	Chronic
Pathological changes	Edema, cellular infiltrates, myocyte damage	Diffuse coronary artery wall thickening (with focal stenosis)
Diagnostic gold standard	Endomyocardial biopsy	Intracoronary ultrasound (coronary angiography)
Reversibility upon treatment	Yes	No
Rest echocardiography	Increase wall thickness/texture/decrease in ejection fraction	Segmental abnormalities, decreased systolic thickening
Stress test	ST depression and no dysfunction	Regional dysfunction
Coronary flow reserve	Reduced	Reduced
Stress echocardiography prognostic value	Possible	Proven

altered repolarization in this population. In addition, the mode of provocation of ischemia is important. Physical exercise may not be adequate, because heart transplant recipients frequently have a reduced exercise capacity due to muscular weakness following long-term deconditioning and corticosteroid immunosuppression. More important, the chronotropic response to physical exercise is limited due to cardiac denervation; the reduced increase in heart rate may therefore not be adequate to reach the ischemic threshold in all heart transplantation patients. The limitations of a physical exercise test in transplantation patients have been shown in combination with various diagnostic techniques such as exercise electrocardiogram, radionuclide angiography, or exercise echocardiography [13–17]. The mainstay of CAV diagnosis is currently still made up of invasive techniques [1]. Coronary angiography only presents a luminogram and may not be able to detect diffuse concentric thickening of the vessel wall. Intravascular ultrasound (IVUS) is the method of choice to detect alterations of the vessel wall and has emerged as the most sensitive invasive method for diagnosing CAV [18]. Although most investigators measure thickness and extension of intimal hyperplasia by IVUS, no commonly accepted cut-off points or standardized IVUS definitions for CAV exist (minimal number of coronary segments and vessels necessary for valid diagnosis, grading by worst affected sites or mean values).

35.2
Pharmacological Stress Echocardiography for Detection of Acute Rejection

The main resting transthoracic echocardiographic variables proposed for diagnosis of acute allograft rejection include increased wall thickness and wall echogenicity, pericardial effusion, left ventricular diastolic dysfunction and regional or global systolic dysfunction [19–21]. In general, the results have not been encouraging and no single echocardiographic variable alone can be used for accurate detection of acute allograft

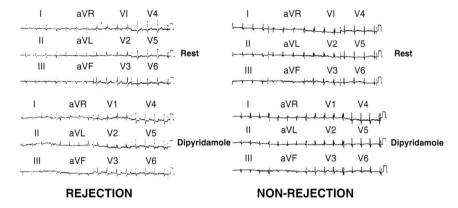

Fig. 35.1 Stress electrocardiogram during acute rejection. The 12-lead electrocardiogram is shown on day 21 after transplantation in resting conditions (*upper panel*) and at peak dipyridamole (*lower panel*). At peak dipyridamole, the electrocardiogram shows a transient ST-segment depression. This patient had bioptic evidence of rejection. (From [14], with permission)

rejection [18]. In acute rejection, coronary flow reserve can be acutely impaired [22] and this is mirrored by transient ST-segment depression during stress, as is typical of microvascular angina [3]. These changes typically occur in the absence of wall motion abnormalities [22] and outline a potential role of coronary flow reserve for the diagnostic evaluation of these patients [23] (Fig. 35.1).

35.3
Pharmacological Stress Echocardiography for Detection of Chronic Rejection

Rest- and stress-induced abnormalities can be detected with pharmacological stress echocardiography using dipyridamole [15, 24, 25] or dobutamine [26–35]. As in native coronary artery disease, both tests have a high feasibility rate and a low incidence of reported limiting side effects [18]. In a series systematically evaluating coronary angiography and intracoronary ultrasound, dobutamine stress echocardiography demonstrated wall motion abnormalities in 40% of patients with an apparently normal angiogram [29]. If angiography is used as a reference method, these findings have to be interpreted as false-positive dobutamine stress tests and would therefore explain the relatively low specificity of the stress tests compared to angiography [28–30]. However, the majority of IVUS studies in patients with a normal angiogram revealed moderate to severe intimal hyperplasia, and two-thirds of normal angiographic studies have an abnormal dobutamine stress test and/or IVUS evidence of CAV [20]. In evaluating noninvasive test results, one should consider that angiography is relatively insensitive in detecting CAV and that a normal angiogram in a heart transplant recipient does not exclude functionally relevant CAV [18, 19], which may be mirrored by functional abnormalities during stress (Figs. 35.2, 35.3). A normal pharmacological stress echocardiography result after heart transplantation has a high predictive value for an uneventful clini-

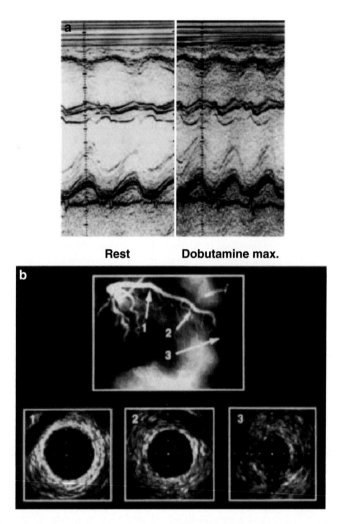

Fig. 35.2 Forty-eight months after transplantation. **a** *M*-mode echocardiogram. Normal systolic wall thickening at rest (*left*) and during maximum dobutamine stress (*right*). **b** Coronary angiogram and intravascular ultrasound (IVUS). Normal left coronary artery by angiography. Absence of significant intimal hyperplasia at three sites (*arrows*) of the left anterior descending artery by IVUS. (From [18], with permission)

cal course [20, 21]. The value of the test seems to be at least comparable to that of a normal angiogram, and a normal pharmacological stress test allows invasive diagnostic procedures to be safely delayed [30–35], especially if coronary flow reserve detectable by transthoracic echocardiography is also above normal (suggested to be 2.7 in these patients) [36]. If the stress test is normal by wall motion and coronary flow reserve criteria, invasive diagnosis is delayed and the next test is scheduled after 12 months [20, 22]: Fig. 35.5. If stress echocardiography shows all motion abnormalities, angiography is performed and, if this test does not yield evidence of CAV, an additional IVUS study might be warranted. This algorithm

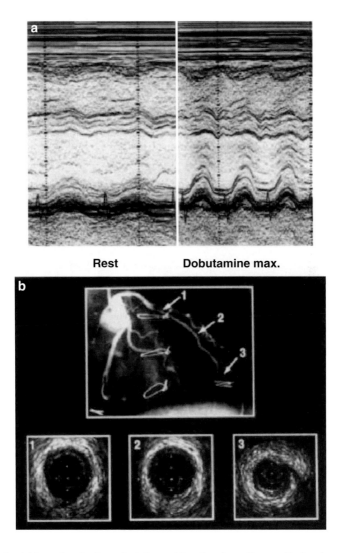

Fig. 35.3 Forty-eight months after transplantation. **a** *M*-mode echocardiogram. Reduced systolic wall thickening at rest (*left*). During maximum dobutamine stress (*right*), septal thickening remains unchanged, whereas posterior wall thickening increases. **b** Coronary angiogram and intravascular ultrasound (IVUS). Contour irregularities without relevant stenosis in left coronary artery by angiography. Severe intimal hyperplasia at three sites (*arrows*) of the left anterior descending artery by IVUS. (From [18], with permission)

helps avoid repeat cardiac catheterization in some patients and leads to a closer surveillance of patients with evidence of functionally relevant and/or progressive CAV [20–22]. This aspect of noninvasive radiation-free follow-up of heart transplant patients is especially important in pediatric patients, in whom dobutamine stress echocardiography was shown to be highly feasible and effective for diagnostic and prognostic purposes [34, 35].

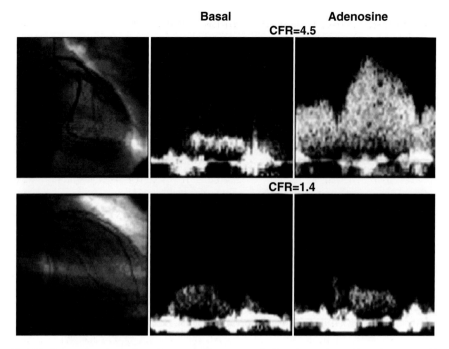

Fig. 35.4 Coronary angiography and coronary flow reserve findings in a patient without (upper panels) and with (lower panels) rejection, which severely reduces coronary flow reserve. (From ref. [23]).

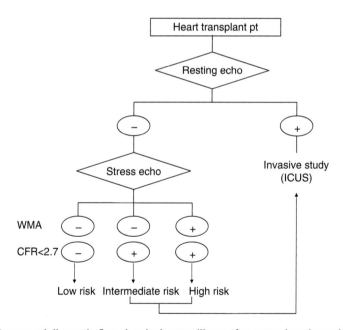

Fig. 35.5 A proposed diagnostic flow-chart in the surveillance of posttransplantation patient. Yearly testing with pharmacological stress echocardiography may help to reduce the need for invasive studies. The reliability of pharmacological stress echocardiography is stronger when the test response shows no wall motion abnormalities and normal coronary flow reserve on left anterior descending artery during transthoracic vasodilation stress echocardiography. CFR, coronary flow reserve; ICUS, intracoronary ultrasound; WMA, wall motion abnormalities

35.4
Pharmacological Stress Echocardiography for Recruitment of Donor Hearts

The heart transplantation is a treatment of heart failure, which is not responding to medications, and its efficiency is already proved: unfortunately, organ donation is a limiting step of this life-saving procedure. Heart donor shortage is a society problem [37]. Patients on the heart transplant waiting list have a 7.3% death rate, and the average waiting time is 2–3 years. As an example, in Italy, approximately 650 patients are on the transplant list and only about 300 transplantations are performed each year. An effective way to solve the current shortage would be to accept an upward shift of the age cutoff limit (from current 45 to 70 years) but age-related high prevalence of asymptomatic coronary artery disease and occult cardiomyopathy severely limit the feasibility of this approach. Recently, Bombardini and coworkers have proposed an alternative approach based on pharmacological stress echocardiography performed at bedside in marginal donors (aged>55 years) [38]. When resting and stress echocardiography results are negative, a prognostically meaningful underlying coronary artery disease or cardiomyopathy can be ruled out and the heart can be rescued and transplanted (Fig. 35.6). Although certainly more data are needed at this point, the appeal of this stress echocardiography-driven way to select hearts "too good

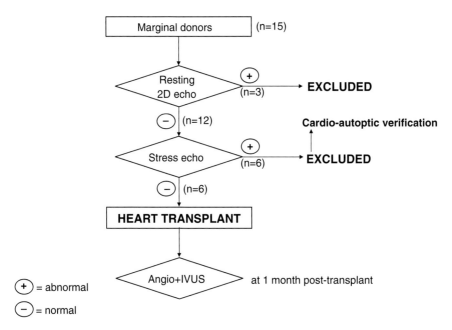

Fig. 35.6 The initial experience with pharmacological-stress echocardiography in recruiting hearts from marginal donors (>55 years). A negative stress echocardiography result deems hearts otherwise lost to donation eligible for donorship. IVUS, intravascular ultrasound (From [39])

Table 35.2 Clinical applications of stress echocardiography in heart transplantation

	Acute rejection	Chronic rejection	Donor recruitment
Unproven	√		
Established		√	
Investigational			√

to die" is exciting for its potential to drastically solve the current mismatch between donor need and supply, with a very favorable cost–benefit profile. The cost of a donor heart is estimated around €200,000 on the "transplant black market." We can recruit otherwise ineligible hearts at the cost of one stress echocardiography (around 500 at the average cost in Europe), with obvious downstream economic benefits.

35.5
Conclusions

Stress echocardiography in cardiac transplantation has three main potential applications: the detection of acute rejection in the first year after cardiac transplantation; the detection of chronic rejection later after cardiac transplantation; and the recruitment of marginal donor hearts as a way to solve the current donor heart shortage (Table 35.2). The three applications have different clinical roles today. Despite the ongoing efforts of old and innovative resting and stress echocardiographic techniques in predicting biopsy-proven acute rejection, endomyocardial biopsies are still regarded as the gold standard for the detection of acute allograft rejection, which is often associated with an acute reduction in coronary flow reserve of potential diagnostic value. Conversely, stress echocardiography is able to identify cardiac graft vasculopathy accurately and has a recognized prognostic value in this clinical setting, where a normal stress echocardiography by wall motion criteria justifies avoiding or delaying invasive studies. In the setting of cardiac allograft vasculopathy, the integration of coronary flow reserve to transthoracic stress echocardiography might further improve the value of the method. Finally, the use of bedside stress echocardiography is still purely investigational, although promising, to select appropriately marginal heart donors with brain death to solve the current shortage of donor heart supply.

References

1. Hunt SA, Haddad F (2008) The changing face of heart transplantation. J Am Coll Cardiol 52:587–598
2. Nitemberg A, Tavolaro O, Loisance D, et al (1989) Severe impairment of coronary reserve during rejection in patients with orthotopic heart transplant. Circulation 79:59–65
3. Picano E, Pálinkás A, Amyot R (2001) Diagnosis of myocardial ischemia in hypertensive patients. J Hypertens 19:1177–1183
4. Camici PG, Crea F (2007) Coronary microvascular dysfunction. N Engl J Med 356:830–840

5. St Goar FG, Pinto FJ, Alderman EL, et al (1992) Intracoronary ultrasound in cardiac transplant recipients. In vivo evidence of "angiographically silent" intimal thickening. Circulation 85:979–987

6. Klauss V, Mudra H, Uberfuhr P, et al (1995) Intraindividual variability of cardiac allograft vasculopathy as assessed by intravascular ultrasound. Am J Cardiol 76:463–466

7. Pflugfelder PW, Boughner DR, Rudas L, et al (1993) Enhanced detection of cardiac allograft arterial disease with intracoronary ultrasonographic imaging. Am Heart J 125:1583–1591

8. Kofoed KF, Czernin J, Johnson J, Kobashigawa J, Phelps ME, Laks H, Schelbert HR (1997) Effects of cardiac allograft vasculopathy on myocardial blood flow, vasodilatory capacity, and coronary vasomotion. Circulation 95:600–606

9. Muehling OM, Wilke NM, Panse P, Jerosch-Herold M, Wilson BV, Wilson RF, Miller LW (2003) Reduced myocardial perfusion reserve and transmural perfusion gradient in heart transplant arteriopathy assessed by magnetic resonance imaging. J Am Coll Cardiol 42:1054–1060

10. Fearon WF, Nakamura M, Lee DP, Rezaee M, Vagelos RH, Hunt SA, Fitzgerald PJ, Yock PG, Yeung AC (2003) Simultaneous assessment of fractional and coronary flow reserves in cardiac transplant recipients: Physiologic Investigation for Transplant Arteriopathy (PITA Study). Circulation 108:1605–1610

11. Weis M, Hartmann A, Olbrich HG, Hör G, Zeiher AM (1998) Prognostic significance of coronary flow reserve on left ventricular ejection fraction in cardiac transplant recipients. Transplantation 65:103–108

12. Rodrigues AC, Frimm Cde C, Bacal F, Andreolli V, Tsutsui JM, Bocchi EA, Mathias W Jr, Lage SG (2005) Coronary flow reserve impairment predicts cardiac events in heart transplant patients with preserved left ventricular function. Int J Cardiol 103:201–206

13. Smart FW, Ballantyne CM, Cocanougher B, et al (1991) Insensitivity of noninvasive tests to detect coronary artery vasculopathy after heart transplant. Am J Cardiol 67:243–247

14. Mairesse GH, Marwick TH, Melin JA, et al (1995) Use of exercise electrocardiography, technetium-99m-MIBI perfusion tomography, and two-dimensional echocardiography for coronary disease surveillance in a low-prevalence population of heart transplant recipients. J Heart Lung Transplant 14:222–229

15. Cohn JM, Wilensky RL, O'Donnell JA, et al (1996) Exercise echocardiography, angiography, and intracoronary ultrasound after cardiac transplantation. Am J Cardiol 77:1216–1219

16. Collings CA, Pinto FJ, Valantine HA, et al (1994) Exercise echocardiography in heart transplant recipients: a comparison with angiography and intracoronary ultrasonography. J Heart Lung Transplant 13:604–613

17. Ciliberto GR, Mangiavacchi M, Banfi F, et al (1993) Coronary artery disease after heart transplantation: non-invasive evaluation with exercise thallium scintigraphy. Eur Heart J 14:226–229

18. Mondillo S, Maccherini M, Galderisi M (2008) Usefulness and limitations of transthoracic echocardiography in heart transplantation recipients. Cardiovasc Ultrasound 6:2

19. Ciliberto GR, Mascarello M, Gronda E, et al (1994) Acute rejection after heart transplantation: noninvasive echocardiographic evaluation. J Am Coll Cardiol 23:1156–1161

20. Ciliberto GR, Pingitore A, Mangiavacchi M, et al (1996) The clinical value of blunting of cyclic gray level variation for the detection of acute cardiac rejection: a two-dimensional, Doppler, and videodensitometric ultrasound study. J Am Soc Echoc 27:142–148

21. Angermann CE, Nassau K, Stempfle HU, et al (1997) Recognition of acute cardiac allograft rejection from serial integrated backscatter analyses in human orthotopic heart transplant recipients. Comparison with conventional echocardiography. Circulation 95:140–150

22. Picano E, De Pieri G, Salerno JA, et al (1990) Electrocardiographic changes suggestive of myocardial ischemia elicited by dipyridamole infusion in acute rejection early after heart transplantation. Circulation 81:72–77

23. Tona F, Caforio AL, Montisci R, Angelini A, Ruscazio M, Gambino A, Ramondo A, Thiene G, Gerosa G, Iliceto S (2006) Coronary flow reserve by contrast-enhanced echocardiography: a new noninvasive diagnostic tool for cardiac allograft vasculopathy. Am J Transplant 6(5 Pt 1):998–1003

24. Ciliberto GR, Massa D, Mangiavacchi M, et al (1993) High-dose dipyridamole echocardiography test in coronary artery disease after heart transplantation. Eur Heart J 14:48–52

25. Ciliberto GR, Parodi O, Cataldo G, Mangiavacchi M, Alberti A, Parolini M, Frigerio M (2003) Prognostic value of contractile response during high-dose dipyridamole echocardiography test in heart transplant recipients. J Heart Lung Transplant 22:526–532

26. Akosah KO, Mohanty PK, Funai JT, et al (1994) Noninvasive detection of transplant coronary artery disease by dobutamine stress echocardiography. J Heart Lung Transplant 13:1024–1038

27. Derumeaux G, Redonnet M, Mouton-Schleifer D, et al (1995) Dobutamine stress echocardiography in orthotopic heart transplant recipients. VACOMED Research Group. J Am Coll Cardiol 25:1665–1672

28. Spes CH, Klauss V, Rieber J, et al (1999) Functional and morphological findings in heart transplant recipients with a normal coronary angiogram: an analysis by dobutamine stress echocardiography, intracoronary Doppler and intravascular ultrasound. J Heart Lung Transplant 18:391–398

29. Spes CH, Klauss V, Mudra H, et al (1999) Diagnostic and prognostic value of serial dobutamine stress echocardiography for noninvasive assessment of cardiac allograft vasculopathy: a comparison with coronary angiography and intravascular ultrasound. Circulation 100:509–515

30. Akosah KO, McDaniel S, Hanrahan JS, et al (1998) Dobutamine stress echocardiography early after heart transplantation predicts development of allograft coronary artery disease and outcome. J Am Coll Cardiol 31:1607–1614

31. Lewis JF, Selman SB, Murphy JD, et al (1997) Dobutamine echocardiography for prediction of ischemic events in heart transplant recipients. J Heart Lung Transplant 16:390–393

32. Derumeaux G, Redonnet M, Soyer R, et al (1998) Assessment of the progression of cardiac allograft vasculopathy by dobutamine stress echocardiography. J Heart Lung Transplant 17:259–267

33. Bacal F, Moreira L, Souza G, Rodrigues AC, Fiorelli A, Stolf N, Bocchi E, Bellotti G, Ramires JA (2004) Dobutamine stress echocardiography predicts cardiac events or death in asymptomatic patients long-term after heart transplantation: 4-year prospective evaluation. J Heart Lung Transplant 23:1238–1244

34. Larsen RL, Applegate PM, Dyar DA, et al (1998) Dobutamine stress echocardiography for assessing coronary artery disease after transplantation in children. J Am Coll Cardiol 32:515–520

35. Pahl E, Crawford SE, Swenson JM, et al (1999) Dobutamine stress echocardiography: experience in pediatric heart transplant recipients. J Heart Lung Transplant 18:725–732

36. Tona F, Caforio AL, Montisci R, Gambino A, Angelini A, Ruscazio M, Toscano G, Feltrin G, Ramondo A, Gerosa G, Iliceto S (2006) Coronary flow velocity pattern and coronary flow reserve by contrast-enhanced transthoracic echocardiography predict long-term outcome in heart transplantation. Circulation 114:I49–I55

37. Zaroff JG, Rosengard BR, Armstrong WF, Babcock WD, D'Alessandro A, Dec GW, Edwards NM, Higgins RS, Jeevanandum V, Kauffman M, Kirklin JK, Large SR, Marelli D, Peterson TS, Ring WS, Robbins RC, Russell SD, Taylor DO, Van Bakel A, Wallwork J, Young JB (2002) Consensus conference report: maximizing use of organs recovered from the cadaver donor: cardiac recommendations, March 28–29, 2001, Crystal City, Va. Circulation 106:836–841

38. Arpesella G, Gherardi S, Bombardini T, Picano E (2006) Recruitment of aged donor heart with pharmacological stress echo. A case report. Cardiovasc Ultrasound 4:3
39. Bombardini T, Arpesella G, Gherardi S, Maccherini M, Serra W, Leone O, Tanganelli P, Pasanisi E, Picano E (2008) Extended donor criteria in heart transplantation with pharmacological stress echocardiography. Eur Heart J 2008 (abstract suppl)

The Emerging Role of Exercise Testing and Stress Echocardiography in Valvular Heart Disease

36

Eugenio Picano, Philippe Pibarot, Patrizio Lancellotti, Jean Luc Monin, and Robert O. Bonow

Major advances in diagnosis and risk stratification, combined with enormous progress in surgical valve replacement and repair, have led to improved outcomes of patients with valvular heart disease over the past 30 years. The most important indication for surgical intervention in patients with hemodynamically significant aortic or mitral valve disease is the development of symptoms, as emphasized in recent guidelines [1–3]. As symptoms may develop slowly and indolently in these chronic conditions, many patients are unaware of subtle changes in effort tolerance, even when questioned directly by their physicians. Hence, recent guidelines of both the American College of Cardiology/American Heart Association (ACC/AHA) and the European Society of Cardiology (ESC) [2, 3] have placed renewed emphasis on the role of exercise testing to provide objective evidence of exercise capacity and symptom status. In addition, while Doppler echocardiography is the method of choice for assessing severity of valvular disease, there is a growing utilization of stress two-dimensional and Doppler echocardiography to assess dynamic changes in hemodynamics in concert with the clinical findings of exercise testing.

Stress echocardiography has become an established method for evaluating patients with coronary artery disease [4–6]. The role of stress echocardiography has been recently expanded to the assessment of the hemodynamic consequences of valvular lesions during stress [7–9]. In a number of clinical conditions, particularly in patients with low-flow, low-gradient aortic valve stenosis (AS), the use of stress echocardiography in the decision-making process has significantly modified the clinical outcome. Evidence accumulated over the last 5 years has led to the incorporation of stress echocardiography in the guidelines of the ACC/AHA [2], the ESC [3], the American Society of Echocardiography [10], and the European Association of Echocardiography [11]. On the basis of the recent recommendations of these scientific organizations, the use of stress echocardiography in valve disease has been ranked as shown in Table 36.1. Applications are either proven (3 stars in the table), probable (2 stars), or possible but not yet established (1 star). Indications of "proven useful" have been incorporated in either one or more of the general cardiology guidelines [2, 3], and those of "probable usefulness" are supported in the stress echocardiography special recommendations [10, 11]. However, indications "of possible value" are not yet supported by the guidelines since they are based only on initial encouraging, but

E. Picano, *Stress Echocardiography*,
© Springer-Verlag Berlin Heidelberg 2009

Table 36.1 Stress echocardiography applications in valvular heart disease

	Aortic gradients (CW)	EF (2D) and SV (2D, PW)	Mitral gradient (CW) PASP (CW)	MR (color), ERO (color; CW), PASP (CW)	Prosthesis gradient (CW) and EOA (2D, PW, CW)	Symptoms
Aortic stenosis						
Low flow, low gradient	√[a]	√[a]				
High flow, high gradient	√[c]					√[b]
Aortic regurgitation						
Asymptomatic, LV dysfunction		√[c]				√[b]
Mitral stenosis						
Symptomatic, mild–moderate			√[a]			√[b]
Asymptomatic, severe			√[a]			
Organic MR						
Symptomatic, mild–moderate				√[b]		√[b]
Asymptomatic, severe				√[a]		√[a]
Ischemic MR						
Symptomatic, mild–moderate		√[b]				√[b]
Pulmonary edema (unknown origin)		√[b]				√[a]
Moderate, before CABG		√[b]				√[b]
Valve Prosthesis						
Symptomatic, equivocal rest findings					√[b]	
Asymptomatic, high gradient					√[b]	√[b]

Color color color Doppler, *CW* continuous-wave Doppler, *EF* ejection fraction, *MR* mitral regurgitation, *EOA* effective orifice area, *ERO* effective regurgitant orifice area, *PASP* pulmonary artery systolic pressure (from tricuspid regurgitant jet velocity), *PW* pulsed-wave Doppler; *SV* stroke volume, *CABG* coronary artery bypass graft
[a] AHA/ACC and/or ESC guidelines
[b] ASE and/or EAE recommendations
[c] Promising reports

limited, experience reported in the literature. The applications of "proven value" should be implemented in daily clinical practice, the applications of "probable value" can be implemented in selected cases, and the applications of "possible value" remain limited to the research domain.

36.1
Aortic Stenosis

Aortic Valve Stenosis with Low Flow, Low Gradient, and Left Ventricular Dysfunction

Patients with severe AS and left ventricular (LV) systolic dysfunction (ejection fraction<40%) often present with a relatively low pressure gradient, i.e., mean gradient less than 40 mmHg (Fig. 36.1). This entity represents a diagnostic challenge because it is difficult to distinguish between patients having true anatomically severe AS from those having pseudo-severe AS. In true severe AS, the primary culprit is the valve disease, and

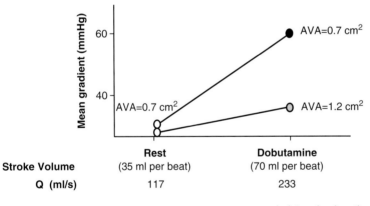

Fig. 36.1 Hemodynamic principles supporting use of dobutamine stress echocardiography in low-flow, low-gradient aortic stenosis. At rest, the mean gradient is low regardless of aortic valve area (*AVA*) because the transvalvular flow rate is low (*white dot*). The stroke volume (*SV*) on the *x*-axis is low at rest (35 ml; *white dot*) and may normalize following dobutamine (70 ml). For a given left ventricular ejection time of 0.3, the mean transvalvular flow rate (*Q*) will increase from 117 to 233 ml s⁻¹. With augmentation of flow with dobutamine, there is a marked increase in gradient (14–57 mmHg in this example) in the case of a true severe stenosis (AVA = 0.7 cm²), whereas there is only a modest increase in gradient (7–19 mmHg) in the case of moderate stenosis (AVA = 1.2 cm²)

the LV dysfunction is a secondary or concomitant phenomenon. The small and relatively fixed aortic valve area (AVA) contributes to raising afterload, decreasing ejection fraction, and reducing stroke volume. In pseudo-severe AS, the predominant factor is myocardial disease, and the severity of AS is overestimated on the basis of AVA because there is incomplete opening of the valve due to reduction in the opening force generated by the weakened ventricle. In both situations, the low-flow state and low-pressure gradient contribute to a calculated AVA that meets criteria for severe AS at rest ($\leq 1.0\,\text{cm}^2$) (Fig. 36.1). Hence, the resting echocardiogram does not distinguish between these two situations. Yet, this distinction is essential since patients with true-severe AS and poor LV function will generally benefit significantly from aortic valve replacement (AVR), whereas the patients with pseudo-severe AS will not.

In patients with low-flow, low-gradient AS and LV dysfunction, it may be useful to determine the transvalvular pressure gradient and to calculate AVA during a baseline resting state and again during low-dose dobutamine stress, to determine whether the stenosis is severe or only moderate [12–20] (Figs. 36.1, 36.2). Side effects are not infrequent with full-dose dobutamine in unselected patients with normal or moderately reduced LV ejection fraction [11, 21], and can occur in one out of five patients with low-flow, low-gradient AS [22]. The main objective of dobutamine stress echocardiography in the context of low-flow AS is to increase transvalvular flow rate while not inducing myocardial ischemia. Hence, a low-dose protocol (i.e., up to $20\,\mu\text{g kg}^{-1}\,\text{min}^{-1}$) should be used for these patients. Moreover, it is preferable to use longer dobutamine stages (5–8 min instead of the 3–5 min generally used for the detection of ischemic heart disease) to ensure that the patient is in a steady-state condition during Doppler echocardiography data acquisition and before proceeding to the next stage. The increase in heart rate should also be taken into consideration given that it may predispose the patient to myocardial ischemia and at one point may override the inotropic effect, thereby limiting the increase in transvalvular flow.

The dobutamine stress approach is based on the notion that patients who have pseudo-severe AS will exhibit an increase in the AVA and little change in transvalvular gradient in response to the increase in transvalvular flow rate [13] (Figs. 36.2, 36.3). In contrast, patients with true severe AS will have no or minimal increase in AVA and a marked increase in gradient when flow is increased because the valve is rigid (Figs. 36.2, 36.4). Several criteria have been proposed in the literature to differentiate pseudo- from true severe AS including a peak stress mean gradient less than 30 or les than 40 mmHg depending on the study, a peak stress AVA greater than 1.0 or greater than $1.2\,\text{cm}^2$, and an absolute increase in effective orifice area (EOA) greater than $0.3\,\text{cm}^2$ during dobutamine stress [14–20]. Although the dichotomization of patients into two categories (true or pseudosevere AS) is convenient, it is an oversimplification, and the classification of the individual patient may not always be as easy as it may appear. The changes in gradient and AVA during dobutamine stress depend largely on the magnitude of the flow augmentation achieved, which may vary considerably from one patient to another. The AVA and gradient are therefore measured at flow conditions that differ dramatically from one patient to another, and the utilization of these indices which are not normalized with respect to the flow increase may lead to misclassification of stenosis severity in some patients. To overcome this limitation,

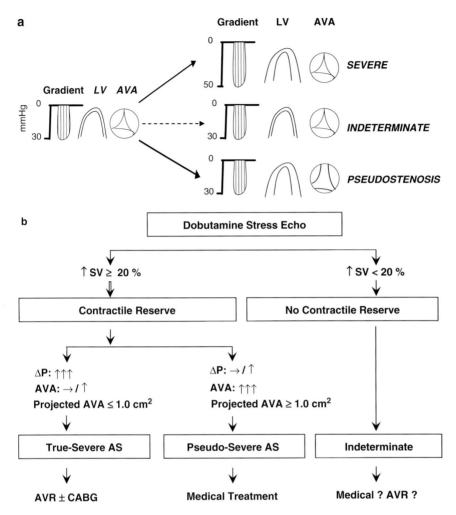

Fig. 36.2 a Hemodynamic principles supporting dobutamine stress echocardiography in low-gradient aortic stenosis (AS) with left ventricular dysfunction. The resting transaortic gradient (<40 mmHg), left ventricular (*LV*) function (<40%), and calculated aortic valve area (*AVA*, <1 cm²) are depicted on the *left*. On the *right*, the three possible responses to dobutamine are shown: in severe AS, the increase in stroke volume (>20%) leads to an increase in gradient with no or only a minimal increase in AVA, but in pseudostenosis, there is only a mild increase in gradient associated with an increase in AVA. The stenosis severity remains "indeterminate" when there is no inotropic response of the left ventricle and thus no significant increase in stroke volume and transvalvular flow rate. **b** Algorithm for the interpretation of the results of dobutamine stress echocardiography in patients with low-flow aortic stenosis. *AVA* aortic valve area, *ΔP* transvalvular pressure gradient, *SV* stroke volume, *AVR* aortic valve replacement, *CABG* coronary artery bypass graft surgery, *sideward arrow* no change, *upward arrow* mild increase, *multiple upward arrows* marked increase

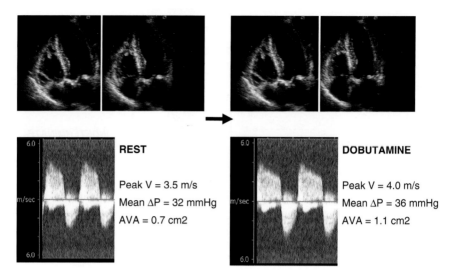

Low flow, low gradient, pseudo-severe aortic stenosis

Fig. 36.3 Pseudosevere aortic stenosis unmasked by dobutamine stress echocardiography in a patient with reduced left ventricular function and low gradient at rest. *Upper panels*: end-diastolic and end-systolic frames at rest (*left*) and after dobutamine (*right*), showing an increase in regional thickening. *Lower panels*: slight increase in pressure gradient (ΔP) and significant increase in aortic valve area (*AVA*)

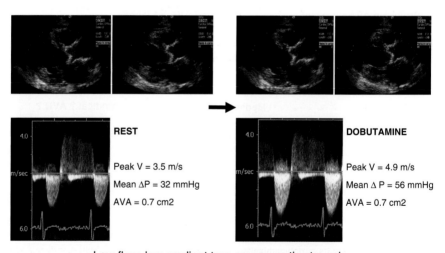

Low flow, low gradient true-severe aortic stenosis

Fig. 36.4 True severe aortic stenosis unmasked by dobutamine stress echocardiography in a patient with reduced left ventricular function and low gradient at rest. *Upper panels*: end-diastolic and end-systolic frames at rest (*left*) and after dobutamine (*right*), showing an increase in regional thickening. *Lower panels*: marked increase in pressure gradient (ΔP) and no increase in aortic valve area (*AVA*)

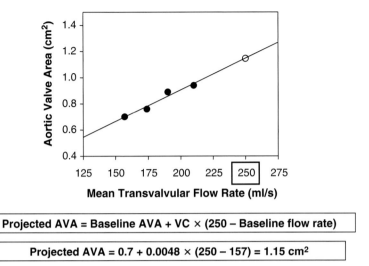

Projected AVA = Baseline AVA + VC × (250 − Baseline flow rate)

Projected AVA = 0.7 + 0.0048 × (250 − 157) = 1.15 cm²

Fig. 36.5 Concept of the projected aortic valve area (*AVA*). Values of AVA obtained at different stages of dobutamine infusion are plotted as a function of flow rate (stroke volume divided by ejection time). The slope of the regression line is the valve compliance (*VC*). The VC can also be obtained using a simplified method by dividing the absolute increase in AVA measured during dobutamine stress by the absolute increase in flow rate. The projected AVA (*open circle*) at a normal flow rate (250 ml s⁻¹) is calculated using the regression equation. In this example, the peak AVA (*) obtained during dobutamine is 0.94 cm², and the absolute increase in AVA is 0.24 cm², which would suggest true severe stenosis. However, calculation of the projected AVA using the baseline values of AVA (0.7 cm²) and flow rate (157 ml s⁻¹) and the valve compliance (0.48 cm² 100 ml⁻¹ s⁻¹) yields a value of 1.15 cm², which is consistent with moderate stenosis

the investigators of the Truly or Pseudo-Severe Aortic Stenosis (TOPAS) multicenter study [23] have proposed a new echocardiographic parameter: the projected AVA at a standardized normal flow rate (Fig. 36.5). A projected AVA of less than 1.0 cm² is considered as an indicator of true severe stenosis [23]. Patients who fail to manifest an increase in stroke volume with dobutamine of 20% or greater have a lack of contractile reserve and have been shown to have a poor prognosis with either medical or surgical management [20]. Moreover, in this subset of patients, it is difficult to determine the true severity of the stenosis. Patients identified as having true severe AS and contractile reserve on dobutamine stress have a much better outcome with AVR than with medical therapy [18, 20]. A number of patients without contractile reserve may also benefit from AVR [20], but decisions in these high-risk patients must be individualized, in the absence of clear guidelines. To this effect, plasma brain natriuretic peptide (<550 pg ml⁻¹) may be useful to identify the patients with lack of contractile reserve who may benefit from AVR [24]. Also, the assessment of aortic valve calcification by multislice computed tomography may be helpful to corroborate the stenosis severity in these patients [25].

In patients with low-flow, low-gradient AS, the indication for dobutamine stress echocardiography is rated as class IIa, with level of evidence B [2], with the caveat that dobutamine stress testing in patients with AS should be performed only in centers with experience in pharmacological stress testing and with a cardiologist in attendance.

36

Asymptomatic Severe Aortic Stenosis with High Gradient

Management of asymptomatic patients with severe AS, defined as peak velocity greater than 4 m s^{-1} and/or mean pressure gradient greater than 40 mmHg and/or AVA less than 1 cm^2 [2, 3], remains a source of debate. The wide interindividual variation in the rate of progression and in the outcome of the disease has recently prompted some authors to recommend early elective surgery in asymptomatic patients with severe AS. The rationale for using this approach is that if one applies a strategy of waiting for symptoms before recommending surgery, the patient may be operated too late in the course of the disease at a stage in which myocardial damage is, at least in part, irreversible.

In this regard, it is also important to emphasize that some patients, and especially elderly patients, may ignore or not report their symptoms, while others may reduce their level of physical activity to avoid or minimize symptoms. The principal role of exercise testing is to unmask symptoms in a significant proportion of patients with AS who claim to be asymptomatic, as these symptoms can predict outcome [26–29]. Reduced exercise tolerance, with development of dyspnea or ST-segment depression, is associated with a worse outcome [27–29]. In this respect, exercise testing is an important tool, and several studies have shown its prognostic value. Moreover, an increase in the mean aortic pressure gradient of more than 20 mmHg during exercise in asymptomatic patients is another predictor of symptom onset in the short term, suggesting that this may also be used as a criterion to recommend early elective surgery (Fig. 36.6) [30]. However, more confirmatory data are

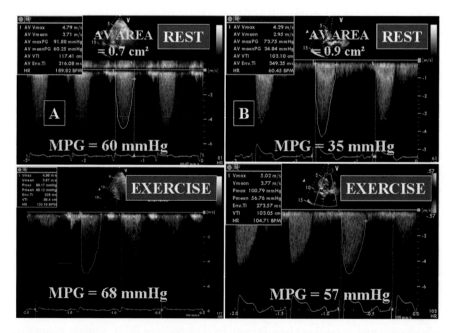

Fig. 36.6 Examples of exercise-induced changes in mean transaortic pressure gradient (*MPG*) in two asymptomatic patients with severe aortic stenosis. **A** Small increase in MPG with exercise. **B** Significant exercise-induced increase in MPG

needed to support the inclusion of this parameter in the routine management of asymptomatic patients with severe AS.

36.2
Aortic Regurgitation

As is the case with AS and chronic mitral regurgitation (MR), development of irreversible LV dysfunction is a major concern in asymptomatic patients with severe aortic regurgitation (AR). In those with normal resting LV systolic function, an increase in LV ejection fraction during either exercise or pharmacologic stress prior to surgery indicates the presence of contractile reserve, and this may predict improvement in LV function after AVR [31]. The assessment of contractile reserve can be extended for the evaluation of patients with AR who have developed LV dysfunction. In these latter patients, exercise tolerance is an important predictor of reversal of LV dysfunction and survival after AVR [32, 33].

The development of symptoms during exercise testing is useful in predicting outcome in patients with severe AR who are apparently asymptomatic at rest. The additional value of stress imaging is unclear. The observed magnitude of change in ejection fraction or stroke volume from rest to exercise is related not only to myocardial contractile function but also to severity of volume-overload and exercise-induced changes in preload and peripheral resistances [2]. The validity of stress echocardiography in predicting outcome of patients with asymptomatic AR is limited mainly by the small number of available studies [34, 35], but is supported by a number of studies using exercise radionuclide angiography [36–39]. Some data supporting the prognostic value of this functional stratification exist in the literature, but they are too few to recommend this specific application for routine clinical use.

To this effect, the ACC/AHA guidelines do not recommend exercise or dobutamine stress echocardiography for routine assessment of LV function in patients with AR [2]. More data are needed to corroborate this application, since the incremental value of stress imaging to LV dimensions and ejection fraction at rest remains unclear [10].

36.3
Mitral Stenosis

A baseline resting transthoracic echocardiography examination is usually sufficient to guide management in asymptomatic patients with mild-to-moderate mitral stenosis (MS) and in symptomatic patients with moderate-to-severe MS who are candidates for either percutaneous balloon valvuloplasty or surgical mitral valve repair or replacement. In some patients, more detailed assessment of valve function and its hemodynamic consequences is needed, particularly when symptoms and Doppler findings are discordant. In asymptomatic patients with severe MS (mean gradient>10 mmHg and mitral valve area<1.0 cm^2), or symptomatic patients with moderate MS (mean gradient of 5–10 mmHg and mitral valve area of 1.0–1.5 cm^2), the measurement of pulmonary artery pressures during exercise or dobutamine stress echocardiography may help distinguish those who could benefit from valvuloplasty or valve replacement from those who should be maintained on medical therapy [2, 40–42]. As is the case with the aortic valve, the transmitral valve pressure gradient is related to the valve orifice area. However, it should be emphasized that the transmitral gradient is much more sensitive to the chronotropic conditions than that of the transaortic gradient and that these conditions may vary extensively from one patient to another. Moreover, for a given valve orifice area, patients with reduced atrioventricular compliance exhibit a more pronounced increase in pulmonary arterial pressure during exercise or dobutamine stress than those with normal compliance [41, 43]. Hence, the resting values of transmitral gradient or pulmonary arterial pressure do not necessarily reflect the actual severity of the disease. Stress echocardiography may therefore be highly useful for confirming the severity of MS and assessing its consequences on the hemodynamic and symptomatic status of the patient under exercise conditions. This test is clearly indicated when there is discordance between the severity of MS as assessed by resting echocardiography and the patient's symptomatic status.

The usually adopted cut-off values, proposed by the ACC/AHA and the ESC guidelines [2, 3], are a peak pulmonary artery systolic pressure greater than 60 mmHg (measured from the tricuspid regurgitant velocity) during exercise (Fig. 36.7) or a mean transmitral pressure gradient greater than 15 mmHg (Fig. 36.8) [2]. Above these threshold values, valvuloplasty or valve replacement is recommended, even for patients with apparently

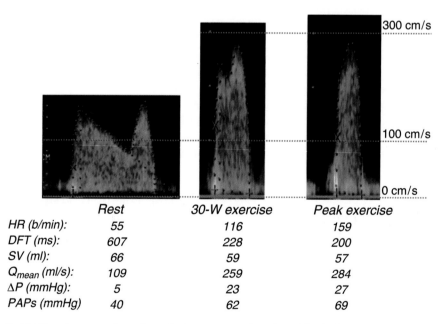

	Rest	30-W exercise	Peak exercise
HR (b/min):	55	116	159
DFT (ms):	607	228	200
SV (ml):	66	59	57
Q_{mean} (ml/s):	109	259	284
ΔP (mmHg):	5	23	27
PAPs (mmHg)	40	62	69

Fig. 36.7 Exercise stress echocardiography in a symptomatic patient with mitral stenosis (mitral valve area: 1.2 cm^2) and relatively low resting mean transmitral pressure gradient (ΔP). With exercise, there is a marked increase in the transvalvular gradient and systolic pulmonary arterial pressure (*PAPs*). In this patient the exercise-induced increase in mean transvalvular flow rate (Q_{mean}) was caused by the dramatic shortening in diastolic filling time (*DFT*). *HR* heart rate, *SV* stroke volume

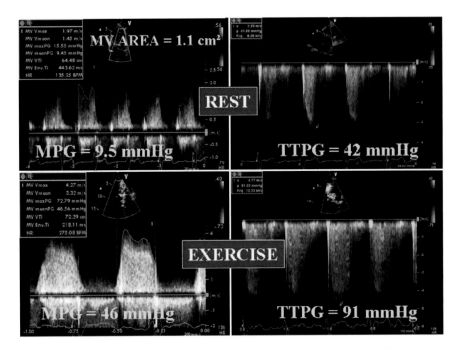

Fig. 36.8 Example of an asymptomatic patient with severe mitral valve stenosis but with moderately elevated mean transmitral pressure gradient (*MPG*) at rest. During exercise, the MPG increases markedly as does the systolic transtricuspid pressure gradient (*TTPG*) indicative of pulmonary hypertension

moderate MS at rest [2, 10, 11]. The use of this stress echocardiography application in MS is rated as class I with level of evidence C for patients with discordant symptoms and stenosis severity [2]. As with other valve conditions, a major role of stress testing in patients with MS is to evaluate exercise capacity and exercise-induced symptoms.

36.4
Mitral Regurgitation

Organic Mitral Regurgitation

The severity of organic MR can be reliably assessed by resting color-flow Doppler echocardiography with the use of semiquantitative or quantitative methods [2, 3, 44]. Such information is useful to predict the development of LV dysfunction and of symptoms [45]. There is presently an important ongoing controversy on whether asymptomatic patients with severe MR should undergo early elective mitral valve repair [45–47]. In selected patients in whom there is a discrepancy between symptoms and severity of MR, and especially in asymptomatic patients with severe MR, exercise stress echocardiography may help to identify patients with subclinical latent LV dysfunction and poor clinical outcome. Worsening of MR severity, a marked increase in pulmonary arterial pressure, the absence of contractile reserve, impaired exercise capacity, and the occurrence of symptoms during stress exercise echocardiography can be useful findings to identify the subset of high-risk patients who may benefit from early surgery. Exercise capacity itself predicts the development of symptoms or LV dysfunction in asymptomatic patients with MR [48]. Recommendations for early surgery in asymptomatic patients should only be made in those who are candidates for mitral valve repair and in experienced centers in which there is a high likelihood (>90%) of successful mitral repair without residual MR [2].

Exercise echocardiography has also been used to unmask the development of severe MR with exercise in patients with rheumatic mitral valve disease and only mild or moderate MR at rest [49]. The spectrum of LV responses to stress is not dissimilar from that described for AR, but the prognostic impact of this functional heterogeneity remains unsettled. Although still relatively unexplored, the assessment of contractile reserve in patients with MR may provide important information for risk stratification and clinical decision making, especially in asymptomatic patients with severe MR. A threshold value of pulmonary artery systolic pressure greater than 60 mmHg during exercise may also identify patients with severe MR who might be referred for surgery [2, 10]. The application of stress echocardiography in asymptomatic patients with severe MR is rated as a class IIa recommendation with level of evidence C [2].

Ischemic Mitral Regurgitation

Exercise stress echocardiography is valuable in identifying hemodynamically significant MR in patients with LV systolic dysfunction, especially when ischemic heart disease is the underlying etiology. Ischemic MR is primarily a disease of the LV myocardium and develops with a structurally normal mitral valve. The magnitude of ischemic MR varies dynamically in accordance with changes in loading conditions, annular size, and the balance of tethering versus closing forces applied on the mitral valve leaflets. Hence, the severity of MR assessed by resting echocardiography does not necessarily reflect the severity under exercise conditions. In patients with ischemic MR, quantitative assessment of exercise-induced changes in the degree of MR may be useful to unmask patients at high risk of poor outcome. An increase in the effective regurgitant orifice area to 13 mm^2 or greater or an increase in the systolic pulmonary arterial pressure to 60 mmHg or greater (Fig. 36.9) at peak exercise stress is predictive of increased morbidity and mortality [50]. Furthermore, the magnitude of increase in effective regurgitant orifice during exercise cannot be predicted from the resting regurgitant orifice. Hence, exercise Doppler echocardiography provides important incremental information over resting echocardiography in patients with ischemic MR.

Pierard and Lancellotti [51–53] have proposed that exercise stress echocardiography in patients with ischemic MR can provide useful information in the following situations: (1) patients with exertional dyspnea out of proportion to the severity of resting LV dysfunction or MR; (2) patients in whom acute pulmonary edema occurs without an obvious cause; and (3) patients with moderate MR before surgical revascularization. Their data also suggest that exercise echocardiography may be helpful in identifying patients at high risk of mortality and heart failure.

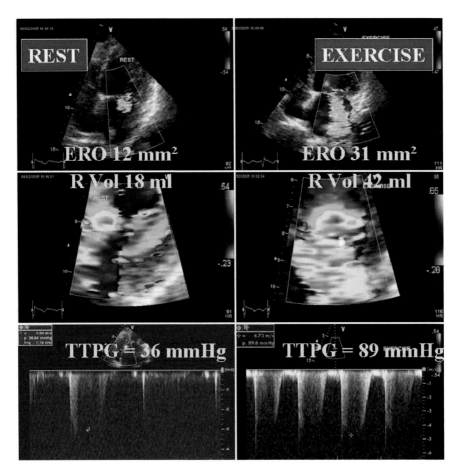

Fig. 36.9 Apical 4-chamber view showing color-flow Doppler and proximal flow-convergence region at rest and during exercise in a patient with a large exercise-induced increase in mitral regurgitation and estimated pulmonary artery systolic pressure. *ERO*, effective regurgitant orifice; *RVol*, regurgitant volume; *TTPG*, systolic transtricuspid pressure gradient

36.5
Prosthetic Heart Valves

Echocardiography is the method of choice for evaluating prosthetic valve function. This evaluation follows the same principles used for the evaluation of native valves with some important caveats [54, 55]. First, imaging of the valve occluder and assessment of transprosthetic flow are limited by reverberations and shadowing caused by the valve components. Second, the fluid dynamics of mechanical prosthetic valves may differ substantially from that of a native valve. The flow is eccentric in monoleaflet valves and is composed of three separate jets in bileaflet valves, with the flow velocity potentially higher in the central orifice jet than in the two lateral orifice jets.

Because most prosthetic valves are inherently stenotic, the EOA of a prosthetic valve is often too small in relation to body size, a phenomenon known as prosthesis–patient mismatch (PPM). In the aortic position, PPM is considered moderate when the indexed EOA is less than or equal to $0.85\,cm^2\,m^{-2}$ and severe when it is less than or equal to $0.65\,cm^2\,m^{-2}$ [55]. In the mitral position, the cut-off values are 1.2 and $0.9\,cm^2\,m^{-2}$, respectively. PPM has been linked to impaired exercise capacity, suboptimal symptomatic improvement, incomplete regression of LV hypertrophy and pulmonary hypertension, and increased cardiac events and mortality following valve replacement [56–60]. PPM is, by far, the most frequent cause of increased transprosthetic gradient. It is important to differentiate this condition from acquired prosthetic stenosis, which may result from leaflet calcification of bioprostheses and pannus overgrowth or thrombus formation on mechanical prostheses.

The presence of increased mean transprosthetic gradient (15–20 mmHg for aortic prostheses and 5–7 mmHg for mitral prostheses) and/or symptoms should prompt further evaluation. In particular, it is important to determine whether the elevated gradient, and eventually the associated symptoms, are due to PPM, an intrinsic stenosis of the prosthesis, or a localized high gradient, a phenomenon that occurs only in bileaflet mechanical valves. Occasionally, an abnormally high jet velocity corresponding to a localized gradient may indeed be recorded by continuous wave Doppler through the smaller central slit-like orifice of bileaflet mechanical prostheses. This phenomenon yields measurement of an abnormally high gradient and low EOA, thus mimicking the findings of intrinsic prosthesis dysfunction.

As normally and abnormally functioning prostheses can produce similar estimated gradients at rest by transthoracic echocardiography, it may be difficult to distinguish between high gradients caused by artifactual phenomena from those caused by prosthetic valve stenosis or PPM. In these situations, stress echocardiography may be valuable in confirming or excluding the presence of hemodynamically significant prosthetic valve stenosis or PPM, especially when there is discordance between the prosthetic valve hemodynamics measured by echocardiography at rest and the patient's symptomatic status [55, 61–65]. In contrast to a normally functioning and well-matched prosthesis (including a bileaflet mechanical valve with a localized high gradient at rest), a stenotic valve prosthesis or PPM is generally associated with a marked increase in gradient with exercise, often associated with pulmonary arterial hypertension, the development of symptoms, and impaired exercise capacity on exercise echocardiography [66–73]. A disproportionate increase in transvalvular gradient (>20 mmHg for aortic prostheses or>12 mmHg for mitral prostheses) generally indicates severe prosthesis dysfunction or PPM (Fig. 36.10). High resting and stress gradients occur more often with biological rather than mechanical prostheses, stented rather than stentless bioprostheses, smaller (≤21 for aortic, and ≤25 for mitral) rather than larger prostheses, and mismatched rather than nonmismatched prostheses. In fact, the behavior of the transprosthetic pressure gradient under exercise conditions is essentially determined by the indexed EOA (Fig. 36.10), which in turn may be influenced by the patient's body size, prosthesis model and size, mismatch between body size and prosthesis size, and pathologic obstruction of the prosthesis caused by leaflet calcification, pannus, or thrombus.

As is the case in native aortic valves that have developed low-flow, low-gradient AS, dobutamine stress echocardiography may be useful in differentiating true prosthesis stenosis from pseudostenosis or PPM in patients with prosthetic valves and low cardiac output. In the case of pseudostenosis with low output, the resting transprosthetic flow rate and

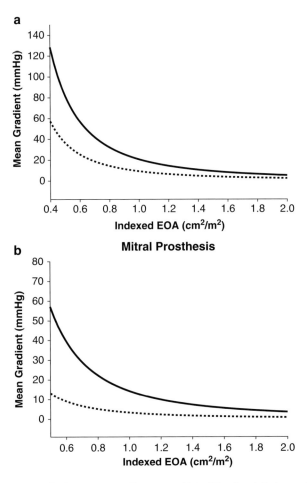

Fig. 36.10 Mean transprosthetic pressure gradient at rest (dotted lines) and during sustained physical exercise (continuous lines) as a function of the indexed effective orifice area (*EOA*) for aortic (**a**) and mitral (**b**) prostheses. Compared to patients no. 2 and 4 who have large prosthetic EOAs, patients 1 and 3 with small EOAs exhibit a major increase in gradient with exercise, thus suggesting the presence of severe prosthetic stenosis or prosthesis–patient mismatch in these latter patients

thus the force applied on the leaflets are too low to completely open the prosthetic valve. During infusion of dobutamine, however, these patients manifest a substantial increase in the prosthesis EOA with the increasing flow rate, with no or minimal elevation in the prosthetic gradient. In contrast, true severe prosthetic stenosis or PPM is associated with no significant increase in EOA and a marked increase in gradient with dobutamine, often with additional diagnostic changes (such as LV dysfunction or marked elevation in pulmonary arterial pressure) and symptoms.

It should be emphasized that exercise or dobutamine stress echocardiography does not distinguish between acquired prosthesis stenosis and PPM, as in both cases the EOA remains small and the gradient increases markedly with stress. In this situation, one should compare the EOA values obtained during stress echocardiography with the normal reference values of EOA for the model and size of the specific prosthesis that has been implanted in the patient [55]. If the measured EOA is substantially lower than the normal reference EOA, one should suspect prosthesis dysfunction. If, on the other hand, the measured EOA is within the normal reference range, and the indexed EOA is low, one should consider the presence of PPM.

In patients undergoing surgical correction of ischemic MR, a restrictive annuloplasty combined with coronary artery bypass grafting is the most common approach. However, this procedure is associated with a relatively high rate of recurrence of MR, and restrictive annuloplasty may result in functional MS in some patients [74]. In patients with postoperative symptoms or evidence of either residual MR or functional MS, exercise testing may be useful to assess symptoms and exercise capacity, and the assessment of exercise hemodynamics with stress echocardiography can provide additional important information regarding the significance of MS and/or of dynamic MR.

There are relatively few studies investigating the added value of stress echocardiography for the management of patients with prosthetic valves or mitral annuloplasty rings, and the available studies are generally based on small numbers of patients. Although stress echocardiography has been shown to be useful in the evaluation of prosthetic valve dysfunction and PPM, its value in risk stratification and prediction of clinical outcomes is not well established. Thus, further studies are needed in this challenging field.

36.6
Coronary Artery Disease and Coronary Flow Reserve

Diagnosis of Coronary Artery Disease in Patients with Valvular Heart Disease

Although stress echocardiography is a widely accepted, accurate, and safe noninvasive technique to diagnose the presence and severity of coronary artery disease in patients without valvular heart disease, relatively few data are available on its accuracy and safety in patients with hemodynamically significant valve disease. In general, one can expect that the sensitivity of stress echocardiography will be similar in patients with and without valvular heart disease but the specificity will be lower [75, 76]. Coronary flow reserve can be severely reduced in patients with AS or AR even when the epicardial coronary arteries are normal [77–79]. For this same reason, the specificity of perfusion imaging is also suboptimal in patients with LV hypertrophy secondary to valvular heart disease [75]. For practical purposes, conventional coronary angiography remains the established investigation for ruling out significant coronary artery disease in the preoperative evaluation of patients awaiting valve surgery, although cardiac computed tomography may also have a role in patients without coronary calcification.

Coronary Flow Reserve in Valvular Heart Disease

In patients with severe AS and normal coronary arteries, the reduced coronary flow reserve is more closely related to the severity of the stenosis than to the degree of LV hypertrophy [80].

The impairment of coronary flow reserve classically observed in AS may be caused by several factors including extravascular compression of the coronary microvasculature due to elevated LV diastolic pressures, a shortening of diastolic perfusion time, and an increase in myocardial metabolic demand resulting from the LV pressure overload.

Following AVR, normalization of coronary flow reserve is directly related to the augmentation in valve EOA [79]. Stentless bioprostheses are associated with greater improvement in coronary flow reserve compared to that of stented bioprostheses or mechanical valves [80], presumably because stentless bioprostheses generally provide a larger EOA for a given annulus size. In the future, the assessment of coronary flow reserve is likely to play an increasingly important role in the assessment of patients with valvular heart disease, especially aortic valve disease, before and after AVR. Positron emission tomography has an established role in quantifying coronary flow reserve, and cardiac magnetic resonance imaging is evolving as another noninvasive method for this assessment [81], with the potential to quantify the transmural gradient of flow reserve across the myocardial wall [82]. Both techniques have been applied to study changes in coronary flow reserve in patients with AS after AVR [79, 80]. Transthoracic echocardiography also has the potential to study coronary flow reserve of the middistal left anterior descending coronary artery [83], and this technique has been applied to patients with AS [84] (Fig. 36.11).

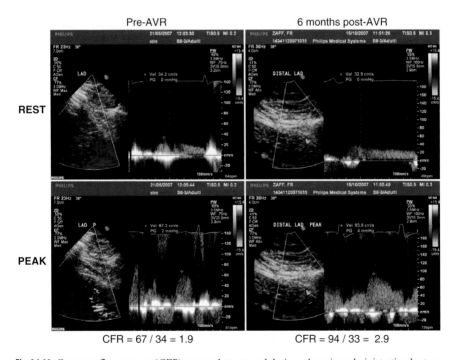

Fig. 36.11 Coronary flow reserve (*CFR*) assessed at rest and during adenosine administration by transthoracic stress echocardiography in a patient with severe aortic stenosis and angiographically normal coronary arteries before (*left panel*) and 6 months after (*right panel*) aortic valve replacement (*AVR*). In the postoperative assessment, left ventricular hypertrophy is not yet regressed but CFR has substantially improved. (Courtesy of Dr. Fausto Rigo, Venice, Italy)

Echocardiography has the obvious advantage of wide availability and relatively low cost, and with further experience, this technique could be added to the standard, routine applications of echocardiography in evaluating valve disease [85, 86].

36.7
Conclusions

Exercise testing has an established role in the evaluation of patients with valvular heart disease that can aid significantly in clinical decision making. Stress echocardiography has emerged as an important component of stress testing, in which the noninvasive assessment of dynamic changes in valve function, ventricular function, and hemodynamics can be coupled with assessment of exercise capacity and symptomatic responses. Surprisingly, this role is much more clearly established in American [2] than European [3] general cardiology guidelines, despite the larger and earlier acceptance of stress echocardiography in the European practice for the diagnosis of coronary artery disease [1, 5, 6]. Stress echocardiography has the advantages of wide availability, low cost, and versatility for the assessment of disease severity [2, 3, 10, 11]. In addition to its established applications in valvular heart disease, transthoracic Doppler echocardiography also has the potential to assess coronary flow reserve. The versatile applications of stress echocardiography can be tailored to the individual patient with aortic or mitral valve disease, both before and after valve replacement or repair. Hence, exercise-induced changes in valve hemodynamics, ventricular function, and pulmonary artery pressure, together with exercise capacity and symptomatic responses to exercise, provide the clinician with diagnostic and prognostic information that can contribute importantly to subsequent clinical decisions.

References

1. Gibbons RJ, Balady GJ, Bricker JT, et al (2002) ACC/AHA 2002 guideline update for exercise testing: summary article. A Report of the American College of Cardiology/American HeartAssociation Task Force on Practice Guidelines (Committee to Update the 1997 Exercise Testing Guidelines). Circulation 106:1883–1892
2. Bonow RO, Carabello BA, Chatterjee K, et al (2006) ACC/AHA 2006 guidelines for the management of patients with valvular heart disease. A report of the American College of Cardiology/American Heart Association Task Force on Practice Guidelines (writing Committee to Revise the 1998 guidelines for the management of patients with valvular heart disease). J Am Coll Cardiol 48:e1–e148
3. Vahanian A, Baumgartner H, Bax J, et al (2007) Guidelines on the management of valvular heart disease. Task Force on the Management of Valvular Heart Disease of the European Society of Cardiology. Eur Heart J 28:230–268
4. Picano E (1992) Stress echocardiography: from pathophysiological toy to diagnostic tool. Point of view. Circulation 85:1604–1612
5. Gibbons RJ, Abrams J, Chatterjee K, et al (2003) ACC/AHA 2002 guideline update for the management of patients with chronic stable angina: summary article. A report of the American College of Cardiology/American Heart Association Task Force on Practice Guidelines

(Committee on the Management of Patients With Chronic Stable Angina). J Am Coll Cardiol 41:159–168

6. Fox K, Garcia MA, Ardissino D, et al (2006) Guidelines on the management of stable angina pectoris: executive summary. Task Force on the Management of Stable Angina Pectoris of the European Society of Cardiology. Eur Heart J 27:1341–1348

7. Schwammenthal E, Vered Z, Rabinowitz B, et al (1997) Stress echocardiography beyond coronary artery disease. Eur Heart J 18:D130–D137

8. Decena BF III, Tischler MD (1999) Stress echocardiography in valvular heart disease. Cardiol Clin 17:555–572

9. Fulps D, Davis C, Shah P (2002) Exercise Doppler echocardiography: utility in obtaining hemodynamic evaluation. Cardiac Ultrasound Today 7/8:118–149

10. Pellikka PA, Nagueh SF, Elhendy AA, Kuehl CA, Sawada SG (2007) American Society of Echocardiography recommendations for performance, interpretation, and application of stress echocardiography. J Am Soc Echocardiogr 20:1021–1041

11. Sicari R, Niohyannopoulos P, Evangelista A, et al (2008) Stress echocardiography consensus statement of the European Association of Echocardiography. Eur J Echocardiogr 9(4):415–437

12. Otto CM, Pearlman AS, Kraft CD, et al (1992) Physiologic changes with maximal exercise in asymptomatic valvular aortic stenosis assessed by Doppler echocardiography. J Am Coll Cardiol 20:1160–1167

13. Grayburn PA (2006) Assessment of low-gradient aortic stenosis with dobutamine. Circulation 113:604–606

14. deFilippi CR, Willett DL, Brickner ME, et al (1995) Usefulness of dobutamine echocardiography in distinguishing severe from non severe valvular aortic stenosis in patients with depressed left ventricular function and low transvalvular gradients. Am J Cardiol 75:191–194

15. Schwammenthal E, Vered Z, Moshkowitz Y, et al (2001) Dobutamine echocardiography in patients with aortic stenosis and left ventricular dysfunction: predicting outcome as a function of management strategy. Chest 119:1766–1777

16. Nishimura RA, Grantham JA, Connolly HM, et al (2002) Low-output, low-gradient aortic stenosis in patients with depressed left ventricular systolic function: the clinical utility of the dobutamine challenge in the catheterization laboratory. Circulation 106:809–813

17. Monin JL, Monchi M, Gest V, et al (2003) Aortic stenosis with severe left ventricular dysfunction and low transvalvular pressure gradients: risk stratification by low dose dobutamine echocardiography. J Am Coll Cardiol 37:2101–2107

18. Monin JL, Quere JP, Monchi M, et al (2003) Low-gradient aortic stenosis: operative risk stratification and predictors for long-term outcome: a multicenter study using dobutamine stress hemodynamics. Circulation 108:319–324

19. Zuppiroli A, Mori F, Olivotto I, et al (2003) Therapeutic implications of contractile reserve elicited by dobutamine echocardiography in symptomatic, low-gradient aortic stenosis. Ital Heart J 4:264–270

20. Quere JP, Monin JL, Levy F et al. (2006) Influence of preoperative left ventricular contractile reserve on postoperative ejection fraction in low-gradient aortic stenosis. Circulation 113:1738–1744

21. Picano E, Mathias W Jr, Pingitore A, Bigi R, Previtali M, on behalf of the EDIC Study Group. (1994) Safety and tolerability of dobutamine-atropine stress echocardiography: a prospective, large-scale, multicenter trial. Lancet 344:1190–1192

22. Bountioukos M, Kertai MD, Schinkel AF, et al (2003) Safety of dobutamine stress echocardiography in patients with aortic stenosis. J Heart Valve Dis 12:441–446

23. Blais C, Burwash IG, Mundigler G, et al (2006) The projected valve area at normal flow rate improves the assessment of stenosis severity in patients with low flow aortic stenosis: the multicenter TOPAS (Truly or Pseudo Severe Aortic Stenosis) Study. Circulation 113:711–721

36

24. Bergler-Klein J, Mundigler G, Pibarot P, et al (2007) B-type natriuretic peptide in low-flow, low-gradient aortic stenosis: relationship to hemodynamics and clinical outcome. Circulation 115:2848–2855

25. Messika-Zeitoun D, Aubry MC, Detaint D, et al (2004) Evaluation and clinical implications of aortic valve calcification measured by electron-beam computed tomography. Circulation 110:356–362

26. Otto CM, Burwash IG, Legget ME, et al (1997) Prospective study of asymptomatic valvular aortic stenosis: clinical, echocardiographic, and exercise predictors of outcome. Circulation 95:2262–2270

27. Amato MC, Moffa PJ, Werner KE, et al (2001) Treatment decision in asymptomatic aortic valve stenosis: role of exercise testing. Heart 86:381–386

28. Alborino D, Hoffmann JL, Fournet PC, et al (2002) Value of exercise testing to evaluate the indication for surgery in asymptomatic patients with valvular aortic stenosis. J Heart Valve Dis 11:204–209

29. Das P, Rimington H, Chambers J (2005) Exercise testing to stratify risk in aortic stenosis. Eur Heart J 26:1309–1313

30. Lancellotti P, Lebois F, Simon M, et al (2005) Prognostic importance of quantitative exercise Doppler echocardiography in asymptomatic valvular aortic stenosis. Circulation 112(suppl I):I-377–I-382

31. Borer JS, Bonow RO (2003) Contemporary approach to aortic and mitral regurgitation. Circulation 108:2432–2438

32. Bonow RO, Picone AL, McIntosh CL, et al (1985) Survival and functional results after valve replacement for aortic regurgitation from 1976 to 1983: influence of preoperative left ventricular function. Circulation 72:1244–1256

33. Bonow RO, Dodd JT, Maron BJ, et al (1988) Long-term serial changes in left ventricular function and reversal of ventricular dilatation after valve replacement for chronic aortic regurgitation. Circulation 78:1108–1120

34. Wahi S, Haluska B, Pasquet A, et al (2000) Exercise echocardiography predicts development of left ventricular dysfunction in medically and surgically treated patients with asymptomatic severe aortic regurgitation. Heart 84:606–614

35. Espinola-Zavaleta N, Gómez-Núñez N, Chávez PY, et al (2001) Evaluation of the response to pharmacological stress in chronic aortic regurgitation. Echocardiography 18:491–496

36. Bonow RO, Lakatos E, Maron BJ, Epstein SE (1991) Serial long-term assessment of the natural history of asymptomatic patients with chronic aortic regurgitation and normal left ventricular systolic function. Circulation 84:1625–1635

37. Tornos MP, Olona M, Permanyer-Miralda G, et al (1995) Clinical outcome of severe asymptomatic chronic aortic regurgitation: a long-term prospective follow-up study. Am Heart J 130:333–339

38. Borer JS, Hochreiter C, Herrold EM, et al (1998) Prediction of indications for valve replacement among asymptomatic or minimally symptomatic patients with chronic aortic regurgitation and normal left ventricular performance. Circulation 97:525–534

39. Tarasoutchi F, Grinberg M, Spina GS, et al (2003) Ten-year clinical laboratory follow-up after application of a symptom-based therapeutic strategy to patients with severe chronic aortic regurgitation of predominant rheumatic etiology. J Am Coll Cardiol 41:1316–1324

40. Hecker SL, Zabalgoitia M, Ashline P, Oneschuk L, O'Rourke RA, Herrera CJ (1997) Comparison of exercise and dobutamine stress echocardiography in assessing mitral stenosis. Am J Cardiol 80:1374–1377

41. Schwammenthal E, Vered Z, Agranat O, Kaplinsky E, Rabinowitz B, Feinberg MS (2000) Impact of atrioventricular compliance on pulmonary artery pressure in mitral stenosis: an exercise echocardiographic study. Circulation. 102:2378–2384

42. Reis G, Motta MS, Barbosa MM, Esteves WA, Souza SF, Bocchi EA (2004) Dobutamine stress echocardiography for noninvasive assessment and risk stratification of patients with rheumatic mitral stenosis. J Am Coll Cardiol 43:393–401

43. Li M, Dumesnil JG, Mathieu P, et al (2005) Impact of valve prosthesis-patient mismatch on pulmonary arterial pressure after mitral valve replacement. J Am Coll Cardiol 45:1034–1040

44. Zoghbi WA, Enriquez-Sarano M, Foster E, et al (2003) Recommendations for evaluation of the severity of native valvular regurgitation with two-dimensional and Doppler echocardiography. J Am Soc Echocardiogr 16:777–802

45. Enriquez-Sarano M, Avierinos JF, Messika-Zeitoun D, et al (2005) Quantitative determinants of the outcome of asymptomatic mitral regurgitation. N Engl J Med 352:875–883

46. Rosenhek R, Rader F, Klaar U, et al (2006) Outcome of watchful waiting in asymptomatic severe mitral regurgitation. Circulation 113:2238–2244

47. Madaric J, Watripont P, Bartunek J, et al (2007) Effect of mitral valve repair on exercise tolerance in asymptomatic patients with organic mitral regurgitation. Am Heart J 154:180–185

48. Supino PG, Borer JS, Schuleri K, et al (2007) Prognostic value of exercise tolerance testing in asymptomatic chronic nonischemic mitral regurgitation. Am J Cardiol 100:1274–1281

49. Tischler MD, Battle RW, Saha M, Niggel J, LeWinter MM (1995) Observations suggesting a high incidence of exercise-induced severe mitral regurgitation in patients with mild rheumatic mitral valve disease at rest. J Am Coll Cardiol 25:128–133

50. Pierard LA, Lancellotti P (2004) The role of ischemic mitral regurgitation in the pathogenesis of acute pulmonary edema. N Engl J Med 351:1627–1634

51. Lancellotti P, Gérard P, Piérard LA (2005) Long term outcome of patients with heart failure and dynamic mitral regurgitation. Eur Heart J 26:1528–1532

52. Pierard LA, Lancellotti P (2006) Dyspnea and stress testing. N Engl J Med 354:871–873

53. Pierard LA, Lancellotti P (2007) Stress testing in valve disease. Heart 93:766–772

54. Gottdiener JS, Bednarz J, Devereux R, et al (2004) American Society of Echocardiography recommendations for use of echocardiography in clinical trials. J Am Soc Echocardiogr 17:1086–1119

55. Pibarot P, Dumesnil JG (2007) Prevention of valve prosthesis–patient mismatch before aortic valve replacement: does it matter and is it feasible? Heart 93:549–551

56. Blais C, Dumesnil JG, Baillot R, Simard S, Doyle D, Pibarot P (2003) Impact of valve prosthesis-patient mismatch on short-term mortality after aortic valve replacement. Circulation 108:983–988

57. Ruel M, Rubens FD, Masters RG, et al (2004) Late incidence and predictors of persistent or recurrent heart failure in patients with aortic prosthetic valves. J Thorac Cardiovasc Surg 127:149–159

58. Mohty D, Malouf JF, Girard SE, et al (2006) Impact of prosthesis-patient mismatch on long-term survival in patients with small St. Jude medical mechanical prostheses in the aortic position. Circulation 113:420–426

59. Bleizifer S, Eichinger WB, Hettich I, et al. (2007) Impact of prosthesis-patient mismatch on exercise capacity in patients after bioprosthetic aortic valve replacement. Heart 94:637–641

60. Magne J, Mathieu P, Dumesnil JG, et al (2007) Impact of prosthesis-patient mismatch on survival after mitral valve replacement. Circulation 115:1417–1425

61. Wu WC, Ireland LA, Sadaniantz A (2004) Evaluation of aortic valve disorders using stress echocardiography. Echocardiography 21:459–466

62. Pibarot P, Dumesnil JG, Jobin J, et al (1999) Hemodynamic and physical performance during maximal exercise in patients with an aortic bioprosthetic valve: comparison of stentless versus stented bioprostheses. J Am Coll Cardiol 34:1609–1617

63. Pibarot P, Dumesnil JG, Jobin J, et al (1999) Usefulness of the indexed effective orifice area at rest in predicting an increase in gradient during maximum exercise in patients with a bioprosthesis in the aortic valve position. Am J Cardiol 83:542–546

64. Pibarot P, Dumesnil JG (2000) Hemodynamic and clinical impact of prosthesis-patient mismatch in the aortic valve position and its prevention. J Am Coll Cardiol 36:1131–1141

65. De Carlo M, Milano AD, Musumeci G, et al (1999) Cardiopulmonary exercise testing in patients with 21 mm St. Jude medical aortic prosthesis. J Heart Valve Dis 8:522–529

66. Tatineni S, Barner HB, Pearson AC, et al (1989) Rest and exercise evaluation of St. Jude Medical and Medtronic Hall prostheses: influence of primary lesion, valvular type, valvular size, and left ventricular function. Circulation 80(suppl I):I-16–I-23

67. van den Brink RB, Verheul HA, Visser CA, Koelemay MJ, Dunning AJ (1992) Value of exercise Doppler echocardiography in patients with prosthetic or bioprosthetic cardiac valves. Am J Cardiol 69:367–372

68. Dressler F, Labovitz A (1992) Exercise evaluation of prosthetic heart valves by Doppler echocardiography: comparison with catheterization studies. Echocardiogr 9:235–241

69. Wiseth R, Levang O, Tangen G, Rein KA, Skjaerpe T (1993) Exercise hemodynamics in small (<21-mm) aortic valve prostheses assessed by Doppler echocardiography. Am Heart J 15:138–146

70. Shigenobu M, Sano S (1995) Evaluation of St. Jude Medical mitral valve function by exercise Doppler echocardiography. J Card Surg 10:161–168

71. Becassis P, Hayot M, Frapier J-M, et al (2000) Postoperative exercise tolerance after aortic valve replacement by small-size prosthesis. J Am Coll Cardiol 36:871–877

72. Minardi G, Manzara C, Creazzo V, et al (2006) Evaluation of 17-mm St. Jude Medical Regent prosthetic aortic heart valves by rest and dobutamine stress echocardiography. J Cardiothorac Surg 1:27

73. Hobson NA, Wilkinson GA, Cooper GH, Wheeldon NM, Lynch J (2006) Hemodynamic assessment of mitral mechanical prostheses under high flow conditions: comparison between dynamic exercise and dobutamine stress. J Heart Valve Dis 15:87–91

74. Magne J, Sénéchal M, Mathieu P, Dumesnil JG, Dagenais F, Pibarot P (2008) Restrictive annuloplasty for ischemic mitral regurgitation may induce functional mitral stenosis. J Am Coll Cardiol 51(17):1692–1701

75. Patsilinakos SP, Kranidis AI, Antonelis IP, et al (1999) Detection of coronary artery disease in patients with severe aortic stenosis with noninvasive methods. Angiology 50:309–317

76. Picano E, Pálinkás A, Amyot R (2001) Diagnosis of myocardial ischemia in hypertensive patients. J Hypertens 19:1177–1183

77. Marcus ML, Doty DB, Hiratzka LF, Wright CB, Eastham CL (1982) Decreased coronary reserve: a mechanism for angina pectoris in patients with aortic stenosis and normal coronary arteries. N Engl J Med 307:1362–1366

78. Rajappan K, Rimoldi OE, Dutka DP, et al (2002) Mechanisms of coronary microcirculatory dysfunction in patients with aortic stenosis and angiographically normal coronary arteries. Circulation 105:470–476

79. Rajappan K, Rimoldi OE, Camici PG, et al (2003) Functional changes in coronary microcirculation after valve replacement in patients with aortic stenosis. Circulation 107:3170–3175

80. Bakhtiary F, Schiemann M, Dzemali O, et al (2007) Impact of patient-prosthesis mismatch and aortic valve design on coronary flow reserve after aortic valve replacement. J Am Coll Cardiol 49:790–796

81. Nagel E, Klein C, Paetsch I, et al (2003) Magnetic resonance perfusion measurements for the noninvasive detection of coronary disease. Circulation 108:432–437

82. Lee DC, Simonetti OP, Harris KR, et al (2004) Magnetic resonance versus radionuclide pharmacological stress perfusion imaging for flow-limiting stenoses of varying severity. Circulation 110:58–65

83. Rigo F, Richieri M, Pasanisi E, et al (2003) Usefulness of coronary flow reserve over regional wall motion when added to dual-imaging dipyridamole echocardiography. Am J Cardiol 91:269–273

84. Hildick-Smith DJ, Shapiro LM (2000) Coronary flow reserve improves after aortic valve replacement for aortic stenosis: an adenosine transthoracic echocardiography study. J Am Coll Cardiol 36:1889–1896

85. Rigo F (2005) Coronary flow reserve in stress-echo lab: from pathophysiologic toy to diagnostic tool. Cardiovasc Ultrasound 3:8

86. Picano E (2004) Sustainability of medical imaging: education and debate. BMJ 328:578–580

Stress Echocardiography in Children

37

Eugenio Picano and Michael Henein

The rationale for applying stress echocardiography in children is not different from application of the technique in adults [1]. Sick children may need cardiac stress imaging, and stress echocardiography is becoming more common in the pediatric population [2]. Obviously, to perform these procedures in the most adequate way, proper training of personnel and staffing of the pediatric stress laboratory are required to ensure the safety of patients and that the desired testing information is obtained. For these reasons, and as recommended by a recent 2006 statement of the American Heart Association (AHA), pediatric testing should remain an integral part of pediatric cardiology training [3]. A focused competence for the pediatric population should ideally be an integral part of the high-volume stress echocardiography laboratory. Diagnostic questions raised by children are extremely variable, and require a versatile approach of highly trained personnel. In our experience, pediatric stress echocardiography is performed in teamwork – between an adult cardiologist trained in stress echocardiography with a pediatric cardiologist directly involved in the treatment of the patient. Together, the two cardiologists discuss the indications, perform the examination, and use the results in light of the clinical context (Table 37.1). In this way, inappropriateness is minimized and the diagnostic yield is optimized.

37.1
Pediatric Coronary Artery Disease

There are several patient populations for whom stress echocardiography can be used to detect ischemia-producing coronary artery stenosis in children. Kawasaki disease (KD) is an acute self-limited vasculitis of childhood that is characterized by fever, bilateral non-exudative conjunctivitis, erythema of the lips and oral mucosa, changes in the extremities, rash, and cervical lymphoadenopathy. Advances in clinical therapies (with intravenous immune globulin and aspirin) have reduced, but not eliminated, the incidence of coronary artery abnormalities in affected children. Today, KD is the most common cause of acquired cardiovascular disease in children in the USA. Coronary artery aneurysms or ectasia develop in 20% of untreated children and may lead to ischemic heart disease or sudden

E. Picano, *Stress Echocardiography*,
© Springer-Verlag Berlin Heidelberg 2009

37

Table 37.1 Application of pediatric stress echocardiography

	Target	Method	Stress	Disease
CAD detection	Regional wall motion abnormalities	2D	Ex (dob, dip)	Kawasaki, transplant CAD, Arterial switch
Valve stenosis	Transvalvular gradients	CW Doppler	Ex (dob)	Native aortic stenosis, native pulmonary stenosis, Prosthetic valves
Pulmonary hemodynamics	PASP	CW Doppler (TR jet)	Ex (dob)	Right ventricular overload
Contractile reserve	Normal base-line function, depressed baseline function	2D	Ex (dob)	Thalassemia
Coronary flow reserve	Coronary macro- and microcirculation	Pulsed Doppler CFR	Dip, ado, cold	Kawasaki, switch, right and left ventricular overload

CAD coronary artery disease, *Ex* exercise, *dob* dobutamine, *dip* dipyridamole, *CW* continuous wave, *PASP* pulmonary artery systolic pressure, *TR* tricuspid regurgitation, *CFR* coronary flow reserve

death [4]. According to 2004 AHA guidelines on KD, cardiac stress testing for reversible ischemia is indicated to assess the existence and functional consequences of coronary artery abnormalities in children with KD and coronary aneurysms (evidence level A). Whichever the chosen stress, diagnostic accuracy for identifying angiographically assessed coronary artery disease is high and comparable, with stress-induced wall motion abnormalities representing a highly specific, and sensitive, marker of coronary artery involvement. More than 100 cases have been published to date with exercise or pharmacological echocardiography, with excellent overall diagnostic accuracy [5–8], comparable to stress scintigraphy. Guidelines conclude that "*the choice of stress modality should be guided by institutional expertise with particular techniques, as well as by the age of the child (e.g., pharmacological stress should be used in young children in whom traditional exercise protocols are not feasible*" [4]. The acute diagnostic benefit is similar between these techniques, but the long-term risk is disproportionately high with ionizing techniques. Therefore, the use of methods such as myocardial scintigraphy [9], computed tomography [10], and systematic coronary angiography [11] should be drastically minimized in these patients [12, 13].

A national survey in Japan on the pediatric cardiologist's clinical approach for patients with KD showed that for high-risk patients, as early as in 2002, more responders favored stress echocardiography when compared with nuclear imaging. For high-risk levels, 60% of pediatric cardiologists perform coronary angiography not on a regular basis but only when coronary symptoms are present or when stress imaging suggests myocardial ischemia [14].

Clearly, more data are needed in this field, but stress echocardiography based on visual assessment of regional wall motion abnormalities will play a key role in surveillance and management of patients with coronary artery residua. To date, alternative echocardiographic approaches based on other, more quantitative markers of ischemia, are available. These include longitudinal function assessment with mitral annulus plane systolic excursion [15], cyclic backscatter variation with tissue characterization techniques [16], and perfusion changes with myocardial contrast echocardiography [17]. Each of these markers has an interesting rationale. Long-axis function can detect minor forms of ischemia, unable to affect radial function and regional systolic thickening, since longitudinal fibers run in the subendocardial layer, thus abnormalities accurately reflect subendocardial ischemic dysfunction. Longitudinal function can be impaired when radial motion is normal or even supernormal [15]. Cyclic backscatter variation is proportional to intramural contractility, and higher in the subendocardium than in the subepicardium, mirroring the well-known intramural contractility gradient. Therefore, minor forms of subendocardial hypoperfusion may impair subendocardial function and blunt cyclic backscatter variation without a detectable impairment in regional systolic thickening [16]. Finally, myocardial contrast echocardiography evaluates myocardial perfusion heterogeneity, which is more sensitive (albeit less specific) than regional wall motion abnormalities as a marker of myocardial ischemia [17]. None of these markers should be exclusively considered for clinically driven applications due to inadequate validation to date. At present, it appears reasonable to propose a very simple diagnostic algorithm in these patients, who must be screened with resting transthoracic echocardiography to detect coronary artery morphological anomalies, which are the cornerstone of diagnosis and risk stratification (from class I, low risk, to V, high risk). A positive stress echocardiography finding is frequently found in the high-risk class, therefore, it appears appropriate to use it in class V patients [8] (Fig. 37.1).

37.2
Transplant Coronary Artery Disease

The leading cause of death after the first year of cardiac transplant is transplant coronary artery disease, occurring in up to 43% of patients at 3 years following transplant [18]. This form of coronary disease, also known as graft coronary disease, differs from classical atherosclerosis in both histologic and angiographic features and it progresses much more rapidly. Because the disease is diffuse and usually involves small vessels it makes coronary arteriography an unreliable diagnostic technique — a matter that turned physicians to other modalities, such as stress echocardiography. A total of five dobutamine echocardiographic studies, including over 100 patients, showed excellent diagnostic value [19–21] and prognostic capability, since patients with positive test results had a sixfold higher risk of subsequent cardiac events [22, 23].

37

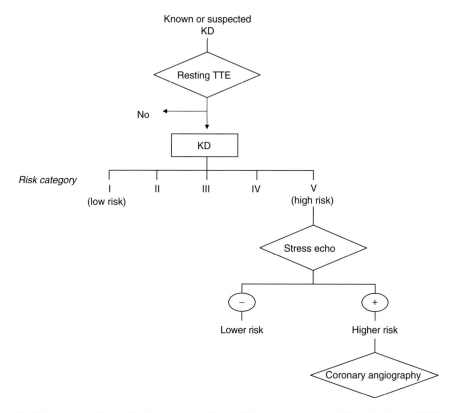

Fig. 37.1 A proposed algorithm in a young patient with known or suspected Kawasaki disease (*KD*). Resting transthoracic echocardiography is essential for the diagnosis and for risk assessment. In patients with high-risk class (AHA grade V), stress echocardiography is warranted. Patients with a positive response belong to a higher risk group warranting further investigation with coronary angiography with the perspective of an ischemia-driven revascularization

37.3
Transposition of Great Arteries After Surgical Repair

The long-term problems that are associated with repaired transposition of the great arteries depend on the type of repair. The oldest patients have intraatrial repair, either Mustard or Senning type, in which venous return is directed to the contralateral left ventricle by means of an atrial baffle. As a consequence, the right ventricle supports the systemic circulation. Relatively young patients undergo an arterial switch operation, to allow the left ventricle to function as the systemic pump through removal of the Mustard/Senning atrial baffles and reconstructing of an atrial septum in patients with complete transposition [24].

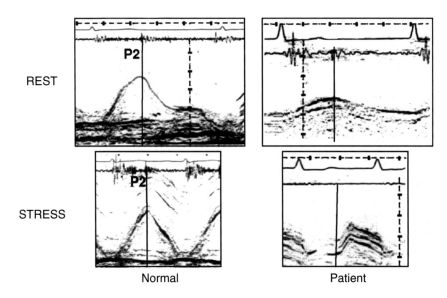

Fig. 37.2 Right ventricular free wall *M*-mode at rest (*top*) and stress (*bottom*) from a normal control and a patient after Mustard repair showing stress-induced incoordination of the patient (*right*) suggesting underlying ischemia. (Modified from [25])

In patients with Mustard or Senning repair, right ventricular dysfunction and pulmonary hypertension are a possible complication. Patients with exertional symptoms, angina-like chest discomfort, or breathlessness could be physiologically assessed by stress echocardiography. There is a close relationship between right ventricular function in these patients and exercise tolerance assessed by cardiopulmonary exercise testing. Furthermore, in these patients, the right ventricular function becomes very abnormal at fast heart rate, demonstrating disturbances similar to those seen in patients with coronary artery disease, suggesting a possible underlying ischemic dysfunction [25]. These findings are consistent with those found in dilated cardiomyopathy (Fig. 37.2).

The arterial switch operation, which includes coronary artery transfer, is the surgical procedure of choice for transposition of the great arteries. Mortality and clinical long-term outcome largely depend on adequate perfusion through the transferred coronary arteries. Late deaths can be related to coronary occlusion, and intravascular ultrasound assessment late after arterial switch operation revealed proximal eccentric intimal thickening in most coronary arteries, suggesting the development of early atherosclerosis in reimplanted coronary arteries [26]. These patients tend to have a consistently reduced coronary flow reserve [27]. Only anecdotal reports present in the literature on a total of 34 patients from two studies – one with dobutamine [28], the other with transesophageal atrial pacing [29] – suggest that a stress-induced regional wall motion abnormality or reduced left ventricular long-axis function portends a negative prognosis.

37.4
Valve and Intraventricular Gradients

Several studies have been performed in native stenotic aortic, pulmonary, and prosthetic valves during high-flow states to unmask an abnormally high increase in gradients. In fact, the transvalvular gradient increases with increasing flow rates, the higher the transvalvular flow, the higher the pressure gradient. A moderately and a severely diseased native valve, and a normal or abnormally functioning prosthesis, may display similar gradients at rest, but the marked rise in mean gradients during stress in the latter is to be distinguished from the fairly flat gradient response of the moderately diseased native or normally functioning prosthetic valves. The rationale of this application is very strong, but systematic data, especially in children, are still conspicuously lacking to date [30]. A similar application evaluates the development of intracardiac gradients in young athletes or patients with hypertrophic cardiomyopathies, in whom dobutamine or exercise can unmask an intraventricular obstruction unapparent at rest and which may have prognostic and therapeutic implications [31].

37.5
Contractile Reserve

Patients with normal ejection fraction at rest can indeed have subtle alteration in left ventricular function. This initial impairment can be detected as a reduction in long-axis function detected by mitral annular plane systolic excursion or tissue Doppler imaging, both in experimental models [32] and in patients [33]. Alternatively, an initial myocardial damage can be detected as a blunted contractile response to an inotropic stress, such as dobutamine or exercise. This pattern has been described in anthracycline-treated long-term survivors of childhood cancer [34–37] or in thalassemic patients at an early stage of disease [38]. At a more advanced stage, left ventricular function can be depressed and the inotropic challenge can restore a normal function in patients who will have less perioperative risk in the case of intervention and better natural history if left on medical therapy [4] (Fig. 37.3).

The assessment of contractile reserve of the right ventricle is of great importance [25]. In patients with Mustard repair for transposition of the great arteries or repaired tetralogy of Fallot [39], impaired exercise tolerance can be predicted by right ventricular long-axis function at baseline and during stress. The lower the contractile reserve of the right ventricle, the lower the exercise capability and the right ventricular stroke volume. Longitudinal function can be assessed by simple long-axis amplitude of motion (from TAPSE for right and MAPSE for left ventricle, 25), or from peak systolic velocity of basal left ventricular segments by tissue Doppler imaging [39]. In patients with repaired tetralogy of Fallot, exercise stress echocardiography unmasks a substantial heterogeneity in right ventricular contractile reserve, pulmonary artery systolic pressure, and right ventricular volume (Fig. 37.4). Those patients with reduced right ventricular contractile reserve also have lower exercise tolerance, higher cardiac peptides plasma levels, and more dilated right ventricle with cardiovascular magnetic resonance [40].

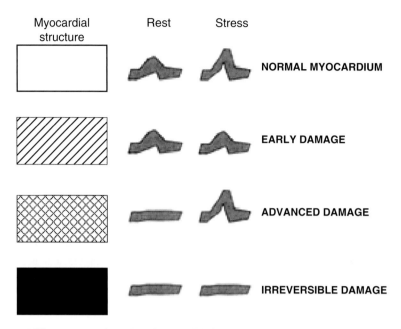

Fig. 37.3 Different stages of severity of myocardial damage in cardiomyopathy, due to, for instance, thalassemia or cardiotoxic chemotherapy

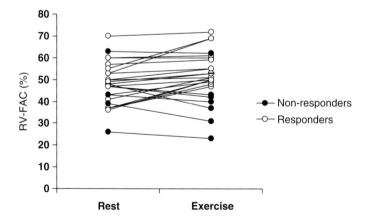

Fig. 37.4 Exercise stress echocardiography results in grown-up congenital heart disease patients with repaired tetralogy of Fallot. There is an obvious heterogeneity in right ventricular fractional area change during exercise. Patients with depressed right ventricular contractile reserve (nonresponders) also show higher BNP values and lower exercise tolerance. BNP, brain natriuretic peptides. (By courtesy of G. Festa et al. [39])

37.6
Coronary Flow Reserve

Coronary flow reserve can be reduced in children with congenital heart disease as a consequence of epicardial coronary artery anomalies due to primary coronary microcirculatory damage or ventricular hypertrophy [41]. Pulsed Doppler transthoracic echocardiography is ideally suited for assessing coronary flow reserve in these patients, both in the mid-distal left anterior descending coronary artery (with >90% feasibility) and in the right coronary posterior descending arteries (with >70% feasibility). High-frequency transducers with second harmonic technology greatly enhance the success rate of the technique in expert hands, often not requiring contrast injection. The employed stressor is usually adenosine or dipyridamole, but the cold pressor test has also been fruitfully proposed in children. The normal increase in coronary flow reserve is about 250% following adenosine (or dipyridamole, which accumulates endogenous adenosine) and about 200% after cold, which mainly acts through a hemodynamically mediated increase in heart rate and blood pressure [42]. Coronary flow reserve could be impaired – even in the absence of anatomic epicardial coronary artery disease – in children 5–8 years after the switch operation, which is mirrored by reduced vasodilation following nitrates, an endothelium-independent vasodilator stimulus [27]. In KD, the impairment in coronary flow reserve is largely independent of epicardial coronary artery lesions and aneurysms, again suggesting primary coronary microcirculation impairment [43]. The reduction of coronary flow reserve can be either diffuse or branch-specific [43–49]. The impairment of coronary flow reserve is an integrated index of epicardial vessel status, myocardial hypertrophy, and coronary microcirculation structural and functional conditions [47, 48]: Fig. 37.5. In adults, the reduction in coronary flow reserve has a clinically relevant prognostic value, above and beyond regional wall motion [49, 50]. Whether this is true also for children remains to be established in future studies.

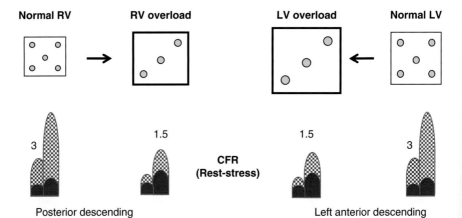

Fig. 37.5 The coronary flow reserve (*CFR*) pattern, as can be visualized by transthoracic vasodilator stress echocardiography, in patients with left ventricular (*right panel*) or right ventricular (*left panel*) overload

37.7
Conclusions

Stress echocardiography should be considered an extension of traditional resting cardiac assessment. The need and value of understanding myocardial function, valvular physiology, and pulmonary hemodynamics in children during stress will promote a growth of this specific field, especially in view of the increasing radiological exposure of children with congenital heart disease from aggressive use of computed tomography and scintigraphy [51–53] (Table 37.2). At the age of 15–20 years, grown-up congenital heart (GUCH) disease patients have already cumulated a dose exposure corresponding to 2,000 chest X-rays [54], with an estimated lifetime extra-risk of cancer of 1 in 10 to 1 in 100, and with a measured 200% increase in micronuclei and chromosome aberrations in circulating lymphocytes [55]. These data are worrying, but not surprising, since it is well known that the radiation damage for any given dose is three- to fourfold higher in children than in adults [56–58]. In spite of this, 30% of stress imaging in children is still done with perfusion imaging [3], which gives a radiation exposure of 500–1,700 chest X-rays (with a risk of cancer greater than 1 in 100 for a 1-year-old girl). This inconvenient situation is perpetuated by the lack of information of specialty guidelines – not even mentioning radiation dose and risk – and by the current very suboptimal awareness of doses and risks by patients [59, 60], pediatricians [59], cardiologists [61], and radiologists [62]. Notwithstanding this escalating radiation exposure, there has been remarkably little public discussion of the need for fundamental changes in our current imaging practice in adults and especially in children [3, 4]. Although we can debate the multiple reasons for this silence, there is no question that with the restoration of radiological awareness, stress echocardiography will become the technique of choice, even more than in adults (Table 37.3), and – when used in tandem with magnetic resonance – will help heart patients to achieve the benefits of the highest diagnostic standards without the long-term oncogenic risks of radiation exposure [63]. This

Table 37.2 Exposure and risks of imaging techniques in children younger than 1 year

	Dose (mSv)	Dose equivalent (chest X-rays)	Cancer risk
64-slice MSCT (with ECG modulation)	15	750	~1 in 100
64-slice MSCT (without ECG modulation)	29	1,450	~1 in 50
Cardiac stress scintigraphy (201-Thallium)	27	1,350	~1 in 50
Cardiac stress scintigraphy (99 m sestamibi)	10	500	~1 in 200
Coronary angiography	5	250	~1 in 500
Cardiovascular magnetic resonance	0	0	0
Echocardiography	0	0	0

MSCT multislice computed tomography

Table 37.3 Stress echocardiography in children vs. adults

	Adults	Children
Stress	Exercise>Pharmacologic	Pharmacologic>Exercise
Evidence available	Established	Initial
Safety concerns	+	+++
Vulnerability to radiation damage	+	++++
Use of cardiac scintigraphy	Declining	Disappearing
Complementary technique	CMR	CMR

CMR cardiovascular magnetic resonance

is important in all patients [64], and should be our dominant thought in planning diagnostic strategies in children.

References

1. Picano E (1992) Stress echocardiography. From pathophysiological toy to diagnostic tool. Point of view. Circulation 85:1604–1612
2. Kimball TR (2002) Pediatric stress echocardiography. Pediatr Cardiol 23:347–357
3. Paridon SM, Alpert BS, Boas SR, et al; American Heart Association Council on Cardiovascular Disease in the Young, Committee on Atherosclerosis, Hypertension, and Obesity in Youth. (2006) Clinical stress testing in the pediatric age group: a statement from the American Heart Association Council on Cardiovascular Disease in the Young, Committee on Atherosclerosis, Hypertension, and Obesity in Youth. Circulation 113:1905–1920
4. Newburger JW, Takahashi M, Gerber MA, et al; Committee on Rheumatic Fever, Endocarditis, and Kawasaki Disease, Council on Cardiovascular Disease in the Young, American Heart Association (2004) Diagnosis, treatment, and long-term management of Kawasaki disease: a statement for health professionals from the Committee on Rheumatic Fever, Endocarditis, and Kawasaki Disease, Council on Cardiovascular Disease in the Young, American Heart Association. Pediatrics 114:1708–1733
5. Pahl E, Sehgal R, Chrystof D, et al (1995) Feasibility of exercise stress echocardiography for the follow-up of children with coronary involvement secondary to Kawasaki disease. Circulation 91:122–128
6. Noto N, Ayusawa M, Karasawa K, et al (1996) Dobutamine stress echocardiography for detection of coronary artery stenosis in children with Kawasaki disease. J Am Coll Cardiol 27:1251–1256
7. Kimball TR, Witt SA, Daniels SR (1997) Dobutamine stress echocardiography in the assessment of suspected myocardial ischemia in children and young adults. Am J Cardiol 79:380–384
8. Zilberman MV, Goya G, Witt SA, et al (2003) Dobutamine stress echocardiography in the evaluation of young patients with Kawasaki disease. Pediatr Cardiol 24:338–343
9. Lim CW, Ho KT, Quek SC. (2006) Exercise myocardial perfusion stress testing in children with Kawasaki disease. J Paediatr Child Health 42:419–422
10. Chu WC, Mok GC, Lam WW, et al (2006) Assessment of coronary artery aneurysms in paediatric patients with Kawasaki disease by multidetector row CT angiography: feasibility and comparison with 2D echocardiography. Pediatr Radiol 36:1148–1153

11. Ogawa S, Ohkubo T, Fukazawa R, et al (2004) Estimation of myocardial hemodynamics before and after intervention in children with Kawasaki disease. J Am Coll Cardiol 43:653

12. Kleinerman RA (2006) Cancer risks following diagnostic and therapeutic radiation exposure in children. Pediatr Radiol 36:121–125

13. Ait-Ali L, Foffa I, Andreassi MG (2007) Diagnostic and therapeutic radiation exposure in children: new evidence and perspectives from a biomarker approach. Pediatr Radiol. 37:109–111

14. Kahwaji IY, Connuck DM, Tafari N, et al (2002) A national survey on the pediatric cardiologist's clinical approach for patients with Kawasaki disease. Pediatr Cardiol 23:639–646

15. Henein MY, Dinarevic S, O'Sullivan CA, et al (1998) Exercise echocardiography in children with Kawasaki disease: ventricular long axis is selectively abnormal. Am J Cardiol 81:1356–1359

16. Yu X, Hashimoto I, Ichida F, et al (2001) Dipyridamole stress ultrasonic myocardial tissue characterization in patients with Kawasaki disease. J Am Soc Echocardiogr 14:682–690

17. Ishii M, Himeno W, Sawa M, et al (2002) Assessment of the ability of myocardial contrast echocardiography with harmonic power Doppler imaging to identify perfusion abnormalities in patients with Kawasaki disease at rest and during dipyridamole stress. Pediatr Cardiol 23:192–199

18. Pahl E (2000) Transplant coronary artery disease in children. Prog Pediatr Cardiol 11:137–143

19. Lewis JF, Selman SB, Murphy JD, et al (1997) Dobutamine echocardiography for prediction of ischemic events in heart transplant recipients. J Heart Lung Transplant 16:390–393

20. Larsen RL, Applegate PM, Dyar DA, et al (1998) Dobutamine stress echocardiography for assessing coronary artery disease after transplantation in children. J Am Coll Cardiol 32:515–520

21. Pahl E, Crawford SE, Swenson JM (1999) Dobutamine stress echocardiography: experience in pediatric heart transplant recipients. J Heart Lung Transplant 18:725–732

22. Donofrio MT, Kakavand B, Moskowitz WB (2000) Evaluation of regional wall motion and quantitative measures of ventricular function during dobutamine stress echocardiography in pediatric cardiac transplantation patients. J Am Soc Echocardiogr 13:932–940

23. Di Filippo S, Semiond B, Roriz R, et al (2003) Non-invasive detection of coronary artery disease by dobutamine-stress echocardiography in children after heart transplantation. J Heart Lung Transplant 22:876–882

24. Li W, Henein M, Gatzoulis M (2008) Echocardiography in adult congenital heart disease. Springer, Heidelberg

25. Li W, Hornung TS, Francis DP, et al (2004) Relation of biventricular function quantified by stress echocardiography to cardiopulmonary exercise capacity in adults with Mustard (atrial switch) procedure for transposition of the great arteries. Circulation 110:1380–1386

26. Pedra SR, Pedra CA, Abizaid AA, et al (2005) Intracoronary ultrasound assessment late after the arterial switch operation for transposition of the great arteries. J Am Coll Cardiol 45:2061–2068

27. Hauser M, Bengel FM, Kühn A, et al (2001) Myocardial blood flow and flow reserve after coronary reimplantation in patients after arterial switch and Ross operation. Circulation 103:1875–1880

28. Hui L, Chau AK, Leung MP, et al (2005) Assessment of left ventricular function long term after arterial switch operation for transposition of the great arteries by dobutamine stress echocardiography. Heart 91:68–72

29. De Caro E, Ussia GP, Marasini M, et al (2003) Transoesophageal atrial pacing combined with transthoracic two dimensional echocardiography: experience in patients operated on with arterial switch operation for transposition of the great arteries. Heart 89:91–95

30. Decena BF III, Tischler MD (1999) Stress echocardiography in valvular heart disease. Cardiol Clin 17:555–572, ix

31. Cotrim C, Almeida AG, Carrageta M (2007) Clinical significance of intraventricular gradient during effort in an adolescent karate player. Cardiovasc Ultrasound 5:39

32. Hartmann J, Knebel F, Eddicks S, et al (2007) Noninvasive monitoring of myocardial function after surgical and cytostatic therapy in a peritoneal metastasis rat model: assessment with tissue Doppler and non-Doppler 2D strain echocardiography. Cardiovasc Ultrasound 5:23

33. Mercuro G, Cadeddu C, Piras A, et al (2007) Early epirubicin-induced myocardial dysfunction revealed by serial tissue Doppler echocardiography: correlation with inflammatory and oxidative stress markers. Oncologist 12:1124–1133

34. De Wolf D, Suys B, Maurus R, et al (1996) Dobutamine stress echocardiography in the evaluation of late anthracycline cardiotoxicity in childhood cancer survivors. Pediatr Res 39:504–512

35. Klewer SE, Goldberg SJ, Donnerstein RL, et al (1992) Dobutamine stress echocardiography: a sensitive indicator of diminished myocardial function in asymptomatic doxorubicin-treated long-term survivors of childhood cancer. J Am Coll Cardiol 19:394–401

36. Lanzarini L, Bossi G, Laudisa ML, et al (2000) Lack of clinically significant cardiac dysfunction during intermediate dobutamine doses in long-term childhood cancer survivors exposed to anthracyclines. Am Heart J 140:315–323

37. De Souza AM, Potts JE, Potts MT, et al (2007) A stress echocardiography study of cardiac function during progressive exercise in pediatric oncology patients treated with anthracyclines. Pediatr Blood Cancer 49:56–64

38. Mariotti E, Agostini A, Angelucci E, et al (1996) Reduced left ventricular contractile reserve identified by low dose dobutamine echocardiography as an early marker of cardiac involvement in asymptomatic patients with thalassemia major. Echocardiography 13:463–472

39. Apostolopoulou SC, Laskari CV, Tsoutsinos A, et al (2007) Doppler tissue imaging evaluation of right ventricular function at rest and during dobutamine infusion in patients after repair of tetralogy of Fallot. Int J Cardiovasc Imaging 23:25–31

40. Ait-ali L, Festa G, Gerbasi E, et al (2008) Semisupine exercise Doppler stress echocardiography in operated Fallot. Eur J Echocardiography (Abstract Supp)

41. Oskarsson G (2004) Coronary flow and flow reserve in children. Acta Paediatr Suppl 93:20–25

42. Noto N, Karasawa K, Ayusawa M, et al (1997) Measurement of coronary flow reserve in children by transthoracic Doppler echocardiography. Am J Cardiol 80:1638–1639

43. Cicala S, Galderisi M, Grieco M, et al (2007) Transthoracic Echo-Doppler Assessment of Coronary Microvascular Function Late after Kawasaki Disease. Pediatr Cardiol 29:321–327

44. Shimada S, Harada K, Toyono M, et al (2007) Using transthoracic Doppler echocardiography to diagnose reduced coronary flow velocity reserve in the posterior descending coronary artery in children with elevated right ventricular pressure. Circ J 71:1912–1917

45. Harada K, Yasuoka K, Tamura M, et al (2002) Coronary flow reserve assessment by Doppler echocardiography in children with and without congenital heart defect: comparison with invasive technique. J Am Soc Echocardiogr 15:1121–1126

46. Hiraishi S, Hirota H, Horiguchi Y, et al (2002) Transthoracic Doppler assessment of coronary flow velocity reserve in children with Kawasaki disease: comparison with coronary angiography and thallium-201 imaging. J Am Coll Cardiol 40:1816–1824

47. Oskarsson G, Pesonen E (2002) Flow dynamics in the left anterior descending coronary artery in infants with idiopathic dilated cardiomyopathy. Am J Cardiol 90:557–561

48. Doty DB, Wright CB, Hiratzka LF, et al (1984) Coronary reserve in volume-induced right ventricular hypertrophy from atrial septal defect. Am J Cardiol 54:1059–1063

49. Cortigiani L, Rigo F, Gherardi S, et al (2007) Additional prognostic value of coronary flow reserve in diabetic and nondiabetic patients with negative dipyridamole stress echocardiography by wall motion criteria. Am Coll Cardiol 50:1354–1361

50. Rigo F, Sicari R, Gherardi S, et al (2008) The additive prognostic value of wall motion abnormalities and coronary flow reserve during dipyridamole stress echo. Eur Heart J 29:79–88

51. Picano E (2004) Sustainability of medical imaging. Education and Debate. BMJ 328:578–580

52. Brenner DJ, Hall EJ (2007) Computed tomography–an increasing source of radiation exposure. N Engl J Med 357:2277–2284
53. Amis ES Jr, Butler PF, Applegate KE, et al; American College of Radiology. (2007) American College of Radiology white paper on radiation dose in medicine. J Am Coll Radiol 4:272–284
54. Ait-Ali L, Bedetti G, Botto N, et al (2007) Cumulative radiation doses from medical testing in grown-up patients with congenital heart disease. Eur Heart J (Abstract Suppl)
55. Andreassi MG, Ait-Ali L, Botto N, et al (2006) Cardiac catheterization and long-term chromosomal damage in children with congenital heart disease. Eur Heart J 27:2703–2708
56. Committee to Assess Health Risks from Exposure to Low Levels of Ionizing Radiation; Nuclear and Radiation Studies Board, Division on Earth and Life Studies, National Research Council of the National Academies (2006) Health Risks From Exposure to Low Levels of Ionizing Radiation: BEIR VII Phase 2. The National Academies Press, Washington, DC
57. ICRP (2007) The 2007 Recommendations of the international commission on radiological protection. Ann ICRP 37:1–332
58. FDA Warning (2001) Center for Devices and Radiological Health. Public health notification: reducing radiation risk from computed tomography for pediatric and small adult patients (2 Nov 2001). Available at: www.fda.gov/cdrh/safety.html (accessed July 28, 2006)
59. Thomas KE, Parnell-Parmley JE, Haidar S, et al. (2006) Assessment of radiation dose awareness among pediatricians. Pediatr Radiol. 2006 May 13
60. Bedetti G, Pizzi C, Gavaruzzi G, et al (2008) Sub-optimal awareness of radiological dose among patients undergoing cardiac stress scintigraphy. J Am Coll Radiol 5:126–131
61. Correia MJ, Hellies A, Andreassi MG, et al (2005) Lack of radiological awareness among physicians working in a tertiary-care cardiological centre. Int J Cardiol 105:307–311
62. Lee CI, Haims AH, Monico EP, et al (2004) Diagnostic CT scans: assessment of patient, physician, and radiologist awareness of radiation dose and possible risks. Radiology 231:393–398
63. Picano E (2003) Stress echocardiography: a historical perspective. Special Article. Am J Med 114:126–130
64. Picano E (2004) Informed consent and communication of risk from radiological and nuclear medicine examinations: how to escape from a communication inferno. Education and debate. BMJ 329:849–853

Section 5

Comparison with Other Imaging Techniques

Stress Echocardiography Versus Stress Perfusion Scintigraphy

38

Thomas H. Marwick and Eugenio Picano

38.1
Nuclear Cardiology, the Land of Our Fathers

Nuclear cardiology is the time-honored offspring of the marriage between nuclear technology and coronary physiology [1]. Several imaging paradigms later endorsed by stress echocardiography were first understood, proposed, and popularized by nuclear cardiology: the merit of imaging cardiac function during stress, in lieu of the simple electrocardiogram; the value of the pharmacological alternative to physical exercise for stressing the heart; the need to assess viability in segments with resting dysfunction; the advantage of routine use of digital handling for data acquisition, storage, and display; and the prognostic impact of extent and severity of stress-induced ischemia [2]. Although the comparison of nuclear cardiology and echocardiography previously involved a fundamental philosophical issue between the diagnosis of coronary disease based on perfusion (hence the possibility of influencing these data on the basis of small-vessel disease, hypertrophy, and other causes of abnormal coronary flow reserve) and evidence of ischemia (hence less sensitivity to mild disease that may engender submaximal attainment of flow without ischemia), recent advances have made it possible for both techniques to offer function and coronary flow reserve data [3]. Each technique is experiencing a "methodological drift" to incorporate information previously monopolized by the other – thus, gated single-photon emission computed tomography (SPECT), ventriculography, and attenuation correction have been added to SPECT, while harmonic imaging, pulsed Doppler coronary flow velocity imaging, myocardial contrast, and real-time three-dimensional (3D) imaging have been added to echocardiography. The benefits of these technical advances may render current comparisons somewhat obsolete.

38.2
SPECT, PET, and PET–CT Imaging: Advantages and Limitations

SPECT imaging in combination with 201 thallium or 99mTc-tracers is a powerful technique for the detection of perfusion abnormalities during hyperemia induced by pharmacological

E. Picano, *Stress Echocardiography*,
© Springer-Verlag Berlin Heidelberg 2009

or physical stress and it also allows assessment of viability [4]. The mechanism of this test – based on the detection of relative hyperemia – is a fundamental distinction from stress echocardiography, which is dependent on the induction of ischemia in a functional and metabolic sense. Hyperemia may be induced directly (by coronary vasodilators) or indirectly (whereby endogenous vasodilators are produced in response to exercise or dobutamine). The presence of preexisting coronary vasodilation induced by antianginal therapy, or limitation of the vasodilator response due to drug therapy or submaximal exercise, may blunt the difference between rest and stress, impairing the detection of less severe stenoses and contributing to lower sensitivity [5]. Nonetheless, antianginal drug therapy has a greater effect on the results of echocardiography [6, 7] because it prevents the development of ischemia.

Advantages

SPECT and positron emission tomography (PET) have a high technical success rate and are relatively operator-independent. SPECT has excellent sensitivity (usually 85–90%) and good-to-moderate specificity (70–80%) for the detection of angiographically assessed coronary artery disease. The accuracy of PET is probably greater, especially in the posterior circulation and in obese subjects, where the inherent attenuation correction of PET is advantageous [8]. The extent and severity of stress-induced perfusion defects have important prognostic implications, now supported by a huge evidence base with SPECT [9, 10] and a smaller evidence base with PET [11].

Limitations

The major limitations of SPECT and PET are economic cost, environmental impact, and high radiation dose. For a cardiac imaging test, with the average cost (not charges) of an echocardiogram equal to 1 (as a cost comparator), the cost of a SPECT study is 3.27×, of PET 14×, and of PET–CT around 20× higher [12]. For stress imaging, compared with the treadmill exercise test equal to 1 (as a cost comparator), the cost of stress echocardio-graphy is 2.1×, of stress SPECT scintigraphy 5.7× [13], and of stress SPECT–CT around 20× higher. This cost assessment does not include the indirect additional costs of radiation-induced cancer and the environmental impact of radioactive tracer production and waste [14]. The older problem of limited availability of PET has been superseded by the problem of greater numbers of scanners but their heavy commitment to oncology work. In addition, PET perfusion imaging has been dependent on pharmacologic stress as PET tracers have a short half-life.

38.3
MPI vs. Stress Echocardiography

Stress echocardiography and myocardial perfusion imaging (MPI) have a very similar pathophysiological rationale, methodological approach (with assessment of perfusion and function), and clinical results (Table 38.1).

Accuracy for Coronary Artery Disease

The sensitivity and specificity of both tests are in the 80–85% range, with greater sensitivity for SPECT (especially for single vessel and left circumflex disease) and greater

Table 38.1 Myocardial radionuclide perfusion imaging: advantages and limitations

	Advantages	Limitations
Operator-independent	++	
Radiation dose		—
Long-standing experience	+++	
Environment impact		—
Convincing display	++	
Low specificity (LBBB, HPT)		—
Extensive prognostic data base	+	
High cost, limited availability		—

Advantages are scored as + good; ++ very good; +++ excellent advantage. Limitations are scored as −
mild; — moderate; —— severe limitation
LBBB left bundle branch block, *HPT* hypertension

specificity for stress echocardiography (especially in women, left ventricular hypertrophy, and left bundle branch block).

The equivalence between stress echocardiography and MPI is often considered surprising in light of the "ischemic cascade," which suggests that because perfusion disturbances precede ischemia, perfusion imaging should be more sensitive than wall motion imaging for the detection of ischemia. However, the results of these noninvasive tests are governed not only by the underlying physiology, but also by their imaging characteristics. The imaging strengths of echocardiography (spatial and temporal resolution, independent assessment of segmental wall motion) may therefore compensate for its current dependence on ischemia.

Beyond Sensitivity and Specificity

The modern application of functional testing has moved on from simply the diagnosis of coronary artery disease to assisting in decision-making, especially regarding the presence, location, and extent of ischemia. In these respects, the sensitivity and specificity for the diagnosis of coronary disease are of limited relevance – for example, in postinfarction patients, this analysis does not discriminate between the diagnoses of scar and ischemia.

The regional accuracy of stress echocardiography and perfusion scintigraphy may be important with respect to decision-making about revascularization. Breast and diaphragmatic attenuation are not the cause of artifacts with echocardiography, but should be readily recognized with nuclear imaging. The posterior wall poses a problem for perfusion scintigraphy (due to lower counts), and the lateral wall with echocardiography (due to overlying lung). Scintigraphy may be more accurate than echocardiography in these segments [15].

Although the assessment of the extent of ischemia appears to be broadly similar with echocardiography and nuclear techniques, stress echocardiography has a problem in defining the presence of multivessel coronary artery disease, with nuclear imaging being significantly more sensitive. Likewise, the detection of ischemia in combination with infarction is simpler with scintigraphy than echocardiography.

38

Prognostic Value for Coronary Artery Disease

The prognostic value of stress echocardiography has been well defined and comparison of the two techniques has shown them to be similar [16, 17]. Cardiac death is uncommon in individuals with stable chronic coronary disease. While ischemia and scar detected by either SPECT or stress echocardiography are predictive of cardiac events, the predictive value of a positive test result has generally been below 20%. For both echocardiography and nuclear tests, the next step in a patient with a positive test result is to substratify the level of risk. Clinical features such as age, diabetes, and symptoms of congestive heart failure are predictive of outcome in stable coronary artery disease, and may be used to select patients for more extensive testing combined with imaging assessment. Similarly, the results of stress testing – expressed, for example, as the Duke treadmill score – are of use in selecting patients for either test. Moreover, both stress echocardiography and myocardial perfusion SPECT [18] appear to be equally useful in substratifying patients at intermediate risk of events.

Interestingly, a cost-effectiveness study showed that outcomes of groups with comparable levels of risk were similar but the imaging and downstream costs of SPECT were greater in the low–intermediate-risk patients. Because of the higher sensitivity of SPECT, this technique was the most cost-effective strategy in intermediate–high-risk patients (e.g., those with known coronary artery disease) [19].

Merits of SPECT and Stress Echocardiography

The advantages of stress perfusion imaging include less operator-dependence, higher technical success rate, higher sensitivity, and better accuracy when multiple resting left ventricular wall motion abnormalities are present [13]. The advantages listed in guidelines for stress echocardiography over stress perfusion scintigraphy include a higher specificity and a greater availability, versatility, and greater convenience [13]. The lower specificity of SPECT may reflect problems of posttest referral bias with an established test technique and false-positive rates related to image artifacts. It should be recognized that recent technical advances, including gated SPECT and attenuation correction, have improved the specificity of SPECT.

Finally, echocardiography provides important anatomic and functional information that is either not provided or is provided poorly by scintigraphy. Valve diseases such as aortic stenosis or ischemic mitral regurgitation are important comorbidities of coronary artery disease, and may merit dynamic evaluation in some circumstances [20]. Likewise, exertional dyspnea may be an important presenting symptom of coronary artery disease [21], but may also be due to diastolic dysfunction. The ability to measure left ventricular filling pressure with exercise may be a useful adjunct to exercise echocardiography [22].

38.4
Current Clinical Indications

The current indications to MPI substantially overlap with stress echocardiography [4, 23]. The technique is especially indicated in patients with nonfeasible, nondiagnostic, or ambiguous exercise ECG stress test results. The use of MPI as a first-line imaging technique (whenever resources permit) is allowed [24] but not recommended by the guidelines. Stress imaging can be used as a first-line test in patients with uninterpretable ECG for baseline left bundle branch block, Wolff–Parkinson–White syndrome, paced rhythms, or alterations on resting ECG. In clinical environments where stress echocardiography expertise is available, MPI should be restricted to patients in whom stress echocardiography is not feasible or has yielded ambiguous results. The performance of both stress imaging tests is of dubious efficiency. A concordantly positive result is highly predictive of a critical coronary artery stenosis and clears the pathway toward an ischemia-driven revascularization. More often, a discordant result is found with stress echocardiography negativity (typical of a high specificity technique) and perfusion imaging positivity (typical of a high sensitivity technique). This patient has the same probability of having normal coronary arteries or mild-to-moderate coronary artery disease. Proceeding to coronary angiography, with unavoidable escalation of costs, risks, and revascularization, has a very questionable prognostic benefit. In these patients we currently perform stress cardiovascular magnetic resonance (CMR) [25, 26], which has at least the same accuracy as scintigraphy for viability and ischemia detection [12, 27], with no radiation burden and no ecological stress. Appropriate indications to MPI as stipulated by recent specialty European guidelines [23] are listed in Table 38.4.

38.5
The Elephant in the Room – Radiation Safety

The radiation burden of stress SPECT and PET ranges from the dose equivalent of 500–1,600 chest X-rays [3, 28] (Table 38.2). In light of dose optimization, which in Europe is also reinforced by the EURATOM law [29] and medical imaging guidelines [30],

Table 38.2 The radiation dose for common nuclear cardiology examinations (from [31])

Procedures	Effective radiation dose (mSv)	Equivalent no. of chest radiographs
Perfusion cardiac rest–stress technetium 99m sestamibi scan	10	500
Perfusion cardiac rest–stress thallium scan	21	1,050
Thallium-201 stress and reinjection (3.0 mCi + 1.0 mCi)	25	1,250
Dual isotope (3.0 mCi Th-201 + 30 mCi Tc-99m) stress	27	1,600
Cardiac PET ^{18}F–FDG	3.5	175
Cardiac PET ^{13}N-ammonium	2.0	100
Cardiac PET ^{15}O-water	4.0	200
CT–PET	25	1,500

it is especially disorienting that in the USA – generally expected to be a reliable site of best medical practice – 35% of the 9.3 million stress scintigraphies in 2002 were performed used 201Tl with 86% of these being dual isotope studies, perhaps because of the relatively fast patient throughput [28]. Thallium is still proposed by authorities as the best tracer for cardiac studies in the USA [28], and yet it has been officially dismissed for its obviously unfavorable radioprotection profile in many European laboratories including the Institute of Clinical Physiology of Pisa.

In addition to the issue of economic cost, discussed above, the main differences between the tests from a societal perspective are the ecological impact and the radiation burden for the patients and the doctors. The additional extra-risk of a cancer is around 1 in 1,000 (for a middle-aged man performing a sestamibi scan) but can be as high as 1 in 300 for a 35-year-old woman undergoing a thallium scan [29, 30]. In terms of population burden, the 10 million scans performed each year in the USA translate into a population risk of 20,000 new cancers per lifetime [4, 27, 28]. With the confidence intervals of the current risk estimates, the risk may be two- to threefold higher (60,000 new cancers) or two- to threefold lower (7,000 new cancers). One must be sure that there is no better way to make an accurate diagnosis of coronary artery disease. The great number (>30%) of inappropriate examinations [31], the frequent unawareness of dose and risks by the referring physician and the practitioner [32], and the provision of limited radiation safety information to the patient [33] set the stage for a perfect medicolegal storm [34, 35], especially in presence of tight regulations existing in the European law and strongly discouraging unjustified use of ionizing testing [30].

PET and SPECT scanners have been linked to computed tomographic (CT) scanners, which are digital radiological systems that acquire data in the axial plane, producing images of internal organs of high spatial and contrast resolution. The combination of PET or SPECT and CT as a single unit provides spatial and pathological correlation of the abnormal metabolic or flow activity, allowing images from both systems to be obtained from a single instrument in one examination procedure with optimal coregistration of images [4]. The resulting fusion images facilitate the most accurate interpretation of both PET and SPECT and CT studies (Fig. 38.1). The recent White Paper on Multimodality Imaging of the European Society of Radiology and the European Association of Nuclear Medicine put forward two indications on multimodality imaging [8]: (1) Diagnosis of coronary artery disease: the major advantage of the integrated approach to the diagnosis of coronary artery disease is the added sensitivity of PET and SPECT and CT angiography. With integrated PET/SPECT–CT systems, the limitations of both techniques can be overcome, leading to improved diagnostic capability. (2) Guiding management of coronary artery disease: Not all coronary artery stenoses are flow limiting, and PET or SPECT stress perfusion imaging complements the anatomical CT data by providing functional information on the hemodynamic significance of such stenoses, thus allowing more appropriate selection of patients who may benefit from revascularization procedures. However, while there are no questions about the diagnostic accuracy and the beauty of SPECT and, even more staggering, of combined PET–CT scans, it is very counterintuitive to accept an extensive use of these techniques in light of their exorbitant costs, high radiation burden, environmental impact, and availability of several nonionizing imaging techniques (such as ultrasound and magnetic resonance imaging) offering comparable information.

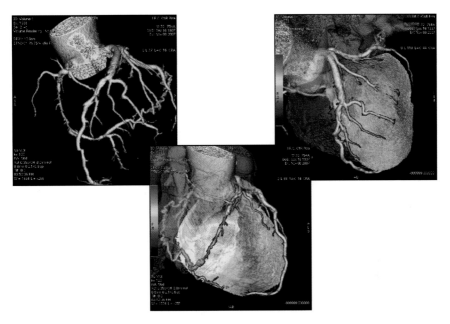

Fig. 38.1 An example of hybrid PET–CT imaging, with simultaneous representation of coronary anatomy (*left*) and perfusion (*right and middle panels*). (Courtesy of Dr. Danilo Neglia, Head of Cardiac PET Lab, Institute of Clinical Physiology, Pisa, Italy)

The long-standing comparison and competition between echocardiography and SPECT has radically changed in the last 5 years, as we have entered the "age of sustainability," i.e., the need to consider economic cost, biological hazards, long-term radiation risks, and environmental impact in our diagnostic flow-charts. (3). In light of this new perspective, the previous attractions of the polychrome, 3D, quantitative, operator-independent approach of nuclear imaging may come to appear a little jaded. Specifically, in centers having the requisite expertise for stress echocardiography, there are limited reasons to add nuclear perfusion imaging for diagnostic and prognostic purposes, and there may be social and ecological reasons why the nuclear alternative is less desirable [36]. If contrast-enhanced stress echocardiography does not salvage the technically difficult stress echocardiography, stress CMR provides an excellent, quantitative and reproducible, alternative for a nonionizing assessment of wall motion, and perfusion reserve, with accuracy at least comparable to MPI for ischemia and viability detection.

Perhaps in part related to competing technologies, the number of perfusion scans in the USA has begun to decline. The approach of ignoring [13], negating [38], or minimizing [23] the risks linked to radiation exposure is changing in a time of increased cultural, regulatory, and legal pressure towards the prescribers to minimize the biological burdens of inappropriate prescriptions. There is also an increasing attention to awareness regarding doses and risks of nuclear cardiology procedures in prescribers, practitioners, and patients [39] (Table 38.3).

38

Table 38.3 Head-to-head comparison between myocardial perfusion imaging (*MPI*) and stress echocardiography

	MPI	Stress echocardiography
Diagnostic parameter	Perfusion (WM)	WM (CFR)
Relative cost	3	1
Sensitivity	Higher	High
Specificity	Moderate	High
Radiation burden (CXr)	500–1500	0
Patient friendliness	Low	High
Operator friendly	Low	High
Environment friendly	Low	High

WM wall motion, *CFR* coronary flow reserve, *CXr* X-ray

38.6
Conclusion

Nuclear perfusion imaging and stress echocardiography show common pathophysiological roots and produce similar clinical fruits. They share a bipartisan imaging strategy to replace an anatomy-driven with a more physiologically oriented approach, referring for coronary angiography for ischemia-driven revascularization only patients with uncontrolled symptoms or a high-risk pattern of stress imaging. They are, more or less, equally reliable "gatekeepers" for more invasive, risky, and costly procedures, and have a recognized similar diagnostic and prognostic accuracy [40–43]. On the basis of these well-established findings, ACC/AHA guidelines concluded that "the choice of which test to perform depends on issues of local expertise, available facilities and considerations of cost-effectiveness" [13]. However, the societal climate surrounding medical practice has become more sensitive to the environmental costs of testing, and recent European guidelines have added that the advantages of stress echocardiography include its "being free of radiation" [24]. However, if we put the choice of cardiac stress imaging in the wider context of medical imaging, the European Commission recommendations clearly state that a nonionizing test should always be preferred when the information is grossly comparable to an ionizing test and both are available [36]. Applying guidelines, whenever a stress imaging test is clinically indicated, stress echocardiography is the first line test; when stress echocardiography is not feasible or yields ambiguous response, stress CMR is an excellent radiation-free option. If stress CMR technology and expertise are not available, stress MPI can be considered (Table 38.4). Although very different practice patterns are today present in high-volume centers, MPI and stress echocardiography are better used as alternative rather than redundant techniques. A good MPI is better than a bad stress echocardiography study, and a good stress echocardiography study is better than a poor MPI – but it is equally obvious that the capability to perform good echocardiography is one of the indicators of the quality of a cardiology division, and that the choice between stress echocardiography and MPI should be made in the context of the environmental, biological, and economic effects (Tables 38.5 and 38.6).

Table 38.4 Appropriate indications to MPI

	Appropriate	Uncertain	Inappropriate
Symptomatic, intermediate pretest probability, unable to exercise, abnormal ECG	√		
Acute chest pain, uncertain diagnosis	√		
Evaluation post-PCI or CABG		√	
Patients capable to exercise, interpretable ECG			√

Appropriate indications to MPI in a cardiological environment without access to stress echocardiography and/or stress CMR

CABG coronary artery bypass graft, *PCI* percutaneous coronary intervention

Table 38.5 The comparable diagnostic and prognostic information of cardiac stress imaging techniques (modified from [2])

	References	Population	Techniques	Results
Diagnostic accuracy for CAD	O'Keefe et al. (1995) [17]	11 studies (808 pts)	Stress echocardiography Perfusion imaging	Sensitivity = 78% Specificity = 86% Sensitivity = 83% (p = ns vs. echocardiography) Specificity = 77% (p = ns vs. echocardiography)
	Fleischmann et al. (1998) [18]	44 studies (5,974 pts)	Exercise echocardiography vs. exercise SPECT	Sensitivity = 85% Specificity = 77% Sensitivity = 87% (p = ns vs. echocardiography) Specificity = 64%
Prognostic value	Gibbons et al. (1999) [21]	9 studies (3,497 pts)	Stress echocardiography	PPV: 14%-66% NPV: 81%-98%
		12 studies (12,589 pts)	Stress myocardial imaging	PPV = 3.8%-41% NPV = 81.2%-100%
Diagnostic value of viability	Bax et al. (1997) [19]	37 studies (1,341 pts)	F-18 fluorodeoxyglucose metabolic imaging	Specificity higher (p < 0.001) for low-dose dobutamine
			Thallium perfusion imaging Dobutamine echocardiography	
Prognostic value of viability	Allman et al. (2002) [20]	24 studies (3,089 pts)	F-18 fluorodeoxyglucose metabolic imaging	No measurable performance difference for predicting revascularization benefit between the three testing techniques
			Thallium perfusion imaging Dobutamine echocardiography	

CAD coronary artery disease, *NPV* negative predictive value, *PPV* positive predicted value, *pts* patients, *ns* not significant

Table 38.6 Broad levels of risk for common X-ray examinations and isotope scans

X-ray examination or nuclear medicine isotope scan	Effective doses (mSv) clustering around a value of:	Equivalent period of natural background radiation	Lifetime additional risk of cancer per examination[a]
Chest X-ray	0.01	A few days	Negligible risk
Skull X-ray	0.1	A few weeks	Minimal risk
			1 in 1,000,000 to 1 in 100,000
Breast (mammography) Lung isotope scan	1.0	A few months to a year	Very low risk 1 in 100,000 to 1 in 10,000
Cardiac gated study Cardiac thallium scan	10	A few years	Low risk 1 in 10,000 to 1 in 1,000

[a] These risk levels represent very small additions to the 1-in-3 chance we all have of getting cancer. The table is summarized from Table 38.2 of "Radiation and your patient: a web module produced by Committee 3 of the International Commission on Radiological Protection (ICRP)".
Typically, environmental radiation amounts to approximately 2–3 mSv per year

References

1. Gould KL, Westcott RJ, Albro PC, et al (1978) Noninvasive assessment of coronary stenoses by myocardial imaging during pharmacologic coronary vasodilatation. II. Clinical methodology and feasibility. Am J Cardiol 41:279–287
2. Berman DS, Hachamovitch R, Shaw LJ, et al (2006) Roles of nuclear cardiology, cardiac computed tomography, and cardiac magnetic resonance: noninvasive risk stratification and a conceptual framework for the selection of noninvasive imaging tests in patients with known or suspected coronary artery disease. J Nucl Med 47:1107–1118
3. Picano E (2003) Stress echocardiography: a historical perspective. Special article. Am J Med. 114:126–130
4. Marcassa C, Bax JJ, Bengel F, et al (2008) on behalf of the European Council of Nuclear Cardiology (ECNC), the European Society of Cardiology Working Group 5 (Nuclear Cardiology and Cardiac CT), and the European Association of Nuclear Medicine Cardiovascular Committee. Clinical value, cost-effectiveness, and safety of myocardial perfusion scintigraphy: a position statement. Eur Heart J 29:557–563
5. Sicari R (2004) Anti-ischemic therapy and stress testing: pathophysiologic, diagnostic and prognostic implications. Cardiovasc Ultrasound 2:14
6. Lattanzi F, Picano E, Bolognese L, et al (1991) Inhibition of dipyridamole-induced ischemia by antianginal therapy in humans. Correlation with exercise electrocardiography. Circulation 83:1256–1262
7. Sicari R, Cortigiani L, Bigi R, et al; Echo-Persantine International Cooperative (EPIC) Study Group; Echo-Dobutamine International Cooperative (EDIC) Study Group (2004) Prognostic value of pharmacological stress echocardiography is affected by concomitant antiischemic therapy at the time of testing. Circulation 109:2428–2431

8. Cuocolo A, Adam A (2007) The "White paper of the European Association of Nuclear Medicine (EANM) and the European Society of Radiology (ESR) on multimodality imaging": a message from the EANM and ESR Presidents. Eur J Nucl Med Mol Imaging 34:1145–1146

9. Sharir T, Germano G, Kavanagh PB, et al (1999) Incremental prognostic value of post-stress left ventricualr ejection fraction and volume by gated myocardial perfusion single photon emission computer tomography. Circulation 100:1035–1042

10. Hachamovitch R, Hayes S, Friedman J, et al (2004) Stress perfusion single-photon emission computed tomography is clinically effective and cost-effective in risk stratification of patients with a high likelihood of coronary artery disease (CAD) but not known CAD. J Am Coll Cardiol 43:200–208

11. Merhige ME, Breen WJ, Shelton V, et al (2007) Impact of myocardial perfusion imaging with PET and (82)Rb on downstream invasive procedure utilization, costs, and outcomes in coronary disease management. J Nucl Med 48:1069–1076

12. Pennell DJ, Sechtem UP, Higgins CB, et al; Society for Cardiovascular Magnetic Resonance; Working Group on Cardiovascular Magnetic Resonance of the European Society of Cardiology (2004) Clinical indications for cardiovascular magnetic resonance (CMR): Consensus Panel report. Eur Heart J 25:1940–1965

13. Gibbons RJ, Abrams J, Chatterjee K, et al; American College of Cardiology; American Heart Association Task Force on practice guidelines (Committee on the Management of Patients With Chronic Stable Angina) (2003) ACC/AHA 2002 guideline update for the management of patients with chronic stable angina–summary article: a report of the American College of Cardiology/American Heart Association Task Force on practice guidelines (Committee on the Management of Patients With Chronic Stable Angina). J Am Coll Cardiol 41:159–168

14. International Atomic Agency(1996) International basic safety standards for protection against ionizing radiations and for the safety of radioactive sources. IAEA Safety Series No 115. IAEA, Vienna

15. Bateman TM, Heller GV, McGhie AI, et al (2006) Diagnostic accuracy of rest/stress ECG-gated Rb-82 myocardial perfusion PET: comparison with ECG-gated Tc-99m sestamibi SPECT. J Nucl Cardiol 13:24–33

16. Poldermans D, Fioretti PM, Boersma E, et al (1994) Dobutamine-atropine stress echocardiography and clinical data for predicting late cardiac events in patients with suspected coronary artery disease. Am J Med 97:119–125

17. Shaw LJ, Marwick TH, Berman DS, et al (2006) Incremental cost-effectiveness of exercise echocardiography vs. SPECT imaging for the evaluation of stable chest pain. Eur Heart J 27:2448–2458

18. Berman DS, Kang X, Slomka PJ, et al (2007) Underestimation of extent of ischemia by gated SPECT myocardial perfusion imaging in patients with left main coronary artery disease. J Nucl Cardiol 14:521–528

19. Shaw LJ, Hachamovitch R, Berman DS, et al (1999) The economic consequences of available diagnostic and prognostic strategies for the evaluation of stable angina patients: an observational assessment of the value of precatheterization ischemia. Economics of Noninvasive Diagnosis (END) Multicenter Study Group.. J Am Coll Cardiol 33:661–669

20. Pierard LA, Lancellotti P (2007) Stress testing in valve disease. Heart 93:766–772 (Review)

21. Abidov A, Rozanski A, Hachamovitch R, et al (2005) Prognostic significance of dyspnea in patients referred for cardiac stress testing. N Engl J Med 353:1889–1898

22. Burgess MI, Jenkins C, Sharman JE, et al (2006) Diastolic stress echocardiography: hemodynamic validation and clinical significance of estimation of ventricular filling pressure with exercise. J Am Coll Cardiol 47:1891–1900

38

23. Brindis RG, Douglas PS, Hendel RC, et al; American College of Cardiology Foundation Quality Strategic Directions Committee Appropriateness Criteria Working Group; American Society of Nuclear Cardiology; American Heart Association. ACCF/ASNC (2005) Appropriateness criteria for single-photon emission computed tomography myocardial perfusion imaging (SPECT MPI): a report of the American College of Cardiology Foundation Quality Strategic Directions Committee Appropriateness Criteria Working Group and the American Society of Nuclear Cardiology endorsed by the American Heart Association. J Am Coll Cardiol 46:1587–1605

24. Fox K, Garcia MA, Ardissino D, et al; Task Force on the Management of Stable Angina Pectoris of the European Society of Cardiology; ESC Committee for Practice Guidelines (CPG) (2006) Guidelines on the management of stable angina pectoris: executive summary: the Task Force on the Management of Stable Angina Pectoris of the European Society of Cardiology. Eur Heart J 27:1341–1381

25. Pingitore A, Lombardi M, Scattini B, et al (2008) Head to head comparison between perfusion and function during accelerated high-dose dipyridamole magnetic resonance stress for the detection of coronary artery disease. Am J Cardiol 101:8–14

26. Sicari R, Pingitore A, Aquaro G, et al (2007) Cardiac functional stress imaging: a sequential approach with stress echo and cardiovascular magnetic resonance. Cardiovasc Ultrasound 5:47

27. Schwitter J, Wacker CM, van Rossum AC, et al (2008) MR-IMPACT: comparison of perfusion-cardiac magnetic resonance with single-photon emission computed tomography for the detection of coronary artery disease in a multicentre, multivendor, randomized trial. Eur Heart J 29:480–489

28. Einstein AJ, Moser KW, Thompson RC, et al (2007) Radiation dose to patients from cardiac diagnostic imaging. Circulation 116:1290–1305

29. Council Directive 97/43/EURATOM of 30 June 1997 on health protection of individuals against the dangers of ionizing radiation in relation to medical exposure and repealing Directive 84/466/Euratom. http://ec.europa.eu/energy/nuclear/radioprotection/doc/legislation/9743_en.pdf

30. Picano E (2004) Sustainability of medical imaging. Education and Debate. BMJ 328:578–580

31. Picano E (2004) Informed consent and communication of risk from radiological and nuclear medicine examinations: how to escape from a communication inferno. BMJ 329:849–851

32. Gibbons RJ, Miller TD, Hodge D, et al (2008) Application of appropriateness criteria to stress single-photon emission computed tomography sestamibi studies and stress echocardiograms in an academic medical center. J Am Coll Cardiol 51:1283–1289

33. Correia MJ, Hellies A, Andreassi MG, et al (2005) Lack of radiological awareness among physicians working in a tertiary-care cardiological centre. International Journal of Cardiology 105: 307–311

34. Bedetti G, Pizzi C, Gavaruzzi G, et al (2008) Suboptimal awareness of radiologic dose among patients undergoing cardiac stress scintigraphy. J Am Coll Radiol 5:126–131

35. Picano E, Vano E, Semelka R, et al (2007) The American College of Radiology white paper on radiation dose in medicine:deep impact on the practice of cardiovascular imaging. Cardiovasc Ultrasound 5:37

36. Bedetti G, Loré C (2007) Radiological informed consent in cardiovascular imaging: towards the medico-legal perfect storm? Cardiovasc Ultrasound 5:35

37. European Commission (2001) Radiation protection 118: referral guidelines for imaging. Office for Official Publications of the European Communities, Luxembourg

38. Abbott BG, Zaret BL (2003) Contemporary cardiology and hysteric nucleophobia. Am J Med 114:131–134

39. Amis ES Jr, Butler PF, Applegate KE, et al; American College of Radiology (2007) American College of Radiology white paper on radiation dose in medicine. J Am Coll Radiol 4:272–284

40. Heijenbrok-Kal MH, Fleischmann KE, Hunink MG (2007) Stress echocardiography, stress single-photon-emission computed tomography and electron beam computed tomography for the assessment of coronary artery disease: a meta-analysis of diagnostic performance. Am Heart J 154:415–423

41. Allman KC, Shaw LJ, Hachamovitch R, et al (2002) Myocardial viability testing and impact of revascularization on prognosis in patients with coronary artery disease and left ventricular dysfunction: a meta-analysis. J Am Coll Cardiol 39:1151–1158

42. Metz LD, Beattie M, Hom R, et al (2007) The prognostic value of normal exercise myocardial perfusion imaging and exercise echocardiography: a meta-analysis. J Am Coll Cardiol 49:227–237

43. Marwick TH (2004) Does the extent of malperfusion or ischemia on stress testing predict future cardiac events? Am J Med 117:58–59

Stress Echocardiography Versus Cardiac CT

39

Eugenio Picano and William Wijns

39.1
Cardiac Imaging in the CTA Era

Several techniques such as stress echocardiography and myocardial perfusion imaging have become available to assess cardiac function and myocardial perfusion. With the arrival of multislice computed tomography coronary angiography (CTA), noninvasive imaging of coronary anatomy has also become possible. The introduction of multidetector row computed tomography (CT) in 1999 led to a significant improvement in the temporal and spatial resolution of CT allowing the visualization of small and rapidly moving structures, such as coronary arteries, to be visualized with good image quality. Although the initial four-slice scanners already showed some promising diagnostic potential, currently 64-slice CT is considered state of the art for cardiac CT imaging, whereas 256-slice systems are being developed [1]. Conceptually, CTA allows one to track the natural history of coronary artery disease with the earliest possible marker, providing unprecedented noninvasive insight into the coronary anatomy and coronary wall structure changes, which anticipate by years, and sometimes decades, the onset of myocardial perfusion or functional changes during stress, which are the cornerstone of current noninvasive diagnosis of coronary artery disease by stress scintigraphy or stress echocardiography [2] (Fig. 39.1). The information content of CTA is very high, in any case higher than invasive angiography, probably equivalent to gray-scale intravascular ultrasound plus angiography. Invasive coronary angiography can identify obstructive as well as complex lesions, but it is restricted to the coronary lumen and is unable to depict the coronary wall. Thus, features such as vessel remodeling or plaque composition are missed. CTA depicts not only a coronary luminogram as coronary angiography does, but also the thickness of the wall and the plaque composition to some extent [3] as ultrasound does [4, 5]. This is especially important in the early diagnosis of coronary artery disease, since the earliest stage of atherosclerosis is the initial positive remodeling with preserved lumen, as plaque accumulates [6] (Fig. 39.1). Several studies showed an increased level of inflammatory markers, high lipid cores, and pronounced medial thinning in positively remodeled vessels [7]. Some of the initial acute presentations of the disease may occur when the adaptive remodeling mechanisms are

E. Picano, *Stress Echocardiography*,
© Springer-Verlag Berlin Heidelberg 2009

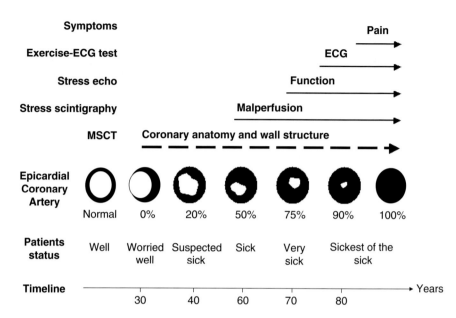

Fig. 39.1 The timeline of atherosclerosis and the disruptive opportunity offered by CTA to image coronary atherosclerotic disease, directly, decades before stress-induced changes in function and perfusion are detectable during stress echocardiography and stress scintigraphy. The information on initial positive remodeling of arterial wall and plaque composition of the plaque is off-limits for invasive coronary angiography and can be obtained with intracoronary ultrasound. (Redrawn and adapted from [2])

exhausted and a threshold mass of plaque (depending on vessel diameter) starts to breach towards the lumen. CTA can also offer insight into the structural composition of plaque which – for any given plaque size – contributes to plaque vulnerability [8], with lipid-rich, high-risk plaques (hypoechoic by ultrasound and hypodense by CT) more prone to rupture and subsequent thrombotic occlusion than calcium-rich, low-risk plaques (hyperechoic with shadowing by ultrasound and hyperdense by CT). This conceptual breakthrough translated into a scientific and commercial explosion with the newer 64-slice generations of multidetector CT scanners, which significantly improved the diagnostic performance for the assessment of coronary artery disease, and decreased the proportion of nonassessable segments [9]. This determined a surge of scientific and clinical interest in the method, destined to grow in the foreseeable future. In the UK, for instance, the growth rate of cardiac CTA is expected to be in the range of +4,800% within the year 2020 when compared to 2006 [10]. Indeed, 72% of US cardiologists order CT angiography procedures every month and many cardiologists plan to purchase the CT equipment necessary for performing this examination in their own practice. The message is clear and simple, and comes straight from scientific journals and lay press [11]: beautiful, easily obtained images of coronary artery stenoses, which otherwise would go undetected, provide an opportunity to intervene early enough and put an end to sudden death, without hospital stay, without catheters inserted into the body, and without heaps of consent forms to be signed informing the patient about the risk of death and myocardial infarction, as is the case with invasive cardiac catheterization [12]. However, if inappropriately used, cardiac CT may become a double-edged sword, with potential to create a huge reservoir of tens of thousands of future cancers in a not-too-distant future [13–15]. In fact, while the radiation dose of a cardiac CT scan is in the same order of magnitude as other diagnostic tests used in cardiology, such as nuclear perfusion scans (with a typical effective dose of 8–25mSv, corresponding to a dose equivalent of 400–1,250 chest X-rays), all possible measures should be taken to keep the dose as low as possible, and considerations as to clinical indications for cardiac CT must always take radiation exposure into account [1, 16, 17]. Clearly, at this point the pros and cons of each imaging technique need to be carefully incorporated in the clinical decision making – also shared with the patient [16] – so that the combination of the various techniques may yield the greatest benefit to the individual patient, while waiting for more data and comprehensive guidelines defining the relative role of different techniques in clinical practice [18].

39.2
Advantages and Limitations of Cardiac CTA

Coronary CTA has wide availability, and – compared with magnetic resonance angiography – higher spatial resolution and more consistent, shorter examination time with better patient adherence. It is also possible with CT to assess the presence and extent of coronary calcification. The amount of coronary calcium correlates moderately closely to the overall atherosclerotic plaque burden, but its place in risk stratification of asymptomatic individuals remains uncertain [1]. It is true that the use of calcium score has quite convincing (non randomized) outcome impact over years [19, 20], but it is equally true that the question remains open on how much incremental information can be obtained by CTA. It is also unclear whether the extra information provided by calcium score assessment is better than that provided by simpler, radiation-free atherosclerosis imaging biomarkers such as carotid intima-media thickness by ultrasound scan [21, 22]. Recent guidelines do not recommend unselected "screening" or patient self-referral in individuals with very low (<1.0% annual risk) or very high risk (>2% annual risk). A beneficial contribution can most likely be expected in individuals who seem to be at intermediate risk for coronary events (1.0–2.0% annual risk), yet this hypothesis has not been prospectively studied so far [1] (Table 39.1).

The main limitation of CTA is ionizing radiation exposure [23]. Coronary CTA can expose the patient to considerably higher amounts of ionizing radiation than standard radiographs, CT calcium scoring, or coronary angiography [24–29] (Table 39.2). For each specific test, there is a wide interinstitutional variability in the dose administered, depending on the type of technology and operator attention paid to dose optimization [30] (Fig. 39.2). The dose is also higher when the dual source technique is used [20] and with hybrid imaging with positron emission tomography (PET) [31]. The corresponding risk of

Table 39.1 Cardiac CT: advantages and limitations

	Advantages	Limitations
Versatility (coronary; embolism; dissection)	+++	
Radiation dose		——
Operator-independent	+++	
Allergic, nephrotoxic iodinated contrast		—
High access	+++	
Stented, calcified plaques		—
Round-the-clock availability	+++	
Irregular rhythm, high heart rate, high body mass index		—

Table 39.2 The average radiation dose of cardiac CT

	Effective dose (mSv)	Equivalent number of chest X-rays
Calcium score	2	100
64-slice MSCT	15	750
64-slice MSCT bypass graft	20	1,000
MSCT–PET (cardiac)	25	1,250
MSCT, 64-slice, no ECG pulsing, yes aorta	29	1,450

MSCT multislice computed tomography, *PET* positron emission tomography

cancer is linearly correlated with the radiation dose, and a CTA with a dose of 15 mSv (750 chest X-rays) carries an estimated cancer risk of 1 in 500 in a 50-year-old man [32]. Another safety concern regards the use of contrast agents (about 100 ml of iodinated contrast) [1]. In addition to nephrotoxicity, intravenous administration of iodinated contrast media may also be associated with anaphylactoid reaction. Coronary CTA is a purely diagnostic test that does not provide an option for immediate intervention. Because the temporal resolution is low, motion artifacts can occur. Predictable visualization of the coronary arteries is not possible at present in patients with atrial fibrillation or frequent ectopy. Coronary artery segments with substantial calcification may not be evaluable with respect to the presence of a hemodynamically relevant stenosis. The coronary lumen is generally not well observed in the region of a coronary stent [28].

39.3
Stress Echocardiography vs. Cardiac CTA

Stress echocardiography and CTA have a completely different – and therefore potentially complementary – pathophysiological rationale, methodological approach, and clinical results, as summarized in Table 39.3. The most important difference is the separation between the anatomic and the functional approach. Comparative studies have demonstrated that anatomic imaging with CTA (Fig. 39.3) may provide information complementary to

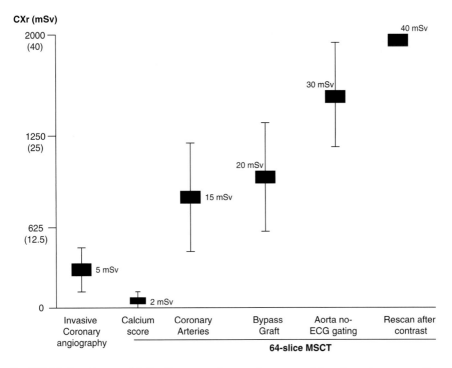

Fig. 39.2 Median doses and indicative ranges (on *y-axis*, expressed in mSv and corresponding equivalent of chest X-rays) for invasive coronary angiography (taken as a reference standard) and cardiac CT with different protocols and methods: calcium scoring; coronary angiography ECG-gated; coronary artery bypass grafting; non-ECG gated coronary angiography and aorta scan. (Adapted from [10], from original data of [14, 16, 17, 19])

Table 39.3 Head-to-head comparison between MSCT and stress echocardiography

	MSCT	Stress echocardiography
Approach	Anatomic	Functional
Direct alternative	Coronary angiography	MPI
Radiation exposure	500–1,500 chest X-rays	Ø
Stress required	No	Yes
Contrast required	Yes	No
Relative cost	3	1
High predictive value	Negative	Positive
Next generation	CT–PET	2D Doppler (CFR)

MSCT multislice computed tomography, *PET* positron emission tomography, *MPI* myocardial perfusion imaging, *CFR* coronary flow reserve

Normal coronary arteries   **LAD stenosis**

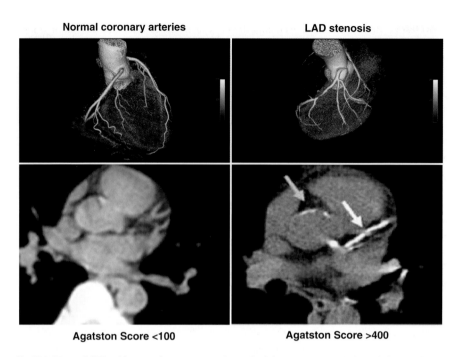

Agatston Score <100   **Agatston Score >400**

Fig. 39.3 Normal CTA with normal coronary arteries and calcium score <100 (*left*); and abnormal CTA with left anterior descending coronary artery stenosis and calcium score >400 (*right*). (Courtesy of Dr. Dante Chiappino and Dr. Paolo Marraccini, Institute of Clinical Physiology, Fondazione Gabriele Monasterio, Pisa and Massa, Italy)

the traditionally used techniques for functional assessment. From these studies can be derived that only approximately 50% of significant stenosis on CTA are functionally relevant; a large proportion of significant (>50%) lesions on CTA do not result in perfusion abnormalities [33]. Alternatively, many patients with normal perfusion show considerable atherosclerosis on CTA. Data with direct comparison of stress echocardiography and CTA are conspicuously lacking to date, but preliminary evidence suggests that the most frequent source of CTA–stress echocardiography mismatch is represented by patients with negative stress echocardiography and positive CTA findings [34]. Therefore, the combined use of these techniques may enhance the assessment of the presence and extent of coronary artery disease. Whether this can be cost-effective and risk-effective remains to be established, and will likely depend on the clinical presentation and specific diagnostic questions.

The aggressive use of CTA for mass screening in asymptomatic subjects will also possibly lead to irresistible triggering of coronary stenting, irrespective of the symptomatic status, functional significance of the stenosis, or any form of prognostic evaluation [12]. Already, and although the clinical cardiologist is offered many options and techniques for noninvasive functional evaluation, up to 71% of percutaneous coronary interventions (PCIs) are being performed in the absence of any sort of functional evaluation [35]. Yet, we know now that in chronic stable angina – and even more in asymptomatic patients – an anatomic stenosis associated with negative stress testing and normal function has a very low risk and should be left untreated, whereas a similar coronary stenosis with high-risk stress test positivity dictates an ischemia-driven revascularization with maximal prognostic benefit [36, 37]. The scenario of anatomy-driven revascularization, often referred to as the oculostenotic reflex, is even more worrisome now that safety concerns associated with late stent thrombosis have been identified and PCI indications have expanded to include patient and lesion subsets in whom coronary bypass surgery was shown to portend a survival benefit over medical therapy. With the recent disclosure of the COURAGE (Clinical Outcomes Utilizing Revascularization and Aggressive Drug Estimation) trial, showing no superiority of PCI over contemporary pharmacologic therapy in patients with stable angina, it was suggested that a number of PCI procedures are, in fact, unnecessarily performed [38]. Taken together, the appropriateness of the explosive growth in revascularization procedures by use of PCI, possibly further fuelled by diagnostic carpet bombing with CTA, is under question. Concerns will only increase if the radiation side of the risk–benefit balance of imaging and interventions is included in the appropriateness assessment, as currently recommended by practice guidelines [39, 40].

39.4
Current Clinical Indications

The Foundation of the American College of Cardiology has responded to the rapid and uncontrolled increase of medical imaging procedures by defining appropriateness criteria for cardiac CTA [39]. Table 39.4 lists indications that are currently viewed as appropriate for performing CT angiography. They closely mirror those of stress echocardiography in many subsets [40].

Table 39.4 Appropriate, uncertain and inappropriate indications to CTA or stress echocardiography (adapted from [28, 29])

	Appropriate	Uncertain	Inappropriate
Chest pain syndrome, intermediate probability of CAD, ECG uninterpretable or patient unable to exercise	√		
Acute chest pain, intermediate pretest probability of CAD, no ECG changes and serial enzymes negative	√		
Postrevascularization with change of symptoms	√		
Asymptomatic ≥5 years after CABG or ≥2 years after PCI		√	
Evaluation of bypass graft and coronary anatomy after CABG in asymptomatic patients			√
Asymptomatic patients with low-to-moderate CHR risk by Framingham Risk Criteria			√
Preoperative evaluation for noncardiac surgery in low-risk surgery and intermediate perioperative risk			√

CAD coronary artery disease, *CABG* coronary artery bypass graft, *PCI* percutaneous coronary intervention, risk by Framingham Risk Criteria

Although it is tempting to obtain in the same patient both anatomic (with CTA) and functional (with stress echocardiography or scintigraphy) insight to have a more integrated pathophysiological and prognostic picture, this practice is today unsupported by the available evidence and will act as a dangerous multiplier of costs and risks [13]. The burden is even increased by the hybrid imaging with cardiac CTA–PET, capable of combining coronary anatomy and flow reserve in a single picture [41] – but with considerable further radiation exposure.

In the individual patient, the expected benefit should be weighed against the acute (dye allergic reaction), subacute (dye nephrotoxic effects), and chronic (long-term cancer risk) risk of CTA. Similarly, the indication to stress echocardiography should consider the risks of the stress (exercise or pharmacological) and, if administered, of the echocardiographic contrast agent [42, 43]. Any intended use of the CTA technique to follow-up serially the atherosclerotic burden or the revascularization outcome should be restrained by consideration of the cumulative radiation burden resulting from serial studies. The use of the technique should also be discouraged in children, in whom it has been proposed to diagnose complex congenital heart disease or, specifically, Kawasaki disease or other conditions involving coronary arteries [44]. The same radiation is three to four more oncogenic in a child [32] – and therefore the technique should be considered in children only if stringently indicated and there is no alternative. In particular, when serial evaluation over time is needed, nonionizing imaging procedures (such as magnetic resonance imaging and echocardiography) should be considered [45].

An important aspect, often neglected in real life, is that the appropriateness of an indication to CTA (as well as to other testing) will have to include a calculated – not guesstimated – European Society of Cardiology or Framingham Heart Study score and pretest probability. At present, the intermediate pretest probability has far too wide boundaries (between 13 and 87% according to estimates of Diamond and Forrester). This will also allow one to calculate the posttest probability of disease, by incorporating the positive and negative likelihood ratio portended by an abnormal or normal test result, respectively. Likelihood ratios are much more clinically useful in the individual patient than "sensitivity" and "specificity." For instance, in a patient with 5% pretest likelihood of disease, a normal CTA will give a 1% likelihood of disease – hardly justifying the test since the level of certainty of the diagnosis is not significantly improved by the test, irrespective of its result [46]. It is also obvious that all our calculations of pre- and posttest likelihood are based on angiographically assessed coronary artery disease, recognized as a "battered gold standard" for decades [47]. The consequence is that we need to retrain our eyes again, new scores need to be designed that have prognostic impact, and that the relation between image and action should be shifted, certainly different from what it is with invasive angiography. Most likely, we simply can no longer afford the reassuring approach of comparing CTA with coronary angiography [18].

39.5
Conclusions

CTA is exploding in beauty, availability, and versatility. It offers unique information, without catheters, on coronary anatomy, calcium content, and general cardiac morphology, including the pulmonary veins and aorta. It is at the crossroads between two disruptive events – one technological and the other conceptual. Truly innovative technology is disruptive of existing practice, and CTA has for the first time made coronary anatomy accessible noninvasively [18]. However, its use has also promoted the diffusion of a new disruptive concept that changed time-honored medical behaviors: long-term radiation risks should be included in the risk–benefit assessment of competing imaging techniques [48]. This obvious concept has long been ignored by physicians [49–51], but is now an integral part of the very definition of appropriateness [39–40] and must be considered for societal as well as for medicolegal reasons [13–16]. Today, the average adult cardiac patient receives 20% of the cumulative radiological dose from CTA [52]. Small individual risks applied to an increasingly large population may create a public health issue some years in the future [53]. About 2% of all cancers in the USA may be attributable to the radiation from CT studies [14]. This has led opinion leaders to express concerns on a deregulated and aggressive screening use of CTA, since *we can't just be screening the population of the worried well who want to have their non-invasive angiogram done, because the population burden of radiation would be unacceptable*" [9]. This concept probably applies to any radiation-based test (thus also to calcium score) which simply does not qualify for screening in the general population. We lack any evidence that CTA is better than calcium score in moderate–high-risk patients, based on the Framingham Heart Study or European Society of Cardiology risk score, and probably we will miss this information for decades, until proper long-term follow-up data become available. Any evidence-based indication in this field will require prospective randomization of thousands of patients followed up for many years, and including as end points not only cardiovascular events – which is the primary target of CTA imaging – but also cancer, whose risk is increased by radiation-based screening. Paradoxically, in this way screening begets screening, since CTA scans for cardiovascular disease will lead to increased risk for cancer, with a vicious circle of domino testing or snowball screening of highly questionable risk–benefit and cost–benefit plausibility.

At the same time, the awareness of radiation-related hazards has stimulated research and technological advances in an attempt to reduce radiation exposure. There are three ways to reduce the overall radiation dose from CT in the individual patient and the population [8]. The first is to optimize doses, in individual studies, which is made easier by the latest-generation automatic exposure–control options. The second is to replace CT use, when practical, with other options. Today, in the cardiac patient with low-to-intermediate pretest probability of disease, this means relying on stress echocardiography as a first-line imaging test instead of cardiac CTA, and possibly considering invasive coronary angiography as a direct option in some other patients with high pretest probability – with less radiation exposure than cardiac CTA [2]. Stress echocardiography has recognized limitations in the subjectivity of reading, dependence on acoustic window, and suboptimal sensitivity, and therefore might be replaced as a first-line imaging test by perfusion scintigraphy, but again this option is limited by the radiation dose of scintigraphy, often repeated serially in the cardiac patient [35]. The third and most effective way to reduce the population dose from CT is simply to decrease the number of CT studies that are inappropriately prescribed [8], for instance, in patients with a high pretest likelihood of disease, in whom the use of CTA will most likely not result in a "negative" scan that would help to avoid invasive angiography and is therefore not recommendable. The most appropriate indication today is the possibility to reliably rule out coronary artery

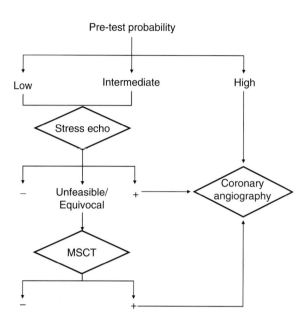

Fig. 39.4 Suggested diagnostic algorithm on the basis of the pr-test probability of disease. In presence of a high pretest probability, a direct invasive coronary angiography can be warranted without further noninvasive testing. In patients with low-to-intermediate probability, stress echocardiography is indicated as a first-line test. In patients with ambiguous results and/or intermediate probability, a cardiac CT may be warranted

disease in patients with intermediate pretest probability of disease, such as in patients with atypical chest pain and ambiguous stress echocardiography results (Fig. 39.4). In the future, diagnostic flow-charts, combining noninvasive anatomic and functional imaging, need to be evaluated in large patient populations to establish their efficacy, safety, and cost-effectiveness. The development of radiation-sparing technology capable of abating by tenfold the current exposure levels of CTA will play a key role in improving the risk–benefit profile of CTA [54], shifting the threshold of application of CTA toward less sick, and possibly worried well, patients (Fig. 39.5). In these patients (right side of the diagram in Fig. 39.5) at present functional evaluation (for instance, with stress echocardiography) prevails over anatomy and serves as gatekeeper. Although CTA is universally acclaimed to offer a unique opportunity to extend our capability to diagnose coronary artery disease with the potential to have an impact on sudden ischemic cardiac death and unheralded myocardial infarction, there is the risk of exacerbating the overuse of suboptimal practices [12] and inducing significant available long-term cancer risks, unless diagnostic workup paradigms are adjusted. It is also inexorable that on the day magnetic resonance imaging will allow coronary imaging with a comparable level of predictability and precision [55], CTA will be reserved only for those patients who cannot enter the magnetic resonance scanner.

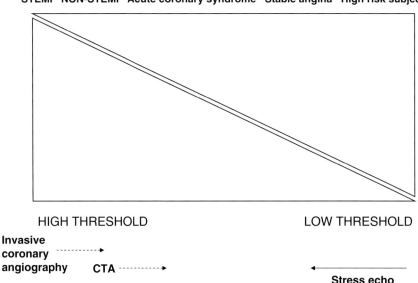

STEMI   NON-STEMI   Acute coronary syndrome   Stable angina   High risk subject

HIGH THRESHOLD   LOW THRESHOLD

Invasive
coronary   ·········►
angiography   **CTA** ·········►
                                              ◄───────────
                                               Stress echo
              Low dose CTA ·········►

Fig. 39.5 Access to coronary anatomy: shift in paradigm. Because knowledge of coronary anatomy required invasive catheterization, patients referred for the examination were either very sick or carefully selected by prior noninvasive functional testing (*right*). By keeping the threshold at a high level, invasive diagnosis was restricted to symptomatic or high-risk subjects. With the emergence of noninvasive coronary angiography, the threshold will be lowered and more patients or even asymptomatic subjects will undergo CTA, often in the absence of prior functional testing. A brake to the inexorable right shift of CTA is the relatively high radiation exposure. With new technologies allowing substantial dose reduction, the threshold of application of CTA will decrease further. The role of noninvasive functional testing will shift from primary diagnostic to prognostic stratification, selecting patients more likely to benefit from an ischemia-driven revascularization. (Modified from [12])

References

1. Schroeder S, Achenbach S, Bengel F, et al (2008) Cardiac computed tomography: indications, applications, limitations, and training requirements: Report of a Writing Group deployed by the Working Group Nuclear Cardiology and Cardiac CT of the European Society of Cardiology and the European Council of Nuclear Cardiology. Eur Heart J 29:531–556
2. Erbel R (1996) The dawn of a new era – non-invasive coronary imaging. Herz 21:75–77
3. Schmid M, Pflederer T, Jang IK, et al (2008) Relationship between degree of remodeling and CT attenuation of plaque in coronary atherosclerotic lesions: an in-vivo analysis by multidetector computed tomography. Atherosclerosis 197:457–464
4. Picano E, Landini L, Distante A, et al (1985). Angle dependence of ultrasonic backscatter in arterial tissue: a study in vitro. Circulation 72:572–576

5. Yamagishi M, Terashima M, Awano K, et al (2000) Morphology of vulnerable coronary plaque: insights from follow-up of patients examined by intravascular ultrasound before an acute coronary syndrome. J Am Coll Cardiol 35:106–111
6. Glagov S, Weisenberg E, Zarins CK, et al (1987) Compensatory enlargement of human atherosclerotic coronary arteries. N Engl J Med 316:1371–1351
7. Virmani R, Kolodgie FD, Burke AP, et al (2000. Lessons from sudden coronary death: a comprehensive morphological classification scheme for atherosclerotic lesions. Arterioscler Thromb Vasc Biol 20:1262–1275
8. Falk E, Shah PK, Fuster V (1995) Coronary plaque disruption. Circulation 92:657–671
9. Vanhoenacker PK, Heijenbrok-Kal MH, Van Heste R, et al (2007). Diagnostic performance of multidetector CT angiography for assessment of coronary artery disease: meta-analysis. Radiology 244:419–4
10. Gershlick AH, de Belder M, Chambers J, et al (2007) Role of non-invasive imaging in the management of coronary artery disease: an assessment of likely change over the next 10 years. A report from the British Cardiovascular Society Working Group. Heart 93:423–431
11. Time Magazine (2005) Cover page. How to stop a heart attack before it happens. Amazingly detailed new Heart Scans help doctors spot trouble without surgery. How technology could save your life. Sept 5, 2005
12. Sechtem UP (2007) Computed Tomography coronary angiography: what is the hype, the reality, and the future? Dial Cardiovasc Med 2123–132
13. Picano E (2004) Sustainability of medical imaging. Education and Debate. BMJ 328:578–580
14. Brenner DJ, Hall EJ (2007) Computed tomography–an increasing source of radiation exposure. N Engl J Med 357:2277–2284
15. Bonow RO (2005) New windows on the heart. Advances in Cardiovascular Imaging. Interview with Anthony N DeMaria. Cardiosource. American College of Cardiology. September 5
16. Picano E (2004). Informed consent and communication of risk from radiological and nuclear medicine examinations: how to escape from a communication inferno. Education and debate. BMJ 329:849–851
17. Thompson RC, Cullom SJ (2006) Issues regarding radiation dosage of cardiac nuclear and radiography procedures. J Nucl Cardiol 13:19–23
18. Wijns W, De Bruyne B, Vanhoenacker PK (2007) What does the clinical cardiologist need from noninvasive cardiac imaging: is it time to adjust practices to meet evolving demands? J Nucl Cardiol 14:366–370
19. Möhlenkamp S, Schmermund A, Lehmann N, et al (2008) Subclinical coronary atherosclerosis and resting ECG abnormalities in an unselected general population. Atherosclerosis 196:786–794
20. Kronmal RA, McClelland RL, Detrano R, et al (2007) Risk factors for the progression of coronary artery calcification in asymptomatic subjects: results from the Multi-Ethnic Study of Atherosclerosis (MESA). Circulation 115:2722–2730
21. Pignoli P, Tremoli E, Poli A, et al (1986) Intimal plus medial thickness of the arterial wall: a direct measurement with ultrasound imaging. Circulation 74:1399–1406
22. Roman MJ, Naqvi TZ, Gardin JM, et al; American Society of Echocardiography; Society of Vascular Medicine and Biology (2006) Clinical application of noninvasive vascular ultrasound in cardiovascular risk stratification: a report from the American Society of Echocardiography and the Society of Vascular Medicine and Biology. J Am Soc Echocardiogr 19:943–954
23. Lee CI, Forman HP (2008) The hidden costs of CT bioeffects. J Am Coll Radiol 5:78–79
24. Hermann F, Martinoff S, Meyer T, et al (2008) Reduction of radiation dose estimates in cardiac 64-slice CT angiography in patients after coronary artery bypass graft surgery. Invest Radiol 43:253–260

25. Delhaye D, Remy-Jardin M, Rozel C, et al (2007) Coronary artery imaging during preoperative CT staging: preliminary experience with 64-slice multidetector CT in 99 consecutive patients. Eur Radiol 17:591–602

26. Morin RL, Gerber TC, McCollough CH (2003) Radiation dose in computed tomography of the heart. Circulation 107:917–922

27. Einstein AJ, Henzlova MJ, Rajagopalan S (2007) Estimating risk of cancer associated with radiation exposure from 64-slice computed tomography coronary angiography. JAMA 298:317–323

28. Alkadhi H, Scheffel H, Desbiolles L, et al (2008) Dual-source computed tomography coronary angiography: influence of obesity, calcium load, and heart rate on diagnostic accuracy. Eur Heart J 29:766–776

29. Semelka RC, Armao DM, Elias J Jr, et al (2007) Imaging strategies to reduce the risk of radiation in CT studies, including selective substitution with MRI. J Magn Reson Imaging 25:900–909

30. Hausleiter J, Meyer T, Hermann F et al (2009) Estimated radiation dose associated with cardiac CT angioplasty. JAMA 301:500–507

31. Brix G, Beyer T (2005) PET/CT: dose-escalated image fusion? Nuklearmedizin 44:S51–S57

32. Committee to Assess Health Risks from Exposure to Low Levels of Ionizing Radiation; Nuclear and Radiation Studies Board, Division on Earth and Life Studies, National Research Council of the National Academies (2006) Health risks from exposure to low levels of ionizing radiation: BEIR VII Phase 2. The National Academies Press, Washington, DC. Available at: http://www.nap.edu/reportbrief/11340rb.pdf

33. Gibbons RJ, Abrams J, Chatterjee K, et al; American College of Cardiology; American Heart Association Task Force on practice guidelines (Committee on the Management of Patients With Chronic Stable Angina). (2003) ACC/AHA 2002 guideline update for the management of patients with chronic stable angina-summary article: a report of the American College of Cardiology/American Heart Association Task Force on practice guidelines. Committee on the Management of Patients With Chronic Stable Angina. J Am Coll Cardiol 41:159K–168K

34. Nixdorff U, Küfner C, Achenbach S, et al (2008) Head-to-head comparison of dobutamine stress echocardiography and cardiac computed tomography for the detection of significant coronary artery disease. Cardiology 110:81–86

35. Fox K, Garcia MA, Ardissino D, et al; Task Force on the Management of Stable Angina Pectoris of the European Society of Cardiology; ESC Committee for Practice Guidelines (CPG) (2006) Guidelines on the management of stable angina pectoris: executive summary: the Task Force on the Management of Stable Angina Pectoris of the European Society of Cardiology. Eur Heart J 27:1341–1381

36. Schuijf JD, Wijns W, Jukema JW, et al (2006) Relationship between noninvasive coronary angiography with multi-slice computed tomography and myocardial perfusion imaging. J Am Coll Cardiol 48:2508–2514

37. Topol EJ, Ellis SG, Cosgrove DM, et al (1993) Analysis of coronary angioplasty practice in the United States with an insurance-claims data base. Circulation 87:1489–1497

38. Boden WE, O'Rourke RA, Teo KK, et al; COURAGE Trial Research Group (2007) Optimal medical therapy with or without PCI for stable coronary disease. N Engl J Med 356:1503–1516

39. Hendel RC, Patel MR, Kramer CM, et al; American College of Cardiology Foundation Quality Strategic Directions Committee Appropriateness Criteria Working Group; American College of Radiology; Society of Cardiovascular Computed Tomography; Society for Cardiovascular Magnetic Resonance; American Society of Nuclear Cardiology; North American Society for Cardiac Imaging; Society for Cardiovascular Angiography and Interventions; Society of Interventional Radiology (2006) 2006 appropriateness criteria for cardiac computed tomog-

raphy and cardiac magnetic resonance imaging: a report of the American College of Cardiology Foundation Quality Strategic Directions Committee Appropriateness Criteria Working Group, American College of Radiology, Society of Cardiovascular Computed Tomography, Society for Cardiovascular Magnetic Resonance, American Society of Nuclear Cardiology, North American Society for Cardiac Imaging, Society for Cardiovascular Angiography and Interventions, and Society of Interventional Radiology. J Am Coll Cardiol 48:1475–1497

40. Douglas PS, Khandheria B, Stainback RF, et al; American College of Cardiology Foundation; American Society of Echocardiography; American College of Emergency Physicians; American Heart Association; American Society of Nuclear Cardiology; Society for Cardiovascular Angiography and Interventions; Society of Cardiovascular Computed Tomography; Society for Cardiovascular Magnetic Resonance (2008) ACCF/ASE/ACEP/AHA/ASNC/SCAI/SCCT/SCMR 2008 appropriateness criteria for stress echocardiography: a report of the American College of Cardiology Foundation Appropriateness Criteria Task Force, American Society of Echocardiography, American College of Emergency Physicians, American Heart Association, American Society of Nuclear Cardiology, Society for Cardiovascular Angiography and Interventions, Society of Cardiovascular Computed Tomography, and Society for Cardiovascular Magnetic Resonance endorsed by the Heart Rhythm Society and the Society of Critical Care Medicine. J Am Coll Cardiol 51:1127–1147

41. Cuocolo A, Adam A (2007) The "White paper of the European Association of Nuclear Medicine (EANM) and the European Society of Radiology (ESR) on multimodality imaging": a message from the EANM and ESR Presidents. Eur J Nucl Med Mol Imaging 34:1145–1146

42. Picano E, Mathias W Jr, Pingitore A, et al (1994) Safety and tolerability of dobutamine-atropine stress echocardiography: a prospective, multicentre study. Echo Dobutamine International Cooperative Study Group. Lancet 344:1190–1192

43. Varga A, Garcia MA, Picano E, International Stress Echo Complication Registry (2006) Safety of stress echocardiography (from the International Stress Echo Complication Registry). Am J Cardiol 98:541–543

44. Newburger JW, Takahashi M, Gerber MA, et al; Committee on Rheumatic Fever, Endocarditis, and Kawasaki Disease, Council on Cardiovascular Disease in the Young, American Heart Association (2004) Diagnosis, treatment, and long-term management of Kawasaki disease: a statement for health professionals from the Committee on Rheumatic Fever, Endocarditis, and Kawasaki Disease, Council on Cardiovascular Disease in the Young, American Heart Association. Pediatrics 114:1708–1733

45. European Commission (2006) Radiation protection 118: referral guidelines for imaging. http://europa.eu.int/comm/environment/radprot/118/rp-118-en.pdf (accessed 10 January 2001)

46. Meijboom WB, van Mieghem CA, Mollet NR, et al (2007) 64-slice computed tomography coronary angiography in patients with high, intermediate, or low pretest probability of significant coronary artery disease. J Am Coll Cardiol 50:1469–1475

47. Marcus ML, Skorton DJ, Johnson MR, et al (1988) Visual estimates of percent diameter coronary stenosis: "a battered gold standard." J Am Coll Cardiol 11:882–885

48. Picano E (2003) Special article. Stress echocardiography: a historical perspective. Am J Med 114:126–130

49. Lee CI, Haims AH, Monico EP, et al (2004) Diagnostic CT scans: assessment of patient, physician, and radiologist awareness of radiation dose and possible risks. Radiology 231:393–398

50. Correia MJ, Hellies A, Andreassi MG, et al (2005) Lack of radiological awareness among physicians working in a tertiary-care cardiological centre. Int J Cardiol 105:307–311

51. Abbott BG, Zaret BL (2003).Contemporary cardiology and hysteric nucleophobia. Am J Med 114:131–134

52. Bedetti G, Botto N, Andreassi MG, et al (2008) Cumulative patient effective dose in cardiology. Br J Radiol May 28
53. Amis ES Jr, Butler PF, Applegate KE, et al; American College of Radiology (2007) American College of Radiology White Paper on Radiation Dose in Medicine. J Am Coll Radiol 4:272–284
54. Husmann L, Valenta I, Gaemperli O, et al (2008) Feasibility of low-dose coronary CT angiography: first experience with prospective ECG-gating. Eur Heart J 29:191–197
55. Bluemke DA, Achenbach S, Budoff M, et al (2008) Noninvasive coronary artery imaging. Magnetic resonance angiography and multidetector computed tomography angiography. A scientific statement from the American Heart Association Committee on Cardiovascular Imaging and Intervention of the Council on Cardiovascular Radiology and Intervention, and the Councils on Clinical Cardiology and Cardiovascular Disease in the Young. Circulation Jun 27

Eugenio Picano and Juerg Schwitter

40.1
Coronary Artery Disease Detection by CMR: The Rich Cardiologist's Super Stress Echocardiography?

Recently, cardiovascular magnetic resonance (CMR) imaging has emerged as a new non-invasive imaging modality providing high-resolution images in any desired plane of the heart, combined with the potential to assess and monitor left and right ventricular function [1, 2]. Although early attempts to use stress CMR, combined with dipyridamole [3] or dobutamine [4] stress, with standard (low-temporal resolution) gradient echo techniques date back to the early 1990s, the scientific and clinical interest in stress CMR rose strikingly in the last 5 years as a consequence of technological improvements (Table 40.1). To assess cardiac function, cine MR imaging is performed with gradient echo pulse sequences. Between 20 and 30 frames with a temporal resolution of 50 ms or less are usually sufficient to evaluate the entire cardiac cycle and are displayed in a cine loop, allowing a dynamic read with the same format, projections, segment assignment (17-segment model), and reading criteria (from 1 = normal to 4 = dyskinetic) as for stress echocardiography [5]. Gradient echo images provide an excellent contrast between intracavitary blood and the endocardium without the use of contrast medium and provide and accurate delineation of the endocardium and epicardium.

Wall motion can be assessed by CMR at rest and during stress. Over the years, the initial standard cine gradient echo images changed into the tremendously improved temporal resolution of new steady-state free precession (SSFP) pulse sequences. Together with technical improvements in patient monitoring within the magnet as well as due to the reduction in imaging time with accelerated pharmacological stress protocols, stress CMR with wall motion analysis has become more feasible and more accurate. CMR also has the potential of assessing myocardial perfusion, by visualizing the first pass of a conventional gadolinium-based MR contrast medium (perfusion CMR) [6–8].

In perfusion CMR, the acquisition is performed during CMR injection while hyperemia is induced pharmacologically (generally by means of adenosine or dipyridamole). This is methodologically and conceptually different from the late gadolinium enhancement

40

Table 40.1 Versatility of CMR for coronary artery disease detection

Method (image mode)	WM rest	WM stress ischemia	Viability	Hyperemia optional: rest	Coronary artery anomalies
			Parameter		
Cine SSFP acquisitions	√	√			
Late gadolinium enhancement (LGE)			√		
Low-dose dobutamine CMR			√		
First-pass perfusion CMR				√	
Rest 3D acquisitions with navigators					√

WM wall motion, *SSFP* steady-state free precession, *LGE* late gadolinium enhancement (imaging 15–20 min after contrast medium injection depending on dose injected)

(LGE) technique for scar detection, which is performed at rest (no stress required) and after several minutes from contrast medium injection, since the redistribution phase in the tissue (and not the first-pass effect in the vessels) is the diagnostic target. CMR visualizes directly myocardial scar as hyperenhanced areas in T1-weighted images [9–11] (Fig. 40.1). The high spatial resolution of contrast-enhanced MR imaging now makes it possible to visualize microinfarcts associated with successful percutaneous coronary intervention, as well as the detection of subendocardial infarcts, which do not exhibit a wall motion abnormality (Fig. 40.2) but still may have prognostic significance [12]. Newer developments for respiratory motion correction possibly in combination with 3-T scanners will hopefully also allow for the assessment of coronary anatomy with an accuracy similar to multislice computed tomography – and without radiation burden or sensitivity to calcium artifacts. To date, clinically useful imaging of the coronary arteries is restricted to identification of the origin and course of anomalous coronary arteries and of bypass grafts [13].

40.2
Stress CMR: Advantages and Limitations

Major advantages of CMR are the radiation-free, nonionizing nature and the tremendous versatility (Table 40.2) of the information supplied, also independent of acoustic window. Another major asset, especially valuable today in research-oriented contexts, is the possibility of quantification of volumes, global function, and scar mass. Due to the high spatial resolution of CMR scar imaging, the transmural extent of scar is easily quantifiable. In some research laboratories, software is available also for regional function quantification [14–17]. Perfusion quantification is currently still demanding with more robust approaches, which

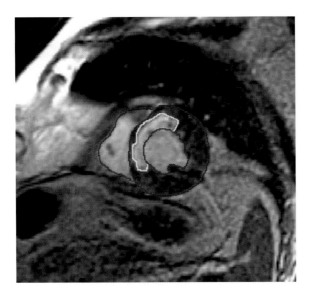

Fig. 40.1 A delayed enhancement image showing a subendocardial scar in the septal and anterior region

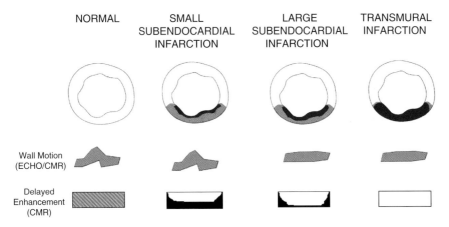

Fig. 40.2 Different levels of transmural myocardial scar induce different levels of echocardiographic and CMR (wall motion) and CMR-specific (delayed enhancement) changes. For 10–30% subendocardial scar involvement, scar is detectable only by CMR and remains functionally silent on the basis of standard conventional regional wall motion changes

also worked in larger studies using, for example, the upslope of the myocardial signal during first pass as a perfusion-linked parameter [7, 18], while absolute quantification of perfusion in ml/min/g tissue is not yet established for coronary artery disease detection by perfusion CMR [7, 19].

Table 40.2 Stress CMR: advantages and limitations

	Advantages	Limitations
Nonionizing energy	+++	
Availability, costs, expertise, skills of operators, personnel		—
Versatility (function, perfusion, scar, viability, flow)	+++	
Stress (dobutamine) stressful		–
Independent of acoustic window	++	
Claustrophobia, metallic clips, pacemakers, etc.		—
Quantification possible for volumes, global function, scar	++	
Contrast medium toxicity (NSF) in renal failure		—

NSF nephrogenic systemic fibrosis. Approximately 250 cases confirmed out of approximately 140 million contrast medium applications. Cyclic contrast medium for magnetic resonance appear not to cause nephrogenic systemic sclerosis (as of June 2007)

The main limitations of CMR include time-consuming data acquisition and analysis and the fact that not all patients can be studied, since pacemakers and metallic clips are still a contraindication for CMR. Additional concern arose regarding the use of contrast medium in patients with impairment of renal function. Paramagnetic contrast media have long been considered absolutely safe and well tolerated. Recently, in May 2007, the FDA (and EMEA) ordered a "boxed warning" on the safety of gadolinium-containing contrast agents, on the basis of 200 cases of nephrogenic systemic fibrosis (NSF) that occurred in patients with kidney failure after administration of some types of gadolinium-based contrast media (linear chelates). In NSF (also called nephrogenic fibrosing dermopathy, NFD), patients develop tight and rigid skin making it difficult to bend joints. NSF/NFD may also result in fibrosis, or sclerosis, of body organs resulting in the inability of body organs to work properly and can lead to death [20]. Cost and safety concerns should lead to a prudent use of contrast media, especially in patients with kidney failure [21]. In this regard, it is important to emphasize that excellent diagnostic accuracy can be reached by CMR simply on the basis of regional wall motion analysis, which does not require contrast medium. Availability of CMR is still a limitation, but the market is growing fast, with a +762% increase of use of cardiac CMR from year 2003 to year 2005 according to Medicare [22].

40.3
Stress Echocardiography vs. Stress CMR

The recent experience with stress CMR for coronary artery disease detection with state-of-the-art technology has been characterized by the attempt to evaluate wall motion (stress dobutamine CMR) [4, 23] and perfusion imaging (stress adenosine or dipyridamole CMR) [3, 7, 24–27]. It is well known from cardiac stress imaging experience over the last 20 years that wall motion and perfusion provide partially different information, and each one has its strengths and weaknesses [28–30]. Regional wall motion abnormalities are more specific, identify trouble-makers in the short run, require true subendocardial myocardial ischemia, and are best suited to assess the effects of medical antiischemic therapy (Fig. 40.3). Perfusion or flow heterogeneity is more sensitive, can identify trouble-makers in the long-run [31–33], does not require true subendocardial ischemia but only perfusion heterogeneity, which may frequently occur with mild-to-moderate coronary stenosis or even with normal coronary arteries and concomitant microvascular disease, and is less affected by concomitant antiischemic therapy at the time of testing [34, 35] (Fig. 40.4). CMR evaluates perfusion by means of contrast medium first-pass kinetics, and stress echocardiography coronary flow reserve through Doppler flow velocity. CMR requires paramagnetic contrast

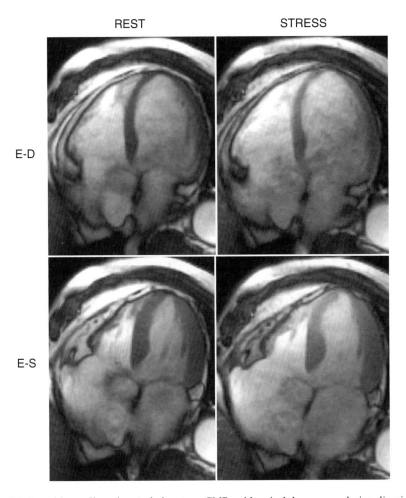

Fig. 40.3 A positive wall motion study by stress CMR, with apical dyssynergy during dipyridamole stress. (Courtesy of Dr. Alessandro Pingitore, modified from [27])

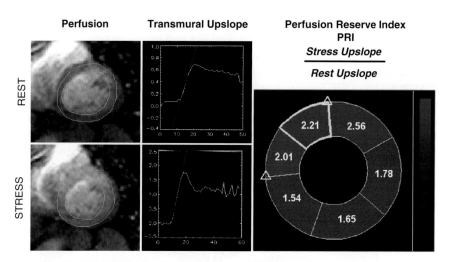

Fig. 40.4 A positive perfusion study with stress CMR, with blunted increase in perfusion in the anteroseptal region. (Courtesy of Dr. Alessandro Pingitore)

medium, whereas ultrasound contrast medium is often not needed with stress echocardiography. A perfusion reserve approach is typically applied when flow is measured in a vessel for which the supply territory is not known, thereby providing some measure of indexing by normalizing hyperemic flow with resting flow. If perfusion in the tissue is measured as, for example, by perfusion CMR, the supply territory is known, as the volume is known in which perfusion is measured (x- and y- resolution time slice thickness). Consequently, "normalization" by resting flow appears unnecessary, and in fact it adds substantial confounding factors which govern resting perfusion (and for which no correction is available) [35]. Not surprisingly, PET perfusion studies repeatedly showed closer correlations between area stenoses in coronary arteries and hyperemic flow than with flow reserve [36, 37]. Other serious concerns regarding a flow reserve approach would need absolute quantification of perfusion, which is currently not possible by CMR and, in addition, geometrical match of myocardial tissue for stress and rest situation (with large differences in heart rate and therefore filling) is difficult. In addition, the multicenter perfusion CMR trials, all with high diagnostic yield, used hyperemic perfusion data only [24, 38]. Direct comparative studies will be needed to answer the questions of whether stress only or stress–rest protocols should be used for perfusion CMR.

An important difference between CMR and echocardiography regards the use of stresses. Ideally, one would like to catch "two birds with one stone," i.e., to assess function and perfusion with only one stress. As a matter of fact, usually dobutamine is used for function assessment, and dipyridamole (or adenosine) for perfusion assessment. With echocardiography, high doses of dipyridamole given with a fast, accelerated infusion protocol allow one to have the same sensitivity as high-dose dobutamine [30, 39] and also to simultaneously assess coronary flow velocity with a maximal hyperemic stimulus [40]. This has been less used with CMR, probably also for a methodological reason, since perfusion CMR is sensitive for motion during data acquisition. This problem can be mitigated by acquiring data during phases of minimal cardiac motion (end-diastole and end-systole) but would become a limiting factor if perfusion data acquisition should take place at high heart rates [7, 41].

In front of largely comparable diagnostic and likely prognostic information, which tends to be better for CMR in patients with difficult acoustic window especially in challenging segments such as the inferior wall [42], there are differences between the two techniques. Echocardiography can be combined with any form of physical (such as exercise) and pharmacological stress, whereas exercise stress (which is the first choice in coronary artery disease patients able to exercise, and the only choice for stress testing in valvular heart disease patients) is currently not feasible in a clinical setting with CMR. The cost of CMR is considerably higher than for echocardiography [1], and the availability is certainly lower for CMR. Stress echocardiography is portable and can be made at the bedside, and this is a crucial advantage in some clinical settings such as patients with acute chest pain. The safety is certainly excellent, for any given stress, in the echocardiography laboratory, since the on-line imaging and hand contact of the sonographer and nurse with the patient in an unrestricted environment, with ECG and blood pressure monitoring, allow for early detection of complications and instantaneous treatment. In the stress CMR laboratory, ischemia during stress is detectable in early stages due to the generally good imaging conditions; however, in the case of emergencies, the scanner environment necessitates special equipment and training of all personnel, and thus, efforts to ensure safe studies in the MR scanner are substantial [43] especially with dobutamine, which is known to be associated with threefold more frequent life-threatening complications compared with dipyridamole or adenosine (1 in 300 vs. 1 in 900) [44, 45]. The safety and cost gap in favor of stress echocardiography is further enhanced by the strict need of paramagnetic contrast in stress CMR to evaluate coronary artery disease. However, for stress echocardiography the contrast is rarely used for enhancement of left ventricular border detection or coronary flow reserve assessment of the left anterior descending artery, and contrast perfusion imaging is not a viable clinical option today for stress echocardiography. A major advantage, especially in research-oriented environments and for scientific protocols, is that stress CMR is much better equipped for a convenient quantification of tissue structure – even in a transmural sense, separating subendocardial from subepicardial layers [46]. For assessment of myocardial function by CMR, reliable (semi)-automatic quantification is still not available, but newer methods, particularly tagging techniques hold promise for achieving this goal in the near future [14–16]. Regarding quantification of myocardial perfusion by CMR, it should be kept in mind that hemodynamically relevant stenosis can be detected with state-of-the art CMR today, implicating that changes in myocardial perfusion in the range of several ml/min/g tissue are detected, for instance, by calculating "upslope" maps and comparing them with normal data [7, 18]. No larger trials are currently available to demonstrate that smaller changes in perfusion, such that might be caused by microcirculatory alterations, are detectable by perfusion CMR, and therefore at least for a clinical application no reliable quantitative CMR methods are available. These quantifications are theoretically possible with echocardiography, for instance, with myocardial velocity imaging, but de facto impossible and/or irreproducible in a clinical setting – although recently developed angle-independent techniques such as speckle tracking or real-time three-dimensional stress echocardiography show some potential in this regard (Table 40.3).

40

Table 40.3 Stress CMR vs. stress echocardiography (*echo*)

	CMR	Stress echo
Cost	+++	+
Availability	+	+++
Portability	No	Yes
Wall motion	Yes	Yes
Perfusion (CMR)/Flow (echo)	Yes	Yes (LAD only)
Contrast material needed	Yes	Usually no
Stress: inotropic	Dob	Ex, dob, dip
Stress: hyperemia	Ado, dip	Dip, ado
Safety profile	Good	Good
Imaging time	>1 h	<30 min
Operator dependence	Yes	Substantial
Dependence on acoustic window	No	Yes
Quantification: LV volumes, global function	Very accurate	Accurate
Quantification: RV volumes, scar	Accurate	Difficult
Absolute quantification: regional function, perfusion	Possible, not (yet) well validated	Difficult
Transmurality visible (perfusion, function, scar)	Possible	Not possible

Ado adenosine; *Dip* dipyridamole; *Ex* Exercise; *LV* left ventricle; *RV* right ventricle

40.4
Clinical Implications

In a high-volume tertiary care referral center for cardiac imaging, stress CMR may play a clinically relevant role today witnessed by the growth of demand in this specific field. Looking at the guidelines of the European Society of Cardiology, published in 2006 and summarized in Table 4, CMR techniques were not yet included for clinical utilization. However, at the time of data collection for these guidelines, the relevant comparative CMR trials were not yet available. In the past few years, several multicenter perfusion CMR trials, in particular the multicenter, multivendor MR-IMPACT I and II [24, 38], demonstrated an excellent performance in detecting coronary artery disease. As these MR-IMPACT trials are also the largest multicenter single-photon emission computed tomography (SPECT) trials utilizing state-of-the-art technology and radioactive tracers, perfusion CMR can be compared with SPECT. In both trials, perfusion CMR outperformed SPECT and it appears reasonable to recommend perfusion CMR, provided the institution features adequate expertise in this technique, as a first-line technique when myocardial perfusion (a high sensitivity, high negative predictive value gatekeeper) is the desired diagnostic end point. When regional wall motion abnormality (a high specificity, high positive predictive

Table 40.4 Appropriate indications for stress CMR (from [29])

1. Detection of coronary artery disease in symptomatic patients
• Evaluation of chest pain syndrome *and*
• Intermediate pretest patient probability of coronary artery disease
2. Detection of myocardial viability
• Left ventricular function <35% *and*
• Viability assessment important for decision-making

value gatekeeper) is the preferred diagnostic option, stress echocardiography is the most cost-effective choice, and functional CMR can still be an excellent second choice when stress echocardiography is unfeasible and/or inconclusive (Fig. 40.5). A similar approach can also be used for the assessment of myocardial viability (Fig. 40.6). In many patients a simple resting transthoracic echocardiography study can show signs of necrosis, in the presence of a thinned, hyperechoic, and dyskinetic wall [47]. In patients with preserved end-diastolic thickness, low-dose dobutamine can show a regional and global inotropic reserve of established prognostic value in predicting a good response to medical therapy, revascularization, and cardiac resynchronization therapy [48–50]. However, in patients with difficult echocardiography studies or ambiguous response, LGE can be an excellent diagnostic option [51], does not require any stress, and today is probably the true gold standard for viability identification and quantification. Low-dose dobutamine CMR can also be performed with the same methodology and interpretation criteria as low-dose do-butamine [52].

Compared with stress echocardiography, stress CMR is more costly and complex, and probably less safe. It is, however, less operator- and patient-dependent, and shares with echocardiography the nonionizing nature of the employed energy, which allows a totally radiation-free noninvasive assessment of the patient. This is a decisive asset for the refer-ring physician and the patient, who will invariably decide to go for CMR when informed of the radiation dose of a stress scintigraphy, ranging from 500 to 1,500 chest X-rays [53, 54]. This is especially important if we consider the societal implications of stress imaging, and the fact that small individual risks multiplied by billion examinations become a significant population risk [55–57]. For instance, today about 10 million stress perfusion scintigraphies are performed every year in the USA. Considering an average dose exposure of 1,000 chest X-rays per exam, this yields a risk of 1 in 500 for a 50-year-old man and a cumulative popu-lation risk of 20,000 new cancers each year [55] (Fig. 40.7). The abatement of long-term oncogenic risk is also important for a correct cost–benefit (not only risk–benefit) assessment. For a resting cardiac imaging test, the average cost (not changes) of an echocardiogram being equal to 1 (as a cost comparator), the cost of a SPECT is 3.2×, and of a cardiovascular magnetic resonance study 5.51× higher [1]. However, long-term downstream costs should also be included in a correct cost-effective analysis, and this makes CMR even more attractive when compared with SPECT [58]. For functional (wall motion) stress imaging, dobutamine CMR should not be used as a "rich doctor's super stress echocardiography," as a first-line tool to evaluate left ventricular function under stress: this would be a waste of resources, in many cases, with no benefit for the patient and the system. It should be used, rather, as the "smart

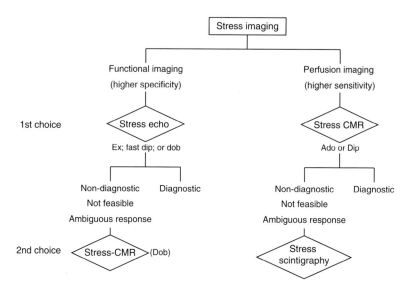

Fig. 40.5 The proposed diagnostic algorithm for the diagnosis of coronary artery disease in a radiation risk-conscious environment

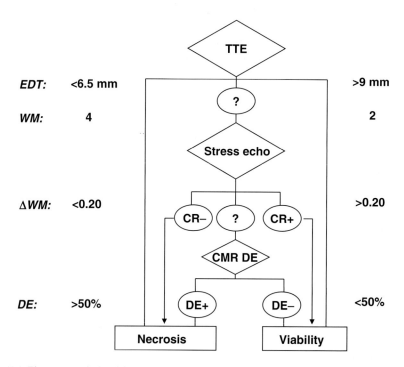

Fig. 40.6 The proposed algorithm for the diagnosis of myocardial viability in a radiation risk-conscious environment. *CR* contractile reserve, *DE* delayed enhancement, *EDT* end-diastolic thickness, *WM* wall motion (from 1 = normal; 2 = hypokinetic; 3 = akinetic; 4 = dyskinetic)

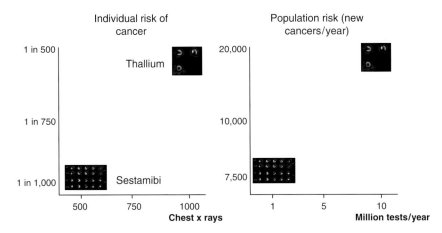

Fig. 40.7 Stress imaging from the individual (*left panel*) and societal (*right panel*) perspective. Each year in the USA 10 million scintigraphy studies are performed. The radiological dose of a stress perfusion scintigraphy ranges from 600 (sestamibi) to 1,600 (thallium or dual isotope) chest X-rays. The average individual risk per exam considering the average dose of 1,000 chest X-rays is 1 cancer every 500 exposed patients (*left panel*) and translates into a population risk of 20,000 new cancers per year (*right panel*)

cardiologist's second choice," when stress echocardiography is not feasible and/or yields ambiguous results. For perfusion imaging, stress CMR (with adenosine or dipyridamole) can already be used as "the smart cardiologists' SPECT." In fact, when compared with stress SPECT, stress CMR has no radiation exposure ("smart patient's SPECT") and at least comparable accuracy. Regarding viability assessment, low-dose dobutamine echocardiography is well established as a specific test to predict recovery of function. In ambiguous situations, particularly with high interventional risk due to severely reduced global left ventricular function, LGE of CMR can add valuable information to predict outcome after surgery [52]. In this way, we reconcile the top priority of granting the patient the highest possible quality of care with the principle of optimizing use of resources and minimizing long-term risks of radiation exposure [61], as recommended today by the European Union EURATOM law [59], European Commission medical imaging referral guidelines [60], and most authoritative scientific societies [61].

References

1. Pennell DJ, Sechtem UP, Higgins CB, et al; Society for Cardiovascular Magnetic Resonance; Working Group on Cardiovascular Magnetic Resonance of the European Society of Cardiology (2004) Clinical indications for cardiovascular magnetic resonance (CMR): Consensus Panel report. Eur Heart J 25:1940–1965
2. American College of Radiology; Society of Cardiovascular Computed Tomography; Society for Cardiovascular Magnetic Resonance; American Society of Nuclear Cardiology; North American Society for Cardiac Imaging; Society for Cardiovascular Angiography

40

and Interventions; Society of Interventional Radiology (2006) ACCF/ACR/SCCT/SCMR/ASNC/NASCI/SCAI/SIR 2006 appropriateness criteria for cardiac computed tomography and cardiac magnetic resonance imaging. A report of the American College of Cardiology Foundation Quality Strategic Directions Committee Appropriateness Criteria Working Group. J Am Coll Radiol 3:751–771

3. Pennell DJ, Underwood SR, Ell PJ, et al (1990) Dipyridamole magnetic resonance imaging: a comparison with thallium-201 emission tomography. Br Heart J 64:362–369

4. Pennell DJ, Underwood SR, Manzara CC, et al (1992). Magnetic resonance imaging during dobutamine stress in coronary artery disease. Am J Cardiol 70:34–40

5. Cerqueira MD, Weissman NJ, Dilsizian V, et al; American Heart Association Writing Group on Myocardial Segmentation and Registration for Cardiac Imaging (2002) Standardized myocardial segmentation and nomenclature for tomographic imaging of the heart. A statement for healthcare professionals from the Cardiac Imaging Committee of the Council on Clinical Cardiology of the American Heart Association. Int J Cardiovasc Imaging 18:539–542

6. Schwitter J (2007) Perfusion cardiovascular magnetic resonance: will it replace SPECT? Dialogues Cardiovasc Med 12:114–122

7. Schwitter J, Nanz D, Kneifel S, et al (2001) Assessment of myocardial perfusion in coronary artery disease by magnetic resonance: a comparison with positron emission tomography and coronary angiography. Circulation 103:2230–2235

8. Nagel E, Thouet T, Klein C, et al (2003) Noninvasive determination of coronary blood flow velocity with cardiovascular magnetic resonance in patients after stent deployment. Circulation 107:1738–1743

9. Kim RJ, Wu E, Rafael A, et al (2000) The use of contrast-enhanced magnetic resonance imaging to identify reversible myocardial dysfunction. N Engl J Med 343:1445–1453

10. Thygesen K, Alpert JS, White HD; Joint ESC/ACCF/AHA/WHF Task Force for the Redefinition of Myocardial Infarction (2007) Universal definition of myocardial infarction. Circulation 116:2634–2653

11. Schwitter J, Saeed M, Wendland MF, et al (1997) Influence of severity of myocardial injury on distribution of macromolecules: extravascular versus intravascular gadolinium-based magnetic resonance contrast agents. J Am Coll Cardiol 30:1086–1094

12. Kwong RY, Chan AK, Brown KA, et al (2006) Impact of unrecognized myocardial scar detected by cardiac magnetic resonance imaging on event-free survival in patients presenting with signs or symptoms of coronary artery disease. Circulation 113:2733–2743

13. Hauser TH, Manning WJ (2008) The promise of whole-heart coronary MRI. Curr Cardiol Rep 10:46–50

14. Garot J, Bluemke DA, Osman NF, et al (2000) Fast determination of regional myocardial strain fields from tagged cardiac images using harmonic phase MRI. Circulation 101:981–988

15. Ryf S, Spiegel MA, Gerber M, et al (2002) Myocardial tagging with 3D-CSPAMM. J Magn Reson Imaging 16:320–325

16. Ryf S, Kissinger KV, Spiegel MA, et al (2004) Spiral MR myocardial tagging. Magn Reson Med 51:237–242

17. Epstein FH (2007) MRI of left ventricular function. J Nucl Cardiol 14:729–744

18. Giang TH, Nanz D, Coulden R, et al (2004) Detection of coronary artery disease by magnetic resonance myocardial perfusion imaging with various contrast medium doses: first European multi-centre experience. Eur Heart J 25:1657–1665

19. Schwitter J (2006) Myocardial perfusion imaging by cardiac magnetic resonance. J Nucl Cardiol 13:841–854

20. Ersoy H, Rybicki FJ (2007) Biochemical safety profiles of gadolinium-based extracellular contrast agents and nephrogenic systemic fibrosis. J Magn Reson Imaging 26:1190–1197

21. Gruppo di lavoro SIRM-SIN-AIRN (2007) Fibrosi nefrogenica sistemica: raccomandazioni per l'uso degli agenti di contrasto a base di gadolinio.www.sirm.org. 30 October 2007 Consensus 2007

22. Levin DC, Rao VM, Parker L, Frangos AJ, et al (2008) Ownership or leasing of MRI facilities by nonradiologist physicians is a rapidly growing trend. J Am Coll Radiol 5:105–109

23. Nagel E, Fleck E (1999) Functional MRI in ischemic heart disease based on detection of contraction abnormalities. J Magn Reson Imaging 10:411–417

24. Schwitter J, Wacker CM, van Rossum AC, et al (2008) MR-IMPACT: comparison of perfusion-cardiac magnetic resonance with single-photon emission computed tomography for the detection of coronary artery disease in a multicentre, multivendor, randomized trial. Eur Heart J 29:480–489

25. Jahnke C, Nagel E, Gebker R, et al (2007) Prognostic value of cardiac magnetic resonance stress tests: adenosine stress perfusion and dobutamine stress wall motion imaging. Circulation 115:1769–1776

26. Bodi V, Sanchis J, Lopez-Lereu MP, et al (2007) Prognostic value of dipyridamole stress cardiovascular magnetic resonance imaging in patients with known or suspected coronary artery disease. J Am Coll Cardiol 50:1174–1179

27. Pingitore A, Lombardi M, Scattini B, et al (2008) Head to head comparison between perfusion and function during accelerated high-dose dipyridamole magnetic resonance stress for the detection of coronary artery disease. Am J Cardiol 101:8–14

28. Picano E (1992) Stress echocardiography. From pathophysiological toy to diagnostic tool. Circulation 85:1604–1612

29. Fox K, Garcia MA, Ardissino D, et al; Task Force on the Management of Stable Angina Pectoris of the European Society of Cardiology; ESC Committee for Practice Guidelines (CPG) (2006) Guidelines on the management of stable angina pectoris: executive summary: the Task Force on the Management of Stable Angina Pectoris of the European Society of Cardiology. Eur Heart J 27:1341–1381

30. Sicari R, Nihoyannopoulos P, Evangelista A, et al; European Association of Echocardiography (2008) Stress echocardiography consensus statement of the European Association of Echocardiography. Eur J Echocardiogr 9:415–437

31. Rigo F, Sicari R, Gherardi S, et al (2008) The additive prognostic value of wall motion abnormalities and coronary flow reserve during dipyridamole stress echo. Eur Heart J 29:79–88

32. Cortigiani L, Bigi R, Sicari R, et al (2006) Prognostic value of pharmacological stress echocardiography in diabetic and nondiabetic patients with known or suspected coronary artery disease. J Am Coll Cardiol 47:605–610

33. Sicari R, Cortigiani L, Bigi R, et al; Echo-Persantine International Cooperative (EPIC) Study Group; Echo-Dobutamine International Cooperative (EDIC) Study Group (2004) Prognostic value of pharmacological stress echocardiography is affected by concomitant antiischemic therapy at the time of testing. Circulation 109:2428–2431

34. Sicari R, Rigo F, Gherardi S, et al (2008) The prognostic value of Doppler echocardiographic assessed coronary flow reserve is not affected by concomitant anti-ischemic therapy at the time of testing. Am Heart J 156(3):573–579

35. Schwitter J, DeMarco T, Kneifel S, et al (2000) Magnetic resonance-based assessment of global coronary flow and flow reserve and its relation to left ventricular functional parameters: a comparison with positron emission tomography. Circulation 101:2696–2702

36. Di Carli M, Czernin J, Hoh CK, et al (1995) Relation among stenosis severity, myocardial blood flow, and flow reserve in patients with coronary artery disease. Circulation 91:1944–1951

37. Picano E, Parodi O, Lattanzi F, et al (1994) Assessment of anatomic and physiological severity of single-vessel coronary artery lesions by dipyridamole echocardiography. Comparison with positron emission tomography and quantitative arteriography. Circulation 89:753–761

38. Schwitter J, Wacker C, Wilke N, et al (2006) Magnetic resonance imaging for myocardial perfusion assessment in coronary artery disease trial (MR-IMPACT II): A phase III multicenter, multi-vendor trial comparing perfusion cardiac magnetic resonance versus single photon emission computed tomography for the detection of coronary artery disease. Circulation 114:II 806

39. Picano E, Molinaro S, Pasanisi E (2008) The diagnostic accuracy of pharmacological stress echocardiography for the assessment of coronary artery disease: a meta-analysis. Cardiovasc Ultra 6:30

40. Rigo F, Murer B, Ossena G, et al (2008) Transthoracic echocardiographic imaging of coronary arteries: tips, traps, and pitfalls. Cardiovasc Ultrasound 6:7

41. Schwitter J (2005) Myocardial perfusion in ischemic heart disease. In: Higgins CB, de Roos A (eds) MRI and CT of the Cardiovascular Systeme. Lippincott Williams and Wilkins, Philadelphia

42. Nagel E, Lehmkuhl HB, Bocksch W, et al (1999) Noninvasive diagnosis of ischemia-induced wall motion abnormalities with the use of high-dose dobutamine stress MRI: comparison with dobutamine stress echocardiography. Circulation 99:763–770

43. Wahl A, Paetsch I, Gollesch A, et al (2004) Safety and feasibility of high-dose dobutamine-atropine stress cardiovascular magnetic resonance for diagnosis of myocardial ischaemia: experience in 1000 consecutive cases. Eur Heart J 25:1230–1236

44. Picano E, Mathias W Jr, Pingitore A, et al (1994) Safety and tolerability of dobutamine-atropine stress echocardiography: a prospective, multicentre study. Echo Dobutamine International Cooperative Study Group. Lancet 344:1190–1192

45. Varga A, Garcia MA, Picano E; International Stress Echo Complication Registry (2006) Safety of stress echocardiography (from the International Stress Echo Complication Registry). Am J Cardiol 98:541–543

46. Ryf S, Rutz AK, Boesiger P, et al (2006) Is post-systolic shortening a reliable indicator of myocardial viability? An MR tagging and late-enhancement study. J Cardiovasc Magn Reson 8:445–451

47. Faletra F, Crivellaro W, Pirelli S, et al (1995) Value of transthoracic two-dimensional echocardiography in predicting viability in patients with healed Q-wave anterior wall myocardial infarction. Am J Cardiol 76:1002–1006

48. Picano E, Sicari R, Landi P, et al (1998) Prognostic value of myocardial viability in medically treated patients with global left ventricular dysfunction early after an acute uncomplicated myocardial infarction: a dobutamine stress echocardiographic study. Circulation 98:1078–1084

49. Sicari R, Picano E, Cortigiani L, et al; VIDA (Viability Identification with Dobutamine Administration) Study Group (2003) Prognostic value of myocardial viability recognized by low-dose dobutamine echocardiography in chronic ischemic left ventricular dysfunction. Am J Cardiol 92:1263–1266

50. Ciampi Q, Villari B (2007) Role of echocardiography in diagnosis and risk stratification in heart failure with left ventricular systolic dysfunction. Cardiovasc Ultrasound 5:34

51. Wagner A, Mahrholdt H, Holly TA, et al (2003) Contrast-enhanced MRI and routine single photon emission computed tomography (SPECT) perfusion imaging for detection of subendocardial myocardial infarcts: an imaging study. Lancet 361:374–379

52. Wellnhofer E, Olariu A, Klein C, et al (2004) Magnetic resonance low-dose dobutamine test is superior to SCAR quantification for the prediction of functional recovery. Circulation 109:2172–2174

53. Picano E (2004) Informed consent and communication of risk from radiological and nuclear medicine examinations: how to escape from a communication inferno. BMJ 329:849–851

54. Bedetti G, Pizzi C, Gavaruzzi G, et al (2008) Suboptimal awareness of radiologic dose among patients undergoing cardiac stress scintigraphy. J Am Coll Radiol 5:126–131

55. Picano E (2003) Stress echocardiography: a historical perspective. Special Article. Am J Med 114:126–130
56. Picano E (2004) Sustainability of medical imaging. Education and Debate. BMJ 328:578–580
57. Brenner DJ, Hall EJ (2007) Computed tomography–an increasing source of radiation exposure. N Engl J Med 357:2277–2284
58. Bedetti G, Pasanisi E, Pizzi C, et al (2008) Economic analysis including long-term risks and costs of alternative diagnostic strategies to evaluate patients with chest pain. Cardiovasc Ultrasound 6:21
59. Council Directive 97/43/Euratom of 30 June 1997 on health protection of individuals against the dangers of ionising radiation in relation to medical exposure, and repealing Directive 84/466/Euratom. Official Journal of the European Communities L 180 1997 Jul 9:0022–7
60. European Commission (2001) Radiation protection 118: referral guidelines for imaging. Luxembourg: Office for Official Publications of the European Communities, 2001
61. Amis ES Jr, Butler PF, Applegate KE, et al; American College of Radiology (2007) American College of Radiology white paper on radiation dose in medicine. J Am Coll Radiol 4:272–284

Appropriateness in the Stress Echocardiography Laboratory

41

Eugenio Picano

Every year five billion imaging tests are performed worldwide, and about half of these are cardiovascular examinations [1]. According to recent estimates, 30–50% of all examinations are partially or totally inappropriate, i.e., risks and costs outweighs benefits [2]. Following the definition of the American College of Cardiology Foundation, an appropriate imaging study is one in which the expected incremental information, combined with clinical judgment, exceeds any expected negative consequences by a sufficiently wide margin for a specific indication that the procedure is generally considered acceptable care and a reasonable approach for the indication [3] (Fig. 41.1). Negative consequences include the risks of the procedure itself (i.e., radiation or contrast exposure) and the downstream impact of poor performance such as delay in diagnosis (false-negative results) or inappropriate diagnosis (false-positive results). This implies potential harm for patients undergoing imaging (who take the risks of an imaging study without a commensurate benefit), excessive delay in the waiting lists for other patients needing the examination, and an exorbitant cost for society, with no improvement and possibly with a reduction in care quality [3]. Health care costs in the USA now exceed a stunning two trillion dollars, representing 16% of the country's gross domestic product by 2016, and, in the words of Alan Greenspan, are on "an unsustainable trajectory." Cardiac imaging greatly contributes to this escalation of costs, and stress imaging tests in particular have increased at an annual rate of 6.1% since 1993 in individuals covered by Medicare. Diagnostic imaging has increased more rapidly than any other component of medical care, and echocardiography is the single most frequently used test in the Medicare population, except for laboratory tests [4]. The volume of cardiovascular services increased 5.5% per capita between 2004 and 2005 in the USA, driven largely by the growth of cardiac imaging services [4]. Although the diagnostic and prognostic information provided by these tests is not without a cost, some studies have shown that the use of noninvasive imaging in appropriately selected patients translates into savings because of more appropriate selection of even more expensive procedures [5, 6]. However, these studies involved patients who were appropriately selected for testing; and the trade-off between costs and benefits will not be the same when studies are performed less appropriately [7]. In order to limit the detrimental consequences of the pandemic of inappropriateness and diagnostic obesity, the UK College of Radiology in 1999 [8], the

E. Picano, *Stress Echocardiography*,
© Springer-Verlag Berlin Heidelberg 2009

41

Risk vs Benefit: The code of appropriateness

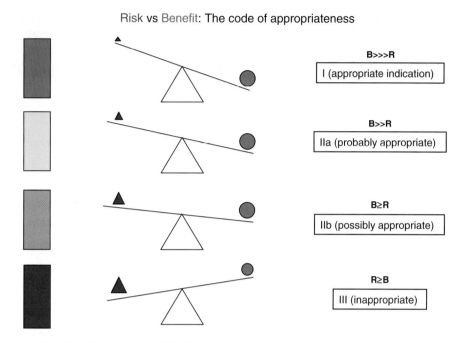

B>>>R

I (appropriate indication)

B>>R

IIa (probably appropriate)

B≥R

IIb (possibly appropriate)

R≥B

III (inappropriate)

Fig. 41.1 The balance between risks (*red triangle*) and benefits (green circle) determining the appropriateness score of testing. The three angles of the red triangle represent acute, subacute, and long-term (radiation) risks. Acute risks occur within seconds and minutes (e.g., death or myocardial infarction during stress or catheterization); subacute risks within days or weeks (e.g., contrast-induced nephropathy); and long-term risks (due to cumulative exposure to ionizing radiation) after years or decades

European Commission in 2001 [9], and more recently the American College of Cardiology [3] have prepared guidelines on appropriateness of general or specialized imaging testing, including stress perfusion scintigraphy [10] and stress echocardiography [11]. The ultimate goal of these documents is to define the appropriate test for the appropriate indication in the appropriate patient: a difficult, elusive, and moving target which is, however, one of the new features, and not the least important, of good-quality medical care [3, 9].

41.1
The Ulysses Syndrome in the Cardiac Imaging Laboratory

The Ulysses syndrome was first described in 1972 by Canadian physician Dr. Mercer Rang, who applied it to the ill effects of extensive diagnostic investigations conducted because of a false-positive or indeterminate result in the course of a routine laboratory screening [12]. Ulysses left Troy in full physical and psychological health. Equipped with a safe ship and a competent crew, he was sure he would return home quickly; instead it turned out that he lost all his crew, his ship, and he was able to make it home only after a journey full of hardship. Today, the most frequent diagnostic investigation is a cardiac imaging test. Mr. Ulysses, a typical middle-aged "worried-well" asymptomatic subject with an A-type coronary personality, a heavy (opium) smoker, leading a stressful life, would be advised to have a cardiological check-up after 10 years of war (Fig. 41.2). The family physician directly refers the patient to the cardiologist (step 2), who suggests a transthoracic echocardiogram (step 3), which is perfectly normal, but with poor visualization of segment 17, the true apex. The patient is again sent to the echocardiography laboratory to repeat the transthoracic echocardiogram with echo-contrast injection (step 4): the apex is perfectly visualized and looks normal. However, just to be on the safe side, the cardiologist suggests a multislice computed tomography (step 5) study. Ulysses accepts enthusiastically since he recently read the front page and cover story of *Time* magazine (5 September 2005) explaining that in this way you can detect asymptomatic life-threatening coronary artery stenosis. The scan shows only minor luminal irregularities of very uncertain pathological meaning. At this point, thallium stress perfusion scintigraphy (step 6) is performed. A very mild, questionable hypoperfusion of the inferobasal wall is documented. The stress echocardiography (step 7) is performed and a very mild apical hypokinesis is observed at peak exercise in presence of marked systolic blood pressure rise. At this point the cardiologist asks for further examinations and Mr. Ulysses becomes increasingly anxious. One after another, Ulysses undergoes a PET-adenosine stress (step 8: marginally positive finding at basal lateral wall) and magnetic resonance imaging with adenosine and gadolinium contrast (step 9: marginally positive finding on the basal inferior septum). The patient is eventually referred for coronary angiography (step 10); the island of Ithaca is crowded with nonsignificant coronary stenoses, unrelated to perfusion defects or wall motion abnormalities, which may, however, trigger the oculostenotic reflex [4] leading to the vicious circle of angioplasty (obviously with drug-eluting stent), imaging test for the diagnosis of silent restenosis, presence of perfusion or wall motion defects, re-angiography, and so on and so forth.

None of these examinations is free, and they all imply a financial and a safety cost. For a resting cardiac imaging test, taking the average cost (not charges) of an echocardiogram as equal to 1 (as a cost comparator), the cost of a CT is 3.1×, of a SPECT 3.2×, of a cardiovascular magnetic resonance imaging 5.51×, of a PET scan 14.03×, and of a right and left heart catheterization 19.95× higher [13]). For stress cardiac imaging, compared with the treadmill exercise test considered as equal to 1 (as a cost comparator), the cost of stress scintigraphy is 2.1×, and of stress SPECT scintigraphy 5.7× higher [14].

There are non-negligible acute risks in several noninvasive imaging techniques. Exercise testing entails a very small but definite risk, and data confirm that there is up to 1 myocardial infarction or death per 2,500 tests [15]. Major, life-threatening side effects (sustained ventricular tachycardia, ventricular fibrillation, and myocardial infarction) occur in about 1 out of 300 dobutamine echocardiography and 1 out of 1,000 dipyridamole echocardiography tests [16, 17]. In general, exercise is safer than pharmacological stress, in which major complications are three times more frequent with dobutamine than with dipyridamole [18, 19].

The use of nephrotoxic contrast agents in large doses with CT imaging is a major concern, since it induces an acute worsening of renal function – not always reversible – in about 10% of patients with impaired renal function [11]. Also with echocardiography, the

41

Ulysses's syndrome

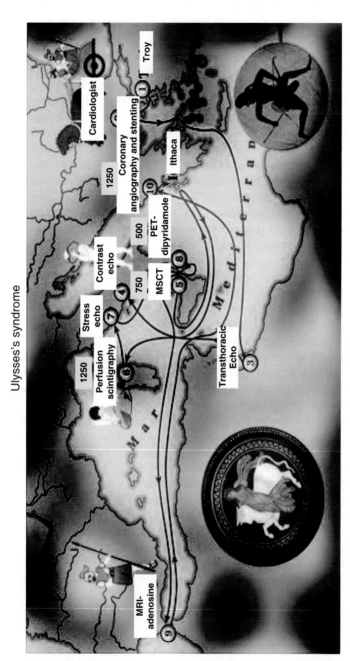

- Total cost: >20,000 €
- Total radio load: 4,000 CXR
- Total serious complication load: 5% (contrast + gadolinium+stress+cath+radiation-induced cancer)

Fig. 41.2 Ulysses' voyage as a metaphor for the diagnostic pathway of the patient with suspected coronary artery disease. At the end of the first round of this odyssey, the cumulative cost is more than 100 times a simple exercise-electrocardiography. The cumulative radiation dose is that of more than 4,000 chest X-rays. The cumulative damage (including acute, subacute, and long-term risks) will cause a serious health detriment (including infarction, renal insufficiency, or cancer) in about 5–10% of patients

use of contrast agents may add an extra risk of about 1 in 10,000 of allergic and life-threatening [20] reactions. Moreover, experimentally, the number of injured cardiomyopathies increased with increasing contrast agent dose and ultrasound exposure [20], possibly due to acoustic cavitation and acoustic current production, which may locally deliver high levels of mechanical energy (higher with increasing power output, mirrored by the mechanical index). Minor side effects (probably due to microembolization of injected bubbles) are frequent in up to 10% of patients, and include headache, nausea and vomiting, dysgeusia, and dyspnea. Major life-threatening side effects are rare but possible, and consist of ventricular tachycardia, pulmonary edema, ventricular fibrillation, and even death. Toxic effects led the FDA to force manufacturers to add a "boxed warning" on Luminity in October 2007, stating that "4 deaths and 110 various nonfatal reactions occurred during or 30 min after the infusion (out of about two million studies)" [21]. Recently, additional concern arose regarding the use of paramagnetic contrast agents during CMR in patients with impairment of renal function. Paramagnetic contrast agents have long been considered absolutely safe and well tolerated. However, in May 2007, the FDA (and EMEA) ordered a boxed warning on the safety of gadolinium-containing contrast agents, on the basis of 200 cases of nephrogenic systemic fibrosis (NSF) that occurred in patients with kidney failure. NSF (also called nephrogenic fibrosing dermopathy, NFD) causes the patient to develop tight and rigid skin making it difficult to bend joints. NSF/NFD may also result in fibrosis, or sclerosis, of body organs resulting in the inability of body organs to work properly and can lead to death [22]. Risks are acute (linked to stress), subacute (linked to contrast use), and long-term (linked to radiation) (Table 41.1).

The rate of complications is obviously higher with invasive imaging procedures. For instance, coronary angiography has a cumulative risk of 1–2% of major complications (including dissection, myocardial infarction, stroke) and 1 in 1,000 risk of death [23]. Contrast-induced nephropathy is the third most common cause of hospital-acquired renal failure, ranging between 3% and 14% in patients with cardiovascular pathology undergoing angiography procedures [24]. All of these risks may be fully acceptable in the presence of a proper indication, but become totally unacceptable if the indication is less than appropriate. More than ten million stress imaging procedures [25] and more than one million coronary angiographies [23] are performed every year in the USA alone. The small individual risk thus becomes an important population burden [26].

Table 41.1 Acute, subacute, and long-term risks in cardiac imaging

	Acute	Subacute	Chronic
Most frequent cause	Stress	Iodinated contrast	Radiation
Timing	Seconds	Days	Years
Examples	Myocardial infarction	Renal failure	Cancer
Cellular target	Endothelium of coronary arteries	Kidney tubular cell	Somatic cells (lung, breast, bone marrow)
Risk per exam	1 in 500 to 1 in 1,000	1 in 50 to 1 in 100	1 in 500 to 1 in 1,000
Cumulative nature	No	No	yes

41

Besides these clearly recognized acute and subacute risks, long-term risks linked to imaging radiation should also be considered. Medical X-rays and γ-rays are a proven human carcinogen [8, 9]. In radiology and nuclear medicine, higher acute doses correspond to higher long-term risks; there are no safe doses, and all doses add up in determining the cumulative risks over a lifetime [8, 9, 27]. Doses of common imaging are reported in yellow in Fig. 41.2, and range from the equivalent of 300 chest X-rays of a coronary angiography to that of 1,250 chest X-rays of a thallium scan [28]. With imaging cumulative doses (radiation expenditure), the patient "buys" increasing risks of developing cancer during their lifetime.

In other words, at the end of the first round of examinations shown in Fig. 41.2, Ulysses paid about 100 times the cost of a simple exercise electrocardiography test – probably all that he needed. He received a 5% cumulative risk of major short-term adverse events (from renal insufficiency to myocardial infarction). He received a cumulative dose exposure of about 4,000 chest X-rays, corresponding to an extra-risk of cancer of 1 in 150. The invasive and interventional procedures that he underwent did not improve his quality of life since he was asymptomatic at the beginning of his cardiological history and the anatomy-driven revascularization will not increase his life expectancy [14, 28, 29]. Periodic follow-up examinations with imaging testing will be scheduled – mostly inappropriately [9] – and the Odyssey will probably last forever.

41.2
Appropriateness in Stress Echocardiography

The proliferation of cardiac stress imaging may represent an added value when appropriate, and an added cost when inappropriate. Unfortunately, the definition of appropriateness is obvious in theory, but not so straightforward on practical grounds. Unlike prevention and treatment strategies supported by evidence-based practice guidelines, the evidence base for imaging is anecdotal, fragmented, and lacking in prospective clinical trials [3]. As a consequence, the process for developing appropriateness criteria is only partially evidence-based and is heavily weighted by expert consensus [3]. On an arbitrary scale of 1 (most inappropriate) to 9 (most appropriate), indications are classified as "appropriate" (score >7, test is generally acceptable and is a reasonable approach for the indication), "uncertain" (score between 4 and 6, test may be generally acceptable and may be a reasonable approach for the indication), and "inappropriate" (score <3, test is not generally acceptable and is not a reasonable approach for the indication). The most frequent appropriate, uncertain, and inappropriate indications met in the clinical practice of high-volume laboratories are listed in Table 41.2 [20]. Following these criteria, only two out of three stress echocardiography (or nuclear stress imaging) tests are appropriate, with similar numbers observed in disparate geographic, cultural, and economic situations – from Italy to Australia [30] to the USA [31] (Fig. 41.3). Of interest, the vast majority of inappropriate studies were restricted to only a few patient indications, with the four most frequent inappropriate indications listed in Table 41.2 accounting for 88% of all inappropriate examinations [31]. This repetitive pattern of inappropriateness points to a need for quality improvement and educational programs to achieve measurable improvement in results [32]. This is

Table 41.2 Most frequent appropriate/uncertain/inappropriate indications in coronary artery disease (*CAD*) detection and/or risk stratification

	Appropriate	Uncertain	Inappropriate
ECG uninterpretable or unable to exercise, or prior stress ECG equivocal	√		
Coronary artery stenosis of unclear significance (CT or angiography)	√		
Postrevascularization not in the early post-procedure period, with change in symptoms	√		
Presurgery, high risk nonemergent, poor exercise tolerance	√		
Viability test in ischemic cardiomyopathy, known CAD, patient eligible for revascularization	√		
Asymptomatic or stable symptoms, repeat stress echo after >5 years		√	
Asymptomatic <5 years after CABG or <2 years after PCI		√	
Asymptomatic, low risk			√
Preop, intermediate risk surgery, good exercise capacity			√
Symptomatic, low pretest probability, interpretable ECG, able to exercise			√

Preop, low-risk surgery, *CT* computed tomography, *CABG* coronary artery bypass graft, *PCI* percutaneous coronary intervention

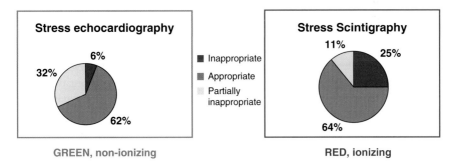

Fig. 41.3 Inappropriateness in stress echocardiography (*left*) and cardiac stress imaging (*right*). Data are derived from [30] (Pisa and Brisbane echocardiography laboratories in Italy and Australia) and [31] (Mayo Clinic nuclear cardiology laboratory in the USA)

especially important today and in view of the projected spectacular rise of cardiac imaging in the next 15 years [33] (Fig. 41.4).

It is certainly good to have multiple imaging tools, which allow us to avoid the contraindications and limitations of each technique and to tailor the best (most effective) test

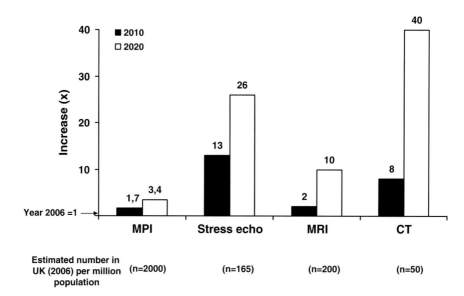

Fig. 41.4 Future trends in the use of cardiac imaging up to the year 2020. (Redrawn from the original data of [33])

in individual patients (Fig. 41.5). The best test choice should also consider the test with the lowest cost – for any given accuracy – and, importantly, the test with the lowest acute, chronic, and long-term risks. This concept is clearly spelled out in guidelines of the UK College of Radiology in 1999 [8], Medical Imaging guidelines in 2001 [9], and the American College of Cardiology guidelines in 2006 [10, 11].

For example, with special regard to the radiation issue, European Union guidelines state that "for instance, because MRI does not use ionizing radiation, MRI should be preferred when both CT and MRI would provide similar information and when both are available." The American College of Cardiology definition of appropriateness defines an imaging study as "one in which the expected incremental information exceeds the negative consequences, which include the risks of the procedure (i.e., radiation or contrast exposure) and the downstream impact of poor test performance."

Imaging technology evolution in the last 30 years was characterized by a shift from one-dimensional (1970s) to a two-dimensional (1980s–1990s) and current three-dimensional representation of the heart provided by all major imaging modalities. The evolution of technology has most likely not always been fully matched by our maturity in using it. We should probably move from a one-dimensional approach to imaging (typical of the 1980s) to the two-dimensional approach (considering cost-effectiveness, not only effectiveness) up to a three-dimensional approach integrating benefit, cost, and risk.

Appropriateness in health care, like quality, can be a moving target and not easy to define. However, it is also true that, as with many quality measures, the very act of having appropriateness criteria and measuring your own appropriateness performance is likely to improve the quality of what is being measured [32]. This needs to be done to improve

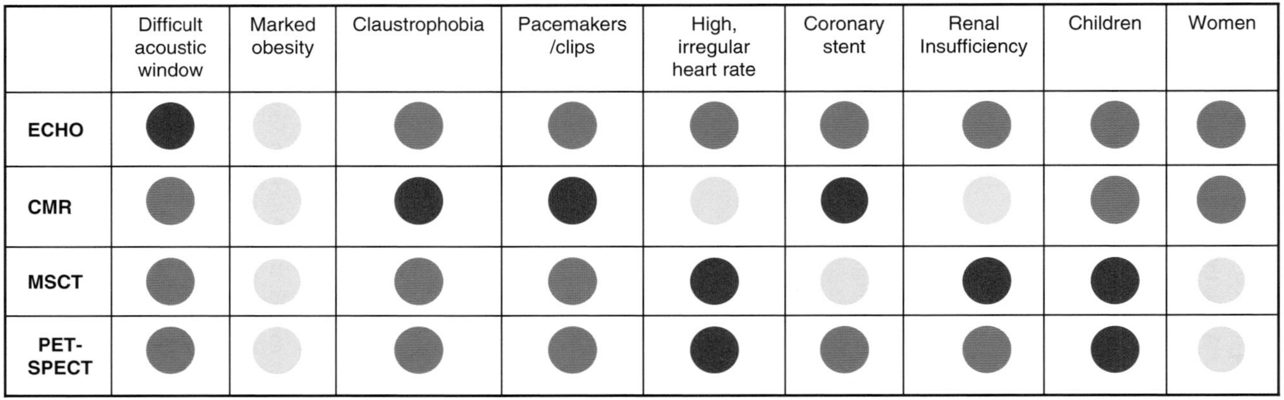

Fig. 41.5 Indications (*green dot*), relative contraindications (*yellow dot*), and contraindications (*red dot*) of different techniques in cardiac imaging

the quality of our profession, to address the existing concerns of those who pay for these services, and to optimize the immense benefits our patients can derive from the appropriate practice of cardiac imaging and stress echocardiography. Cardiac imaging must not become another chapter of the medical nemesis [33, 34]. Ivan Illich wrote in 1976 (the beginning of the imaging era): "Act so that the effect of your action is compatible with the permanence of genuine human life. Very concretely applied this could mean: Do not raise radiation levels unless you know that this action will not be visited upon your grandchild." The contemporary practice of imaging seems to ignore this sound advice. Cardiac imaging studies that expose patients to ionizing radiation should be ordered only after thoughtful consideration of the potential benefit to the patient, and in keeping with established appropriateness criteria [35].

References

1. Picano E (2005). Economic and biological costs of cardiac imaging. Cardiovasc Ultrasound 3:13
2. Herzog C, Rieger CT (2004) Risk of cancer from diagnostic X-rays. Lancet 363:340–1
3. Patel MR, Spertus JA, Brindis RG, et al; American College of Cardiology Foundation (2005). ACCF proposed method for evaluating the appropriateness of cardiovascular imaging. J Am Coll Cardiol 46:1606–13
4. Redberg RF (2007). The appropriateness imperative. Am Heart J 154:201–2
5. Shaw LJ, Hachamovitch R, Berman DS, et al (1999) The economic consequences of available diagnostic and prognostic strategies for the evaluation of stable angina patients: an observational assessment of the value of precatheterization ischemia. Economics of Noninvasive Diagnosis (END) Multicenter Study Group. J Am Coll Cardiol 33:661–9
6. Shaw LJ, Marwick TH, Berman DS, et al (2006) Incremental cost-effectiveness of exercise echocardiography vs. SPECT imaging for the evaluation of stable chest pain. Eur Heart J 27:2448–58
7. Ayanian JZ (2006) Rising rates of cardiac procedures in the United States and Canada: too much of a good thing? Circulation 113:333–5
8. Good Practice Guide for Clinical Radiologists. Ref No: BFCR(99)11. Board of Faculty of Clinical Radiology. The Royal College of Radiologists
9. European Commission. Radiation protection 118: referral guidelines for imaging. http://europa.eu.int/comm/environment/radprot/118/rp-118-en.pdf (accessed 10 January 2001)
10. Hendel RC, Wackers FJ, Berman DS, et al; American Society of Nuclear Cardiology (2006). American Society of Nuclear Cardiology consensus statement: Reporting of radionuclide myocardial perfusion imaging studies. J Nucl Cardiol 13:e152–6
11. Douglas PS, Khandheria B, Stainback RF, et al; American College of Cardiology Foundation Appropriateness Criteria Task Force; American Society of Echocardiography; American College of Emergency Physicians; American Heart Association; American Society of Nuclear Cardiology; Society for Cardiovascular Angiography and Interventions; Society of Cardiovascular Computed Tomography; Society for Cardiovascular Magnetic Resonance (2008). ACCF/ASE/ACEP/AHA/ASNC/SCAI/SCCT/SCMR 2008 appropriateness criteria for stress echocardiography: a report of the American College of Cardiology Foundation Appropriateness Criteria Task Force, American Society of Echocardiography, American College of Emergency Physicians, American Heart Association, American Society of Nuclear Cardiology, Society for Cardiovascular Angiography and Interventions, Society of Cardiovascular Computed

Tomography, and Society for Cardiovascular Magnetic Resonance: endorsed by the Heart Rhythm Society and the Society of Critical Care Medicine. Circulation 117:1478–97

12. Rang M (1972). The Ulysses syndrome. Can Med Assoc J 106:122–3

13. Pennell DJ, Sechtem UP, Higgins CB, et al; Society for Cardiovascular Magnetic Resonance; Working Group on Cardiovascular Magnetic Resonance of the European Society of Cardiology (2004). Clinical indications for cardiovascular magnetic resonance [CMR]: Consensus Panel report. Eur Heart J 25:1940–65

14. Gibbons RJ, Abrams J, Chatterjee K, et al; American College of Cardiology; American Heart Association Task Force on practice guidelines (Committee on the Management of Patients With Chronic Stable Angina) (2003). ACC/AHA 2002 guideline update for the management of patients with chronic stable angina-summary article: a report of the American College of Cardiology/American Heart Association Task Force on practice guidelines. [Committee on the Management of Patients With Chronic Stable Angina]. J Am Coll Cardiol 41:159–68

15. Picano E, Mathias W Jr, Pingitore A, et al (1994). Safety and tolerability of dobutamine-atropine stress echocardiography: a prospective, multicentre study. Echo Dobutamine International Cooperative Study Group. Lancet 344:1190–2

16. Picano E, Marini C, Pirelli S, et al (1992). Safety of intravenous high-dose dipyridamole echocardiography. The Echo-Persantine International Cooperative Study Group. Am J Cardiol 70:252–8

17. Varga A, Garcia MA, Picano E; International Stress Echo Complication Registry (2006). Safety of stress echocardiography (from the International Stress Echo Complication Registry). Am J Cardiol. 98:541–3

18. Marcassa C, Bax JJ, Bengel F, et al; European Council of Nuclear Cardiology (ECNC); European Society of Cardiology Working Group 5 (Nuclear Cardiology and Cardiac CT); European Association of Nuclear Medicine Cardiovascular Committee (2008). Clinical value, cost-effectiveness, and safety of myocardial perfusion scintigraphy: a position statement. Eur Heart J 29:557–63

19. Sicari R, Nihoyannopoulos P, Evangelista A, et al; European Association of Echocardiography (2008) Stress echocardiography expert consensus statement: European Association of Echocardiography (EAE) (a registered branch of the ESC). Eur J Echocardiogr 9:415–37

20. Lester SJ, Miller FA Jr, Khandheria BK (2008) Contrast echocardiography: beyond a black box warning? J Am Soc Echocardiogr 21:417–8

21. Stiles S (2008) FDA backpedals on warnings in Echo-contrast labelling. Heartwire. Nedscape Today

22. Ersoy H, Rybicki FJ (2007). Biochemical safety profiles of gadolinium-based extracellular contrast agents and nephrogenic systemic fibrosis. J Magn Reson Imaging 26:1190–7

23. Bashore TM, Bates ER, Berger PB, et al; American College of Cardiology. Task Force on Clinical Expert Consensus Documents. American College of Cardiology/Society for Cardiac Angiography and Interventions Clinical Expert Consensus Document on cardiac catheterization laboratory standards (2001). A report of the American College of Cardiology Task Force on Clinical Expert Consensus Documents. J Am Coll Cardiol 37:2170–214

24. Schrader R (2005). Contrast material-induced renal failure: an overview. J Interv Cardiol 18:417–23

25. Brindis RG, Douglas PS, Hendel RC, et al; American College of Cardiology Foundation Quality Strategic Directions Committee Appropriateness Criteria Working Group; American Society of Nuclear Cardiology; American Heart Association (2005). ACCF/ASNC appropriateness criteria for single-photon emission computed tomography myocardial perfusion imaging (SPECT MPI): a report of the American College of Cardiology Foundation Quality Strategic Directions Committee Appropriateness Criteria Working Group and the American

41

Society of Nuclear Cardiology endorsed by the American Heart Association. J Am Coll Cardiol 46:1587–605

26. Picano E (2003). Stress echocardiography: a historical perspective. Special Article. Am J Med 114:126–30
27. Picano E (2004). Sustainability of medical imaging. Education and Debate. BMJ 328:578–80
28. Picano E (2004). Informed consent and communication of risk from radiological and nuclear medicine examinations: how to escape from a communication inferno. Education and Debate. BMJ 329:849–51
29. Boden WE, O'Rourke RA, Teo KK, et al; COURAGE Trial Research Group (2007). Optimal medical therapy with or without PCI for stable coronary disease. N Engl J Med 356:1503–16
30. Picano E, Pasanisi E, Brown J, et al (2007). A gatekeeper for the gatekeeper: inappropriate referrals to stress echocardiography. Am Heart J. 154:285–90
31. Gibbons RJ, Miller TD, Hodge D, et al (2008). Application of appropriateness criteria to stress single-photon emission computed tomography sestamibi studies and stress echocardiograms in an academic medical center. J Am Coll Cardiol 51:1283–9
32. Bonow RO (2008). Is appropriateness appropriate? J Am Coll Cardiol 51:1290–1
33. Gershlick AH, de Belder M, Chambers J, et al (2007). Role of non-invasive imaging in the management of coronary artery disease: an assessment of likely change over the next 10 years. A report from the British Cardiovascular Society Working Group. Heart 93:423–31
34. Smith R (2002). Book Review. Limits to Medicine. Medical Nemesis: The Expropriation of Health. BMJ 324:923
35. Gerber TC, Carr JJ, Arai AE, et al (2009) Ionizing Radiation in Cardiac Imaging. A Science Advisory From the American Heart Association Committee on Cardiac Imaging of the Council on Clinical Cardiology and Committee on Cardiovascular Imaging and Intervention of the Council on Cardiovascular Radiology and Intervention. Circulation. Feb 2. [Epub ahead of print]

Index

Heterozonal, 76, 249, 250
Hibernation, 50, 51, 273–276, 280, 281, 287
Hierarchy of testing, 69–70, 244
High body mass index, 556
High energy phosphates, 43, 44, 273
Highest diagnostic standards, 15, 531
High-frequency transducers, 130, 530
High heart rate, 52, 82, 160, 224, 329, 335,
    367, 575
High lipid cores, 553
High radiosensitivity of breast, 415
High-risk patients, 309, 419, 505, 510, 524,
    542, 561
High-risk plaques, 554
High-risk surgery, 421
Historical and societal perspective, 3–15
Historical background, 125–128, 159–160,
    175, 189–192, 207–208, 221, 273–274,
    343–345, 376–378
History of infarction, 471
Homocysteine, 61, 210
Homozonal, 76, 250
Hormones, 383
Hybrid PET-CT imaging, 545
Hydrogen ions, 44, 58, 241, 242
Hyperemia, 34, 49, 110, 125, 129, 192, 208,
    345, 377, 381, 382, 407, 539, 540, 569
Hyperhomocysteinemia, 384
Hyperkinesis, 83, 96, 99, 260, 325, 436
Hypertension, 22, 37, 84, 108, 112–116, 118,
    160, 161, 169, 170
Hypertensives, 197, 297, 376
Hypertrophic cardiomyopathy, 22, 27, 37, 133,
    137, 138, 261, 366, 418, 430, 432, 467,
    479–485,
Hyperventilation, 57, 58, 99, 131, 200, 229,
    241–244, 269, 301, 443
Hypokinesis, 39, 77, 96, 99, 249, 355, 587
Hypoperfusion of the inferobasal wall, 587
Hypotension, 60, 178, 179, 194, 209, 212,
    253, 254, 262, 268, 297, 382, 420
Hypoxia, 115, 208

I

Identification of myocardial viability, 10, 180,
    183, 200, 262, 276–278, 398
Idiopathic dilated cardiomyopathy, 137, 199,
    405, 468
Images of coronary artery stenoses, 554
Imaging equipment and techniques, 147–148
Imaging modalities using ionizing radiation, 13
Imaging technology, 7, 110, 349, 353
Imaging technology evolution, 592

Inappropriate imaging testing, 15
Inappropriate use of stress testing, 269–270
Inappropriateness, 523, 585, 590
Inappropriateness in stress echo, 591
Incomplete recovery, 249, 253
Increased chronotropy, 60
Increased contractility, 175
Increased demand, 60–62
Increased inotropy, 60
Indications, 116, 169, 182–183, 199–201,
    215–216, 227, 236, 259–270, 288, 289,
    296, 299, 355–356, 398, 419, 421, 499,
    523, 542–543, 544, 547, 555, 559, 577,
    590, 591, 593
Indications for stress testing, 268–269
Indications in coronary artery disease, 591
Induced ischemia severity, 253–254
Inducible ischemia, 35, 117, 181, 268, 283,
    285, 287, 303, 306–310, 312, 366, 368,
    398, 399, 418, 441
Inducible wall motion abnormalities, 39, 40,
    100, 138, 215, 254, 298, 368, 442, 444,
    451, 460, 480, 482
Infarction, 3, 23, 36, 51, 52, 75, 106, 110,
    125–127
Inferior vena cava diameter, 112
Inferobasal wall, 587
Inflamed bronchial mucosa, 208
Inosine, 209
Inotropism, 176
Intermediate risk surgery, 421, 591
Intermediate stenosis, 138, 159
Interpretation, 57, 71, 82, 137, 145, 149, 151,
    160, 163, 222–224, 259, 260, 269, 319,
    324, 327, 329, 332, 337, 345, 381, 408,
    434, 503, 544, 577
Interstitial lung edema, 84, 366
Interventional radiology, 12
Interventricular obstruction, 179
Intra-arterial nitroprusside 378
Intracellular biochemical events, 44
Intracoronary catheter placement, 127
Intracoronary injection of nitroglycerin, 234
Intracoronary ultrasound (ICUS) 26, 27, 82,
    441, 489, 492, 554
Intramyocardial pressure (IMP), 129, 406
Intravascular thrombosis, 21
Intravenous immune globulin, 523
Intraventricular dyssynchrony, 336, 471–473
Intraventricular gradients, 436, 484, 528
Intraventricular pressure gradient, 254, 436,
    482, 483
Investigational, 116, 348, 356, 494

Printing and Binding: Stürtz GmbH, Würzburg